OBSTETRICS & GYNECOLOGY ON CALL

First Edition

Edited by

Ira R. Horowitz, MD, FACOG
Director of Gynecologic Oncology
Associate Professor
Department of Gynecology and Obstetrics
Emory University School of Medicine
Atlanta, Georgia

Series Editor

Leonard G. Gomella, MD
Assistant Professor of Urology,
Jefferson Medical College of
Thomas Jefferson University,
Philadelphia, Pennsylvania

APPLETON & LANGE
Norwalk, Connecticut

Copyright © 1993 by Appleton & Lange
Simon & Schuster Business and Professional Group

98 99 00 01 / 10 9 8 7 6

Prentice-Hall International (UK) Limited, *London*
Prentice-Hall of Australia Pty. Limited, *Sydney*
Prentice-Hall Canada, Inc., *Toronto*
Prentice-Hall Hispanoamericana, S.A., *Mexico*
Prentice-Hall of India Private Limited, *New Delhi*
Prentice-Hall of Japan, Inc., *Tokyo*
Simon & Schuster Asia Pte. Ltd., *Singapore*
Editora Prentice-Hall do Brasil, Ltda., *Rio de Janeiro*
Prentice Hall, *Englewood Cliffs, New Jersey*

ISBN: 0-8385-7174-3
ISSN: 1063-8644

Acquisitions Editor: Martin Wonsiewicz
Production Editor: Sheilah Holmes
Cover Designer: Kathleen D. Hornyak

PRINTED IN THE UNITED STATES OF AMERICA

ISBN   0-8385-7174-3

90000

9 780838 571743

Dedicated to my parents, my wife Julie, and our daughters Andrea and Rebecah, who have supported me through my career and the writing of this book.

IRH

Contents

Associate Editor

Marianne Billeter, PharmD
Assistant Professor of Clinical Pharmacy,
College of Pharmacy, Xavier University of Louisiana,
New Orleans, Louisiana

Contributors

Fouad Abbas, MD
Assistant Professor of Gynecology and Obstetrics,
Division of Gynecologic Oncology,
University of Maryland School of Medicine,
Baltimore, Maryland

Jean Anderson, MD
Assistant Professor of Gynecology and Obstetrics,
Division of Gynecology,
The Johns Hopkins University School of Medicine,
Baltimore, Maryland

Marianne Billeter, PharmD
Assistant Professor of Clinical Pharmacy,
College of Pharmacy,
Xavier University of Louisiana,
New Orleans, Louisiana

Nancy Callan, MD
Associate Professor of Obstetrics and Gynecology,
Division of Maternal Fetal Medicine,
The Johns Hopkins University School of Medicine,
Baltimore, Maryland

Jude Crino, MD
Assistant Professor of Obstetrics and Gynecology,
Division of Maternal Fetal Medicine,
University of Texas Health Sciences Center,
Houston, Texas

Gary A. Dildy, MD
Department of Obstetrics and Gynecology,
Division of Maternal Fetal Medicine,
Baylor College of Medicine,
Houston, Texas

Michelle R. Dudzinski, MD
Assistant Professor of Gynecology and Obstetrics,
Division of Gynecologic Oncology,
The Johns Hopkins University School of Medicine,
Baltimore, Maryland

Sebastian Faro, MD, PhD
Professor and Chairman,
Department of Obstetrics and Gynecology,
University of Kansas Medical Center,
Kansas City, Kansas

Terry Feng, MD
Assistant Professor of Gynecology and Obstetrics,
Division of Maternal Fetal Medicine,
The Johns Hopkins University School of Medicine,
Baltimore, Maryland

David Foster, MD
Assistant Professor of Gynecology and Obstetrics,
Director, Division of Gynecology,
The Johns Hopkins University School of Medicine,
Baltimore, Maryland

Doug Fraker, MD
Senior Staff, Surgery Branch,
National Cancer Institute, National Institutes of Health,
Bethesda, Maryland

Steven Friedman, MD
Department of Obstetrics and Gynecology,
University of Tennessee,
Memphis, Tennessee

Leonard G. Gomella, MD
Assistant Professor of Urology,
Jefferson Medical College of
Thomas Jefferson University,
Philadelphia, Pennsylvania

Tricia Gomella, MD
Attending in Neonatology,
Francis Scott Key Medical Center,
Part-Time Instructor in Pediatrics,
The Johns Hopkins University School of Medicine,
Baltimore, Maryland

Steven A. Haist, MD
Assistant Professor of Medicine,
Division of General Medicine and Geriatrics,
Department of Medicine,
University of Kentucky College of Medicine,
Lexington, Kentucky

Terre Holden-Currie, RN
Oncology Nurse,
Department of Gynecology and Obstetrics,
Division of Gynecologic Oncology,
The Johns Hopkins University School of Medicine,
Baltimore, Maryland

Ira R. Horowitz, MD
Director of Gynecologic Oncology
Associate Professor
Department of Gynecology and Obstetrics
Emory University School of Medicine
Atlanta, Georgia

Mary Jo Johnson, MD
Assistant Professor of Obstetrics and Gynecology,
Division of Maternal Fetal Medicine,
University of Maryland School of Medicine,
Baltimore, Maryland

Timothy RB Johnson, MD
Associate Professor of Gynecology and Obstetrics,
The Johns Hopkins University School of Medicine,
Baltimore, Maryland

Debbie Kulp-Hugues, MD
Senior Resident,
Department of Urology,
Thomas Jefferson University,
Philadelphia, Pennsylvania

Brian Kirshon, MD
Assistant Professor of Obstetrics and Gynecology,
Division of Maternal Fetal Medicine,
Baylor College of Medicine,
Houston, Texas

Jonathan F. Leake, MD
Gynecologic Oncologist,
Department of Obstetrics and Gynecology,
Providence Hospital,
Sandusky, Ohio

Alan T. Lefor, MD
Assistant Professor of Surgery and Oncology,
Department of Surgery,
University of Maryland School of Medicine,
Baltimore, Maryland

Maurizio Maccato, MD
Assistant Professor of Obstetrics and Gynecology,
Section of Infectious Diseases,
Baylor College of Medicine,
Houston, Texas

David McGinnis, MD
Chief Resident, Department of Urology,
Jefferson Medical College of Thomas Jefferson University,
Philadelphia, Pennsylvania

Denise Murray, MD
Instructor, Department of Obstetrics and Gynecology,
The Johns Hopkins University School of Medicine,
Baltimore, Maryland

Nicholas A. Pavona, MD
Assistant Professor of Surgery,
Benjamin Franklin University,
Sewell, New Jersey

Mark Pearlman, MD
Assistant Professor of Obstetrics and Gynecology,
University of Michigan Medical School,
Ann Arbor, Michigan

Janet S. Rader, MD
Assistant Professor of Obstetrics and Gynecology,
Washington University School of Medicine,
St. Louis, Missouri

Alex Reiter, MD
Assistant Professor of Obstetrics and Gynecology,
Division of Maternal Fetal Medicine,

Baylor College of Medicine,
Houston, Texas

John T. Repke, MD
Associate Professor of Obstetrics and Gynecology and
of Reproductive Biology,
Harvard Medical School,
Boston, Massachusetts

John B. Robbins, MD
Assistant Professor of Medicine,
Division of General Internal Medicine and Geriatrics,
Department of Medicine,
University of Kentucky Medical Center,
Lexington, Kentucky

Valerie Robbins, RN
Clinical Nurse Specialist,
Department of Obstetrics and Gynecology,
The Johns Hopkins University School of Medicine,
Baltimore, Maryland

J. Courtland Robinson, MD
Assistant Professor of Gynecology and Obstetrics,
The Johns Hopkins University School of Medicine,
Baltimore, Maryland

Eric R. Sargent, MD
Resident, Department of Urology,
University of Iowa Hospitals and Clinics,
Iowa City, Iowa

Leon G. Smith, Jr., MD
Assistant Professor of Obstetrics and Gynecology,
Division of Maternal-Fetal Medicine,
Baylor College of Medicine,
Houston, Texas

Benjamin Stahr, MD
Asociate Pathologist,
Atlanta Dermatopathology and Pathology Associates,
Atlanta, Georgia

Eric Wiebke, MD
Assistant Professor of Surgery,
Indiana University School of Medicine,
Indianapolis, Indiana

Preface

Obstetrics and Gynecology On Call provides a finger-tip reference to assist the practicing clinician, house officer, and medical student. The material is organized in a concise, problem-oriented format. The most common problems encountered in obstetrics and gynecology are presented. Each problem is followed by immediate questions, differential diagnosis, physical examination findings, pertinent laboratory values, radiologic evaluation, and treatment plan.

Commonly performed procedures in obstetrics and gynecology are also illustrated. This will assist house officers and medical students in surviving the rigors of the clinical arena. Also present are chapters reviewing fluid and electrolyte management, blood component therapy, ventilator management, and commonly used medications.

I am grateful to Tricia Gomella, MD, for providing the "On-Call" concept originally used in her book *Neonatology: Basic Management, On Call Problems, Diseases and Drugs,* published by Appleton & Lange in 1988. In addition, I am thankful to the editors of the preceding two books in this series: Leonard G. Gomella, MD, and Alan T. Lefor, MD, editors of *Surgery On Call* (Appleton & Lange, 1990), and Steven A. Haist, MD, John B. Robbins, MD, and Leonard G. Gomella, MD, who edited *Internal Medicine On Call* (Appleton & Lange, 1991). These texts provided a format for the problems presented in *Obstetrics and Gynecology On Call.*

I would like to thank Appleton & Lange for providing us the forum to present a unique approach to the education of medical students and house officers through these publications.

Finally, I extend my appreciation to Johnsie C. Faith for her dedicated secretarial support during the past two years, which made this text possible.

IRH

1   On Call Problems

OBSTETRICS

1. ABDOMINAL PAIN

I. Problem. A 23-year-old patient of 24 weeks' gestation is complaining of abdominal pain, nausea, and vomiting. Nausea and vomiting had been present earlier in the pregnancy but the pain is a new symptom.

II. Immediate Questions

    A. What are the vital signs? Fever indicates an inflammatory process. Hypotension and tachycardia may indicate shock due to sepsis or hemorrhage. Fever may be absent in those patients receiving antipyretic medications.

    B. Where is the pain located? This is only a general guide to the diagnosis of abdominal pain, since early in the course of the illness pain may be "shifted" away from the actual site of the pathologic process, then become generalized late in the course. The classic example is appendicitis, in which discomfort is initially periumbilical or epigastric and later becomes localized in the right lower quadrant. In the pregnant patient, the right lower quadrant localization of appendicitis moves upward to right mid abdomen as gestational age progresses (Figure 1–1). If the process goes unchecked, generalized peritonitis may result. Referred pain to the groin can be seen with ureteral colic, and referred back pain with pancreatitis or a ruptured abdominal aneurysm. Uterine pain occurs with labor, chorioamnionitis, and infarcted myoma. Inguinal pain can be associated with "round ligament syndrome" (Figures 1–2 and 1–3).

    C. What is the status of the fetus? Fetal heart rate, perceived fetal activity (if > 20 weeks' gestation), and status of membranes (ruptured or unruptured)?

    D. When did the pain start? Acute, explosive pain is typical of a perforated viscus, ruptured aneurysm, ruptured abscess, or ectopic pregnancy. Pain intensifying over 1–2 hours is typical of acute cholecystitis, infarcting leiomyoma, acute pancreatitis, strangulated bowel, mesenteric thrombosis, proximal small bowel obstruction, or renal or ureteral colic. Vague pain that in-

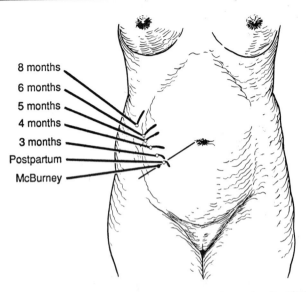

8 months
6 months
5 months
4 months
3 months
Postpartum
McBurney

Figure 1–1. Changes in position of the appendix as pregnancy advances. (month = calendar month. (*From Pernoll ML, Benson RC [eds]:* Current Obstetric and Gynecologic Diagnosis and Treatment, *6th ed. Norwalk, Connecticut, Appleton & Lange, 1987.*)

plicated peptic ulcer disease, and various gynecologic and genitourinary conditions (see Figure 1–3).

E. What is the quality of the pain? (For example, dull, sharp, burning, intermittent, constant, the worst pain ever experienced.) Classically described patterns include "burning" (peptic ulcer disease), "searing" (ruptured uterus or ruptured aortic aneurysm), "intermittent" (renal or ureteral colic), and "cramping" (uterine) (see Figure 1–3). Have the patient scale the severity of the pain from 1 (least painful) to 10 (most painful). This gives a guide to follow the course more objectively.

F. What makes the pain better or worse? Pain that increases with deep inspiration is associated with diaphragmatic irritation (pleurisy, inflammatory lesions of the upper abdomen). Food often relieves the pain of peptic ulcer disease. Narcotics will relieve colic but will do little to ease the pain of strangulated bowel or mesenteric thrombosis. Bending forward often relieves the pain of pancreatitis.

G. What are the associated symptoms? Vaginal discharge is

G. What are the associated symptoms? Vaginal discharge is seen in premature rupture of membranes or pelvic inflammatory disease. Bleeding occurs with abruptio placentae or early labor. Vomiting with the onset of pain is seen in peritoneal irritation or perforation of a hollow viscus. It is a prominent feature of upper abdominal diseases such as Boerhaave's syndrome, acute gastritis, or pancreatitis. In distal small bowel or large bowel obstruction, nausea is usually present long before vomiting begins. **Hematemesis** suggests upper GI bleeding (ulcer disease, Mallory-Weiss syndrome). **Diarrhea,** if severe and associated with abdominal pain, suggests infectious gastroenteritis, and if bloody, may represent ischemic colitis, ulcerative colitis, Crohn's disease, or amebic dysentery. **Constipation** alternating with diarrhea may be seen with diverticular disease or irritable bowel syndrome. Although constipation is often nonspecific, **obstipation** (absence of passage of both stool and flatus) is strongly suggestive of mechanical bowel obstruction. **Hematuria** suggests a genitourinary cause such as stone or infection.

H. What is the character of the emesis? "Coffee ground" vomitus suggests gastric or small bowel bleeding above the ligament of Treitz. Bright red bleeding suggests location above the stomach such as in Mallory-Weiss syndrome.

I. When did the patient last eat? This allows assessment of the time course of the illness and is particularly important if anesthesia is planned.

J. What is the patient's past medical and surgical history? History of prior cesarean section (especially classic) carries an increased risk of uterine rupture (2%). Knowledge of a history of ulcers, gallstones, alcohol abuse, previous operations, and a list of current medications will aid in establishing the cause. A history of blunt abdominal trauma 1–3 days prior to the onset of pain may signify uterine trauma, uterine rupture, subcapsular hemorrhage of the liver, or spleen or kidney trauma.

III. Differential Diagnosis. Abdominal pain has intra-abdominal and extra-abdominal sources and can be associated with both medical and surgical diseases. The list is too long to reproduce in its entirety here, but Table 1–1 lists some of the more frequently encountered causes.

A. Intra-abdominal
   1. Uterine. Degenerating leiomyomas, adnexal torsion or rupture, pelvic inflammatory disease, chorioamnionitis, ectopic pregnancy.
   2. GI. Viral or bacterial enteritis, inflammatory bowel disease,

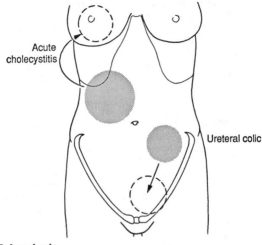

Acute
cholecystitis

Ureteral colic

Referred pain

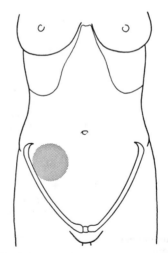

Shifting pain

Figure 1–2. Referred pain and shifting pain in the acute abdomen. Solid circles indicate the site of maximum pain and dashed circles, the sites of lesser pain. *continued*

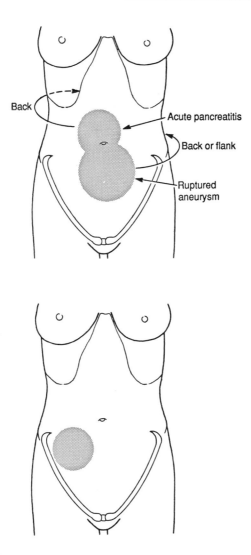

Figure 1-2. cont'd (*From Boey JH: Acute Abdomen. In Way LW [ed]:* Current Surgical Diagnosis and Treatment, *8th ed. San Mateo, California, Appleton & Lange, 1988.*) (*From Gant NF:* Basic Obstetrics and Gynecology. *Norwalk, Connecticut, Appleton & Lange, 1992.*)

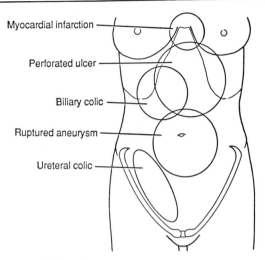

Abrupt, excruciating pain

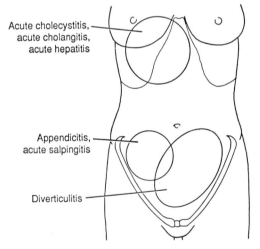

Gradual, steady pain

Figure 1–3. The location and character of the pain are useful in the differential diagnosis of acute abdomen. *continued*

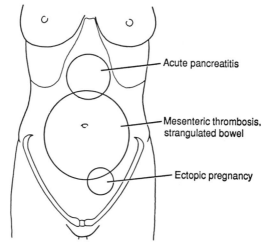

Rapid onset of severe, constant pain

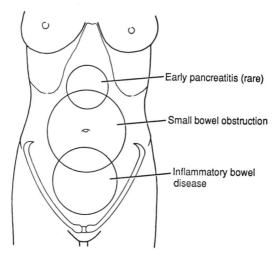

Intermittent, colicky pain, crescendo with free intervals

Figure 1–3. cont'd (*From Boey JH: Acute Abdomen. In Way LW [ed]:* Current Surgical Diagnosis and Treatment, *8th ed. San Mateo, California, Appleton & Lange, 1988.*)

TABLE 1–1. COMMON CAUSES OF ACUTE ABDOMEN. CONDITIONS IN ITALIC TYPE OFTEN REQUIRE URGENT OPERATION.

Gastrointestinal tract disorders
  Appendicitis
  Small and large bowel obstruction
  Strangulated hernia
  Perforated peptic ulcer
  Bowel perforation
  Meckel's diverticulitis
  Boerhaave's syndrome
  Diverticulitis
  Inflammatory bowel disorders
  Mallory-Weiss syndrome
  Gastroenteritis
  Acute gastritis
  Mesenteric adenitis

Liver, spleen, and biliary tract disorders
  Acute cholecystitis
  Acute cholangitis
  Hepatic abscess
  Ruptured hepatic tumor
  Spontaneous rupture of the spleen
  Splenic infarct
  Biliary colic
  Acute hepatitis

Pancreatic disorders
  Acute pancreatitis

Urinary tract disorders
  Ureteral or renal colic
  Acute pyelonephritis
  Acute cystitis
  Renal infarct

Gynecologic disorders
  Ruptured ectopic pregnancy
  Twisted ovarian tumor
  Ruptured ovarian follicle cyst
  Acute salpingitis
  Dysmenorrhea
  Endometriosis

Vascular disorders
  Ruptured aortic and visceral aneurysms
  Acute ischemic colitis
  Mesenteric thrombosis

Peritoneal disorders
  Intra-abdominal abscesses
  Primary peritonitis
  Tuberculous peritonitis

Retroperitoneal disorders
  Retroperitoneal hemorrhage

From Way LW (ed): Current Surgical Diagnosis and Treatment, *8th ed. Norwalk, Connecticut, Appleton & Lange, 1988.*

  hyperemesis gravidarum, cholecystitis, hepatitis, omental infarction.
  3. **GU.** Renal stone, mechanical ureteral obstruction due to pregnancy, pyelonephritis, a cystitis, lower urinary tract obstruction (commonly due to incarcerated uterus).
  4. **Musculoskeletal.** Round ligament syndrome, pelvic joint laxity.
  5. **Vascular.** Ruptured aneurysm, dissecting aneurysm, mesenteric thrombosis or embolism, splenic or hepatic rupture—usually post-traumatic or secondary to toxemia or hepatic adenoma.

B. **Extra-abdominal.** These may rarely present as pain "referred" to the abdomen, such as from sickle cell crisis, pneumonia (especially lower lobe), myocardial infarction, and rarely, diabetic ketoacidosis. These tend to be "medical" diseases, and surgery is not generally indicated.

C. Other. Blunt trauma may cause injuries to solid viscera (spleen, liver, kidney, pancreas) or to fixed structures such as the duodenum. **Penetrating trauma** may injure any intra-abdominal structure.

IV. Database

A. Physical examination key points. Table 1–2 lists the physical findings associated with various causes of acute abdomen.

1. **Overall appearance.** A patient writhing in agony is typical of colic, while a motionless patient is typical of peritoneal irritation.
2. **Lungs.** Listen for basilar rales or rhonchi indicating possible pneumonia. Dullness to percussion may represent pleural effusion or consolidation.
3. **Heart.** Look for evidence of cardiac decompensation, especially in a patient with preexisting coronary disease (distended neck veins, S3 gallop, peripheral edema), which may direct attention toward a myocardial infarction or atrial fibrillation to suggest emboli.
4. **Abdomen**
   a. **Inspection.** Note the presence of distention (obstruc-

TABLE 1–2. PHYSICAL FINDINGS WITH VARIOUS CAUSES OF ACUTE ABDOMEN.

Condition	Helpful Signs
Perforated viscus	Scaphoid, tense abdomen; diminished bowel sounds (late); loss of liver dullness, guarding or rigidity.
Peritonitis	Motionless; absent bowel sounds (late); cough and rebound tenderness; guarding or rigidity.
Inflamed mass or abscess	Tender mass (abdominal, rectal, or pelvic); punch tenderness; special signs (Murphy's, psoas, or obturator).
Intestinal obstruction	Distention; visible peristalsis (late); hyperperistalsis (early) or quiet abdomen (late); diffuse pain without rebound tenderness; hernia or rectal mass (some).
Paralytic ileus	Distention; minimal bowel sounds; no localized tenderness.
Ischemic or strangulated bowel	Not distended (until late); bowel sounds variable; severe pain but little tenderness; rectal bleeding (some).
Bleeding	Pallor, shock; distention; pulsatile (aneurysm) or tender (eg, ectopic pregnancy) mass; rectal bleeding (some).

From Way LW (ed): Current Surgical Diagnosis and Treatment, 8th ed. Norwalk, Connecticut, Appleton & Lange, 1988.

tion, ileus, ascites), flank ecchymoses (hemorrhagic pancreatitis), surgical scars (adhesions, tumor).

   b. Auscultation. Listen for bowel sounds (absent with obstruction or ileus, hyperperistaltic with gastroenteritis, "rushes" with small bowel obstruction).

   c. Percussion. Tympany is associated with distended loops of bowel, dullness and a fluid wave with ascites; loss of liver dullness is associated with free air.

   d. Palpation. Uterine tenderness, fetal number, position, presence of uterine contraction. Guarding, rigidity, and rebound tenderness are hallmarks of peritonitis. Localized tenderness is often seen with cholecystitis, appendicitis, salpingitis, and diverticulitis. Costovertebral angle tenderness is common with pyelonephritis. **Murphy's sign** (inspiratory splinting with palpation of the gallbladder) suggests acute cholecystitis. Pain with active hip flexion (**psoas sign**) can represent a retrocecal appendix or psoas abscess. The **obturator sign** (pain on internal and external rotation of the flexed thigh) can be found with a retrocecal appendix or obturator herniation. Look especially for uterine irritability, uterine contractions (frequency and duration), and uterine irregularity, which suggests the presence of leiomyomas.

5. **Rectal examination.** A mass suggests a rectal carcinoma, multiple fissures suggest Crohn's disease, and unilateral right-sided tenderness is suggestive of appendicitis (usually retrocecal) or an abscess. If stool is present, evaluate for occult blood.

6. **Fetal heart rate.** Normal (120–180) baseline rate may be higher in earlier gestation. Be especially vigilant for extreme variability in rate, especially decelerations below 100.

7. **Pelvic examination.** Look for the presence of blood per os cervix suggesting cervical dilatation and effacement, evidence of purulent or foul-smelling discharge, evidence of frank tissue per os cervix, evidence of instrumentation or trauma, and drainage of amniotic fluid grossly or thorough check for ferning and nitrazine positivity (see page 348). **Note:** If a history of bleeding is given in the second or third trimester, manual exam should be deferred until placenta previa is ruled out by ultrasound.

8. **Examine for Alder's sign.** After the point of maximum pelvic tenderness is located, turn the patient onto her left side. If tenderness is significantly reduced in intensity, the source of pain is probably uterine or adnexal.

9. **Costovertebral angle tenderness.** This suggests pyelonephritis, perinephric abscess, or ureteral obstruction with stone. Pyelonephritis is more commonly right-sided in pregnancy.

10. **Skin.** Look for jaundice. Spider angiomas may be seen normally in pregnancy, in contrast to nonpregnant status where angiomas suggest liver disease. Cool, clammy skin from peripheral vasoconstriction is an ominous sign of severe hypotension.

B. Laboratory data

1. **Hemogram.** Anemia may indicate hemorrhage from an ulcer, colon cancer, ruptured ectopic, ruptured ovarian cyst, etc. Leukocytosis indicates the presence of inflammation. A low white count is more typical of viral infections such as gastroenteritis or mesenteric adenitis.

2. **Urinalysis.** Hematuria (especially in a catheterized specimen) may indicate nephrolithiasis; pyuria and hematuria can be present in urinary tract infections.

3. **Urine culture and sensitivity.** > 100,000 colonies/mm^3 positive on clean catch or 10, 000 colonies/mm^3 on a catheterized specimen indicates urinary tract infection.

4. **Liver function tests.** Determine bilirubin, SGOT (AST), SGPT (ALT), 5'-nucleotidase. Elevated total and direct bilirubin suggests obstructive biliary disease. Alkaline phosphatase can be elevated due to placental alkaline phosphatase, and 5'-nucleotidase is a better assay for obstructive jaundice.

5. **Amylase.** Markedly elevated levels are associated with pancreatitis. Amylase can also be elevated with perforated ulcer and small bowel obstruction; occasionally, a pseudocyst or hemorrhagic pancreatitis may be present with a normal amylase level.

6. **Cervical culture.** Send specimen specifically for gonorrhea and chlamydia if pelvic inflammatory disease is suspected.

7. **Arterial blood gases.** Hypoxia is often an early sign of sepsis. Acidosis may be present in ischemic bowel disease.

8. **Serum electrolytes, BUN, creatinine.** Bowel obstruction with vomiting can cause hypokalemia, dehydration, or both. Dehydration is suggested by a BUN/creatinine ratio > 20 : 1.

C. Radiologic and other studies

1. **Ultrasound.** Studies may reveal gallstones, ectopic pregnancy, ureteral dilatation, fetal status (over 28–30 weeks), and the presence of a uterine lesion.

2. **Fetal monitoring.** Documentation of presence of contractions, variability in fetal heart rate, fetal arrhythmia. Nonstress test can be performed > 28–30 weeks (see procedure 6, page 351).

3. **Flat and upright chest films.** The radiation dose from a chest x-ray series is of very low risk to the fetus, especially in gestations beyond the first trimester. X-rays may reveal

pneumonia, widened mediastinum (dissecting aneurysm), and pleural effusion or elevation of a hemidiaphragm (subdiaphragmatic inflammatory process). Free air under the diaphragm suggests a perforation and is most often seen on the upright chest film.

4. **Flat and upright abdominal films.** If the patient is debilitated, a lateral decubitus view may be substituted for the upright film. Observe for the following key elements: gas pattern, bowel dilatation, air-fluid levels, presence of air in the rectum, pancreatic calcifications, subdiaphragmatic air, loss of psoas margin, gall and renal stones, portal vein air, aortic calcifications.

5. **Magnetic resonance imaging.** A new imaging technique, of low risk in pregnancy. Fetal movement may result in artifact.

6. **Endoscopic studies.** Cystoscopy, colonoscopy, esophagogastroduodenoscopy (EGD), laparoscopy as indicated.

7. **Fern and nitrazine testing.** Ferning can be checked by applying a sample of vaginal pool to a glass slide and letting it dry. The microscopic pattern is characteristic for amniotic fluid (see Procedure 2, page 347). it has been suggested that blood increases the chance of a false negative result.

V. **Plan.** Abdominal pain in any patient can present a diagnostic dilemma. The surgeon's goal is to determine if abdominal pain requires surgical treatment in order to prevent further morbidity. Severe pain that has been present for 6 or more hours and does not improve is likely to have a cause requiring surgical intervention. Many cases of abdominal pain have no definite diagnosis before laparotomy. A brief period of observation may ultimately point to the cause, but operation is safer in most cases. The use of analgesics remains controversial, but most clinicians now believe moderate doses of pain medicine will not mask symptoms while making the patient much more comfortable. Specific types of therapy and operations for each possible diagnosis cannot be described here but can be found in surgical and medical textbooks. It is essential to recognize that certain conditions are life threatening and usually require urgent operation (see Table 1–11, page 117).

A. **Determine the fetal status;** in particular, rule out intrauterine sepsis and fetal distress.

B. **Keep the patient NPO and prepare for exploratory laparotomy** with appropriate lab tests. Start an IV and run fluid adequately to treat preexisting dehydration if present.

C. **Exploratory laparotomy** is indicated for appendicitis, ruptured ectopic pregnancy, perforated viscus, splenic or hepatic injury, uterine rupture, or fetal distress in a salvageable fetus (can depend upon estimation of fetal size and weight by ultrasound correlated with estimated gestational age).

REFERENCES

Burnakis TG, Hildebrandt NB: Pelvic inflammatory disease: a review with emphasis on antimicrobial therapy. *Rev Infect Dis* 8:86, 1986.
DeCherney AH, Jones EE: Ectopic pregnancy. *Clin Obstet Gynecol* 28:365, 1985.
Kumazawa T: Sensory innervation of reproductive organs. *Prog Brain Res* 67:115, 1986.
Laguardia KD et al: A 10-year review of maternal mortality in a municipal hospital in Rio de Janeiro: a cause for concern. *Obstet Gynecol* 75:27–32, 1990.
Lee CH, Raman S, Sivanesaratnam V: Torsion of ovarian tumors: a clinicopathologic study. *Int J Gynecol Obstet* 28:21–25, 1989.
Procacci P, Zoppi M, Maresca M: Clinical approach to visceral sensation. *Prog Brain Res* 67:21–28, 1986.

2. BREAST PROBLEMS POSTPARTUM

I. **Problem.** You are called to see a breast-feeding patient with the complaint of sore breasts on the third postpartum day.

II. **Immediate Questions**

A. **Is the patient breast- or bottle-feeding?** If the patient is bottle-feeding, you may want to consider lactation suppression.

B. **Is the patient febrile?** It is important to rule out mastitis in a patient with sore breasts and fever.

C. **Is her pain associated with nursing?** Problems with "latching on" may lead to nipple pain.

D. **Are there other symptoms of malaise or myalgias?** The patient who feels systemically ill may have either mastitis or breast abscess.

III. **Differential Diagnosis**

A. **Breast engorgement.** Milk production usually begins on the second or third postpartum day. The breasts may become very hard, swollen, and tender.

B. **Mastitis.** Usually has its onset in the first or second postpartum week, but may also occur when the baby is beginning to space out feeding intervals 5–6 weeks postpartum.

C. **Breast abscess.** This localized complication of mastitis will require incision and drainage.

    D. Nipple soreness. Temporary soreness can be quite severe and is associated with the baby latching on to the breast.

    E. Clogged duct. One or more of the milk ducts can be obstructed at any time during nursing, which will result in localized engorgement and pain.

IV Database

A. Physical examination key points

1. **Vital signs.** Check for fever. Although breast engorgement may be associated with fever, it is important to rule out a breast infection, or mastitis.
2. **Breast.** Engorgement usually involves both breasts and, except for temperature elevation, will be without systemic symptoms. Tender nipples should be examined for cracks and fissures. A V-shaped, erythematous, tender segment of the breast is indicative of localized cellulitis or mastitis. The patient is often febrile with systemic symptoms of malaise and myalgias. A clogged duct will result in a tender lump but can be differentiated from breast abscess by lack of systemic symptoms and resolution with nursing.

B. Laboratory data

1. **Hemogram.** An elevated white blood cell count is present with a breast abscess and occasionally with mastitis.
2. **A sample of expressed milk may be cultured,** although it will rarely affect clinical management. *Staphylococcus aureus,* transmitted from the baby's nasopharynx, is the most common organism isolated.

C. Radiologic and other studies. Usually not needed.

V. Plan

A. Breast engorgement.
Treatment of breast engorgement will depend on the mode of feeding. The breast-feeding patient should allow her baby to feed on demand and should avoid supplemental formula or dextrose water feeds. She should also wear a well-supporting bra and may be given analgesics such as Tylenol. In contrast to the bottle-feeding patient, she may also alleviate engorgement by taking a warm shower and by expressing milk either manually or by pump prior to nursing.

B. Mastitis.
Early antibiotic treatment of mastitis is mandatory to prevent formation of a breast abscess. A penicillinase-resistant penicillin or cephalosporin may be used, eg, dicloxacillin 250 mg q6h for a 10-day course. Erythromycin or sulfonamides may be used in the patient with penicillin allergy. The patient should be encouraged to continue nursing and be assured that neither the

infection nor the prescribed antibiotic will adversely affect her baby. Drainage of the affected breast is important in preventing a breast abscess.

C. **Clogged duct.** Treatment of a clogged duct consists of gentle massage of the affected area while nursing to encourage drainage of the duct. The affected breast should be offered to the baby first so that it will be drained more completely. Prevention of this problem includes varying positions while nursing and avoiding a restrictive bra.

D. **Breast abscess.** Treatment of a breast abscess is incision and drainage. Again, the baby need not stop nursing; however, if the breast is too tender, the mother may prefer pumping with a mechanical device.

E. **Sore nipples.** Sore nipples are a common problem during the first week of nursing. Drying agents such as soap or alcohol should be strictly avoided; lanolin or vitamin A&D ointment may be applied after nursing. The mother should be encouraged to nurse in different positions so the baby will attach to her nipple at different areas.

F. **Lactation suppression.** Can be accomplished by avoiding suckling and milk expression during the postpartum period. Well-supported bras, analgesics, and ice packs will decrease the symptoms of breast engorgement. Hormonal therapy may be started immediately after labor with testosterone enanthate 90 mg and estradiol valerate 4 mg (approximately 50% efficient). The most widely accepted pharmacologic therapy is bromocriptine 2.5 mg twice daily for two weeks (80% efficiency).

REFERENCES

Bowes WA Jr: Postpartum Care. In Gabbe SG, Niebyl JR, Simpson JL (eds): *Obstetrics, Normal and Problem Pregnancies.* New York, Churchill Livingstone, 1986, pp 623–647.
Creasy RK, Resnik R (eds): *Maternal Fetal Medicine.* Philadelphia, WB Saunders, 1984, p 628.
Eiger MS, Olds SW: *The Complete Book of Breast Feeding.* New York, Workman Publishing, 1972.

3. CONTRACTIONS (PREMATURE, TERM)

I. **Problem.** A pregnant 23-year-old woman presents to Labor and Delivery complaining of contractions.

II. **Immediate Questions**

A. **What is the gestational age?** Determining the gestational age is essential for formulation of a management plan. In general, a gestational age of ≥ 37 weeks is considered term and 20–37 weeks is preterm. The gestational age should be assigned by best obstetric estimate based on clinical criteria and laboratory determinations. The patient's prenatal records should be examined whenever possible. The most reliable clinical estimator of gestational age is an accurate last normal menstrual period.

B. Does the patient give a history suspicious for ruptured membranes? The patient with ruptured membranes may give a history of sudden loss of fluid or of a persistent slow leak.

C. Does the patient have vaginal bleeding or spotting? Vaginal bleeding or spotting may be a sign of cervical change or of abruption or placenta previa.

D. What is the patient's past obstetric history? If the patient has had a previous preterm delivery or poor obstetric outcome, she is at risk for these complications during her current pregnancy. If the patient has had a previous cesarean section, the type of uterine scar should be documented by reviewing the operative note.

E. Has the patient had any problems complicating her current pregnancy? Many medical and obstetric complications occurring earlier in the pregnancy may put the patient at risk for preterm labor or affect the management of both preterm and term labor.

F. What medications is the patient receiving? The patient's medications may reveal a medical problem which she has failed to mention. Certain medications, such as insulin, may need to be administered intravenously during labor. Appropriate drug levels (eg, antiseizure medications) should be obtained.

G. Has the patient used any street drugs? Cocaine, in particular, has been associated with preterm labor and placental abruption.

H. What are the vital signs? Hypertension may be indicative of preeclampsia. Fever may suggest an infectious process such as urinary tract infection or chorioamnionitis.

III. Differential Diagnosis

A. Term labor. If the gestational age is 37 weeks or greater and there is evidence of progressive cervical change by serial pelvic examinations, the diagnosis is labor at term (see Table A–5, page 596).

B. False labor. Uterine contractions which may be uncomfortable but do not cause cervical dilatation or effacement are termed "false labor." This may develop at any time during pregnancy but is observed most commonly late in pregnancy and in parous women. The contractions of false labor are characteristically irregular in occurrence and of brief duration. This diagnosis should be made with extreme caution, especially if the patient is preterm. The patient should be carefully evaluated with serial pelvic examinations by the same examiner over a period of several hours before her contractions are dismissed as false labor. Contractions which are increasing in frequency, duration, or intensity most likely represent prodromal labor, even if a cervical change cannot be documented.

C. Preterm labor. If the gestational age is 20–37 weeks, the diagnosis of preterm labor may be made if there is evidence of cervical change or if the patient is having regular uterine contractions occurring every 10 minutes or less. The cause of preterm labor in most patients is unknown. However, the following conditions have been shown to be associated with preterm labor:

1. **Urinary tract infection.** The incidence of preterm labor is increased not only in patients with pyelonephritis, but also in patients with infections confined to the lower urinary tract, even when asymptomatic.
2. **Ruptured membranes.** Preterm labor is commonly preceded by rupture of the membranes.
3. **Amniotic fluid infection.** There is a growing body of evidence to support chorioamnionitis, both overt and subclinical, as a significant etiologic factor in preterm labor. As many as one-third of preterm deliveries have been associated with evidence of chorioamnionitis.
4. **Overdistended uterus.** Multiple gestations and hydramnios are known to significantly increase the risk of preterm labor.
5. **Anomalies of conception.** Fetal and placental malformations and karyotypic abnormalities are associated with a high incidence of preterm labor and delivery.
6. **Fetal death in utero.** Spontaneous labor commonly follows preterm fetal demise by a variable period of time.
7. **Serious maternal disease.** Severe systemic maternal diseases such as hypertensive disorders, cardiac disease, collagen vascular disease, renal disease, and hemoglobinopathies are associated with an increased risk of preterm labor.
8. **Dehydration.** Severe maternal dehydration has been associated with the onset of preterm labor.
9. **Retained intrauterine device.** Pregnancy with a retained intrauterine device is associated with a high incidence of preterm labor.
10. **Uterine anomalies.** Any congenital uterine anomaly, including those resulting from in utero DES exposure, predisposes the patient to preterm labor. Leiomyomas have also been associated with an increased incidence of preterm labor

IV. Database

A. Physical examination key points

1. **Vital signs.** Fever suggests an infectious process. Hypertension may be indicative of preeclampsia.
2. **Lungs.** Auscultation may reveal evidence of pneumonia, asthma, or other maternal pulmonary disease.
3. **Abdomen.** The fundal height should be carefully measured as a clinical estimator of gestational age (see Figure A–4 in the Appendix). Unless the patient is morbidly obese, uterine contractions should be palpable. Intensity of contractions may be assessed by attempting to indent the uterus digitally during a contraction. Uterine tenderness should be assessed by palpation between contractions. Note whether the uterus is diffusely tender or if the tenderness is localized, which may be indicative of placental abruption.
4. **Pelvic examination.** A sterile speculum examination should be performed initially on all preterm patients and on any patient giving a history suspicious for ruptured membranes. The amount and source of any bleeding should be noted. A visual estimation of cervical dilatation should also be performed. Digital cervical examination should be performed following the sterile speculum examination unless the diagnosis of premature rupture of the membranes or placenta previa has been made. Dilatation, effacement, station, and presentation should be documented. Uterine size prior to 16 weeks' gestation is helpful in assessment of gestational age.
5. **Fetal heart tone.** As a general rule, fetal heart tones are audible using electronic Doppler by 12–14 menstrual weeks, and by 19–20 weeks using a nonelectronic fetoscope.
6. **Extremities.** Look for edema, which may be indicative of preeclampsia. In addition, check for varicosities and for areas of tenderness or palpable cords, which would suggest deep vein thrombosis.
7. **Neurologic examination.** Look for hyperreflexia, which is seen in preeclampsia (see Problem 18, page 76).

B. Laboratory data

1. **Hemogram.** Leukocytosis with a left shift may be secondary to contractions alone but may also suggest an infectious process.
2. **Urinalysis.** High specific gravity indicates dehydration. Positive nitrites or leukocyte esterase on dipstick suggest urinary tract infection, as do white blood cells and bacteria on microscopic examination.
3. **Type and screen.** Should be obtained on all patients admitted to Labor and Delivery to identify Rh status and provide available blood for transfusion.

4. **Toxicology screen (urine, blood, or both).** Consider obtaining this evaluation for the presence of street drugs on patients in preterm labor or with evidence of placental abruption.

5. **Pregnancy test.** Biochemical studies such as serum or urine human chorionic gonadotropin pregnancy tests may be helpful in confirming the clinical assessment of gestational age if the test is positive during the first 6 weeks after the beginning of the last normal menstrual period.

6. **Cervical cultures.** A cervical culture for beta streptococci and gonococci should be obtained.

7. **Lung maturity studies.** If the membranes are grossly ruptured and the patient is preterm, collect 5–10 mL of vaginal pool fluid for lecithin/sphingomyelin ratio (L/S) and phosphatidylglycerol levels (PG) (see Procedure 23, page 382).

C. **Radiologic and other studies**

1. **Sonogram.** If indicated, a sonogram may be helpful in confirming the gestational age, evaluating for fetal anomalies, and assessing amniotic fluid volume in patients with suspected ruptured membranes or hydramnios, and for determining the presentation if this cannot be established by pelvic examination. When using ultrasound measurements to estimate gestational age, it is important to remember that the standard deviation increases with increasing gestational age.

2. **Fern and nitrizine test.** A fern test and nitrizine test should be performed to evaluate for ruptured membranes (see Procedure 3, page 348).

V. **Plan.** The plan of management depends on the gestational age and diagnosis.

A. **Labor at term.** The patient who is in labor at term with evidence of cervical change should be admitted to Labor and Delivery and her labor managed according to the local standards of care.

B. **False labor.** The patient who is having contractions without evidence of cervical change should be advised that these contractions may progress to the effective contractions of true labor. The signs and symptoms of labor should be discussed with her (eg, bloody show; increased vaginal discharge; contractions increasing in frequency, duration, and intensity), and she should be instructed to return should any of these signs or symptoms develop.

C. **Preterm labor**

1. IV access should be obtained in all patients with preterm

labor, and IV hydration begun with an initial fluid bolus of 500–750 mL unless contraindicated due to medical factors.

2. The aggressiveness and extent of tocolytic therapy depends upon the gestational age, status of the membranes, presence of contraindications to tocolysis, and local custom. In general, most clinicians will institute intravenous tocolysis in patients having a gestational age of < 34 weeks with intact membranes and no contraindications to tocolysis.

   a. The most common tocolytic agents today are **ritodrine** and **magnesium sulfate** (see Chapter 7). Most clinicians approach the management of preterm labor at 34–37 weeks on an individualized basis.

   b. A combination of intravenous hydration and **terbutaline** 0.25 mg subcutaneously q3h may be effective in stopping uterine contractions that are not well established.

   c. It remains controversial whether intravenous tocolysis should be undertaken in the presence of ruptured membranes.

   d. Some authors recommend that amniocentesis be performed on patients in preterm labor to rule out chorioamnionitis and assess fetal lung maturity. (see Procedure 1, page 339).

   e. In all cases of preterm labor, therapy should be initiated for any treatable condition that may be a causative factor (eg, urinary tract infection).

REFERENCES

American College of Obstetricians and Gynecologists: Assessment of fetal maturity prior to repeat cesarean delivery or elective induction of labor. ACOG Tech Bull 72. Washington, DC, ACOG, 1989.

American College of Obstetricians and Gynecologists: Preterm labor. ACOG Tech Bull 133. Washington, DC, ACOG, 1989.

Carpenter RJ Jr: Preterm labor: cause and management. *Comp Ther* 8:37, 1982.

Cunningham FG, MacDonald PC, Gant NF: *William Obstetrics*, 18th ed. Norwalk, Connecticut, Appleton & Lange, 1989.

4. CORD PROLAPSE

I. Problem. During artificial rupture of membranes at vertex/minus 2 station (Figure 1–4), a pulsatile cord descends into the vaginal cavity in front of the head.

II. Immediate Questions

A. What is the status of the fetal heart rate and maternal vital signs? If the fetal heart rate is < 60 beats per minute (bpm), fetal

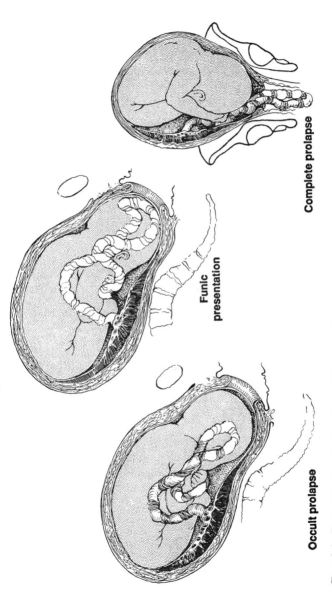

Occult prolapse

Funic presentation

Complete prolapse

Figure 1-4. Types of prolapsed cords. (*From Benson RC [ed]: Current Obstetrics and Gynecologic Diagnosis and Treatment, 5th ed. San Mateo, California, Lange, 1984.*)

distress is present and cesarean section should be performed. Decelerations may be due to another cause such as head manipulation, transition to second stage, or maternal hypotension.

B. Is the cord palpable vaginally and is it pulsating? A nonpulsating cord is usually secondary to intrauterine fetal death.

C. Are contractions occurring? How frequently? Are the contractions being augmented by oxytocin? If the patient is having her contractions augmented by oxytocin, the drip should be discontinued. If there is any possibility of a cord prolapse, the last thing you would want is augmented labor.

III. Differential Diagnosis

A. Malpresentation of a hand or foot can make the diagnosis of cord prolapse a challenge. Careful examination of shape and presence of pulsation of fetal structures in the abnormal presenting part is of primary importance.

B. Nuchal cord and "occult prolapse." Severe variability of fetal heart rate or sudden prolonged bradycardia, in the absence of a palpable cord, can suggest occult cord prolapse or a tight nuchal cord.

C. Prolapse of second twin cord. A rare occurrence with monochorionic-monoamniotic twins, the cord of the second twin can prolapse prior to or following delivery of the first twin. Care must be taken not to clamp off the wrong cord with delivery of the first twin.

IV. Database

A. Physical examination key points

1. **Fetal and maternal vital signs**

   a. Look for repetitive severe variable decelerations (< 60 bpm for > 1 minute per deceleration) or prolonged bradycardia without recovery as evidence of significant compromise of fetal circulation.

   b. Maternal blood pressure is important to maintain at all times. Watch for supine hypotension, which can aggravate an already serious problem by decreasing uterine blood flow.

2. **Pelvic examination.** The umbilical cord is palpated on vaginal examination. Pulseless cords are indicative of intrauterine fetal death. Presenting parts must also be palpated.

V. Plan

A. Procedures to decompress the presenting part from the cord should include Trendelenburg or knee-chest position and elevation of the presenting part by a hand within the vagina until delivery by cesarean section. If intrauterine fetal demise has occurred, vaginal delivery should be attempted.

B. Support the patient. Administer oxygen at 4–6 L/min by mask and maintain adequate IV fluid administration (rapid infusion of IV fluids is not helpful in this situation).

C. Expeditious delivery should be considered. Once the diagnosis of cord prolapse is made, delivery is the primary objective. Cesarean section is usually the most appropriate route.

D. If delivery is not possible, labor should be inhibited with terbutaline 0.25 mg IV bolus.

E. Anesthesia options should be considered including cesarean with local infiltration and parenteral analgesics.

F. Most importantly, anticipation of such a problem is the best defense against disaster. A "double setup" within the delivery room, prepared for cesarean section, should be arranged prior to AROM (artificial rupture of membranes) when the presenting parts are not engaged.

G. If the patient is at full dilatation with a vertex presentation visible, a low forceps delivery can be considered. Otherwise, delivery is best managed abdominally.

REFERENCES

Koonings PP, Paul RH, Campbell K: Umbilical cord prolapse: a contemporary look. *J Reprod Med* 35:690, 1990.
Russell KP: The course and conduct of normal labor and delivery. In Pernoll ML, Benson RC (eds): *Current Obstetrics & Gynecologic Diagnosis & Treatment,* 6th ed. Norwalk, Connecticut, Appleton & Lange, 1987, pp 178–203.

5. FEVER DURING PREGNANCY

I. Problem. A 24-year-old primigravida presents to the emergency room with a temperature of 39°C (102.6°F).

II. Immediate Questions

A. Does she complain of abdominal pain? Although nonspecific, abdominal pain does focus the physical examination as well as the differential diagnosis. The absence of abdominal pain eliminates with reasonable certainty appendicitis, cholecystitis, ruptured viscus, and other serious intra-abdominal lesions.

B. Does she complain of uterine cramping? Although this complaint does not necessarily implicate the uterus as the site of origin (eg, urinary tract infections can cause uterine cramping), it does focus the differential diagnosis.

C. Has there been any significant change in fetal activity? Beyond 18–19 weeks, the time most primigravidas will first note fetal activity, any remarkable change in the pattern of uterine activity may be an indicator of fetal compromise.

D. Does the patient have a cough or sputum production? Respiratory infections are not uncommon during pregnancy. The presence of a cough may implicate the respiratory tract. The presence and characteristics of the sputum (color, viscosity) give some clue to the organisms responsible (see IIIB).

E. Are there urinary symptoms? The presence of dysuria, **increased** frequency (most women normally have frequency during pregnancy), or urgency point to the urinary tract as a possible source of fever. The presence of significant fever with a urinary source almost always indicates upper tract disease; that is, simple cystitis rarely causes high fever. The finding of costovertebral tenderness along with fever and dysuria is helpful to incriminate the upper urinary tract (see Problem 25, page 98).

F. Are other constitutional symptoms present (nausea, vomiting, myalgias, lethargy, diarrhea)? Although these are nonspecific complaints, the presence of significant nausea, vomiting, or diarrhea should prompt evaluation of the patient's volume and electrolyte status.

G. Has she noticed a rash? Rashes during pregnancy are particularly worrisome because certain viral exanthems may have profound implications for the fetus (eg, rubella, parvovirus, varicella).

H. Has there been recent surgery? Operative site infections should be considered.

 I. Has there been recent travel? Certain infections are endemic to particular regions in the United States (eg, coccidioidomycosis in the San Joaquin Valley, histoplasmosis in the Missouri Valley) or elsewhere.

J. Does the patient have sickle cell disease or trait? Functional asplenia develops after numerous bouts with sickle cell crisis, placing the patient at increased risk for serious infections. Sickle cell **trait** confers an increased risk of pyelonephritis during pregnancy.

K. Is there a history of illicit drug use, particularly needle use?
This would place the patient at increased risk for acute and sub-acute endocarditis as well as AIDS and its complications.

L. Are there any HIV risk factors? HIV seroprevalence in the United States is estimated at 1 to 2 million. The HIV-seropositive gravida is at risk for a host of opportunistic infections which may be life threatening.

III. **Differential Diagnosis.** The complete differential diagnosis for fever is incredibly long and tiresome. The list that follows focuses only on infectious causes of fever, and is limited to the more common entities seen in the reproductive age group as well as infectious processes of particular interest to the obstetrician.

A. **Chorioamnionitis.** The most frequent finding in chorioamnionitis is fever (temp > 38.0 °C or 100.4 °F). In addition to fever, any two of the following should be present to make the diagnosis: leukocytosis, foul-smelling or purulent amniotic fluid, maternal and/or fetal tachycardia, or uterine tenderness.

B. **Pneumonia.** Community-acquired pneumonias complicate up to 1% of all pregnancies. The two most common organisms are *Mycoplasma pneumoniae* and *Streptococcus pneumoniae.* Their presentations are generally quite different: *M. pneumoniae* usually has an insidious onset, persistent nonproductive cough, low-grade fever, no rigors, and vague constitutional symptoms (myalgias, fatigue, etc), whereas *S. pneumoniae* classically presents with sudden onset of a single episode of rigors, high fever, cough productive of rust-colored sputum, and pleuritic chest pain. Other bacterial causes of pneumonia (*Legionella* sp., *Hemophilus influenzae, Moraxella catarrhalis, Staphylococcus aureus*) occur much less frequently in the young, healthy host. There are also numerous viruses which can cause pneumonia (see H-7, Other viruses).

C. **Pharyngitis.** Viral causes of pharyngitis are most frequent, but "strep throat" (ie, pharyngitis caused by group A streptococci) has serious potential sequelae including rheumatic fever and glomerulonephritis. It is important to differentiate between these causes. The finding of anterior cervical adenopathy, tonsillar exudate, and pharyngeal erythema characteristic of "strep throat" can also be produced by viral pharyngitis. The only reliable way to distinguish between bacterial and viral pharyngitis is by culture or rapid group A strep screening (enzyme immunoassay). Infectious mononucleosis caused by the Epstein-Barr virus can also cause a severe pharyngitis. Posterior cervical adenopathy, a positive heterophil agglutination test, and atypical lymphocytosis on peripheral WBC smear are clues to help in making this diagnosis.

D. Appendicitis. Fever, abdominal pain, and leukocytosis are clinical clues; neither the fever nor the leukocytosis need be very impressive. Historically, anorexia is almost always present, and if the patient is hungry one can nearly always exclude this diagnosis. The enlarging uterus progressively displaces the appendix cephalad (hence the tenderness) such that, during the third trimester, appendiceal pain may present in the right upper quadrant.

E. Cholecystitis. Gallbladder problems occur more frequently among females in the reproductive age group. Most cases of cholecystitis are chronic and noninfectious, and are not accompanied by fever. Acute cholecystitis is less common, is inflammatory, and is associated with low-grade fever (rarely > 38.0 °C). Acute suppurative cholangitis is due to complete obstruction of the common bile duct. The patient presents acutely ill, often with Charcot's triad (biliary colic, jaundice, and spiking fevers). Acute suppurative cholangitis is a surgical emergency with death the universal outcome if surgery is not performed.

F. Meningitis. The signs and symptoms of meningitis during pregnancy are very similar to those in the nongravid state. Severe headache, nuchal rigidity, fever, and photophobia all suggest the diagnosis. A lumbar puncture is necessary to make the diagnosis (see Laboratory Data).

G. Oral infections. Periodontal abscesses are commonly overlooked, and a physical examination must include careful inspection of the oral cavity. Proper dental referral should follow the finding of an oral abscess.

H. Viral illnesses of obstetric interest
  1. Cytomegalovirus (CMV). Most cases of CMV infection are asymptomatic, but in about 10% an acute mononucleosis-like presentation occurs. The relative risk of fetal sequelae is small: of the approximately 50% of fetuses infected during acute maternal infection, only 5–10% will actually develop neurologic symptoms. If the fetus is affected, however, it can be devastating. Mental retardation, cerebral calcification, hydrocephalus or microcephaly, and chorioretinitis is a common constellation of findings when there is neurologic involvement.
  2. Rubella. Infection with this virus can cause the congenital rubella syndrome (hearing loss, cataracts, and patent ductus arteriosus are the most frequent findings). Overall, maternal infection during the first trimester confers an approximate 50% risk to the fetus; this drops to about 30% in the

second trimester (mostly deafness), and third-trimester infection rarely causes fetal abnormalities.

3. **Varicella (chickenpox).** Varicella is uncommon in adults. Infection in early pregnancy can cause the congenital varicella syndrome (cutaneous scarring, limb hypoplasia, mental retardation, and cerebral atrophy). Maternal infection late in gestation (within 5 days of delivery), before production of protective maternal IgG, places the fetus at risk for neonatal varicella after delivery with an associated 30% mortality. Maternal varicella pneumonia is a very serious process with a mortality rate as high as 50%.

4. **Herpes simplex virus** (see Problem 42, page 162).

5. **Erythema infectiosum (fifth disease).** This is a viral exanthem caused by parvovirus. It infects mostly children and usually occurs in late winter or spring. Typically, a prodromal flulike illness lasts several days. A characteristic "slapped cheek" rash then develops after an intervening asymptomatic period (about one week). The fetus of an infected gravida may develop hydrops fetalis, probably on the basis of profound hemolysis.

6. **Acute viral hepatitis.** This is a systemic infection which affects predominantly the liver. The two most important agents are hepatitis A and hepatitis B virus. Prodromal symptoms include nausea and vomiting, headache, photophobia, myalgias, low-grade fever (more often with A than B), headache, and anorexia. These precede the onset of jaundice by 1–2 weeks. One to 5 days before jaundice appears, dark urine and clay-colored stools are often noted.

7. **Other viruses.** The common cold viruses (adenovirus, rhinovirus) usually produce a self-limited illness lasting 24–96 hours. If the volume status is adequate and there are no serious electrolyte disturbances, it rarely threatens the health of the gravida or her fetus. On the other hand, influenza is a more serious illness, characterized by high fever, extreme prostration, myalgias, and malaise. Pneumonia occurs not infrequently and may be due to a primary influenza pneumonia or secondary bacterial infection (usually *S. aureus, S. pneumoniae,* or *H. influenzae*).

I. **Urinary tract infections.** These are very common and important problems during pregnancy (see problem 40, page 157, for details).

J. **Infectious diarrheas.** Aside from viral causes, the four most common bacterial causes of diarrhea are *Salmonella, Shigella,* enterotoxigenic *Escherichia coli,* and *Campylobacter.* Pseudomembranous colitis due to *Clostridium difficile* is uncommon in the outpatient setting but may follow antibiotic use. Recent travel, food ingestion, or sick family members are helpful clues.

K. Salpingitis. Pelvic inflammatory disease is uncommon during pregnancy, and presents almost exclusively in the first trimester. It is nearly always followed by (septic) abortion.

IV. Database

A. Physical examination key points

1. **Vital signs.** Tachycardia in the face of hypotension is a sign of impending sepsis and must be addressed immediately. Fetal heart tones should be considered a routine part of the patient's vital signs.

2. **Heart.** The finding of a new murmur in a febrile patient should always raise the question of endocarditis, particularly in IV drug users or those with preexisting valvular disease.

3. **Lungs.** Abnormal breath sounds (rales, rhonchi, tubular breath sounds) should generally be followed by chest x-ray to confirm the diagnosis of pneumonia.

4. **Abdomen.** The abdomen often becomes the center of attention when the gravida is febrile. A systematic approach is necessary to ensure both thoroughness and accuracy. Right upper quadrant tenderness is seen with cholecystitis (Murphy's sign), third-trimester appendicitis, or hepatitis (tender liver edge). Signs of peritoneal irritation are less reliable in late gestation. Uterine tenderness may be due to chorioamnionitis, degenerating leiomyomas, or abruptio placentae. Fever should exclude abruptio, and with chorioamnionitis the uterus is usually diffusely tender. To differentiate between uterine tenderness and visceral tenderness, use the **Apt test.**

   a. Examine the patient supine and mark the point of maximal tenderness (PMT).

   b. Place the patient in the lateral decubitus position and reexamine.

   c. If the PMT has moved substantially, it is likely due to visceral illness (eg, appendicitis) since the bowel moves more freely than the tethered uterus. Determine if the uterus is irritable (contracts when palpated), which suggests either infection or abruption.

5. **Skin.** The finding of a rash with concurrent fever suggests a viral illness, some of which are important to consider during pregnancy. Although a diagnosis cannot always be made by examination, the typical appearance of each of the viral exanthems is discussed in Table 1–3.

6. **Rectal examination.** Significant peritonitis associated with

TABLE 1–3. TYPICAL APPEARANCE OF VIRAL EXANTHEMS.

Disease	Rash Characteristics	Prodromal Symptoms
Erythema infectiosum	The rash begins as bilateral erythema of cheeks ("slapped cheeks") followed by a maculopapular rash of the trunk and extremities that clears centrally, leaving a lacy, reticular appearance.	Yes, followed by an asymptomatic period for about 1 week before the rash develops.
Varicella	Begins as a maculopapular rash that becomes vesicular, then pustular, and spontaneously drains, crusts over, and heals. Lesions are in different stages of development, appear in crops, and begin on the head and scalp.	None.
Rubella	A pink macular rash begins on the face and spreads rapidly to the trunk.	Yes, begins several days before the rash.

appendicitis can be demonstrated on rectal examination. Masses (eg, posterior degenerating leiomyomas) can often be appreciated only on rectal exam.

7. **Pelvic examination.** Look for herpetic lesions. In the first trimester, consider pelvic inflammatory disease (tenderness on cervical motion or adnexal tenderness, possibly associated with a mass).

8. **HEENT.** Examine the oral cavity to eliminate oral infections. See if there is significant pharyngeal injection or exudate. Examine the tympanic membranes to exclude otitis media.

9. **Neck.** Determine if there is nuchal rigidity, especially if the patient is complaining of headache. Lymphadenopathy is typically anterior cervical with group A strep throat and posterior cervical with mononucleosis. Thyromegaly might suggest a thyroid storm, an uncommon cause of fever (see Problem 13, page 59).

B. **Laboratory Data**

1. **Hemogram.** Leukocytosis is normal during pregnancy (up to 15, 000/mm^3) and labor (up to 25, 000/mm^3), and must be interpreted carefully.

2. **Urinalysis, culture and sensitivity.** Urinalysis is a good screen to eliminate the urinary tract as a cause of the fever. An entirely normal urinalysis essentially eliminates the urinary tract as a source of infection (exception: obstructive pyelonephritis).

3. **Blood cultures** should be obtained in the febrile patient. Two sets from two different sites is usually adequate.

4. **Sputum culture and gram stain** are important first steps in

evaluating the febrile patient with cough. If *M. pneumoniae* is being considered, cold agglutinin serology is helpful.

5. **Electrolytes** should be evaluated, especially potassium in patients with nausea and vomiting or diarrhea.

6. **Cervical cultures.** Group B strep, *Chlamydia trachomatis,* and *Neisseria gonorrhoeae* cultures should be obtained in preterm labor, rupture of membranes, or chorioamnionitis.

7. **Herpes cultures.** If the patient is symptomatic or lesions are present (crops of vesicles), herpes cultures must be taken. Unroof the lesion, collect a cellular specimen on a swab, and send in viral transport media.

8. **Liver function tests and hepatitis screen.** If the patient has right upper quadrant tenderness or jaundice, check a hepatitis screen (HBsAg, HAA), SGOT (AST) and GGTP (elevated predominantly in parenchymal disease such as hepatitis), and alkaline phosphatase (elevated predominantly in obstructive disease such as cholecystitis).

9. **Arterial blood gases.** Blood gases should be obtained in all acutely ill patients or those with respiratory distress (see Procedure 7, page 352, and Problems 30, 31, and 39 on pages 117, 121, and 153 respectively).

10. **Lumbar puncture.** If meningitis is considered, it should be definitively diagnosed by lumbar puncture (see Procedure 21, page 000).

11. **Amniocentesis and cultures.** Whenever fever is unexplained, amniocentesis will provide helpful results more often than it will cause problems (see Procedure 1, page 339). Gram stain and culture of the fluid (aerobic, anaerobic, *Ureaplasma urealyticum, Mycoplasma hominis*) are the most useful tests; WBCs without bacteria on gram stain are not specific for infection.

12. **Stool cultures.** If the clinical situation suggests a more serious gastroenteritis, cultures for *Salmonella, Shigella,* and *Campylobacter* are appropriate. Also, stool should be examined for leukocytes and the presence of blood should be excluded (guaiac). If the patient has received antibiotics recently, *C. difficile* toxin should be obtained.

C. **Radiologic and other studies**

1. **Chest x-ray** is required if the patient has respiratory symptoms and a clinical picture of pneumonia. Abdominal shielding is necessary.

2. **Abdominal x-ray** is necessary if intestinal perforation or obstruction is considered.

3. **Abdominal ultrasound** may be used to scan the gallbladder for stones or duct abnormalities. For pyelonephritis un-

responsive to antibiotics, use ultrasound to exclude obstructive pyelonephritis.
   4. **Electronic fetal and uterine monitoring** should be done if over 20–24 weeks.

V. Plan

A. **General.** Successful treatment of fever during pregnancy is dependent on achieving the proper diagnosis. The specific treatment for each diagnosis is listed below. Before therapy is started, it is important to guarantee that the gravida is adequately hydrated and oxygenated. Also, high fever (> 38.5 °C) should be controlled during pregnancy (with acetaminophen and a cooling blanket, if necessary).

B. **Specific**
   1. **Pneumonia.** The general treatment of pneumonia is similar regardless of the putative organism. Except for the mildest cases, the patient should be hospitalized. Adequate oxygenation and hydration is the key, and may require supplemental oxygen. Rarely, intubation with positive pressure ventilation is required. PO_2 should be (at minimum) 70 mm Hg. Specific therapy is dictated by the presentation.
      a. "Atypical" presentation (insidious onset, nonproductive cough, low-grade fever, nonhomogeneous infiltrate on x-ray) is usually due to *Mycoplasma,* and is treated with erythromycin 500 mg IV q6h.
      b. Conversely, a sudden onset with high fever, shaking chills, productive cough, and lobar infiltrate is most frequently due to *S. pneumoniae,* and treatment with ampicillin 1–2 g q6h is indicated. The penicillin-allergic patient can receive erythromycin.
      c. Other presentations are less common.
         (1) Varicella pneumonia should be treated with acyclovir.
         (2) Nosocomial pneumonia may be treated with either an extended-spectrum penicillin with a beta-lactamase (eg, Timentin 3 g IV q6h or Unasyn 3 g IV q6h) or an aminoglycoside with a third-generation cephalosporin. Aspiration pneumonia can be treated with either penicillin G (4 million units IV q4h) or clindamycin (900 mg IV q8h).
         (3) Pneumonia due to influenza should be treated with amantadine 100 mg PO q12h. Ribavirin inhalation therapy is also useful.
         (4) Pneumonia that occurs following influenza is usually due to *S. aureus.* Treatment is with nafcillin (1–2 g

q4h) or a first-generation cephalosporin (cefazolin 1–2 g q8h).

2. **Pyelonephritis** (see Problem 40, page 157).

3. **Appendicitis.** The basic treatment for appendicitis is surgical with broad-spectrum perioperative antibiotic therapy (eg, Cefotetan, Timentin). In late gestation, tocolysis is frequently necessary postoperatively and $MgSO_4$ is the preferred agent.

4. **Cholecystitis.** Most gallbladder disease during pregnancy can be managed medically, but acute cholecystitis frequently requires surgery. Broad-spectrum antibiotic coverage, NPO status, nasogastric suction, correction of volume, and electrolyte status are all necessary prior to surgery. Acute suppurative cholangitis (as suggested by Charcot's triad) indicates an immediate need for surgery.

5. **Chorioamnionitis.** Once the diagnosis is made, antibiotics should be started (ampicillin and an aminoglycoside are used most frequently) and efforts begun to effect delivery. The vaginal route is safer and preferred.

6. **Diarrhea.** Hydration and electrolyte status are the immediate concerns when managing infectious diarrheas. If many leukocytes are seen in the stool or gross blood is present, Bactrim is effective for *Salmonella* and *Shigella.* Pseudomembranous colitis can be treated with either vancomycin (125 mg PO q6h for 10 days) or metronidazole (250 mg PO q6h for 10 days).

7. The characteristics and management of three potentially troublesome viral illnesses during pregnancy are summarized in Tables 1–3 and 1–4.

REFERENCES

Gilstrap LC, Faro S: *Infections in Pregnancy.* New York: Allan R. Liss, 1990.

Maccato ML: Pneumonia and pulmonary tuberculosis in pregnancy. *Obstet Gynecol Clin North Am* 16:417, 1989.

Pearlman M: Chorioamnionitis: a logical approach to treatment. *Clin Adv Infec,* May 1990.

6. FETAL HEART RATE ABNORMALITIES

I. **Problem.** You are called to evaluate a patient because of an abnormal fetal heart rate. Normal heart rate is between 120 and 160, although the limits probably should be 110–160 (Table 1–5).

II. **Immediate Questions**

A. **What are the maternal and fetal complications?** Are membranes ruptured or intact? Maternal infections or amnionitis can

TABLE 1–4. DIAGNOSIS AND TREATMENT OF VIRAL ILLNESSES.

Disease	Diagnosis	Management
Erythema infectiosum	Parovirus-specific IgM.	Weekly ultrasound. If evidence of hydrops, consider fetal transfusion.
Rubella	If prenatal rubella titer ≥ 1 : 16, the patient is immune. If unknown, measure IgG level at the time of exposure. If ≥ 1 : 16, patient is immune. If ≤ 1 : 8, measure again in several days. Acute infection is suggested if the titer has increased sharply. Measure IgG again in 3 weeks, run simultaneously with first specimen. If titer increases > 4-fold, this is diagnostic of acute infection. If exposure was several weeks prior to presentation (or atypical illness) and IgG ≥ 1 : 64, check if IgM is present.	Immune globulin is generally *not* effective and should not be administered routinely for exposure. Counseling should be based on definitive diagnosis and gestational age at exposure or illness.
Varicella	Usually made clinically. Tzanck smear from base of vesicle will reveal multinucleated giant cells. Viral isolation is rarely necessary.	Varicella zoster immune globulin (VZIG) may be administered within 48–72 hours of exposure (if negative past history of maternal varicella infection). If maternal status is uncertain, measure maternal serum IgG at the time of exposure. If present, patient is immune. Give acyclovir (5–10 mg/kg IV q8h) for pneumonia or immunocompromised with disseminated infection.

result in fetal heart rate abnormalities including tachycardia and late decelerations.

B. Does the patient have bradycardia, tachycardia, decreased beat-to-beat variability, or decelerations? These may be potentially life threatening. For details see Differential Diagnosis.

C. Is the patient receiving oxytocin? Oxytocin should be stopped: it can cause uterine hypercontractility and result in fetal bradycardia and decelerations.

D. Is the patient in the lateral position? If the patient is lying on her back, supine hypotension secondary to aortocaval compression can cause fetal hypoxia and decelerations.

E. Is the patient well oxygenated and not hypotensive? Mater-

TABLE 1-5. DIFFERENTIAL DIAGNOSIS OF ACUTE FETAL DISTRESS.

	Normal	Possible Fetal Distress	Probable Fetal Distress	Fetal Distress
FHR in beats per minute	120–160	Tachycardia (probably normal)	Tachycardia (or normal)	Tachycardia (or normal) or bradycardia
Beat-to-beat variability	Present	Present but may be decreased	Decreased or absent; rarely, increased	Absent
Response of FHR to uterine contraction	None, or, if membranes ruptured, mild to moderate early deceleration (acceleration with stimulation)	Mild variable decelerations	Prolonged or increasingly severe variable deceleration; (nonconsistent) late deceleration	Severe variable deceleration, late deceleration, or combined patterns
Fetal scalp blood pH anticipated	≥ 7.25	7.20–7.24	7.20–7.24	≤ 7.20
Meconium (term pregnancy)	Usually none	Perhaps	Often present	Often present
Probable fetal condition	Satisfactory	Mildly compromised	Compromised	Often critical

From Pernoll ML, Benson RC (eds): Current Obstetric and Gynecologic Diagnosis and Treatment, 6th ed. Norwalk, Connecticut, Appleton & Lange, 1987.

nal hypoxia and hypotension can cause fetal hypoxia and a.-rhythmias.

F. Are fetal heart accelerations present? Heart rate accelerations after fetal movement are indicative of a healthy fetus.

III. Differential Diagnosis

A. Fetal tachycardia (heart rate > 160 bpm). Causes to check include maternal fever and infection. Without a known cause, fetal arrhythmias and tachycardia may be secondary to fetal heart disease and conduction abnormalities. Tachycardia may also be due to drugs, especially tocolytic drugs.

B. Fetal bradycardia (heart rate < 120 bpm). The causes of bradycardia include fetal distress and congenital heart block. Moderate bradycardia in the 100–120 range is not that abnormal in some situations.

C. Decreased beat-to-beat variability. Decreased variability may be secondary to fetal hypoxia and occasionally the only sign of a dying fetus. Narcotics can cause decreased beat-to-beat variability, and it can also occur in the immediate period after epidural dosing.

D. Early decelerations. These occur and are synchronous with contractions. Early decelerations are secondary to fetal head compression. They are usually present only when the membranes are ruptured and are not a sign of fetal distress (Figure 1–5).

E. Late decelerations. These are consistent with uteroplacental insufficiency and are most often seen in chronic disease states such as intrauterine growth retardation. Late decelerations should be seen at least two-thirds of the time and be repetitive to be of significance. Fifty percent of the time they will respond to therapy (see Figure 1–5).

F. Variable decelerations. These are cord compression and vagal nerve mediated. Variable decelerations occur with decreased amounts of amniotic fluid (see Figure 1–5).

G. If accelerations are present, this is a strong sign of fetal well-being.

IV. Database

A Physical Examination Key Points
  1. Vital signs
    a. Temperature. Maternal infection such as chorioamnionitis or pyelonephritis may manifest itself with increased temperature.

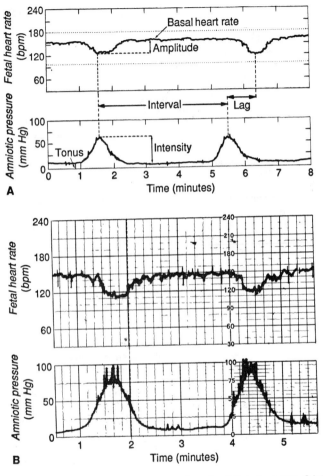

Figure 1–5. Fetal heart rate tracings. *A:* Schematic tracing. *B:* Early deceleration. *C:* Late deceleration. *D:* Variable deceleration.

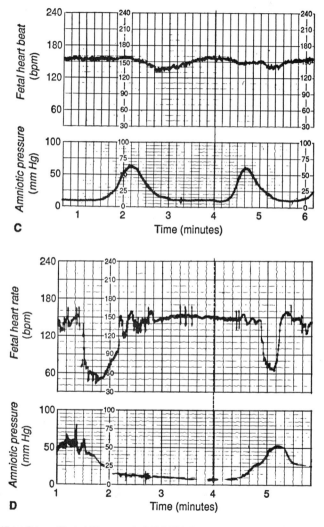

(*From Babson SG et al:* Management of High-Risk Pregnancy and Intensive Care of the Neonate, *3rd ed. St. Louis, Mosby, 1975.*)

    b. **Blood pressure.** Hypotension secondary to hypovolemia, drugs, epidural anesthesia, or maternal blood loss can cause fetal hypoxia and arrhythmias.

2. **Uterus.** The gestational age may be estimated by measuring the fundal height. Umbilical level is equivalent to 20 weeks with each additional fingerbreadth equal to 2 weeks. The uterus should also be evaluated for hyperstimulation. More than fetal heart rate should be auscultated. Also palpate for rigidity and localized tenderness (see Appendix).

3. **Vagina or cervix.** The fetal scalp may be stimulated by the gloved, Betadine-coated examining finger. The presence of fetal heart rate accelerations may be reassuring. Cervical dilatation and effacement should be documented and used in planning the appropriate method of delivery. The presenting part should be identified as well as possible cord prolapse.

B. Laboratory Data

1. **Hemogram.** The white count will be elevated with a severe maternal infection. WBCs are also increased during the second stage of labor. The hematocrit is helpful in evaluating maternal anemia and possible blood loss.

2. **Scalp pH.** (see Procedure 26, page 387). A pH < 7.20 is suggestive of impending fetal death, and the patient requires emergent delivery.

C. Radiologic and other studies

1. **Ultrasound.** Evaluation of fetal gestational age, placental grade, and volume of amniotic fluid is imperative when assessing a fetus with an abnormal heart rate. Ultrasound can also confirm an absent or abnormal heart rate identified on auscultation.

2. **Biophysical profiles** should be obtained to evaluate fetal well-being (see Procedure 6, page 351).

3. **Fetal heart tracing.** Apply a scalp electrode (see Procedure 18, page 371) to obtain a tracing if the head is engaged (Table 1–6). Apply a scalp electrode if:

    a. Membranes are ruptured.

    b. An external tracing is not satisfactory (always evaluate the tracing first: the tocobelt may be poorly placed).

    c. Consider the potential effect of rupturing membranes if severe variables or breech presentation or floating head is found. An external monitor is not as accurate.

4. **Internal uterine pressure monitor (IUPM).** IUPM enables the practitioner to align the deceleration with contraction in addition to identifying hypercontractility (see Procedure 19, page 372).

TABLE 1–6. FETAL HEART RATE PATTERNS.

			Rates in Beats per Minute
	Normal		120–160
Basal FHR	Tachycardia	Moderate	161–180
		Marked	181 or more
	Bradycardia	Moderate	100–119
		Marked	90 or less
Transitory FHR changes	Variability		5–15 beats/min amplitude
	Accelerations		Increased by 15 or more
	Decelerations Early Late Variable		Decreased by 10–40 Decreased by 5–60 Decreased by 10–60, occasionally more

From Pernoll ML, Benson RC (eds): Current Obstetric and Gynecologic Diagnosis and Treatment, 6th ed. Norwalk, Connecticut, Appleton & Lange, 1987.

V. Plan

A. **Position** the patient on her left side to decrease aortocaval compression.

B. **Administer oxygen** to the mother.

C. **Discontinue oxytocin:** uterine contraction may be causing the fetal heart rate changes.

D. **Tocolysis** with terbutaline 0.25 mg SQ should be administered if uterine hypercontractility is present. Tocolytic agents should not be administered if a placental abruption is diagnosed.

E. **Hydrate** the patient with Ringer's lactate, Plasmalyte, or normal saline.

F. **Transfuse** if the patient is actively losing blood secondary to an abruption or placenta previa.

G. **Emergent delivery.** If fetal pH < 7.20 or severe decelerations and bradycardia are present, the patient should be delivered emergently via forceps or cesarean section (see Figure A–3, page 594).

REFERENCE

Gabbe SG, Niebyl JR, Simpson JL (eds): *Obstetrics: Normal and Problem Pregnancies,* 2nd ed. New York, Churchill Livingstone, 1991.

7. HYPERGLYCEMIA IN PREGNANCY

I. **Problem.** A 30-year-old primigravid diabetic presents at 30 weeks' gestation dehydrated with confusion and disorientation.

II. **Immediate Questions**

A. **What is the patient's diabetic therapy?** Is the patient on insulin? If so, how much does she administer daily and when was her last dose? Is the patient on any other medication?

B. **Over what period of time has the problem developed?** When did the patient develop polyuria and polydipsia? This will give an idea of the duration and degree of the problem.

C. **Does the patient have any symptoms to indicate a source of infection, ie, urinary, upper respiratory tract, or gastrointestinal symptoms, fever, or chills?** Infection is commonly a precipitating event for the development of diabetic ketoacidosis (DKA).

D. **Does the patient have an underlying medical condition of any organ system that could predispose to the problem?** Urinary tract infection, asthma, or any other medical condition could precipitate DKA.

E. **Has the patient had similar episodes and, if so, how frequently?** This will give some indication of the degree of diabetic control.

F. **Is the patient under any form of stress?** Any stress factor (surgical, septic, or emotional) can precipitate DKA.

G. **Is there a history of trauma?** Any head or central nervous system trauma could result in confusion.

III. **Differential Diagnosis**

A. **Diabetes**

1. **Insulin dependent (type I) (formerly called juvenile diabetes).** Insulin-dependent diabetics require insulin.

2. **Non-insulin-dependent (type II) (formerly called adult-onset diabetes, or AODM).** Surgical stress often aggravates diabetes. Thus, patients are controlled with diet or oral hypoglycemic agents.

3. **A modified White's classification** of diabetes mellitus appears in Table 1–7.

B. **Diabetic ketoacidosis.** This is the most common cause of dehydration and confusion in a diabetic.

C. **Hyperosmolar nonketotic state.** Hyperglycemia with coma in a patient without ketosis.

TABLE 1–7. MODIFIED WHITE'S CLASSIFICATION OF DIABETES MELLITUS.

Class A:	Chemical diabetes diagnosed *before* pregnancy; managed by diet *alone;* any age of onset or duration.
Class B:	Insulin treatment necessary *before* pregnancy; onset after age 20; duration of less than 10 years.
Class C:	Onset at age 10–19; or duration of 10–19 years.
Class D:	Onset before age 10; or duration of 20 or more years; or chronic hypertension; or background retinopathy.
Class F:	Renal disease.
Class H:	Coronary artery disease.
Class R:	Proliferative retinopathy.
Class T:	Renal transplant.

From Pernoll ML, Benson RC (eds): Current Obstetric & Gynecologic Diagnosis & Treatment, *6th ed. Norwalk, Connecticut, Appleton & Lange, 1987.*

   D. Central nervous system infection. Meningitis or encephalitis could result in confusion and dehydration.

IV. Database

A. Physical examination key points

1. **Vital signs.** Fever and tachycardia suggest infection and hypotension suggests sepsis. Kussmaul respiration (deep, rapid respiratory pattern) may be seen with severe ketoacidosis.
2. **HEENT.** Fruity odor on the breath may signify ketoacidosis.
3. **Lungs.** Listen for evidence of pneumonia.
4. **Abdomen.** Exclude intra-abdominal causes of sepsis.
5. **Neurologic examination.** Obtundation may indicate deterioration of a diabetic condition and development of ketoacidosis.

B. Laboratory data. Significantly elevated fingerstick glucose measurements should be confirmed with a serum glucose determination.

1. **Hemogram.** Infection with leukocytosis may cause a previously well controlled diabetic to develop extremely high blood sugars.
2. **Serum electrolytes.** Potassium and phosphorus must be monitored closely in DKA. Chloride may be low if vomiting has been present. CO_2 will be low in the face of acidosis and hyperventilation.
3. **Arterial blood gases.** Any suspicion of sepsis or DKA should be followed up with a determination of serum pH and PO_2.

4. **Lactic acid measurements** may be useful in DKA.
5. **Hgb A$_1$C** provides a measurement of previous glucose control.
6. **Urinalysis** should be done to look for ketones and glucose. Thresholds for spilling glucose in the urine can vary widely; confirm with a serum glucose if any doubt exists. Glucosuria occurs in pregnancy and is not an accurate measurement of hyperglycemia. The urine should also be evaluated for evidence of infection.
7. **Cultures of blood, urine, central lines, etc,** should be done if infection is suspected.

C. **Radiologic and other studies**
   1. These studies should be selected based on the clinical impression. For example, infection in the postoperative hyperglycemic patient may be evaluated with a chest x-ray if a pulmonary source is suspected, or an abdominal CT scan or ultrasound if an intra-abdominal abscess is considered.
   2. **Fetal assessment.** It is conceivable that there is fetal demise (50%). If the fetus is alive, there may be distress with late decelerations. Following correction of the maternal acidosis in DKA, the fetal state should improve.

V. **Plan.** The basics of management include (1) controlling serum glucose quickly and safely, and (2) treating predisposing infection appropriately.

A. **Sliding-scale insulin**
   1. Small doses of subcutaneous regular insulin can be given every 6 hours based on rapid, automated evaluation of blood sugars using Chemsticks.
   2. Acutely, serum glucose < 200 mg/dL is considered adequate control in the nonpregnant patient and < 100 mg/dL in the pregnant patient.
   3. A typical sliding scale will give no insulin with serum glucose determinations < 180 mg/dL, 3–5 U from 180–240 mg/dL, 6–10 U from 240–400 mg/dL, and 9–15 U for > 400 mg/dL. Any Chemstick > 300 mg/dL should be confirmed with a stat serum measurement from the lab. Patients who have not received insulin previously will need smaller doses until their own response to insulin is assessed.

B. **Diet modification** is needed in diabetic patients, with caloric restriction in the obese patient being important.

C. **Oral hypoglycemic agents.** Many type II diabetics who are receiving these medications may require insulin supplements after an operation, but are usually discharged on the same oral agent. **These drugs are contraindicated in the pregnant patient.**

D. **Severe glucose intolerance due to DKA.** These patients require aggressive therapy, usually in an ICU setting. DKA is usually manifest as tachypnea, dehydration, ketones on the breath, and abdominal pain with hyperglycemia, hyperketonemia, and metabolic acidosis.

1. **Precipitating factors.** In the surgical patient, infection precipitates severe glucose intolerance. It should be appropriately treated.

2. **Dehydration.** Typically patients become volume depleted, often due to severe glycosuria. Rehydrate the patient initially with dextrose-free saline. Increased urine output in these patients may be due to osmotic diuresis and not a reflection of the true volume status. Volume status must be assessed by other means such as a central venous pressure line.

3. **Potassium.** Potassium levels will go down as DKA improves. The potassium ions become intracellular, thus decreasing serum levels. However, total body potassium is actually depleted.

4. **Phosphate.** If hypophosphatemia is present, then potassium can be replaced as potassium phosphate (10 meq/h). Phosphorus is usually not required in the recovery phase.

5. **Bicarbonate.** Doses of 20 meq/h can be administered in DKA with good urine output. Correction of severe acidosis with bicarbonate is sometimes needed. Insulin must be continued until the bicarbonate normalizes. This may mean using both insulin and glucose intravenously. Bicarbonate should be administered if pH is < 7.1.

6. **Insulin.** Start with a 10–20 U IV bolus and follow with a continuous drip. The infusion rate will vary but should be approximately 2–5 U/h initially and adjusted as needed.

7. **Dextrose.** IV fluids should be changed to those containing 5% dextrose when serum glucose levels reach 300 mg/dL.

8. **Maintenance insulin.** Once IV therapy has controlled severe hyperglycemia, maintenance insulin will be needed. Subcutaneous administration should be performed twice a day to achieve better control, often with a combination of NPH and regular insulin. Patients on hyperalimentation can receive maintenance insulin by adding it directly to the solution.

REFERENCES

Coustan DR, Felig P: Diabetes mellitus. In Barrow GN, Ferris TF (eds): *Medical Complications during Pregnancy,* 3rd ed. Philadelphia, WB Saunders, 1988.

Creasy RK, Resnik R (eds): *Maternal Fetal Medicine: Principles and Practice,* 2nd ed. Philadelphia, WB Saunders, 1989.

Phelps RL, Metzger BE, Freinkel N: Medical management of diabetes in pregnancy. In Sciarra JJ, Depp R, Eschenbach DA (eds): *Gynecology and Obstetrics,* Vol 3. Philadelphia, JB Lippincott, 1990.

Thorn GW et al (eds): *Harrison's Principles of Internal Medicine,* 8th ed. New York, McGraw-Hill, 1977.

8. HYPERTENSION IN PREGNANCY

I. Problem. You are called to the emergency room to see a 25-year-old patient who is 12 weeks pregnant with a blood pressure of 150/100.

II. Immediate Questions

A. Is the patient taking any current medications, and is there a suspicion of substance use or abuse? A history as well as a toxicology screen can help to assess whether or not there may be any underlying reason for this patient's elevated blood pressure. The history of essential hypertension would make this unlikely, but nonetheless it should be screened.

B. Has an intrauterine pregnancy been established? While audible fetal heart tones would suggest an intrauterine pregnancy, ultrasound confirmation could be helpful. Hydatidiform mole, complete or partial, has been associated with elevated blood pressure. A normal ultrasound confirming an intrauterine pregnancy would be helpful in eliminating these diagnostic possibilities.

C. Does the patient have any headaches or visual disturbances? Symptoms of persistent headache or scotomas may also be of concern, especially if the patient's blood pressure is poorly controlled, suggesting possible rupture of a berry aneurysm or arteriovenous malformation.

III. Differential Diagnosis

A. Hydatidiform mole. Ultrasound examination or auscultation of the fetal heart, or the two combined, should be able to rule this out effectively. Hydatidiform moles are secondary to dispermic fusion with an egg during fertilization. The mole produces human chorionic gonadotropin (HCG) and can result in a hyperthyroid state and hypertension.

B. Substance use. The use of illegal substances, particularly cocaine, may result in transient elevations of blood pressure.

    C. Collagen vascular disease. Collagen vascular disorders frequently occur in young women of reproductive age and not infrequently complicate pregnancy. Flareups of collagen vascular disease are frequently seen during pregnancy and may present as hypertension.

    D. Preeclampsia (see Problem 18, page 76).

    E. Thyrotoxicosis. Thyroid disease, particularly Graves' disease, is not uncommon among women of reproductive age (see Problems 6 and 13, pages 32 and 59).

    F. Pheochromocytoma. This is an extremely rare cause of hypertension but can be fatal if overlooked.

    G. Essential hypertension. This is a diagnosis of exclusion. Once made, a treatment regimen should be outlined and implemented.

    H. Miscellaneous. Additional causes of hypertension complicating pregnancy include renal vein thrombosis, renal artery stenosis, and other less common medical disorders. Clinical index of suspicion should guide the physician in evaluating the patient for these disorders.

IV. Database

    A. Physical examination key points

        1. Vital signs. Blood pressure should be monitored prior to and throughout treatment. It must increase 30 mm Hg systolic or 15 mm Hg diastolic for the patient to be considered to have mild pregnancy-induced hypertension (PIH). If no previous pressure was recorded, a blood pressure of 140/90 after 20 weeks' gestation is considered PIH. The patient's pulse may be elevated secondary to thyroid or adrenal disease.

        2. HEENT. Evidence of thyroid enlargement is suggestive of thyroid disease. Malar rashes are indicative of systemic lupus erythematosus. Signs of hyperthyroidism should be looked for and include smooth, velvety, warm, dry skin with thinning hair, proximal muscle weakness, lid lag, proptosis, and exophthalmos. Particular attention should be paid to the ophthalmologic examination to detect evidence of chronic hypertensive retinal changes or retinal hemorrhages.

    B. Laboratory data

        1. Hemogram and coagulation studies. A baseline coagulation profile consisting of prothrombin time, partial thromboplastin time, and serum fibrinogen may be obtained, although these tests are more useful in evaluating the patient with hypertension complicating pregnancy in the third trimester. A peripheral smear looking for evidence of hemolysis may also be helpful.

2. **Electrolytes and chemistry panel.** Particular attention should be focused on glucose, liver function, and renal function. Hypertension in pregnancy is more common among patients with glucose intolerance or frank diabetes and in patients with underlying renal disease.

3. **Thyroid function tests.** Specifically, serum thyroid-stimulating hormone (TSH) and serum free thyroxin should be determined. TSH and free thyroxin are utilized during pregnancy because their values do not change with respect to the pregnant state. In contrast, total thyroxin or T_3 resin uptake are both dependent on thyroid-binding globulin, which changes during pregnancy.

4. **Urine metanephrine and vanillylmandelic acid.** These substances are the metabolites of norepinephrine and epinephrine and will be markedly elevated in pheochromocytoma.

5. **24-hour urine.** A quantitative assessment of urinary protein should be obtained via a 24-hour urine collection. Creatinine clearance may also be calculated at this time. Kidney function can be altered by preeclampsia, vascular disease, and essential hypertension.

6. **Additional tests.** Collagen vascular screen (antinuclear antibody) and toxicology screen for illicit substance abuse may be appropriate.

C. **Radiologic and other studies**

1. **Chest x-ray.** An abdominal shield is frequently used when obtaining a chest x-ray in a pregnant patient. There is no harm in doing this, but it should be recognized that most x-ray exposure to the fetus is via scatter through the axial skeleton rather than through the air.

2. **Ultrasound.** Assessment of gestational age is essential in formulating the management plan for a pregnant hypertensive. In addition, the diagnosis of a hydatidiform molar pregnancy may be made.

3. **ECG.** Cardiac abnormalities such as infarction, ventricular hypertrophy, and arrhythmias may be present in the patient with exacerbation of essential hypertension.

V. **Plan.** The acute management of a pregnant patient with hypertension depends primarily on two factors: (1) the absolute blood pressure and whether or not it represents a hypertensive emergency and

(2) the gestational age. A true hypertensive emergency represents a danger to the mother and must be dealt with quickly.

A. **Gestational age < 20 weeks**
  1. **Hydralazine.** Begin with a 5 mg intravenous bolus. The drug may be readministered every 10 minutes for two additional doses. If there is no dramatic response, 10 mg IV q20min may be given until the blood pressure is stabilized. An alternative regimen is to begin a continuous hydralazine infusion starting at approximately 2 mg/h. Blood pressure is continuously measured and the infusion may be increased by 1 mg/h q5min until an acceptable blood pressure is reached. Most patients will be controlled at a hydralazine infusion rate of 6–8 mg/h.
  2. **Alpha-methyldopa.** This remains the drug of first choice for treatment of chronic hypertension during pregnancy. An initial dose of 250 mg PO tid is employed. Alpha-methyldopa is associated with drug-induced hepatitis in approximately 0.5–1% of cases.
  3. **Atenolol/labetalol.** An alternative regimen consists of either atenolol or labetalol. Atenolol is a somewhat cardioselective beta-blocking agent that can be begun at a dose of 50 mg qd in a single dose; 100 mg qd is usually sufficient to control most patients with mild to moderate hypertension. An alternative agent is labetalol, which can generally be begun at 200 mg PO bid. Most patients with mild to moderate hypertension will be controlled with a total daily labetalol dose of 400–800 mg.
  4. **Diuretics.** Diuretics have also been used to treat mild to moderate chronic hypertension. There remains considerable controversy relative to using diuretics during pregnancy. Generally, they are avoided.
  5. **Calcium.** Supplemental calcium has also been used as adjunctive therapy for lowering mild to moderate hypertension. The oral dose is 1–2 g of elemental calcium per day.

B. **Gestational age > 20 weeks.** If preeclampsia has been effectively ruled out (see Problem 18, page 76), then antihypertensive therapy may begin as stated earlier. Certainly after 24 weeks, attention must be paid to the condition of the fetus during initiation of any antihypertensive therapy. The goal of therapy is to maintain the patient's blood pressure at about 140/90. To drop the pressure below this level may result in uteroplacental insufficiency and possible fetal death. In the patient who is beyond 24 weeks' gestation, continuous fetal monitoring should accompany all of these pharmacologic manipulations. Also, intravascularly volume depleted patients may be particularly sensitive to the addition of a second peripheral vasodilator. This should be recognized when managing a patient who is refractory to parenteral hydralazine and who may require one of the other agents such as a calcium channel blocker.

REFERENCES

Anderson GD, Sibai BM: Hypertension in pregnancy. In Gabbe SG, Niebyl JR, Simpson JL (eds): *Obstetrics: Normal and Problem Pregnancies.* New York, Churchill Livingstone, 1986.
Repke JT: The pharmacologic management of hypertension in pregnancy. In Niebyl JR (ed): *Drug Use in Pregnancy.* Philadelphia, Lea & Febiger, 1988.

9. HYPOGLYCEMIA IN PREGNANCY

I. **Problem.** A 29-year-old diabetic presents at 15 weeks' gestation with anxiety and tremulousness. A blood glucose measurement at home was noted to be 40 mg/dL.

II. **Immediate Questions**

   A. **What are the most recent blood glucose measurements?** If the patient measures blood glucose at home either with Chemstrips or by glucometer, the most recent values and trends should be reviewed.

   B. **What type of diabetes does she have, type I or type II?** One of every 100 pregnant women requires insulin administration for the control of glucose intolerance during pregnancy. Hypoglycemia is the most common complication that occurs in the pregnant diabetic. Type I or "brittle" diabetics are more likely to experience episodes of hypoglycemia during pregnancy, especially between 6 and 16 weeks of gestation and during the postpartum period.

   C. **What is her current insulin regimen?** The current insulin regimen should be noted as well as any recent alterations in dosage.

   D. **When was her last insulin dose?** Both the type and amount of her most recent doses are important, as is the elapsed time since administration.

   E. **When was her last meal, and what did it consist of?** Missed meals and inconsistent eating habits may contribute to hypoglycemic incidents.

   F. **Does the patient have any other acute illnesses?** Other chronic disease states and acute illnesses such as viral syndromes can cause extreme swings in glucose levels.

   G. **Are there any other stress factors presently?** The removal of stress factors (surgical, septic, or emotional) may induce hypoglycemia.

H. Has there been any significant change in her level of physical activity, especially any increase? Changes in general physical activity or moderate to vigorous exercise without adequate carbohydrate consumption may be of etiologic importance.

I. Did her symptoms occur gradually, or did mentation deteriorate rapidly? Symptoms of hypoglycemia depend upon the rate of decline in blood glucose, the absolute glucose level, and the duration of exposure to exogenously administered insulin. Glycogenolysis is stimulated by epinephrine and glucagon. Rapid declines in blood glucose result in the release of epinephrine, causing anxiety, tremors, palpitations, hunger, and perspiration. More gradual falls in blood glucose may result in only cerebral symptoms such as confusion, headache, blurred vision, irritability, and loss of consciousness.

J. What is her gestational age, and what is the status of the fetus? Hypoglycemia occurs most often in the first half of pregnancy and in the postpartum period, and can be detrimental to the fetus. The best therapy for the fetus is to treat the maternal cause.

III. Differential Diagnosis

A. Overinsulinization. Excessive insulinization, often due to an overzealous physician or patient, is the most common cause of hypoglycemia during pregnancy. This in turn may be affected by abnormal insulin absorption, decreased carbohydrate intake, changes in activity or exercise, hormonal changes of pregnancy, or termination of pregnancy.

B. Medication use. Drugs other than insulin and sulfonylurea can induce hypoglycemia. Salicylates, propranolol, disopyramide, pentamidine, and quinine are several of the many pharmacologic agents that may play a role in a hypoglycemic episode.

C. Ethanol use. In occasional cases, alcohol abuse can result in symptomatic hypoglycemia. This possibility may be evident from the history or clinical signs.

D. Insulinoma. This is a very rare cause of hypoglycemia during pregnancy. Serum insulin levels should be checked.

E. Factitious. Nondiabetic individuals who secretly take insulin or sulfonylureas are often women in their 20's or 30's who work in health care fields. Suspicion should be raised when documented hypoglycemia is encountered in a nondiabetic with an otherwise negative workup.

F. Acute fatty liver of pregnancy. Severe, persistent, and often life-threatening hypoglycemia may complicate this rare entity, which occurs during the third trimester of pregnancy and may be a variant of pregnancy-induced hypertension.

G. Sudden discontinuation of TPN. This is more theoretical than an actual problem. In fact, most patients can easily tolerate sudden discontinuation of hyperalimentation.

H. Retroperitoneal sarcoma. These rare tumors can cause hypoglycemia.

I. Paraneoplastic syndrome. Hypoglycemia can be caused by the secretion of insulin or insulin-like substances by tumors, especially small cell carcinoma of the lung.

J. Alimentary hypoglycemia. This occurs in 5–10% of patients who have undergone partial to complete gastrectomy and results from rapid gastric emptying time.

K. Hormone deficiencies. Low levels of glucocorticoids, growth hormone, thyroid hormone, and glucagon as well as panhypopituitarism can all cause hypoglycemia.

L. Miscellaneous. Other causes include sepsis, alcoholism, or severe malnutrition.

IV. Database

A. Physical examination key points

1. **Vital signs.** Tachycardia may be caused by an adrenergic response to decreasing glucose levels that results in release of epinephrine.
2. **Skin.** Diaphoresis is also an adrenergic response.
3. **Neurologic examination.** Orientation and level of consciousness may be altered.

B. Laboratory data

1. **Serum glucose.** The most important diagnostic test is the serum glucose level. Values less than 50 mg/dL are diagnostic in the presence of symptoms. Rapid glucose measurements using reagent strips, glucometers, and fingerstick blood samples may be helpful but should be confirmed with a serum level.
2. **Urine glucose levels.** These are usually of little help in this setting.
3. **Serum insulin levels.** Temperature will be elevated if insulinoma is present.
4. **C-peptide levels.** This test detects endogenous insulin pro-

duction. Elevated levels with increased serum insulin suggests insulinoma. If serum insulin is increased and the C-peptide level is decreased, insulin overdosage or surreptitious insulin administration is likely.

V. Plan

A. Initial management. The first steps include taking a history and performing a physical exam. A rapid blood glucose determination should also be performed by fingerstick and a portable glucose monitoring device while awaiting lab confirmation of a serum sample.

B. Mild hypoglycemia. If glucose < 70 mg/dL and the patient is able to follow commands, encourage reversal via oral diet (ie, 8 ounces of low-fat milk with bread or crackers should be given every 15 minutes). Low-fat milk is preferred over beverages containing simple sugars because the latter can result in an initial hyperglycemic response followed by hypoglycemia.

C. Severe hypoglycemia. The following steps should be taken if the patient is unable to cooperate in taking carbohydrate orally.

    1. Parenteral. Give 1 ampule of D50 (dextrose 50%) by IV push. If there is no change, repeat the ampule of 50% dextrose. Some physicians recommend starting with glucagon.

    2. Failure to respond at this point should lead one to question the diagnosis, especially if the results of a serum glucose determination are not back yet to prove hypoglycemia as the cause of the problem.

    3. Glucagon, a polypeptide hormone secreted by the pancreas, results in glycogenolysis with release of glucose. Administer glucagon 1–2 mg IM or SQ into the upper outer thigh near the abdomen. A second injection is given if an adequate response is not achieved after 15 minutes.

    4. Start maintenance D5W at 50–100 mL/h IV to help prevent recurrence of hypoglycemia, and follow up with serial glucose measurements after the initial episode.

    5. Other adjuncts such as subcutaneous epinephrine and intravenous hydrocortisone may be required in severe refractory cases.

D. Prevention. In the pregnant diabetic patient, calorically consistent meals should be scheduled at routine times and snacks allowed between meals, especially before exercise. Frequent monitoring of blood glucose with a glucometer before meals, fasting, at bedtime, and during symptomatic periods is essential. Snacks as well as glucagon should be on hand at all times. The best treatment for hypoglycemia is prevention.

E. **Workup of hypoglycemia.** After the acute episode has been treated, diagnostic tests are required to evaluate the patient for the cause of the hypoglycemia. Serum insulin levels, C-peptide levels, liver function tests, glucose tolerance test, and appropriate radiographic tests should be considered.

REFERENCES

Hollingsworth DR, Moore TR: Diabetes and pregnancy. In Creasy RK, Resnik R (eds): *Maternal-Fetal Medicine: Principles and Practice.* Philadelphia, WB Saunders, 1989.

Hypoglycemia due to insulin and the sulfonylurea agents. In Waife SO (ed): *Diabetes Mellitus.* Indianapolis, Eli Lilly and Company, 1980, p 140.

Olefsky JM: Diabetes mellitus. In Wyngaarden JB, Smith LH Jr (eds): *Cecil Textbook of Medicine,* 19th ed. Philadelphia, WB Saunders, 1992, pp 1291–1309.

Schneider JM, Kitzmiller JL: Medical management of diabetes mellitus during pregnancy. In Brody SA, Ueland K (eds): *Endocrine Disorders in Pregnancy.* Norwalk, Connecticut, Appleton & Lange, 1989.

10. LEG PAIN AND SWELLING (See Problem 68, page 263)

11. LUPUS FLARE

I. **Problem.** A 30-year-old G_5P_{1031} presents with complaints of joint pain, fever, and facial rash. During the initial obstetric visit a VDRL showed a 1 : 2 dilution "weakly reactive."

II **Immediate Questions**

A. **Does she have a history of a similar presentation?** Systemic lupus erythematous (SLE) is a chronic multisystemic inflammatory disease of undetermined origin. The disease occurs for the first time during pregnancy or the postpartum period in up to 14% of all cases. Frequent initial manifestations include arthritis, severe rash, fever, neuropsychiatric disorders, nephritis, pleurisy, and pericarditis. The course is often unpredictable with variable periods of exacerbation and remission.

B. **What is the patient's ethnic background?** SLE is approximately three times more common among blacks than caucasians. Certain Native American tribes have an even greater predilection toward SLE.

C. **What is her obstetric history?** Many authors report normal fertility in SLE patients. However, patients with hypertension and renal disease have increased fetal wastage, preterm labor, and intrauterine growth retardation. Lupus anticoagulant, an IgG or IgM immunoglobulin that has been identified in some patients with SLE, is associated with fetal death. Anticardiolipin antibody, found in 61% of patients with SLE, is also implicated in fetal wastage.

D. What medications is the patient receiving? Drug-induced lupus has been cited with antihypertensive medications such as hydralazine and alpha-methyldopa, cardiac medications such as procainamide and quinidine, and anticonvulsants such as phenytoin and phenobarbital.

E. Is there a family history of collagen vascular disease? If a family member has SLE, the likelihood of SLE increases (approximately 70% risk in identical twins and 5% for other first-degree relatives).

F. What are the vital signs? Patients with SLE frequently have fever during flares. A source of infection should always be ruled out. An elevated blood pressure may be the result of renal manifestations of SLE.

G. Have family members noted any change in the patient's mental status? Neurologic manifestations of SLE include seizures, memory deficits, cerebrovascular lesions, and psychosis.

H. Does the patient have a propensity for bruising? The combination of capillary fragility, thrombocytopenia, and lupus anticoagulant can produce clinically evident clotting problems.

III. Differential Diagnosis

A. Lupus flare. Patients with SLE may present with a number of symptoms. In addition to the classic presentation of butterfly rash, mucosal ulcers, and leukopenia, a fever of unknown origin may herald the onset of SLE. Lupus patients can experience multisystem failure including nephritis, nephrotic syndrome, hypertension, psychosis, seizures, hemolytic anemia, leukopenia, thrombocytopenia, pleurisy, and pericarditis. It is imperative that the hypertensive patient with proteinuria be screened to rule out an exacerbation of SLE, which carries a poorer prognosis.

B. Rheumatoid arthritis and other collagen vascular diseases. Antinuclear antibodies (ANA) will often be positive in these disease states but the clinical manifestations will be different. Rheumatoid factor for patients with SLE may be positive in 20% of cases, but only weakly so.

C. Spirochetal diseases. Secondary syphilis can produce a syndrome very similar to a lupus flare. The fluorescent treponemal antibody absorption (FTA-ABS) test and microhemagglutination assay for palladium (MHA-TP) should be positive only in patients with syphilis. Lyme disease can be differentiated based upon the characteristic skin lesions, called erythema chronicum migrans.

Rocky Mountain spotted fever can produce a syndrome similar to SLE but without renal and hematologic abnormalities. ANA and rheumatoid factor should also be absent with Rocky Mountain spotted fever and Lyme disease.

D. Gonococcal arthritis-dermatitis syndrome can be differentiated from SLE based upon migratory joint pain, painful papules or pustules of the distant extremities, and gram stain and culture of the blood, cervix, synovial fluid, or skin.

E. Lupus nephritis is difficult to distinguish from some forms of preeclampsia. Also, CNS involvement and SLE may culminate in convulsions similar to those of eclampsia. However, differentiation can be made when active urinary sediment and extrarenal manifestations strongly suggest lupus nephritis.

F. AIDS. Bizarre clinical manifestations of AIDS must always be considered in patients with a rash and fever of unknown cause. The laboratory abnormalities found in lupus, such as antinuclear and anti-DNA antibodies, should be negative in patients with AIDS.

IV. Database

A. Physical examination key points

1. **Vital signs.** Blood pressure elevation may indicate renal disease or preeclampsia. Fever may represent a lupus flare or infection.

2. **HEENT.** Conjunctivitis is seen in 10% of patients. Transient blindness may occur secondary to retinal artery spasms.

3. **Heart.** Cardiac examination may reveal a systolic murmur. Occasionally a murmur of mitral or aortic regurgitation may be heard on auscultation, suggesting Libman-Sacks endocardial lesions (verrucous endocarditis complicated with lupus erythematosus disseminatus). Pericarditis or pericardial effusion may be represented by a pericardial friction rub.

4. **Lung.** Most often, if abnormalities are present, a small to moderate-sized unilateral pleural effusion or scattered rales are detected.

5. **Abdomen.** Although the abdomen is generally not involved, an occasional sterile peritonitis with intestinal infarct has been described.

6. **Skin.** Skin lesions range from the characteristic butterfly eruption to macular bullous lesions or vasculitic ulcers. The classic butterfly rash occurs across the cheeks and bridge of the nose.

7. **Extremities.** Symmetric arthritis is most often seen. Most commonly involved are the proximal interphalangeal joints

followed by the wrist, knees, and ankles. Joint effusions can occur; mild muscle atrophy and tenderness of the hand may also be present. Marked ecchymoses may be secondary to clotting abnormalities.

8. **Neuropsychiatric examination.** Peripheral neuropathies have been seen in 10–15% of patients with SLE. Seizures, often grand mal, are common. Psychiatric problems such as psychosis and personality disorders have been described.

B. Laboratory data

1. **Hemogram.** Normocytic normochromic anemia may be present. Leukopenia with WBCs < 500/mm^3 occurs in 46% of patients. Thrombocytopenia is seen in 10–15% of cases.

2. **Urinalysis.** Protein of > 3.5 g/d or cellular casts are indications of active lupus nephritis.

3. **Electrolytes.** A creatinine of 1.6 or greater is associated with > 50% fetal loss.

4. **Serologic tests.** ANA is virtually always positive. An anti-DNA antibody to double-stranded DNA correlates with disease activity, especially with lupus nephritis.

5. **Complement.** Depression of C3, C4, or total hemolytic complement correlates well with active SLE.

6. **Rheumatoid factor.** This is present in 20% of patients with SLE, but in low titers.

7. **Anti-SS-A (Ro) and anti SS-B (La) antibodies.** These correlate with neonatal lupus and congenital heart block.

8. **Lupus anticoagulant** is associated with decidual vasculopathy, placental infarction, fetal growth retardation, recurrent abortion, and fetal death. **Anticardiolipin antibody** is associated with pulmonary hypertension and thrombocytopenia.

C. Radiologic and other studies

1. **Chest x-ray.** Chest films often may show a pleural effusion, pleural thickening, vasculitis, pulmonary infiltrates, or pericardial effusion.

2. **Electrocardiogram.** The ECG may show ST wave elevation and T wave changes of pericarditis.

3. **Biopsy.** Skin biopsy with immunofluorescent staining is performed to detect immunoglobulin deposits in the dermal-epidermal junction. Renal biopsy with immunofluorescent staining is also available.

V. Plan

A. Antepartum

1. **Corticosteroids.** The usual starting dose is prednisone 60 mg qd for up to 2–3 weeks. After symptoms resolve, the

daily dose can be tapered by 5–10 mg at weekly intervals. The response of lupus nephritis to steroids varies based upon the histologic diagnosis. Focal glomerulonephritis responds better to steroids than does membranous or diffuse glomerulonephritis.

2. **Immunosuppressive agents.** Azathioprine has been shown to be effective adjuvant therapy with steroids. The usual dose is 1–2 mg/kg/d.

3. **Antepartum testing**
   a. Obtain nonstress testing and biophysical profiles twice weekly starting at 30 weeks' gestation.
   b. Ultrasound monitoring of fetal growth at 18–22 weeks, 30–32 weeks, and 36–38 weeks should be done routinely.

4. **Other drug therapies.** Both aspirin and heparin separately have been shown to reduce fetal wastage in patients with lupus anticoagulant. Aspirin should be used cautiously because of concern for premature closure of the ductus arteriosus and alterations in neonatal hemostasis.

B. Labor

1. Libman-Sacks heart lesions require antibiotic prophylaxis before labor ensues.

2. **Corticosteroids.** Because chronic steroid therapy suppresses the hypothalamic-pituitary axis, women may not be able to tolerate the stress of labor. When labor begins, cortisone acetate 100 mg IM should be given q8h until completion of the second stage of labor. A cesarean section or any other major operation requires cortisone acetate 100 mg IM, followed by hydrocortisone succinate 100–200 mg IV during surgery. Twenty-four hours prior to elective cesarean section, an additional 100 mg of cortisone acetate should be given IM.

3. **Delivery.** The method of delivery is entirely based upon obstetric indications. The neonatologist should be alerted to the possibility of congenital heart block.

C. Postpartum

1. **Corticosteroids.** The patient should be given an additional 100 mg of hydrocortisone succinate IV if signs of adrenal insufficiency are present, ie, abdominal pain, vomiting, or hypotension. Prophylactic steroid therapy after delivery for asymptomatic patients remains controversial. Steroids can occasionally be decreased if organ failure is improving.

2. **Biopsy.** A renal biopsy 6 weeks after delivery should be considered in any patient with uncertain renal status.

3. **Laboratory follow-up.** C3 and C4 complement levels every

other day for 1 week, then weekly for 6 weeks, may be helpful in gauging therapy.

REFERENCES

Out HJ, Derksen RHWM, Christiaens GCML: Systemic lupus erythematosus and pregnancy. *Obstet Gynecol Surv* 44:585, 1989.
Lockshin MD: Lupus pregnancy. *Clin Rheum Dis* 11:611, 1985.

12. MAGNESIUM TOXICITY

I. Problem. You are called to the labor and delivery unit to evaluate a preeclamptic patient who has just delivered by cesarean section with a general anesthetic. On her arrival in the recovery room she was noted to be very lethargic, somnolent, not easily arousable, and breathing at a rate of approximately 10 breaths per minute.

II. Immediate Questions

A. What dose of magnesium sulfate was the patient receiving? Most patients receive 1–2 g $MgSO_4$ IV every hour. This dose is regulated by following serum levels and changes in physical examination such as decreased patellar reflexes, which are suggestive of high serum magnesium levels. Magnesium sulfate used in patients with premature labor may require doses of up to 3 g/h.

B. What was her last serum magnesium level? Clinically significant hypermagnesemia can begin to be seen at levels as low as 4 mEq/L. Most patients who are being maintained on magnesium sulfate for the prevention of eclampsia will be held at 4–6 mEq/L.

C. What medications had she received as part of her general anesthesia regimen or during her hospitalization? The most likely explanation for this patient's lethargy relates to magnesium toxicity, possibly complicated by depolarizing agents administered during general anesthesia. This not uncommon clinical problem is one that all clinicians caring for patients with preeclampsia receiving magnesium sulfate therapy would be aware of. Additionally, medications that may contribute to the neuromuscular effects of magnesium sulfate should be evaluated.

D. What is the patient's fluid status, including a summary of her entire intake and output since the beginning of her hospitalization? Assessment of recent urinary output is imperative since magnesium is primarily excreted via the kidneys. Preeclampsia is not uncommonly accompanied by oliguria, and pronounced oliguria may contribute to the magnesium toxicity.

III. Differential Diagnosis

A. Magnesium toxicity. Toxicity usually occurs at levels > 6 mEq/L. Lethargy, somnolence, respiratory depression, and cardiotoxicity can be manifested (see IV-B2).

B. Cerebrovascular accident (CVA). In any patient who is manifesting signs of lethargy, the possibility of a CVA must be considered. This is especially true in a preeclamptic patient who has just undergone a surgical procedure under general anesthesia. It is well known that transient hypertension occurs with induction of general anesthesia, and the vasculature of a preeclamptic patient may be particularly sensitive to this phenomenon. Any evidence of focal neurologic signs to suggest a CVA should be carefully evaluated in conjunction with a neurologist.

C. Deplorizing agents. Essential will be to review all medications that the patient received in the hospital. Besides aminoglycoside antibiotics, this will include depolarizing agents given during general anesthesia that may potentiate the toxic side effects of magnesium therapy.

D. Narcotics. Large doses of narcotics during the operative procedure and immediate postoperative period may be responsible for the patient's presentation.
6

IV. Database

A. Physical examination key points

1. **Vital signs.** Hypertension may be secondary to poorly controlled preeclampsia and places the patient at increased risk for CVA and eclampsia. Respiratory depression and irregular heart rates may be present with magnesium toxicity. Hypermagnesemia may also result in hypotension.

2. **HEENT.** Evaluation of pupils and their reactivity with a light source will enable you to rule out a CVA.

3. **Neurologic examination.** An early sign of toxicity is reduced to absent patellar reflexes.

B. Laboratory data

1. **Electrolytes,** including serum calcium, ionized calcium, and serum potassium. Abnormalities in any of these cations can exacerbate clinical hypermagnesemia.

2. **Magnesium.** Toxicity may be seen at levels as low as 4 mEq/L. Most patients are maintained at 4–6 mEq/L to prevent eclampsia. Respiratory depression can appear at magnesium levels of 8–10 mEq/L, and cardiotoxicity, while not usually seen until levels exceed 10 mEq/L, can occur at any serum magnesium level.

C. Radiologic and other studies

      1. Electrocardiogram. Obtain a baseline study. Hypermagnesemia may manifest itself as a shortened Q-T interval up through complete heart block.

V. Plan
A. Initial
    1. Calcium gluconate. Administer 1 g IV over approximately one minute while waiting for serum magnesium and electrolyte values. If calcium administration improves the patient's status, then magnesium toxicity is most likely the correct diagnosis: magnesium is a calcium antagonist, and calcium should reverse its toxicity.

    2. Naloxone. One ampule (0.1–0.4 mg) of naloxone should be given IV if a narcotic cause is being entertained.

    3. Urine output. Magnesium is secreted by the kidneys. Urine output should be maintained at a minimum of 30 mL/h. Decreased output may be secondary to worsening of the patient's preeclampsia, decreased colloid oncotic pressures, or decreased intravascular volume.

B. Follow-up
    1. Maintain serum magnesium, ionized calcium, and potassium within the normal ranges to optimize outcome. (Magnesium should be in the therapeutic range for preeclampsia management, ie, 4–6 mEq/L).

    2. Keep urine output > 30 mL/h with IV fluids.

    3. Hourly clinical assessments of patients on magnesium sulfate therapy should include neurologic evaluation to assess the patellar reflex and respiratory rate. Ideal respiratory rate is 15 breaths per minute or greater.

REFERENCES

Gilman AG et al (eds): *The Pharmacological Basis of Therapeutics,* 7th ed. New York, Macmillan, 1985.
Cunningham FG, MacDonald PC, Gant NF (eds): *Williams Obstetrics,* 18th ed. Norwalk, Connecticut, Appleton & Lange, 1989.

13. MATERNAL TACHYCARDIA

I. Problem. A 28-year-old patient at 30 weeks' gestation complains of a "racing heart."

II. Immediate Questions

    A. What are the vital signs? A normal resting heart rate in pregnancy is 10–15 beats per minute faster than in the nonpregnant state. Blood pressure and respiratory rate are generally increased in physiologic tachycardia due to stress or pain. Temperature elevation may suggest an infectious cause. Conversely, hypothermia and hypotension may indicate either septic shock or primary cardiovascular shock.

B. Is the patient bleeding? Hypovolemia and profound anemia are important and correctable causes of tachycardia. Vaginal bleeding in pregnancy may be due to placenta previa, abruption, or labor.

C. Does the patient have a history of cardiac disease or other preexisting medical problems? Tachycardia may be a significant marker for impending crisis in a chronic process such as hypoglycemia in an insulin-dependent diabetic or thyroid storm in a patient with hyperthyroidism.

D. What drugs is the patient taking? Beta-mimetic agents such as those used in preterm labor and asthma, eg, terbutaline and aminophylline, and over-the-counter cold preparations (pseudoephedrine), caffeine, nicotine, cocaine, etc, should be considered.

E. Was the onset abrupt or gradual? Physiologic cardiac response to stress (ie, sinus tachycardia) tends to be gradual in onset and resolution. Abrupt onset and termination of tachycardia should alert the physician to such pathologic processes as paroxysmal atrial tachycardia (PAT), atrial fibrillation, atrial flutter, or paroxysmal ventricular tachycardia (PVT).

F. What, if anything, seemed to precipitate or terminate the tachycardia episode? The onset of tachycardia associated with exertion, pain, emotional stress, or labor may be a purely physiologic response, and therapy should be directed at the precipitating cause. Vagal maneuvers such as vomiting or carotid massage have a gradual slowing effect with return to previous rate in sinus tachycardia or atrial fibrillation, yet will have no effect or will abruptly terminate the tachycardia in PAT or PVT. **Note:** Carotid massage should not be used if digitalis toxicity is suspected, since dangerous arrhthymias can be evoked.

III. Differential Diagnosis

   A. Physiologic response
       1. Exercise
       2. Anxiety
       3. Pain
       4. Excitement
       5. Labor

B. Cardiopulmonary causes

1. **Hypovolemia.** Dehydration or acute blood loss may cause hypovolemia with compensatory tachycardia. Intravascular volume depletion, as in preeclampsia, may have a similar effect.
2. **Anemia or hypoxia.** Lack of end organ oxygenation can cause tachycardia.
3. **Sepsis or shock.** Decreased peripheral vascular resistance with resulting relative hypovolemia leads to compensatory tachycardia.
4. **Ectopic tachycardia.** Conduction defects or ectopic pacemakers may lead to tachyarrhythmia. Underlying silent cardiac anomalies may become manifest due to external factors such as hypovolemia or hypoxia, as in the PAT of Wolff-Parkinson-White (WPW) syndrome.
5. **AV shunts.** Sometimes these are anatomic, such as atrioventricular or ventriculoseptal defects, but more commonly they are functional as in ventilation/perfusion mismatching due to adult respiratory distress syndrome, asthma, atelectasis, and bronchopulmonary disease.
6. **Valvular disorders.** Aortic regurgitation, valvular stenosis, prolapse, and regurgitation may all be associated with tachycardia, especially as pregnancy advances.
7. **Congestive heart failure or myocardial infarction.** These are rare causes of tachycardia in pregnancy.
8. **Pneumonia.** It can result in maternal fever, hypoxia, and tachycardia.
9. **Pulmonary embolism.** This must be part of the differential diagnosis whenever a patient experiences unexplained tachycardia.

C. Metabolic causes

1. **Fever.** Temperature elevation with tachycardia may be due to neoplasm or autoimmune disease, but infection is the most common cause in pregnant women.
2. **Hypoglycemia.** Hyperemesis may lead to hypoglycemia with tachycardia. Insulin overdose in gestational diabetes is an infrequent but potentially serious cause of tachycardia.
3. **Hypokalemia.** Diuretic therapy, steroid or tocolytic therapy, potassium-wasting nephropathy, adrenocortical dysfunction, or diarrhea may cause severe hypokalemia and tachyarrhythmia.

D. Endocrine causes

1. **Thyrotoxicosis.** Tachycardia in the face of resting tremor, exophthalmos, weight loss, or failure to gain appropriate weight during pregnancy may suggest hyperthyroidism. Findings such as enlarge⌐⌐ thyroid and abnormal thyroid

function tests help to confirm the diagnosis. If untreated, other metabolic stresses may precipitate a life-threatening episode of thyroid storm.

2. Pheochromocytoma. Recurrent paroxysms of tachycardia, especially if accompanied by flushing and diaphoresis, may suggest pheochromocytoma. Tests of urinary vanillylmandelic acid (VMA) will aid in the diagnosis.

E. Pharmacologic causes

1. Beta-mimetic agents. Terbutaline, aminophylline, caffeine, and nicotine are common causes of sinus tachycardia.

2. Exogenous thyroid. Thyroxine preparations may increase resting heart rate.

3. Digitalis. Although digitalis is rarely used in pregnancy, its toxicity leads to tachyarrhythmia.

IV. Database

A. Physical examination key points

1. Vital signs. Elevated blood pressure is consistent with physiologic tachycardia as well as most metabolic and endocrine causes of tachycardia, whereas decreased blood pressure is seen with sepsis, shock, severe hypovolemia, or cardiovascular decompensation. Elevated temperature suggests an infectious origin but can also be seen with drug effects, exertion, and endocrine causes of tachycardia. Conversely, subnormal body temperature may be seen in septic shock. Respiratory rate may be elevated in severe anemia, AV shunts, hypoxia, pain, and exertion.

2. Skin. Flushing may be secondary to fever or pheochromocytoma. Dry skin with poor turgor may suggest dehydration and hypovolemia.

3. Head and neck. Exophthalmos and enlargement of the thyroid may accompany thyrotoxicosis. Dry mucous membranes and decreased skin turgor suggest hypovolemia and dehydration. Pale sclerae may be a sign of severe anemia. Jugular venous pulsations (JVPs) are normal in sinus tachycardia, but cannon A waves may be seen in PAT or atrioventricular junctional tachycardia. Flutter waves are seen in atrial flutter and irregular pulsations with atrial fibrillation. Jugular venous distention may represent cardiac decompensation.

4. Heart. Auscultation of the heart will reveal normal heart sounds in sinus tachycardia. S_1 varies in intensity with atrial fibrillation and S_2 is widely split in PVT. Tachycardia may impair the auscultation of murmurs.

5. **Lungs.** Rales may suggest pulmonary edema. Wheezing is indicative of reactive airway disease, and tachycardia may be due to hypoxia or bronchodilators used for treatment. Decreased breath sounds regionally, bronchial breath sounds, egophony, and fremitus suggest pneumonia.

6. **Abdomen.** Tenderness, rebound, and guarding are consistent with acute abdomen. Palpation of the gravid uterus for contractions can help to rule out labor as a cause of the tachycardia.

7. **Pelvis.** Cervical dilation suggests labor.

8. **Rectum.** Tarry or bloody stool is consistent with gastrointestinal bleeding. Screen the stool for occult blood.

9. **Extremities.** Cyanosis is indicative of hypoxemia and clubbing points to longstanding pulmonary disease. Hyperreflexia and nondependent edema are found in preeclampsia, which can cause intravascular volume depletion. Pulses that are weak and thready are consistent with hypotension and shock.

B. **Laboratory data**
  1. **For immediate evaluation**
     a. **Hemogram.** Low hemoglobin and hematocrit reflect anemia. Leukocytosis suggests infection, while leukopenia with relative lymphocytosis is common in thyrotoxicosis.
     b. **Blood urea nitrogen and creatinine.** Elevated values, especially with BUN disproportionately increased, indicates prerenal azotemia from dehydration and hypovolemia.
     c. **Glucose.** Hypoglycemia is an easily correctable cause of tachycardia. Hyperglycemia may suggest diabetic ketoacidosis.
     d. **Arterial blood gases.** Abnormal values can delineate ventilation and perfusion anomalies, such as pulmonary embolus, which may lead to tachycardia.
     e. **Electrolytes.** A large anion gap may result from the metabolic acidosis of sepsis. Hypokalemia may lead to tachycardia.
     f. **Creatine phosphokinase.** CPK can demonstrate myocardial damage if cardiac fractions are drawn.
     g. **Occult blood.** Examine the stool for occult blood. If positive, this may indicate a GI bleed.
  2. **For further evaluation**
     a. **Blood cultures.** Obtain cultures to determine the presence, type, and sensitivities of organisms causing septicemia.

   b. **Thyroid studies.** When hyperthyroidism is suspected, thyroid-stimulating hormone, T_4, and T_3 resin uptake should be checked.
   c. **Urine for VMA and metanephrines.** A 24-hour urine collection for these metabolites can confirm the diagnosis of pheochromocytoma.
   d. **Toxicology screen.** This may reveal pharmacologic agents which cause tachycardia.

C. **Radiologic and other studies**
   1. **Chest radiograph.** A chest film may reveal evidence of cardiac or pulmonary disease such as congestive failure.
   2. **Ventilation/perfusion (V/Q) scan.** This is useful when there is a high index of suspicion for pulmonary embolism.
   3. **Electrocardiogram.** The ECG may help to further define the specific type of tachyarrhythmia.
   4. **Carotid massage test.** This test should always be performed with electrocardiographic monitoring and is contraindicated in heart block, digitalis intoxication, or cerebrovascular disease. In sinus tachycardia, atrial fibrillation, and many cases of multifocal atrial tachycardia there will be gradual slowing of the heart rate with slow return to the previous rate. PAT will often terminate abruptly and PVT will not respond to carotid massage. To perform, place the fingers over the carotid and gently massage.

V. **Plan**
   A. **Identify and correct potentially dangerous underlying causes of tachycardia.** Continuous cardiac monitoring should be initiated.
      1. **Hypovolemia.** Give IV crystalloid (eg, lactated Ringer's solution) to expand intravascular volume.
      2. **Severe anemia.** Give a transfusion of packed red blood cells. Recommendations for the minimum acceptable hematocrit vary with institutions.
      3. **Sepsis/shock.** Increase intravascular volume with crystalloid and blood initially. If hypotension and tachycardia are still problems, consider pressor agents to raise systemic vascular resistance. Also begin appropriate antibiotic therapy. (see problem 54, page 199).
      4. **Hypoxia.** Give supplemental oxygen and ventilatory support as required.
      5. **Hypoglycemia.** This may be corrected with PO feeding if tolerated, but 25 g D50 followed by D5-containing IV fluids may be required in many circumstances (see Problem 50, page 188).

    6. Hypokalemia (see Problem 51, page 188).

    7. Pharmacologic cause. Withdraw the offending agent(s).

    8. Fever/infection. Short-term lowering of core temperature is achieved as follows.

      a. Apply a cooling blanket or ice packs.

      b. A fluid bolus of 500 to 1000 mL or room-temperature IV fluid may be helpful.

      c. If the patient is receiving mechanical ventilator assistance, core temperature can be lowered by reducing the temperature of the inspired air.

      d. Give Tylenol tablets or suppositories 650 mg q3–4h.

B. Specific treatments for tachycardia

    1. Atrial flutter, atrial fibrillation, and premature beats

      a. Usually these arrhythmias require no treatment unless the patient has significant ventricular dysfunction and is reliant on the atrial contractility for ventricular filling or has severe mitral stenosis.

      b. Direct-current (DC) cardioversion is rarely used. A better strategy in the pregnant patient is to control the ventricular rate, if need be, and wait for the paroxysm to self terminate. Cardiac glycosides (digoxin), beta blockers (propranolol), or calcium channel blockers (verapamil) may be used. All are pregnancy category C: "Risk cannot be ruled out. Human studies are lacking, and animal studies are either positive for fetal risk, or lacking as well. However, potential benefits may justify the potential risk." *Physicians' Desk Reference, 46th ed, 1992.)*

      c. Anticoagulation is indicated if atrial fibrillation or flutter accompanies mitral valve disease or if there is a history of thromboembolic disease (see Problem 68, page 263). In these cases, the patient should receive anticoagulants for at least 1 week prior to any attempts at cardioversion.

    2. Sinus tachycardia. Sinus tachycardia will usually remit spontaneously as the underlying causes are corrected. In prolonged tachycardia that is not compensatory, beta blockers may be employed if need be.

    3. Wolff-Parkinson-White syndrome. The same treatment principles apply to WPW as for paroxysmal supraventricular tachycardia except that DC cardioversion is the preferred therapy. Digitalis is contraindicated, as are beta blockers and calcium channel blockers. Refractory WPW may require surgical resection of the anomalous pathways.

    4. Ventricular tachyarrhythmias. Most cases of asymptomatic ventricular arrhythmia require no treatment despite the fact that ventricular premature beats may be the harbingers of sudden cardiac death. Ventricular tachycardia may be converted to sinus rhythm with lidocaine (pregnancy category B). If medical cardioversion fails or if the tachycardia is poorly tolerated, urgent electric cardioversion may be indicated. Ventricular fibrillation is a cardiovascular catastrophe and requires emergent treatment via the appropriate advanced cardiac life support (ACLS) protocol.

C. **Treatment protocols for specific disease processes with tachycardia**
  1. **Postpartum hemorrhage**
     a. **General treatment strategy.** Minimize blood loss and hypovolemia.
     b. **Specific interventions**
        (1) Perform bimanual examination of the uterus to rule out atony.
        (2) Explore and perform curettage of the uterus to rule out retained placental fragments.
        (3) Examine the vagina and cervix for laceration, and repair as need be.
        (4) If uterine atony is present, proceed in this order:
            (a) Firmly compress the uterus bimanually.
            (b) Infuse oxytocin 40 units in 1 L D5 lactated Ringer's IV.
            (c) Inject methylergonovine maleate 0.2 mg IM (unless the patient is hypertensive or has preeclampsia).
            (d) Inject 15-methylprostaglandin F_2 alpha 250 μg IM.
            (e) Ligate the uterine arteries bilaterally.
            (f) Ligate the hypogastric arteries bilaterally.
            (g) Perform hysterectomy.
  2. **Hypovolemic shock** (see Problem 54, page 199)
     a. **General treatment strategy**
        (1) Eliminate the source of hemorrhage.
        (2) Maintain systolic blood pressure > 90 mm Hg urine output > 30 mL/h.
        (3) Avoid pulmonary edema due to overly aggressive volume replacement.
     b. **Specific interventions**
        (1) Establish IV access with a large-bore catheter.
        (2) Infuse D5 lactated Ringer's solution at high rate until blood products are available.
        (3) Place the patient in Trendelenburg position.
        (4) Administer supplemental oxygen via face mask.
        (5) Infuse packed red blood cells or whole blood when available (fresh-frozen plasma should be infused only if fibrinogen is low or prothrombin time and par-

tial thromboplastin time are prolonged; platelets should be given if platelet count is < 50, 000/mL).

    (6) Eliminate the hemorrhage at its source.

    (7) Consider invasive hemodynamic monitoring if the patient does not respond appropriately to volume replacement.

3. Thyroid storm

a. General treatment strategy

    (1) Identify and treat precipitating factors such as infection, inadequate doses of propylthiouracil, or propranolol for preexisting thyroid disease, undiagnosed gestational trophoblastic disease, or thyroid abnormality (ie, Graves' disease or Hashimoto's thyroiditis).

    (2) Control hypotension, tachycardia, hyperthermia, cardiac dysrhythmias, and congestive heart failure.

    (3) Control the synthesis and release of thyroid hormone.

b. Specific interventions

    (1) Begin rapid hydration with crystalloid.

    (2) Decrease the temperature with acetaminophen per rectum and a cooling blanket.

    (3) Monitor with continuous electrocardiographic monitoring.

    (4) Give propylthiouracil 600 mg PO, then 300 mg PO q6h.

    (5) Give propranolol 1–2 μg/min IV up to 10 μg q4h; may switch to 40–80 mg PO q4h.

    (6) Give sodium iodide 0.5–1.0 g q8h IV. (Caution should be used in the pregnant patient since iodine passes the placenta.)

    (7) Give hydrocortisone 100 mg IV q8h.

    (8) Examine for precipitating cause. If infection is suspected, begin broad-spectrum antibiotics empirically until culture results are available.

REFERENCES

Briggs GG, Freeman RK, Yaffee SJ (eds): *Drugs in Pregnancy and Lactation.* Baltimore, Williams & Wilkins, 1984.

Wilson JD et al (eds): *Harrison's Principles of Internal Medicine,* 12th ed. New York, McGraw-Hill, 1991.

14. MECONIUM

   I. Problem. A patient in early labor presents to the delivery room with meconium-stained fluid.

II. Immediate Questions

   A. What is the gestational age? Meconium passage occurs in 6–11% of all deliveries. It occurs rarely prior to 34 weeks, but as GI maturity occurs it may be present in up to 40% of postdate pregnancies.

   B. What is the nature of the meconium? Meconium-stained amniotic fluid may be classified as light, moderate, or thick ("pea-soup," particulate). Thick meconium occurs more frequently when oligohydramnios is present. If the meconium is noted to be "formed," suspect a breech presentation.

   C. What is the fetal heart rate pattern? Acidemia is seen more commonly in association with meconium when baseline and periodic fetal heart rate abnormalities are present. Decreased fetal heart rate variability or late decelerations are suggestive of fetal hypoxia and acidemia.

   D. Are there risk factors for asphyxia? Meconium passage occurs more commonly in the postdates pregnancy and in pregnancies complicated by intrauterine growth retardation, hypertension, and substance abuse.

III. Differential Diagnosis

   A. Maturation theory. Meconium passage may simply represent GI maturation and motility in late gestation.

   B. Fetal distress. The relationship of meconium passage to fetal distress is unclear. Hypoxia and parasympathetic stimulation secondary to cord compression have been theorized to cause meconium passage. Evidence of chronic stress and meconium are frequently seen in the severely growth retarded fetus.

   C. Intestinal hormones. Motilin and other intestinal hormones have been postulated to stimulate meconium passage.

IV. Database

   A. Physical examination key points

   1. **Pelvic examination.** Meconium-stained fluid (yellow to dark green) may be directly observed by speculum exam or by external exam in the patient with spontaneous or artificially ruptured membranes. It may also be detected at the time of amniocentesis; its presence in amniotic fluid may falsely decrease the lecithin/sphingomyelin (L/S) ratio but will not affect phosphatidylglycerol determination.

   B. Laboratory tests

   1. **Scalp pH.** Scalp sampling for pH analysis should be con-

sidered if the fetal heart rate strip is non-reassuring. A pH < 7.20 or a downward trend may be suggestive of fetal hypoxia.

C. Radiologic and other studies
   1. Fetal heart rate. When meconium is detected, the fetus should be monitored for evidence of decreased beat-to-beat variability, baseline changes, or decelerations.

V. Plan

A. Intrapartum. If meconium is detected during delivery, the fetus should have continuous electronic fetal monitoring.

B. The patient should be informed of the diagnosis, the need for controlled delivery of the fetal head with adequate time for suction, and the need for immediate evaluation by a pediatrician.

C. The pediatrician/neonatologist should be informed about the patient and called to the delivery room prior to delivery. Appropriate resuscitative equipment should be available including laryngoscope, endotracheal tubes, suction apparatus, and oxygen.

D. The fetus should have de Lee suctioning of the nasopharynx and oropharynx prior to delivery of the shoulders, to prevent meconium aspiration syndrome. The cord should be clamped and cut promptly and the baby handed to the awaiting pediatrician.

E. Cord blood gas analysis should be obtained to allow acid-base assessment of the neonate after delivery.

REFERENCES

Carson BS et al: Combined obstetric and pediatric approach to prevent meconium aspiration syndrome. *Am J Obstet Gynecol* 126:712, 1976.
Creasy RK, Resnik R (eds): *Maternal Fetal Medicine.* Philadelphia: WB Saunders, 1984, page 361.
Yeomans ER et al: Meconium in the amniotic fluid and fetal acid-base status. *Obstet Gynecol* 73:175, 1989.

15. PERINATAL GRIEVING

I. Problem. Following a stillbirth delivery, a 28-year-old patient presents on postpartum day 3 with complaints of anorexia, episodic crying, and insomnia.

II. Immediate Questions

A. Are these classic grieving behaviors? If there is verbal acknowledgment of the infant's death and indications of a struggle for emotional acceptance of the loss, these symptoms are probably related to a normal grief reaction.

B. What medications is the patient receiving? Assess dosage and frequency of medications the patient has received since delivery. In a misguided attempt to lessen the patient's distress, physician and nursing staff may be providing maximum narcotic analgesia or inappropriately timed sleep medication and sedation. Over time, this can disrupt normal activity patterns and may actually impair coping abilities by delaying acute grief responses.

C. Has a bereavement protocol been implemented? Many institutions have written guidelines to assist the staff to interact appropriately with grieving patients and families.

III. Differential Diagnosis

A. Normal acute grieving. Major alterations in normal patterns of daily living are very common in the first days or weeks (and sometimes months) following a significant loss.

B. Morbid grief patterns. Suicidal ideation or attempt, delusional thoughts, paranoia, or violent behavior may indicate aberrant grieving or psychosis.

C. Postpartum psychosis (see Problem 17, page 74).

D. Medication side effects. If symptoms are a result of excessive analgesia or sedation, the effects will probably diminish with decreased dosage and frequency of administration. However, some patients may exhibit aberrant behavior with the smallest doses of medications.

IV. Database

A. Physical examination key points
  1. Compare the patient's behaviors to the following grief reactions.
    a. Somatic distress, ie, sighing respirations, fatigue, sleeplessness, and digestive disturbances.
    b. Preoccupation with feelings of guilt.
    c. Preoccupation with the image of the deceased.
    d. Hostile reactions toward other people.
    e. Loss of normal patterns of daily living activities.

B. Laboratory data. None are required.

C. Radiologic and other studies
  1. Chart review. Prior to meeting the patient, review the hospital chart with particular note of the following.
    a. History of previous reproductive loss.

    b. Antepartum diagnosis of fetal demise or compromise.
    c. The patient's response to events occurring in labor and delivery.
    d. The patient's support network.
    e. Progress to date related to elements of the bereavement protocol.
    f. Current or planned involvement of other hospital resources, ie, social worker, chaplain.

V. Plan. Interventions should be directed to supporting the patient's grieving. She and her family should be reassured that her somatic and emotional distress are part of the grieving process necessary for eventual resolution of this crisis situation.

A. Immediate intervention

1. Initiate bereavement protocol (if not already in place). Elements include:
   a. Does the family wish to see or hold the baby?
   b. Do they want to name the baby?
   c. Do they want any remembrances (photo, baby blanket, etc)?
   d. Does the family desire an autopsy?
   e. Do they want a baptism?
   f. Will the family plan a funeral, or do they wish the hospital to dispose of the baby to avoid inappropriate reference to a live infant?

B. Additional interventions

1. Allow the patient to verbalize her feelings. Avoid statements that minimize her loss, such as "Maybe it's better this way" or "You can always have another baby."
2. If the family named the baby, always refer to the deceased by name.
3. Provide additional support if needed by referring to social worker, chaplaincy, compassionate friends (community group), etc.
4. Mild sedation may be helpful in some cases of severe acute distress.
5. Recognize that the patient is probably experiencing guilt and self blame. Encourage staff to "check in" frequently with her to avoid her feeling "abandoned."
6. Provide for discharge follow-up.

REFERENCES

Grief Related to Perinatal Death. OGN Nursing Practice Resource, No. 13, June 1985.

Kowalski K: Managing perinatal loss. *Clin Obstet Gynecol* 23:1113, 1980.
Stirman ED: Emotional aspects of perinatal death. *Clin Obstet Gynecol* 23:4, 1980.

16. POSTPARTUM HEMORRHAGE

I. Problem. A woman has just had a vaginal delivery with spontaneous delivery of the placenta. You notice an excessive amount of blood coming from the vagina.

II. Immediate Questions

A. What are the vital signs? Maternal vital signs may not change until 1200–1500 mL (20–25%) of total volume has been lost. Maternal tachycardia, tachypnea, or a narrow pulse pressure (< 30 mm Hg) indicates significant loss of blood volume.

B. What was the most recent hematocrit? A baseline hematocrit will be needed to assess the amount of blood loss.

C. Is the blood coming from above the cervix? Postpartum hemorrhage is most commonly the result of uterine atony, retained placenta, or genital tract trauma. Genital trauma can rapidly be ruled out by inspection.

D. Is the patient hypertensive? Some of the medications used to treat postpartum hemorrhage are contraindicated in patients with preeclampsia or chronic hypertension.

III. Differential Diagnosis

A. Genital tract trauma. Genital tract trauma causing excessive postpartum bleeding can result from episiotomy, cervical laceration, or vaginal laceration, and should be of special concern after operative vaginal delivery.

B. Uterine bleeding. Risk factors for postpartum atony include hydramnios, multiple gestation, previous postpartum atony, prolonged oxytocin stimulation, halogenated anesthetics, and uterine distention secondary to blood clots. Uterine rupture as a cause of postpartum hemorrhage has been associated with previous uterine scar, hyperstimulation, grand multiparity, and intrauterine manipulation. Abnormal placentation is another cause of bleeding originating from the uterus. The most common problems are retained placenta, placenta accreta, placenta increta, placenta percreta, and a succenturiate lobe.

C. Coagulopathy. Disorders of coagulation associated with abruptio placentae, amniotic fluid embolism, sepsis, or severe preeclampsia may also lead to postpartum hemorrhage.

IV. Database

A. Physical examination key points

1. **Vital signs.** Increased pulse pressure, tachycardia, and tachypnea are early signs of hypovolemia.

2. **Pelvic examination.** Careful visualization of the cervix and vagina to rule out genital tract trauma is very important. Uterine exploration should be done next using a gauze wrap over the first two fingers. Special attention is needed to rule out uterine rupture or retained placenta.

B. Laboratory data

1. **Hemogram.** The patient's hematocrit and platelets should be followed.

2. **Coagulation profile.** Prothrombin time, partial thromboplastin time, fibrinogen, and fibrin split products are needed to evaluate if the patient has a consumption coagulopathy or factor abnormality.

V. Plan

A. **The senior obstetric staff** should be available in case medical therapy fails.

B. **Anesthesia personnel** should be present to facilitate uterine exploration and possible exploratory laparotomy.

C. **Adequate ancillary help** including OR personnel and messenger service to the blood bank and laboratory needs to be available.

D. **Evaluate the uterus for retained products.** Manually explore the uterine cavity for a retained placenta. Ultrasound may provide a less invasive method to evaluate the uterus.

E. **Uterine atony** accounts for approximately 80% of all postpartum hemorrhages.

1. Place a Foley catheter immediately to assess renal perfusion.

2. Administer 4L/min oxygen to the mother.

3. Perform bimanual uterine massage by placing one hand in the vagina and the other abdominally on the uterine fundus.

4. Institute medical therapy while vigorous bimanual massage is performed. In order of preference:

   a. Administer oxytocin/(pitocin) 20–40 units/1000 mL, which may be run in at 250–500 mL over a 10 to 20-minute period. Some obstetricians have recommended injecting 10 units of Pitocin directly into the uterine muscle to treat atony after a cesarean section.

   b. Give methylergonovine maleate (Methergine) 0.2 mg IM

q2–4h prn. Use this drug with caution in patients with preeclampsia, hypertension, vascular, renal, or hepatic disease.

  c. Give 15-methylprostaglandin F_2 alpha 0.25 mg IM, which may be repeated in 20 minutes if no effect is seen. Maintenance doses every 90 minutes may then be instituted up to a total of six injections.

  d. Some physicians have reported minimal success in using hot uterine packs.

5. Surgical therapy. If medical therapy and uterine massage fail, it is imperative that the decision to implement surgical therapy be made quickly. The most senior obstetrician available should be involved in this decision, which includes (see Appendix, Figure A–1):

  a. Uterine artery ligation.

  b. Hypogastric artery ligation.

  c. Ovarian artery ligation (although successful in controlling hemorrhage, the ovaries may be compromised).

  d. Selective arterial embolization by a trained invasive radiologist.

  e. Hysterectomy should be performed only if all conservative measures have failed.

REFERENCES

Benedetti TJ: Obstetric hemorrhage. In Gabbe S, Niebyl J, Simpson J (eds): *Obstetrics, Normal and Problem Pregnancies.* New York, Churchill Livingstone, 1986.

Cunningham FG, MacDonald PC, Gant NF. *Williams' Obstetrics,* 18th ed. Norwalk, Connecticut, Appleton & Lange, 1989.

Schwartz PE: The surgical approach to severe postpartum hemorrhage. In Berkowitz RL (ed): *Critical Care of the Obstetric Patient,* New York, Churchill Livingstone, 1983, chap 10, p 285.

17. POSTPARTUM PSYCHOSIS

I. Problem. A 30-year-old primigravida, status post cesarean section, is reported to be extremely melancholic and refusing to care for her newborn infant.

II. Immediate Questions

  A. When did the patient deliver? Emotional lability and insecurity about mothering abilities may be normal adjustment behavior in the first few days after delivery. Persistence and severity of symptoms may indicate a more serious problem.

  B. Does the patient have a previous psychiatric history? Pregnancy and childbirth are considered situational crises and may exacerbate coping disorders or reactivate unresolved emotional conflicts.

C. **Is the patient threatening to harm the baby or having difficulty with reality testing?** Evidence of acute affective psychosis requires immediate psychiatric intervention, and probable psychotherapeutic medication.

III. Differential Diagnosis

A. **Postpartum Blues.** Transitory emotional distress in the first few postpartum days is estimated to occur in 50–80% of all postpartum patients. "The blues" is probably a normal reaction to childbirth and adjustment to the parental role.

B. **Postpartum Depression.** This disorder is differentiated from postpartum blues by the duration, severity, and number of symptoms. It is experienced in a mild to moderate form by as many as 20% of all postpartum patients.

C. **Postpartum Psychosis.** This disorder involves markedly impaired reality testing. Bizarre behavior is often associated with hallucinations, delusions, and disorganized thought.

IV. Database

A. **Physical examination key points**
   1. **Behavioral observations**
      a. **Postpartum blues.** The patient experiences transitory depression, tearfulness, fatigue, insomnia, and anxiety about her own or her infant's health. Symptoms usually resolve by day 7 postpartum.
      b. **Postpartum depression.** This is characterized by crying, despondency, labile mood, feelings of inadequacy, inability to cope, and unusual irritability or fatigue. It is differentiated from nonpuerperal depressions by the content of the depressive thoughts (focused mainly on parental or nurturing abilities or ambivalence regarding the infant).
      c. **Psychosis.** Florid affective episodes usually begin within 2 weeks of delivery and are associated with hallucinations, extreme emotional lability, and often significant manic symptoms.
   2. **Historical contributing factors**
      a. A history of previous psychiatric illness may predispose the patient to recurrence with subsequent pregnancies.
      b. The health of the newborn may impact on the patient's ability to make a smooth transition into parenthood.

        c. The quality of the patient's support system may be less than ideal.

        d. The patient's feelings regarding the pregnancy may be relevant ie, was it planned or desired, was it a difficult pregnancy.

    B. Laboratory data. None needed.

    C. Radiologic and other studies. None needed.

V. Plan. Interventions will be based on the severity of the psychologic difficulty.

    A. Postpartum blues. Reassure the patient that her symptoms are probably temporary and related to the normal adjustment to delivery and parenthood. Encourage adequate rest and gradual increases in infant care activities if possible. Involve the patient's support network and offer hospital resources if needed (ie, chaplain, social worker).

    B. Postpartum depression. Treatment depends on the severity of the depression. Consultation with the psychiatry service aids in establishing an appropriate diagnosis. Severe depressions may require antidepressants, electroconvulsive therapy (ECT), or antipsychotic medications. Milder depression may respond to brief psychotherapy or enhanced support from family and friends.

    C. Postpartum psychosis. This always necessitates psychiatric referral and generally requires use of antipsychotics, perhaps followed with ECT if no improvement is seen within a week. Acute manic episodes should be managed with antipsychotic medication (ie, imipramine 150–300 mg/d) then followed up with interpersonal psychotherapy, usually on an inpatient basis initially.

REFERENCES

Frank E et al: Pregnancy related affective episodes among women with recurrent depression. *Am J Psychiatry* 143:288, 1987.
Harding J: Postpartum psychiatric disorders: a review. *Compr Psychiatry* 30:109, 1989.
Hopkins J et al: Postpartum depression: a critical review. *Psychol Bull* 95:498, 1984.
Munoz R: Postpartum psychosis as a discrete entity. *J Clin Psychiatry* 46:182, 1985.
Vandenberg R: Postpartum depression. *Clin Obstet Gynecol* 23:1105, 1980.

18. PREECLAMPSIA (Pregnancy-induced Hypertension)

I. Problem. You are called to see a 17-year-old, nulliparous patient who presents to Labor and Delivery at approximately 29 weeks' gestation with a blood pressure of 160/110 and 4+ proteinuria.

II. Immediate Questions

A. Is the maternal condition stable? The mother's health takes priority over the fetus in most situations.

B. Is the fetus viable? If not, additional time is available to stabilize the mother.

C. Is the gestational age of the fetus correct? Various forms of intervention may be dictated by the gestational age.

D. Are there any underlying reasons why this patient may be hypertensive or have proteinuria? (See Problem 8, page 44.)

E. Has the patient seized? Seizure may indicate intracranial hemorrhage or eclampsia (see Problem 21, page 88).

III. Differential Diagnosis

A. Preeclampsia (see Tables 1–8 and 1–9).

B. Hypertension in pregnancy (see Problem 8).

C. Seizures (see Problem 21).

D. HELLP syndrome. This is a syndrome characterized by Hemolytic anemia, Elevated Liver enzymes, and Low Platelets. In general, this manifestation of preeclampsia may be treated as severe preeclampsia. It is important to recognize the HELLP syndrome when it occurs and, equally important, to recognize that these patients may be somewhat atypical in their presentation, occasionally not manifesting the hypertension or proteinuria until relatively late in the course of the disease.

TABLE 1–8. CRITERIA FOR DIAGNOSING PREECLAMPSIA (PIH).

Determination	Mild	Severe
BP systolic[a]	> 140 mm Hg or increase of 30 mm Hg	> 160 mm Hg
BP diastolic[a]	> 90 mm Hg or increase of 15 mm Hg	> 110 mm Hg
Proteinuria[a]	> 300 mg in a 24-hour urine	> 5 g in a 24-hr urine
	Trace, 1+, or 2+ semiquantitative	3+ or 4+ semiquantitative
Oliguria		> 400 mL/24h
Pitting edema	1+	>2+

[a]Values must be duplicated at least 6 hours apart from the initial reading.
PIH = Pregnancy-induced hypertension.

TABLE 1–9. SYMPTOMS OF PREECLAMPSIA (PIH).

Symptom	Mild	Severe
Headache	–	+
Visual disturbances		+
Cerebral disturbances	–	+
Seizures (eclampsia)		+
Serum creatinine	Normal	Increased
Thrombocytopenia	–	+
Hyperbilirubinemia	–	+
SGOT elevation	N/–	0
Fetal growth retardation	–	+
Epigastric pain	–	+

+ present, – not present, N normal.
Adapted from Visscher HC, Rinehart RD (eds): Precis III, An Update in Obstetrics and Gynecology. Washington, DC, American College of Obstetricians and Gynecologists, 1986.

IV. Database

A. Physical examination key points

1. **Vital signs.** The blood pressure should be monitored closely. Blood pressure must increase 30 mm Hg systolic or 15 mm Hg diastolic for the patient to be considered to have mild pregnancy-induced hypertension (PIH). If no previous pressure was recorded, a blood pressure of 140/90 after 20 weeks' gestation is considered PIH.

2. **HEENT.** A funduscopic examination should be done to look for segmental arteriolar narrowing, a classic finding in the preeclamptic patient. The conjunctivas, and mucous membranes should be inspected for evidence of cyanosis.

3. **Lungs.** Pulmonary edema should be identified and treated aggressively. Patients with preeclampsia have a decreased colloid osmotic pressure and are at great risk for pulmonary edema.

4. **Abdomen.** In addition to evaluating uterine size and gestational age, particular attention should be directed toward right upper quadrant pain or epigastric tenderness, which may indicate the HELLP syndrome (see IIID).

5. **Extremities.** Patients with preeclampsia have edema secondary to decreased oncotic pressure and third spacing.

6. **Reflexes.** Preeclampsia presents with hyperreflexia. These reflexes are also used to monitor toxicity from magnesium sulfate.

B. Laboratory data

1. **Hemogram.** In addition to evaluating initial hematocrit and white blood cell count, be aware that patients with preeclamp-

sia may have decreased platelets. A peripheral smear looking for any evidence of intravascular hemolysis should be performed. Platelets are $< 100 \times 10^3/mm^3$ in HELLP.

2. Coagulation studies. Fibrinogen may be decreased and disseminated intravascular coagulation present in the preeclamptic patient.

3. Serum chemistries. The following abnormalities may be seen with preeclamptic and HELLP.

  a. Uric acid levels are increased.

  b. SGOT is elevated (> 72 IU/L in HELLP).

  c. LDH is elevated (> 600 IU/L in HELLP).

  d. Bilirubin is elevated (> 1.2 mg/dL in HELLP).

  e. Total protein and albumin are decreased.

  f. Calcium, phosphate, and magnesium may be altered in preeclampsia.

V. Plan. If the patient's blood pressure is not controlled or the fetus is compromised, moves should be made to effect delivery.

  A. Magnesium sulfate. Administer a 4–6 g bolus IV over approximately 20 minutes, then a continuous infusion at a rate of 2–3 g/h.

    1. Check hourly deep tendon reflexes, respiratory rate, blood pressure, pulse, and urine protein; strict recording of fluid intake and urine output is essential.

    2. Maintain continuous fetal monitoring.

    3. Maintain serum magnesium level at 4–6 meq/L; magnesium levels, while a useful guide, should not be substituted for careful, frequent clinical assessment. (Magnesium toxicity is discussed in Problem 12, page 57.)

  B. Acute management of hypertension (see Problem 8, page 44).

  C. Management of Delivery

    1. Vaginal delivery is preferred.

    2. Use regional anesthesia if these five basic criteria are fulfilled:

      a. The patient has a normal coagulation profile.

      b. There is good IV access with invasive central monitoring in those cases of severe preeclampsia in which accurate cardiovascular information is necessary.

      c. A reproducible means of evaluating the patient's blood pressure is available; automated sphygmomanometers or an arterial line may be helpful.

      d. The patient must be able to undergo hydration prior to the block. This is necessary since many preeclamptic patients are intravascularly depleted, and the sympathectomy that occurs with lumbar epidural anesthesia may produce profound hypotension if intravascular volume status is not restored.

   e. There must be a skilled team of anesthesiologists available who have experience in regional anesthesia during pregnancy.

  3. If the above criteria cannot be met, a balanced general anesthesia for the preeclamptic patient undergoing cesarean section is recommended.

D. **Postpartum or postoperative management.** Once the patient with preeclampsia has delivered, continue with convulsion prophylaxis (magnesium sulfate) for 24 hours after delivery. In some cases, this may be extended if the disease process has not seemed to reverse itself as manifested by reduction in blood pressure accompanied by brisk diuresis. In the postoperative or postpartum period, the same parameters are measured on an hourly basis. Signs and symptoms of magnesium toxicity must still be watched for carefully.

REFERENCES

Anderson GD, Sibai BM: Hypertension in pregnancy. In Gabbe SG, Niebyl JR, Simpson JL (eds): *Obstetrics: Normal and Problem Pregnancies*. New York, Churchill Livingstone, 1986.
Repke JT: The pharmacologic management of hypertension in pregnancy. In Niebyl JR (ed): *Drug Use in Pregnancy*. Philadelphia, Lea & Febiger, 1988.

19. PREMATURE RUPTURED MEMBRANES

  I. **Problem.** A 25-year-old pregnant woman is complaining of leakage of fluid from her vagina.

 II. **Immediate Questions**

    A. **What is the gestational age?** Management and counseling of the patient will depend on the gestational age of the fetus. A pregnancy involving a premature fetus without evidence of infection may be followed expectantly.

    B. **Are fetal heart tones present and is there normal rate and beat-to-beat variability? Are periodic decelerations present?** Evidence of fetal distress will necessitate urgent intervention. Infection may be evidenced by poor variability, fetal tachycardia, or late decelerations.

    C. **Is the patient in labor?** Patients in labor should be monitored. Labor may be indicative of infection. The use of tocolytics in patients with preterm ruptured membranes is controversial.

    D. What are the vital signs? Maternal fever or tachycardia may suggest chorioamnionitis. Hypertension with evidence of pre-eclampsia may indicate the need for immediate delivery.

    E. Is there vaginal bleeding? This may suggest the presence of a placental abruption or partial placenta previa. Both of these clinical entities require careful monitoring and perhaps urgent delivery.

    F. What is the fetal position and size, and are there fetal anomalies? Fetal position will alter the delivery mode if delivery is indicated. The presence of intrauterine growth retardation may require earlier delivery. The type and severity of the fetal anomaly will dictate whether expectant management is appropriate and also the mode of delivery.

III. Differential Diagnosis

    A. Premature rupture of membranes (PROM). A sudden gush or slow leakage of amniotic fluid is expelled through the vagina. Contractions and labor are not always present.

    B. Urinary incontinence. This may be mistaken for premature ruptured membranes. Although the urine may be basic on nitrazine test and vaginal pooling may be present, ferning will be negative (see Procedure 3, page 348).

    C. Vaginal discharge. Vaginitis such as monilia, trichomonas, or bacterial vaginosis may present as a profuse fluid discharge from the vagina. Cervical mucus or a mucus plug may also be confused with PROM.

IV. Database

    A. Physical examination key points

        1. Vital signs. Fever may represent an infectious process. While this may indicate chorioamnionitis, other sources for fever should be sought. Maternal and fetal tachycardia may be indicative of infection.

        2. Heart. Maternal tachycardia may indicate infection.

        3. Lungs. Auscultation may reveal the presence of pneumonia or other pulmonary process to account for a maternal fever.

        4. Abdomen. Uterine contractions or uterine tenderness may indicate chorioamnionitis. Other abdominal processes such as appendicitis, pyelonephritis, or cystitis may lead to positive findings on abdominal exam and also premature labor and ruptured membranes.

        5. Pelvic examination. If preterm ruptured membranes are suspected, a sterile speculum exam should be performed with direct visualization of cervical dilatation. Digital exam should not be done because of the increased risk of infection. A cervical culture should be obtained. Signs of ruptured membranes include pooling of amniotic fluid in the posterior fornix, ferning of fluid on a glass slide, and a basic pH on nitrazine paper (see Procedure 3, p 348).

B. Laboratory data

1. **Hemogram.** Left shift and leukocytosis may suggest infection.

2. **Urinalysis.** Bacteria, white cells, and positive leukocyte esterase suggest a urinary tract infection.

3. **Cervical culture.** Group B beta-hemolytic streptococcus colonization should be treated with oral antibiotics and intravenous antibiotics during labor.

4. **Amniotic fluid culture.** Amniocentesis may be performed for culture, gram stain, and lung maturity studies (see pages 345, 367). Positive cultures have been correlated with chorioamnionitis. The presence of bacteria on gram stain correlates with positive amniotic fluid cultures.

5. **Lecithin/sphingomyelin (LS) and phosphatidyglycerol (PG).** Vaginal pool LS and PG have been shown to be reliable indicators of fetal lung maturity (see Procedures 1 and 23, pages 339 and 382).

C. Radiologic and other studies

1. **Obstetric ultrasound.** An ultrasound study is obtained in the management of preterm ruptured membranes to determine fetal number, position, gestational age, estimated fetal weight, and presence of fetal anomalies and to assess placental localization and amniotic fluid volume.

2. **Fetal heart rate monitoring.** This should be carried out for a prolonged period with an external monitor. If there is no evidence of labor or fetal distress, the patient may be managed expectantly with careful monitoring for labor or evidence of infection.

3. **Antepartum testing.** A variety of testing protocols have been described. Biophysical profiles and nonstress tests have been used (see Procedure 6, page 351). Expectant management of preterm ruptured membranes requires frequent evaluation of fetal well-being.

V. Plan. The management of preterm ruptured membranes depends on gestational age and whether there is evidence of infection or labor. The use of tocolysis and corticosteroids to enhance lung maturity remains controversial. It is essential that any plan include tests to determine infection or fetal distress, which would necessitate delivery.

A. Initial management. Fetal heart rate should be monitored immediately upon admission using fetal monitors. Intravenous access should be established. With evidence of infection, fetal lung maturity, or a term fetus, delivery should be considered. If rupture of membranes occurs in a pregnancy with a previable fetus, the patient should be counseled regarding the increased risk of extreme prematurity and complications of prolonged fetal compression with expectant management.

B. Specific treatment plans. Infection and fetal distress must be ruled out. A common treatment plan includes the following:

1. In-hospital bed rest.
2. Daily evaluation for infection, labor, or evidence of fetal distress using physical exam, white blood cell counts, and antepartum testing as well as biophysical profiles.
3. Pelvic exams should be minimized to avoid infection.
4. The use of prophylactic antibiotics, tocolysis, and corticosteroids remain controversial.
5. Those patients without evidence of fetal maturity may be managed expectantly until there is evidence of infection, labor, fetal distress, or lung maturity.
6. Labor and delivery are managed so as to minimize the risk of infection and fetal distress. If chorioamnionitis is suspected, broad-spectrum antibiotics are begun. If there is cervical colonization by group B beta-hemolytic streptococcus, intravenous antibiotics such as ampicillin are given during labor.

REFERENCES

American College of Obstetricians and Gynecologists: Assessment of fetal maturity prior to repeat cesarean delivery or elective induction of labor. ACOG Committee Opinion 72. Washington, DC, ACOG, 1989.
American College of Obstetricians and Gynecologists: Preterm labor. ACOG Tech Bull 133. Washington, DC, ACOG, 1989.
Carpenter RJ Jr: Preterm labor: cause and management. *Compr Ther* 8:37, 1982.
Cunningham FG, MacDonald PC, Gant NF: *Williams Obstetrics,* 18th ed. Norwalk, Connecticut, Appleton & Lange, 1989.

20. PROLONGED SECOND STAGE OF LABOR

I. Problem. The labor room nurse informs you that your patient has been complete and pushing for the last 2 ½ hours without progress.

II. **Immediate Questions**

A. **How long has your patient been in the second stage of labor?** The second stage of labor begins when dilation of the cervix is complete and ends with delivery of the infant. The second stage normally averages 20 minutes for a multipara and 50 minutes for a primipara. A second stage is usually considered prolonged if it lasts for more than 120 minutes (see Appendix, Figure A–5).

B. **Are there any signs of fetal distress?** Fetal heart rate decelerations due to head or cord compression are common during the second stage of labor. Prolonged, uninterrupted pushing can cause acute fetal distress with signs of deterioration of the fetal heart tones.

C. **Are maternal vital signs stable?** Severe hypotension might suggest severe dehydration or hypovolemia secondary to bleeding. Maternal tachycardia might suggest chorioamnionitis. Both conditions might cause inefficient pushing efforts.

D. **Are the expulsive forces strong enough to complete the delivery?** The main forces involved in the second stage of labor are uterine contractions and the "pushing effort." The latter is produced by increased intraabdominal pressure, created by contraction of the abdominal muscles and expiratory effort with closed glottis. Adequate pushing is usually quantified by its effect on descent and expulsion of the fetus. Conditions that limit pushing include excessive anesthesia, severe maternal cardiac disease, and maternal neuromuscular disease.

E. **What is the presenting part and its position?** Abnormal head presentation (brow or face), abnormal positions (occipitotransverse and persistent occipitoposterior), or severe asynclitism (oblique presentation) are usually associated with prolonged second-stage labor.

F. **How big is the baby?** If the estimated fetal weight is > 4500 g, suggesting macrosomia, the physician should be concerned about the possibility of cephalopelvic disproportion (CPD).

G. **Are there any fetal anomalies?** Fetal malformations such as hydrocephaly, encephalocele, and soft tissue tumors may obstruct the descent of the presenting part and cause a prolonged second stage of labor. With the increased use of prenatal ultrasonography, undiagnosed fetal malformations are less frequent.

III. **Differential Diagnosis**

A. **Hypotonic uterine contractions.** The intensity of contractions can be quantified only by an intrauterine pressure catheter

(IUPC). An adequate first stage of labor includes a wide range of uterine activities with contractions every 2–4 minutes of an amplitude between 25 and 75 mm Hg and achieving 95–395 Montevideo Units. In the second stage of labor, the presence of frequent contractions every 2–3 minutes suggests good uterine activity while less frequent contractions might indicate hypotonic uterine activity.

B. Inappropriate voluntary expulsive forces (the pushing effort). Good pushing during uterine contractions is indirectly quantified by its effect on descent and expulsion of the fetus. Direct quantitation of the pushing effort is difficult, but most women will generate pressures exceeding 100 mm Hg during the second stage of labor. Short, superficial pushing might be a sign of maternal exhaustion, excessive anesthesia, or high epidural block.

C. Abnormal cephalic presentation. If the baby is in cephalic presentation but the head is overextended instead of flexed, the presentation will be face instead of vertex. The presenting part in face presentation is the *chin* (mentum). If the fetal head is in an intermediate position between hyperextension (face presentation) and flexed (occiput presentation), then the presentation is brow with palpable parts being frontal sutures, anterior fontanel, orbital ridges, eyes, and root of the nose. This is usually an unstable presentation that will change with the head engagement to either face or occiput.

D. Abnormal occiput positions. Occiput positions other than occipitoanterior may be associated with difficult labor and a prolonged second stage.

E. Severe asynclitism. This occurs when the sagittal suture does not lie midway between the symphysis and the sacral promontory. The fetal head is laterally deflected to a more anterior or posterior position.

F. Cephalopelvic disproportion
   1. Fetal causes for CPD
      a. Fetal macrosomia (> 4500 g). Ultrasound evaluation is usually not accurate in this range.
      b. Fetal head abnormalities. Hydrocephalus, encephalocele, and large neck tumors might slow down or even obstruct the descent of the fetal head.
   2. Maternal causes for CPD. Contracted pelvis.

IV. Database

  A. Physical examination key points
    1. Vital signs. Fever might denote chorioamnionitis with poor

uterine contractions and severe maternal weakness. Hypotension may be secondary to sepsis or hypovolemia.

2. **Abdomen.** Abdominal palpation of uterine activity is very accurate in establishing the frequency of contractions. Estimate fetal weight.

3. **Pelvic examination**
   a. **Vaginal examination.** Do this to establish the engagement of the presenting part, its position, and whether asynclitism is present.
   b. **Clinical pelvimetry.** Perform qualitative clinical pelvimetry by checking the concavity of the sacral hollow and the opening of the pubic arch. The diagonal conjugate (lower margin of the symphysis pubis to the promontory of the sacrum), if greater than 11.5 cm, rules out a contracted pelvic inlet (see Appendix, Figure A–7).

B. **Laboratory data**
   1. **Fetal scalp pH.** Obtain pH if the fetal heart tracing is suggestive of distress (see Procedure 26, page 387).

C. **Radiologic and other studies**
   1. **Ultrasound.** Echo is done to evaluate fetal size and position.
   2. **Fetal heart tracing** (see Problem 6, page 32).
   3. **Intrauterine pressure catheter.** The IUPC provides a quantitative and qualitative measurement of uterine contractions (see Procedure 19, page 372).

V. **Plan**

A. **Fetal distress.** If the second stage of labor is associated with obvious signs of fetal distress, immediate delivery is mandatory. This can be accomplished by either cesarean section or forceps/vacuum if the latter can be safely performed.

B. **Maternal exhaustion.** Treatment consists of either a brief period of rest followed by renewed pushing or vaginal delivery assisted by a vacuum extractor or low forceps. In the presence of deep anesthesia, one might wait until the effect on the patient's ability to push has abated.

C. **Uterine hypotonia.** In the absence of regular uterine contractions and within the tolerance of the fetus, IV oxytocin augmentation should be started (0.5 mIU/min, increased to a maximum dosage of 20 mIU/min).

D. **Treatment of abnormal presentation.** Abnormalities of fetal head position or asynclitism can be approached either manually or by forceps application and rotation, depending on the experience and skills of the attendant. With traction, the vacuum extractor may also result in spontaneous rotation. When such a malposition cannot be corrected manually or instrumentally, cesarean delivery is appropriate.

E. **Face presentation.** This might be a sign of a contracted pelvis. Vaginal delivery can occur only in the mentum anterior position. In the mentoposterior position a cesarean section is indicated unless the baby is very small, and then a vaginal delivery might be achieved (very rare).

F. **Brow presentation.** Ordinarily, term brow presentation must be converted to either vertex or face presentation in order for a vaginal delivery to occur. Vaginal delivery may be possible, with a very small premature baby.

G. **Persistent occipitoposterior position.** Spontaneous vaginal delivery can occur if the pelvis is large and the perineum is well relaxed. Other possibilities are:
   1. Forceps delivery in occipitoposterior position.
   2. Forceps rotation to occipitoanterior position and then delivery.
   3. Manual rotation to occipitoanterior position followed by spontaneous vaginal delivery. If spontaneous vaginal delivery in the occipitoposterior position does not occur and the above manipulations cannot be easily done, cesarean section is indicated.

H. **Persistent occipitotransverse position.** This is usually only a transitory situation secondary to hypotonic uterine contractions, but it might also occur in a contracted pelvis. In the second case, delivery can be accomplished by cesarean section only. Otherwise:
   1. Manual rotation to occipitoanterior or occipitoposterior position followed by delivery in that position.
   2. Forceps rotation (by Kielland's forceps) to an occipitoanterior or occipitoposterior position followed by delivery in that position.

I. **Abnormalities of fetal head position or asynclitism.** Often these can be corrected either manually or by forceps application and rotation. When the position cannot be easily corrected, cesarean delivery is appropriate.

REFERENCES

American College of Obstetricians and Gynecologists: Dystocia. ACOG Tech Bull 137. Washington, DC, ACOG, 1989.
Cunningham FG, MacDonald PC, Gant NF: *Williams Obstetrics,* 18th ed. Norwalk, Connecticut, Appleton & Lange, 1989.

21. SEIZURES

I. **Problem.** A 28-year-old primigravida patient in early labor is reported to have had a seizure.

II. Immediate Questions

A. **Did the patient have a true seizure?** Many conditions can simulate seizures. Questioning the patient and any witnesses to the event usually helps to rule out migraine, narcolepsy, and cardiovascular syncope (eg, vasovagal episode or cardiac arrhythmia). ECG or Holter monitoring may rule out hemodynamically significant arrhythmias. Knowledge of true seizure characteristics and presence of incontinence may help to exclude pseudoseizures (hysterical seizures), which often can be quite difficult to distinguish from true seizures.

B. **Have basic supportive measures been taken?** During a seizure, the most important function of witnesses is to prevent injury to the patient. Important measures include prevention of aspiration, maintaining the airway, and minimizing trauma (see V–A).

C. **Does the patient have a history of preeclampsia?** (see Problem 18, page 76).

D. **What are the vital signs?** In addition to determining the need for immediate therapy such as fluid resuscitation or antihypertensive medication, the vital signs may aid in diagnosing the cause of the seizure. Elevated blood pressure may suggest eclampsia, fever may suggest infection, etc.

E. **Does the patient have a history of seizures?** If so, is she currently being treated with an anticonvulsant? The dosage required to maintain adequate serum anticonvulsant levels ordinarily increases during pregnancy, and inadequate serum anticonvulsant levels are a frequent cause of breakthrough seizures in late pregnancy. In addition, oral medications may be inadvertently omitted during labor.

F. **Is the patient diabetic?** When a diabetic patient enters labor, her nutritional intake may be insufficient to counteract the insulin administered previously. In addition, labor and oxytocin administration may further decrease her insulin requirements. Both factors may result in hypoglycemic seizures, which can be treated simply and effectively (see Problem 7, page 40).

G. **Did the patient exhibit signs typical of seizures?** Features which are frequently, although not invariably, associated with true seizures should be sought (Table 1–10).

H. **What type of seizure did the patient have?** For diagnostic,

TABLE 1–10. SEIZURES.

Feature	Absence (Petit Mal)	Focal	Generalized (Grand Mal)
Onset and resolution	Abrupt	Abrupt	Abrupt
Duration	5–30 sec	10 sec–2 min	10 sec–2 min
Incontinence	Absent	Absent	Present
Loss of consciousness or awareness	Present	Absent	Present
Stereotyped behavior	Staring, facial twitching	Repetitive movements	Tonic rigidity followed by clonic jerking

prognostic, and therapeutic purposes, try to determine whether the patient had a partial seizure, a partial seizure with generalized spread, a generalized tonic-clonic seizure, or an absence seizure. A general rule is that partial seizures (with or without generalized spread) usually represent focal disease, whereas primary generalized seizures usually do not.

III. **Differential Diagnosis**

A. **True seizure**

1. **Eclampsia.** Approximately 2–4% of patients with preeclampsia will ultimately have seizures. Usually, but not always, these patients will develop hypertension (blood pressure > 140/90 mm Hg), proteinuria (> 1+ on dipstick), and edema prior to seizures. The patient may complain of headache, visual changes, and epigastric or right upper quadrant pain. The cause of eclamptic seizures remains speculative.

2. **Inadequate anticonvulsant levels.** A patient with preexisting epilepsy frequently will be found to have subtherapeutic serum anticonvulsant levels late in pregnancy.

3. **Metabolic disturbance.** Hypoglycemia, hyponatremia, and hypocalcemia may cause seizures, which can be reversed with replacement of the deficient substance. Hyponatremia may result from the administration of large amounts of oxytocin and free water.

4. **Drug or alcohol abuse.** In the substance abuser, withdrawal or intoxication may be the cause of seizures. Most commonly, seizures may result from cocaine or amphetamine intoxication or from alcohol or barbiturate withdrawal.

5. **Medications.** Local anesthetics which are inadvertently injected into the maternal circulation may cause seizures. In addition, normeperidine, a metabolite of meperidine (Dem-

erol), may accumulate in patients with poor renal function and cause seizures.

6. **Trauma.** Subdural and epidural hematomas may develop secondary to closed head trauma, for example after an automobile accident or a fall. Depending on the severity of the injury, loss of consciousness followed by a lucid interval, progressive obtundation, seizures, and hemiparesis may occur. Epidural and acute subdural hematomas constitute true neurosurgical emergencies.

7. **Infection.** Meningitis and encephalitis are frequently associated with seizures. Acute meningitis—bacterial or viral—classically presents with fever, headache, stiff neck, and mental status change. Viral encephalitis may present similarly but with additional evidence of parenchymal involvement such as focal neurologic signs. The diagnosis of bacterial meningitis is of paramount importance, since morbidity and mortality are directly correlated with the interval between onset of disease and administration of antibiotic therapy.

8. **Stroke.** Ischemic strokes (secondary to thrombosis or embolism) or hemorrhagic strokes (hypertensive intracerebral hemorrhage or subarachnoid hemorrhage resulting from ruptured aneurysm or arteriovenous malformation) may result in new-onset seizures.

9. **Cerebral venous thrombosis.** Thrombosis of the sagittal and lateral sinuses can occur during the first four postpartum weeks but may occur before delivery as well. The typical presenting signs and symptoms are severe headache, papilledema, and seizures. Thrombosis may progress and result in paralysis, aphasia, and coma.

10. **Amniotic fluid embolus.** This rare disorder results when a bolus of amniotic fluid enters the maternal circulation and can occur at any time in the peripartum period. The clinical presentation is that of dyspnea, cyanosis, and shock followed by hemorrhage, coagulopathy, and sometimes seizures. Maternal mortality is reportedly > 80%.

11. **Thrombotic thrombocytopenic purpura (TTP).** This rare clinical syndrome consists of thrombocytopenic purpura, microangiopathic hemolytic anemia, renal dysfunction, fever, and neurologic manifestations including seizure. It should be considered in the differential diagnosis of eclampsia and stroke.

12. **Neoplasm.** Neoplasms originating in the CNS (astrocytoma, other gliomas, meningioma) or elsewhere (breast, lung, lymphatic system) may cause new-onset seizures. Vascular malformations may also be responsible.

13. **Idiopathic.** In any patient without a history of seizures, it is possible that the first seizure represents the initial manifesta-

tion of true epilepsy. This is a diagnosis of exclusion, however, and should not be made without a thorough evaluation and consultation with a neurologist.

B. Migraine. In most cases, migraine can be distinguished from seizures with little difficulty. Ordinarily, migraine does not result in loss of consciousness or postictal confusion. In one variant, basilar artery migraine, loss of consciousness does occur and may appear similar to a seizure.

C. Narcolepsy. The characteristic features of narcolepsy include sleep attacks, cataplexy, sleep paralysis, and hypnogogic hallucinations. Distinguishing narcolepsy from seizures is usually possible on clinical grounds alone (including a careful history).

D. Cardiovascular syncope. Cardiovascular syncope denotes loss of consciousness secondary to an acute decrease in cerebral blood flow. One complicating factor is that a prolonged episode of syncope may result in seizures. Nevertheless, other than loss of consciousness, characteristic features of seizures are usually absent. Likely causes of syncope include vasovagal episodes, arrhythmia, and cardiac valvular disease (aortic stenosis). It is important to distinguish syncope from seizures, since treatment of one condition may exacerbate the other.

E. Pseudoseizures (hysterical seizures). A poor imitation of seizures is easily discerned, but a good imitation presents a difficult problem. A normal EEG is helpful but does not rule out true seizures. Furthermore, some patients with true seizure disorders also have pseudoseizures. It has been noted that injuries and incontinence, frequent characteristics of true seizures, rarely occur during pseudoseizures.

IV. Database

A. Physical examination key points

Note: If spinal injury during the seizure appears possible, do not attempt to move the patient (even for examination purposes) until spine films have been obtained and reviewed.

1. **Vital signs.** Significantly elevated blood pressure suggests eclampsia or stroke, while markedly reduced blood pressure points to a vasovagal episode or amniotic fluid embolus. Bradycardia is also seen in vasovagal episodes. Fever suggests infection but may also be seen with eclampsia and TTP.

2. **HEENT.** Examine for signs of trauma. Determine whether visual fields are intact and whether the patient is photophobic. Pupillary light reflexes are lost in generalized convulsions. Mydriasis (pupillary dilatation) occurs in cocaine and am-

phetamine intoxication, and light reflexes may be asymmetric in stroke. Perform a funduscopic examination, looking especially for retinal arteriolar spasm (eclampsia), retinal hemorrhages (stroke), and papilledema (sagittal or lateral sinus thrombosis, tumor).

3. **Neck.** Examine for nuchal rigidity (meningitis).
4. **Heart.** Arrhythmia may be the cause of syncope.
5. **Lungs.** It is important to ensure that the patient is able to ventilate adequately both during and after a seizure. Pulmonary edema may be seen in conjunction with eclampsia.
6. **Abdomen.** Note whether there is right upper quadrant (liver) tenderness or uterine tenderness (placental abruption).
7. **Back.** Examine for spinal tenderness.
8. **Pelvic examination.** Note antepartum vaginal bleeding (placental abruption), or excessive postpartum bleeding (secondary to coagulopathy from eclampsia, TTP, or amniotic fluid embolus).
9. **Extremities.** Look for evidence of injury during the seizure or needle marks indicating drug abuse.
10. **Skin.** Examine for purpura.
11. **Neurologic examination.** Perform a careful neurologic examination, including the cranial nerves, looking especially for focal or lateralizing signs. Hyperreflexia is seen commonly in eclampsia. Spasm of the facial muscles in response to tapping on a branch of the facial nerve (Chvostek's sign) is seen with hypocalcemia. The presence of a postictal (Todd's) paralysis suggests that the seizure was focal, at least initially.

B. **Laboratory data**
   1. **Hemogram.** Elevated hematocrit (hemoconcentration) is consistent with eclampsia. Reduced hematocrit suggests hemolysis (TTP, HELLP syndrome [problem 18, page 76]) or bleeding source. Leukocytosis is indicative of infection. Thrombocytopenia is consistent with eclampsia, trauma, infection, amniotic fluid embolus, and TTP.
   2. **Serum electrolytes.** Hyponatremia, hypokalemia, and hypocalcemia all may cause seizures (see Problems 49, 51, and 53, pages 185, 188, and 195 respectively).
   3. **Blood urea nitrogen and creatinine.** These may be elevated in eclampsia, infection, and TTP.
   4. **Blood glucose.** Hypoglycemia is a likely cause of seizures in diabetics.
   5. **Liver function tests.** Elevations are most likely due to eclampsia.
   6. **Toxicology screen including blood alcohol level.**
   7. **Serum anticonvulsant levels.** If the patient is a known ep-

ileptic maintained on anticonvulsant medication, serum measurements will demonstrate the presence of adequate or inadequate levels.

8. **Urinalysis.** Note especially the presence of proteinuria, one of the hallmarks of eclampsia.

9. **Arterial blood gases.** If the patient appears cyanotic or septic, or if a hypoxic insult is the suspected cause of the seizure(s), arterial blood gas determinations may be helpful.

C. Radiologic and other studies

1. **Magnetic resonance imaging (MRI) and computed tomography (CT).** One or both of these tests should be performed in the same clinical setting that demands an electroencephalogram:

   a. Seizure without an obvious cause or prolonged postictal period.

   b. Lateralizing signs on the neurologic examination or suggestion of a mass lesion also requires imaging of the brain.

   c. True eclamptic seizures refractory to anticonvulsant therapy should also be evaluated with CT or MRI.

   d. The choice of which test to obtain may be dictated by the preference of the consulting neurologist or by the availability of the test at a particular time.

2. **Electroencephalogram (EEG).** In a patient who has a seizure without an obvious underlying cause (such as eclampsia or hypoglycemia) or a prolonged postictal period, an EEG should be performed. It should be noted that the absence of EEG abnormalities during the interictal period does not absolutely rule out true seizures or epilepsy, and the presence of spike patterns does not necessarily rule them in. As with most laboratory tests, the EEG must be interpreted in its clinical context.

3. **Lumbar puncture.** Obtain cerebrospinal fluid for protein, glucose, cell count, syphilis serology, gram stain, and cultures. Lumbar puncture is contraindicated in the presence of a mass lesion (suggested by papilledema or progressive onset of focal neurologic deficit) or signs of herniation (see Procedure 21, page 377).

V. Plan. The general plan should be to stabilize the patient, identify and treat the underlying cause of the seizure, and then treat with an anticonvulsant if indicated.

    A. Stabilize the patient. As noted earlier, the initial steps to be taken are aimed at protecting the patient from harming herself during the seizure.

1. Position the patient's head lower than her body and turned to the side, if possible, to prevent aspiration.
2. Maintain an airway by gently placing a padded tongue depressor or plastic airway in the patient's mouth. Never use force, since forceful application of these maneuvers may lead to increased airway obstruction or injury.
3. Protect the patient from trauma by cushioning her head and padding the bed rails as much as possible. Do not forcibly restrain the patient, since this may cause additional trauma.

B. **Identify and treat the underlying cause of the seizure.** Through history, physical examination, and laboratory evaluation, an underlying cause for most seizures will be found.

1. **Eclampsia.** Standard therapy in North America is magnesium sulfate, which may be administered intravenously. Intravenous phenytoin has also been used in this setting (See C2).
2. **Inadequate anticonvulsant levels.** An epileptic patient with inadequate serum anticonvulsant levels should receive additional doses of her usual medication in order to achieve therapeutic levels. It should be remembered, however, that some epileptics, no matter what pharmacologic attempts are made, have their seizures under control but are never completely seizure free. A single typical seizure in such a patient, in the face of therapeutic serum levels, may demand no further therapy.
3. **Metabolic disturbance.** Correction of the metabolic abnormality alone is usually adequate treatment.
4. **Substance abuse.** Alcohol withdrawal seizures, which usually occur 12–30 hours after the last drink, should be prevented or treated in pregnancy with phenytoin. If rapid administration is necessary, intravenous phenytoin may be used; otherwise, the patient may receive oral phenytoin (see C2). Barbiturate withdrawal seizures may be treated with phenytoin or, when severe, with phenobarbital (see C3). Seizures resulting from cocaine or amphetamine intoxication may be treated with intravenous diazepam (see C4) followed by phenytoin.
5. **Medications.** If toxic levels of local anesthetics are the cause of seizures, they may be treated with intravenous diazepam. If meperidine administration in a patient with renal compromise is the cause, meperidine should be discontinued and substituted with morphine.
6. **Infection.** If meningitis is diagnosed, the patient should be treated with antibiotics immediately after appropriate cul-

tures have been sent. Ordinarily, seizure prophylaxis is not necessary after a single, self-limited seizure. During pregnancy, however, it seems reasonable to institute anticonvulsant therapy for a limited time after even a single seizure. Phenytoin may be used as above.

7. **Focal CNS process.** If stroke, cerebral venous thrombosis, or neoplasm is believed to be the cause of seizures, treatment is at the discretion of the consulting neurologist. Prior to delivery, it seems reasonable to treat even a single seizure or to initiate prophylactic therapy in patients believed to be at risk for seizures.

8. **Amniotic fluid embolus.** Treatment for this catastrophic disorder is usually supportive. Anticonvulsant therapy with phenytoin may be used.

9. **TTP.** Again, treatment is largely supportive, although newer modalities (eg, plasmapheresis) may be useful. Seizures may be treated with phenytoin.

C. **Treat with an anticonvulsant if indicated.** The following regimens may be used when anticonvulsant therapy is indicated in a pregnant patient.

1. **Magnesium sulfate.** Give 4–6 g IV bolus over 15 minutes followed by continuous infusion of 2 g/h. The infusion rate may be adjusted to achieve a therapeutic serum level of approximately 4–8 meq/L (4.8–9.6 mg/dL). Check patellar reflexes and respirations frequently, and discontinue the infusion if reflexes are absent or respirations are < 12/min. The toxic effects of magnesium may be reversed by slow IV infusion of 10–20 mL of 10% calcium gluconate and administration of nasal oxygen.

2. **Phenytoin**

   a. **Intravenous.** One protocol recommends administering an initial IV dose of 1000, 1250, or 1500 mg for patients who weigh < 50, 50–70, or > 70 kg respectively. The rate of infusion is 25 mg/min for the first 750 mg and 12.5 mg/min for the remainder. Frequent blood pressure measurement is mandatory and cardiac monitoring is prudent while the rate of infusion is 25 mg/min. The therapeutic serum level is 10–20 µg/mL. Levels may be checked 1 hour after the infusion is completed and every 12 hours thereafter. Phenytoin should always be mixed into a solution and administered through an intravenous line that does not contain dextrose.

   b. **Oral.** Give 2 doses of phenytoin 500 mg 2 hours apart. Additional doses may be given as needed to achieve the therapeutic serum levels noted above.

3. **Phenobarbital.** Phenobarbital may be administered as an

initial dose of 120 mg IV followed by 60 mg IV q10–15min, up to a maximum of 500 mg, until seizures stop.

4. **Diazepam.** Intravenous doses of 5 mg may be administered q5min, up to a maximum of 20–30 mg, until seizures stop.

REFERENCES

Bellur SN: Neurologic disorders in pregnancy. In Gleicher N (ed): *Principles of Medical Therapy in Pregnancy.* New York, Plenum, 1985, pp 916–932.
Donaldson JO: *Neurology of Pregnancy.* Philadelphia, WB Saunders, 1989.
Solomon GE, Kutt H, Plum F: *Clinical Management of Seizures: A Guide for the Physician.* Philadelphia, WB Saunders, 1983.

22. SHORTNESS OF BREATH (See Problem 39, page 153)

23. SHOULDER DYSTOCIA

I. **Problem.** You are called to Labor and Delivery by the resident staff for assistance in delivering a fetus whose shoulders cannot pass through the pelvic outlet. The head is pulled back against the perineum; the patient is in a lithotomy position.

II. **Immediate Questions**

A. **How large were the patient's previous babies?** If the estimated fetal weight is similar to previous pregnancies, the fetus may have a skeletal or spinal anomaly.

B. **Has an episiotomy been performed, and is it optimal?** If possible, the episiotomy should be extended and a fourth-degree extension created.

C. **Is there adequate help in the room?** Nursing, neonatal, and anesthesia support should be summoned.

III. **Differential Diagnosis**

A. **Shoulder dystocia.** Shoulder dystocia occurs when the fetus's delivery through the birth canal is impaired by lodging of the shoulders in the pelvis. The problem may be secondary to a macrosomic fetus, contracted pelvis, or inadequate episiotomy. Seventy percent of infants delivered with shoulder dystocia weigh more than 4000 g. Diabetes, post-term pregnancy, increased maternal age, excess maternal weight gain, and prolonged second stage increase the risk of shoulder dystocia.

B. **Fetal anomaly.** Occasionally, massive hydrops or a fetal mass such as sacrococcygeal teratoma may be present. If fetal anomaly is a possibility, the infant should be intubated and ventilated because delivery will be extremely difficult.

C. Contracted pelvis. The patient may have a contracted pelvis that does not permit passage of the term fetus.

IV. Database

A. Physical examination key points
1. Pelvic examination
a. Identify the presenting part.
b. Evaluate the pelvis for outlet obstruction. A narrow pubic arch, shortened diagonal conjugate, and decreased intertuberous diameters predispose to dystocia.
c. Evaluate the episiotomy site for possible extension into the rectum or in a mediolateral direction.

B. Laboratory tests. None needed.

C. Radiologic and other studies. None needed. Ultrasound is of limited value with the infant's head already delivered and a shoulder deep in the pelvis.

V. Plan

A. Obtain assistance in the form of experienced nursing help or other physician support.

B. Extend the episiotomy to permit passage of the fetus.

C. Suprapubic (not fundal) pressure can be exerted with pressure placed above the symphysis pubis.

D. The **McRoberts-Gonick maneuver,** taking the patient's legs out of the stirrups and flexing her knees, is the next step that should be undertaken. It can generally assist with delivery of the head and the body.

E. If this is not successful, a **corkscrew maneuver** trying to turn the fetus by rotating the posterior shoulder 180 degrees under the public ramus can then be attempted.

F. Deliver the posterior arm.

G. Assistance in the form of suprapubic pressure and the Mc-Roberts maneuver is often successful. If not, then preparations to replace the head and perform emergency cesarean section might be considered.

REFERENCES

Acker DB, Sach BP, Friedman EA: Risk factors for shoulder dystocia in the average-weight infant. *Obstet Gynecol* 67:164, 1986.

Gross TL et al: Shoulder dystocia: a fetal physician risk. *Am J Obstet Gynecol* 156:1408, 1987.
Sandberg EC: The Zavanelli maneuver extended: progression of a revolutionary concept. *Am J Obstet Gynecol* 158:1347, 1988.

24. THYROID STORM (see Problem 13, page 59)

25. URINARY TRACT INFECTION (See problem 40, page 157)

26. UTERINE INVERSION

I. **Problem.** Upon removal of the placenta, a 35-year-old multipara passes a large tissue mass through her vagina and begins to hemorrhage.

II. **Immediate Questions**

A. **Is there adequate intravenous access?** Life-threatening hemorrhage may occur. Ideally two intravenous lines are begun. Volume must be replaced aggressively.

B. **Is an anesthesiologist available?** Anesthesia, especially halothane, which provides for uterine relaxation, is helpful in reducing the inversion.

C. **Are adequate blood products available?** The patient may hemorrhage excessively, and blood products need to be available in the hospital blood bank.

D. **Is a coagulopathy present?** This may develop with extensive blood loss, and may account for continued bleeding.

E. **Are there other causes for postpartum hemorrhage in this patient?** Placenta accreta, vaginal or cervical lacerations, retained products of conception, uterine atony, or uterine rupture may cause hemorrhage.

III. **Differential Diagnosis**

A. **Uterine inversion.** Inversion occurs in 1 of 2000 deliveries. The uterus is prolapsed through the cervix and passes out of the vaginal introitus.

B. **Vaginal, cervical, or uterine lacerations.** This problem requires careful inspection of the vagina and cervix. In the case of lacerations, bleeding continues despite a contracted uterus.

C. **Uterine atony.** Atony responds to uterine massage and oxytocin or prostaglandin.

    D. Retained products of conception. This situation responds to evacuation of the tissue by curettage.

    E. Placenta accreta. In this condition the placenta adheres abnormally to the myometrium. Attempts at removal of the placenta may result in hemorrhage.

    F. Prolapsed myoma. A cervical or submucosal myoma may prolapse through the vagina and give the appearance of a uterine inversion.

IV. Database

    A. Physical examination key points

        1. Vital signs. Hypotension and tachycardia reflect severe blood loss.

        2. Abdominal examination. With total inversion of the uterus, the uterine fundus may be absent on abdominal palpation. With partial inversion, palpation may reveal an indentation at the top of the uterine fundus.

        3. Pelvic examination. Bimanual exam will reveal a bulge within the vagina. With complete inversion, a mass may be seen at or prolapsing through the introitus. The placenta may or may not still be attached to the uterus.

    B. Laboratory data

        1. Hemogram. While acute blood loss may not be immediately reflected in the hematocrit, volume replacement should be geared to maternal vital signs. However, the hemogram should be obtained serially following treatment to assess the need for additional blood products.

V. Plan.

In the case of uterine inversion, blood loss may be massive and requires prompt volume replacement. Any delay in treatment will increase maternal morbidity and mortality and make it more difficult to replace the inverted uterus.

    A. Initial management

        1. Large-bore (16-gauge) intravenous lines should be placed, and blood products should be obtained.

        2. Immediately request assistance, including an anesthesiologist.

        3. If the placenta remains attached to the uterine fundus, do not remove it until the IV access is established and all is ready for replacement of the uterine fundus, since this may increase maternal bleeding. Some authors would recommend not removing the placenta prior to replacing the fundus.

4. If the uterus is recently inverted and the placenta is separated, the fundus can often be replaced promptly.
5. The inverted fundus is replaced by pushing upward using the palm and fingers. Halothane and tocolytic agents such as terbutaline and ritodrine have been used to assist in replacement of the fundus by providing uterine relaxation (see Chapter 7).
6. After the inversion is reduced, oxytocin or prostaglandin is given to contract the uterus. Any agent given to relax the uterus is discontinued.
7. If the uterus cannot be replaced transvaginally, laparotomy has been proposed to place traction sutures in the uterine fundus to assist in treatment.

B. **Following intervention**
1. Serial hemogram and coagulation studies will assist in volume replacement.
2. The patient should be examined vaginally to assure that the inversion does not recur.

REFERENCES

Cunningham FG, MacDonald PC, Gant NF: *Williams Obstetrics,* 18th ed. Norwalk, Connecticut, Appleton & Lange, 1989, pp 422–423.
Thiery M, Delbeke L: Acute puerperal uterine inversion. Two step management with a β-mimetic and prostaglandin. *Am J Obstet Gynecol* 153:891, 1985.

27. VAGINAL BLEEDING IN PREGNANCY (First, Second, or Third Trimester)

I. **Problem.** You are called to evaluate a pregnant woman with vaginal bleeding.

II. **Immediate Questions**

A. **What are the patient's vital signs?** Check for hemodynamic compromise, hypotension, or tachycardia. If these are present, initiate resuscitation with fluid, blood products, or both. Follow urine output. If the patient is in shock, consider monitoring with a central venous pressure or Swan-Ganz catheter to guide fluid replacement.

B. **What is the rate of bleeding, and how much blood has been lost?** Assess this by the patient's history and by observation of her perineum and clothing. In acute blood loss, the hematocrit may not change until later.

C. **What was the most recent hematocrit or hemoglobin?** This value is useful as a baseline in estimating blood loss.

D. **What is the estimated gestational age, and are fetal heart tones present?** Assess gestational age by last menstrual period and uterine size; if patient is in her third trimester, obtain fetal heart rate.

III. Differential Diagnosis

A. **First- and second-trimester bleeding**
1. **Threatened abortion.** Pain is absent or minimal. The cervix is closed and uneffaced.
2. **Inevitable abortion.** Vaginal bleeding is accompanied by pain and cervical dilatation.
3. **Incomplete abortion.** Products of conception protrude through the cervical os.
4. **Gestational trophoblastic disease (GTD).** The patient may present with a size or date discrepancy and vaginal bleeding. Ultrasound evaluation will reveal a "snow storm" pattern without an intrauterine pregnancy. The serum level of human chorionic gonadotropin (HCG) will also be elevated for appropriate gestational age (see page 314).
5. **Ectopic pregnancy.** Irregular bleeding and abdominal pain are usually present. A prior history of ectopic pregnancy, infertility, or tubal surgery is common. An adnexal mass on pelvic exam is suggestive.
6. **Cervical lesions or genital trauma.** Cervical carcinoma as well as infections can cause vaginal bleeding during pregnancy.

B. **Third-trimester bleeding**
1. **Abruptio placentae.** This is defined as premature separation of the normally implanted placenta. Signs and symptoms usually include uterine tenderness and irritability and hypertonic contractions. It is associated with high parity, hypertension, and past history of abruptio placentae. Trauma and sudden decompression of overdistended uterus are other possible causes. The amount of vaginal bleeding may not represent the total blood volume lost. Thus, the patient may exhibit evidence of hypovolemia out of proportion to the observed external blood loss.
2. **Placenta previa.** This occurs when the placenta completely or partly covers the internal cervical os. It is associated with increasing parity, increasing maternal age, post cesarean delivery, and prior history of placenta previa. Painless vaginal bleeding is the most common presentation. Also, on **Leopold maneuvers** (see Appendix, Figure A–6), the presenting part is not engaged and the fetus may present in breech,

oblique, or transverse lie. Some patients report contractions with the bleeding episode.

3. **Cervical lesions or genital trauma.**

4. **Heavy "show."** This is a diagnosis of exclusion. With a heavy show, a large amount of blood is passed with cervical mucus.

5. **Vasa previa.** This occurs when the velamentous insertions of fetal vessels occur in front of the internal cervical os. If the vessels rupture, rapid fetal hemorrhage usually occurs.

C. **Coagulopathy.** This can occur during all trimesters. Patients with a fetal demise, retained products, and placental abruption are at an increased risk for disseminated intravascular coagulation (DIC). Idiopathic (immunologic) thrombocytopenic purpura (ITP) may result in a coagulopathy secondary to antiplatelet antibodies. More than 90% are IgG and can pass through the placenta, causing a transient ITP in the newborn.

IV. **Database**

A. **Physical examination key points**

1. **Vital signs.** Blood pressure and pulse should be monitored to diagnose a hypovolemic state. The blood pressure will decrease and the pulse increase to compensate for a large blood loss.

2. **Abdomen.** Uterine size can be used as a quick estimator of gestational age (the umbilicus is 20 weeks with each finger diameter equal to 2 additional weeks). Uterine tenderness and increased tone are usually present in abruptio placentae. Fetal presentation may be abnormal in placenta previa. Fetal heart tones should be assessed.

3. **Pelvic examination.** Do not perform digital cervical examination if placenta previa is suspected. Careful speculum examination to rule out genital lacerations or cervical lesions is appropriate. In the first or second trimester, cervical dilatation is associated with inevitable or incomplete abortions.

B. **Laboratory data**

1. **Hemogram.** Serial hematocrit and hemoglobin determinations are helpful in assessing the severity of hemorrhage. White blood cell count with differential is useful if an infectious process is suspected.

2. **Clotting studies.** Prothrombin time, partial thromboplastin time, platelets, fibrinogen, and fibrin split products may reveal coagulation disorders or DIC.

3. **Type and cross-match.** If the patient is Rh negative and unsensitized, Rh immunoglobulin may be indicated.

4. **Beta human chorionic gonadotropin (β-HCG).** In the case

of first-trimester bleeding, serial determinations of the beta subunit of HCG will help to confirm viability of the pregnancy. Serial titers should show a rise of 66% or more every 2 days.

C. Radiologic and other studies

  1. **Ultrasonography.** An echo study is helpful in locating and dating the pregnancy and in evaluating placental location and fetal viability. A gestational sac should be visible at 6 weeks' gestation, fetal cardiac activity by 7–8 weeks.

  2. **External fetal heart monitoring.**

V. Plan

A. Stabilize the maternal condition, then identify and treat the underlying cause of bleeding. If bleeding is hemodynamically significant, large-bore 16-gauge IV lines should be placed and resuscitation with fluid, blood, or both started while further assessment of the patient is completed.

B. First-trimester bleeding. If an abortion is in progress, suction, sharp curettage, or a combination of the two is the treatment of choice.

C. Second-trimester bleeding. If an abortion is in progress, curettage, prostaglandins, or both have been used to complete evacuation of the uterus (see Procedure 29, page 392).

D. Cervical lesions or genital lacerations. Treatment will depend on the location and cause of the lesion. If cervical bleeding occurs, cytologic sampling and cultures for *Chlamydia trichomatis* and *Neisseria gonorrhoeae* are indicated. Evaluate for cervical neoplasia and biopsy suspicious lesions.

E. Placenta previa. If the mother is stable, the goal is to achieve fetal maturity without increasing maternal risk. Therefore, expectant management is indicated unless the fetus is mature, there are obstetric reasons to terminate the pregnancy (ie, pregnancy-induced hypertension, Rh isoimmunization, the fetus is dead or has anomalies incompatible with life), or active labor or excessive bleeding occurs.

F. Abruptio placentae

  1. If the mother is stable and the fetus is alive, close monitoring of the fetal status is necessary.

  2. Cesarean delivery is indicated if there is evidence of fetal distress, excessive bleeding, or any obstetric contraindication to labor.

  3. If the fetus is dead, vaginal delivery should be attempted unless labor is contraindicated.

4. Amniotomy and oxytocin supplementation, if needed, should be performed.
5. Be prepared to vigorously treat hypovolemia and coagulopathy.
6. Postpartum atony is another common complication.
7. Be aware of possible ischemic damage to distant organs, namely the kidney (acute tubular or cortical necrosis) and the anterior pituitary in the mother.

REFERENCES

Cotton DB et al: The conservative aggressive management of placenta previa. *Am J Obstet Gynecol* 137:687, 1980.
Hurd WW et al: Selective management of abruptio placentae: a prospective study. *Obstet Gynecol* 61:467, 1983.
LaFerla JJ: Spontaneous abortion. *Clin Obstet Gynecol* 13:105, 1986.

GYNECOLOGY

28. ABDOMINAL DISTENTION

I. **Problem.** A 42-year-old woman is complaining of abdominal bloating.

II. **Immediate Questions**

A. **Has the patient recently had an operation?** Immediate postoperative abdominal distention is common and may be related to ileus, gastric distention, or obstruction. Retroperitoneal surgery may also cause an ileus.

B. **Is a nasogastric tube in place?** Nasogastric and Cantor tubes can relieve gastric and small bowel distention but will be of little use in draining colonic gas. Verify that the tube is functioning (see Problems 59 and 60, pages 224 and 226).

C. **What medications is the patient receiving?** Certain medications such as narcotics (eg, codeine, morphine, and Lomotil), anticholinergics (atropine, belladonna), and tocolytics (magnesium sulfate, ritodrine) will slow intestinal motility. Diuretic (ie, furosemide) induced hypokalemia may also cause decreased motility.

D. **What previous operations has the patient had?** The cause of the distention may be obstruction from adhesions or tumor.

E. **What are the vital signs?** Abdominal distention may restrict pulmonary function, causing tachypnea or even respiratory failure in patients with severe pulmonary disease. Fever may suggest an infectious process such as peritonitis, pyelonephritis, or pneumonia, which can cause a reflex ileus. Tachycardia and hypotension may indicate severe sepsis or hypovolemia.

F. When was the most recent bowel movement or flatus?
Bowel movements and the passage of flatus are useful indicators of bowel activity. Their absence suggests ileus, which can be mechanical (obstruction) or functional (adynamic ileus) in origin.

G. Has the patient been vomiting? Vomiting is often a sign of obstruction. The character of the material may aid in diagnosing the site of obstruction. In gastric outlet obstruction there is little, if any, bile in the emesis, whereas distal small bowel obstruction tends to be bilious.

H. When was the last menstrual period? The gravid uterus or hemoperitoneum secondary to a ruptured ectopic pregnancy or ruptured ovarian cyst can cause increased abdominal girth. Abdominal bloating is a common symptom associated with premenstrual syndrome (PMS).

III. Differential Diagnosis

A. Gastrointestinal tract obstruction

1. **Stomach.** Gastric outlet obstruction by tumor, ulcer, or gastric atony secondary to surgery can lead to gastric dilatation and a sensation of bloating.

2. **Small intestine.** Adhesions after previous surgery and other mechanical causes such as intraluminal obstruction (foreign body, gallstone, etc) or extraluminal obstruction from tumors (especially ovarian cancer) commonly cause small bowel obstruction. Internal hernias and strangulated or incarcerated external hernias can also cause small bowel obstruction.

3. **Large intestine.** Causes include intrinsic or extrinsic tumors, volvulus, and fecal impaction (particularly in elderly, bedridden patients).

4. **Non-GI tract.** Rarely, other tumors such as retroperitoneal sarcomas, lymphomas, or genitourinary malignancies may cause obstruction.

B. Intestinal ischemia. This is usually diagnosed by acidosis, elevated WBC count, and "pain out of proportion to physical findings."

C. Paralytic ileus (adynamic ileus). This is frequently seen in the postoperative period after abdominal or retroperitoneal surgery. It also occurs after blunt abdominal trauma, can be caused by medications, and can be secondary to intra-abdominal infection (peritonitis) or inflammatory processes (pancreatitis, cholecystitis). "Reflex" ileus is often associated with pneumonia, urinary tract infection (pyelonephritis), or genital tract infections (chorio-amnionitis, endomyometritis, pelvic inflammatory disease, and tubo-ovarian abscess).

D. **Intussusception.** It is most often found at the ileocecal valve and can be due to tumors as the lead point which leads to obstruction.

E. **Organomegaly.** Massive hepatomegaly and splenomegaly may be confused with distention.

F. **Intra-abdominal mass.** A variety of lesions such as cysts (mesenteric, ovarian, renal), tumors, or aneurysms, and even an unrecognized pregnancy, can lead to complaints of distention.

G. **Hemoperitoneum.** Among sexually active women of reproductive age, ruptured ectopic pregnancy is the most common cause of intraperitoneal hemorrhage. Ruptured ovarian cyst is another cause. Postoperative bleeding, either surgical or medical (disseminated intravascular coagulopathy), are further considerations.

H. **Bladder distention.** Urine retention, usually caused by bladder and urethral surgery or a nonfunctional Foley catheter, can cause massive bladder distention. Bladder outlet obstruction, most often due to tumor, radiation stricture, or neurogenic bladder from spinal cord injury, may also cause bladder distention.

I. **Abdominal wall or groin hernia.** This may cause an obstructed loop of bowel which may also be strangulated and thus ischemic.

J. **Hirschsprung's disease.** Also known as aganglionic megacolon, the disorder is usually diagnosed early in life and causes intermittent constipation with bloating and vomiting.

K. **Ascites.** Usually a chronic condition related to liver diseases (alcoholic cirrhosis) or carcinoma (malignant ascites), ascites may be produced by ovarian or fallopian tube carcinomas or sarcomas. Gynecologic tumors that rarely produce ascites are cervical and endometrial carcinomas as well as lymphomas.

L. **Ogilvie's syndrome.** Pseudo-obstruction of the colon in the absence of an obstructing lesion, it is usually seen in bedridden patients with severe extra-abdominal diseases such as respiratory or renal insufficiency or vertebral fractures.

M. **Premenstrual syndrome.** Abdominal bloating is one of many symptoms associated with PMS. Others include headache, breast swelling or tenderness, edema of extremities, increased thirst or appetite, food cravings, acneiform eruptions, constipation, and diarrhea. These symptoms are cyclic, typically occurring 7–10 days prior to menses, and cease during the 24 hours after onset of menses.

IV. Database

A. Physical examination key points

1. **Vital signs.** Fever suggests an inflammatory process, and tachypnea may represent respiratory comprise. Tachycardia may be secondary to infection, hypovolemia, or pain. Hypotension suggests severe infection or hypovolemia.

2. **Heart.** Atrial fibrillation can lead to intestinal embolization and ischemia.

3. **Lungs.** Auscultation may reveal evidence of pneumonia.

4. **Abdomen.** Perform auscultation, percussion, inspection, and palpation. Direct special attention to the left upper quadrant for evidence of gastric distention such as tympany. Evaluate for the presence of bowel sounds (usually absent with peritonitis, increased and high-pitched with small bowel obstruction). Note any old surgical scars and palpate for tenderness that suggests peritoneal irritation (generalized with peritonitis and hemoperitoneum, or localized with other causes of an acute abdomen such as cholecystitis, appendicitis, pelvic inflammatory disease, tubo-ovarian abscesses, or ectopic pregnancy; see Problem 1, page 1). Abdominal wall herniation may be present, and a gravid uterus, large pelvic mass, or omental tumor mass may be appreciated. Costovertebral angle tenderness suggest an inflammatory process involving the diaphragm, liver, spleen, or kidney. A fluid wave is seen in ascites.

5. **Rectal examination.** Digital exam may reveal fecal impaction, pelvic mass, or rectal tenderness. Determine the presence of occult blood on a fecal sample.

6. **Inguinal examination.** Check for hernias in the groin and femoral areas as well as lymphadenopathy.

7. **Skin.** Changes consistent with alcohol abuse, such as spider angiomas or palmar erythema, may go along with ascites.

8. **Peripheral vasculature.** Look for signs of embolization that may have accompanying abdominal emboli leading to intestinal ischemia (absent pulses in the lower extremities).

9. **Pelvic examination.** Adnexal masses or tenderness may suggest pelvic malignancy or pelvic inflammatory disease.

B. Laboratory data

1. **Hemogram.** Left shift and leukocytosis may suggest an infectious process. Marked anemia indicates possible hemorrhage.

2. **Serum electrolytes.** Severe hypokalemia or hypomagnesemia may cause an ileus.
3. **Liver function tests.** Tests that can evaluate for liver disease include bilirubin, alkaline phosphatase, SGOT, and
   SGPT.
4. **Urinalysis.** White cells and positive leukocyte esterase suggest a urinary tract infection.
5. **Serum amylase.** Typically elevated with pancreatitis, it may
   also be increased with a perforated viscus (including ruptured tubal pregnancy), intestinal obstruction, or mesenteric
   ischemia.
6. **Arterial blood gases.** Acidosis may help to diagnose overwhelming sepsis such as from a ruptured tubo-ovarian abscess or ischemic intestine.
7. **Beta human chorionic gonadotropin (β-HCG).** A negative
   test excludes intrauterine or extrauterine pregnancy. An intrauterine pregnancy is usually identified at levels of 6000
   mIU.
8. **Urine and cervical cultures.** These can identify specific urinary or genital tract pathogens.
9. **Gynecologic tumor markers.** HCG, AFP, CEA, and CA-
   125 are associated with certain pelvic malignancies (see
   Chapter 2).

C. **Radiologic and other studies**
   1. **Abdominal x-rays.** Supine and upright abdominal films are
      ordered in all patients with abdominal distention and a neg-
      ative pregnancy test. (**Note:** An upright chest x-ray should
      always be included in the evaluation; see below.) A "ground
      glass" appearance is seen with ascites, air-fluid levels on the
      upright film occur with ileus, and a large gastric bubble may
      suggest postoperative gastric atony or gastric outlet obstruc-
      tion. If the cecum is markedly dilated (> 10–12 cm across),
      cecal perforation may result and emergent intervention is
      needed.
   2. **Chest x-ray.** An upright chest x-ray is often the best film to
      detect free air under the diaphragm. Free air may be normal
      in the immediate postop period following laparotomy, or else
      this may suggest a perforation. Pneumonia may also be di-
      agnosed. Pleural effusion directs attention to a subdia-
      phragmatic inflammatory process or ascites.
   3. **Barium studies.** If obstruction is suspected, these should
      not be obtained without very careful consideration. In the
      case of an intussusception, however, a barium enema may
      be curative as well as diagnostic. These are particularly haz-
      ardous in the presence of a perforation, since extrava-
      sated barium is a terrible complication ("barium peritonitis").

Water-soluble contrast media (meglumine diatrizoate [Gastrografin]) is a good alternative if there is any chance of perforation.

4. **Ultrasound, MRI, and CT scan.** These studies can help establish the diagnosis, especially if a tumor, ascites, or organomegaly is suspected. Cholelithiasis with resulting cholecystitis may be detected on ultrasound. Intrauterine and extrauterine pregnancy can usually be distinguished by 6 weeks' gestation using abdominal and transvaginal ultrasound, and as such should be a primary screening tool in patients with positive pregnancy tests.

5. **Culdocentesis.** This test can be extremely helpful if the diagnosis of ruptured ectopic pregnancy or ruptured ovarian cyst with resultant hemoperitoneum is being entertained. A positive test yields nonclotting blood.

V. Plan. Relieve the distention first, then identify and treat the underlying cause. Excessive distention of the cecum may result in perforation. Gastric distention can lead to vomiting with pulmonary aspiration, dehydration, electrolyte abnormalities, or forceful emesis, which may cause esophageal rupture. Thus, distention itself can lead to serious consequences.

A. Initial management. In most cases, keeping the patient NPO with adequate intravenous hydration is acceptable initial therapy while the workup is in progress (see Chapter 4 for fluid and electrolyte management).

B. Nasogastric intubation. When gastrointestinal obstruction is the cause or severe vomiting is present, a functioning nasogastric tube is essential. In the absence of gastric distention, a nasogastric tube may be less useful at relieving distention, but should be used empirically (see Procedure 16, page 368).

C. Fluid balance. Carefully monitor fluid intake and output, especially if a nasogastric tube is in place.

D. Specific treatment plans. The underlying cause must be clearly identified and appropriately treated. Common treatment plans include:

1. Correct any electrolyte abnormalities, especially hypokalemia and hypomagnesemia. Use IV potassium chloride and IV magnesium sulfate.

2. Review medications and dosing intervals for any agents that may slow intestinal motility, and adjust accordingly.

3. Clear fecal impaction with gentle digital extraction.

4. Benign ascites is usually managed medically (sodium re-

striction, spironolactone) with paracentesis used therapeutically if respiratory comprise is present.

5. Malignant ascites is usually managed surgically with paracentesis used preoperatively if respiratory comprise is present.

6. Postoperative ileus usually clears spontaneously unless complications such as infection intervene.

7. Urine retention responds to placement of a patent Foley catheter.

8. Operative intervention is indicated in many cases of abdominal distention including bowel ischemia, obstruction, hemoperitoneum secondary to ruptured ectopic pregnancy, ruptured ovarian cyst, surgical bleeding, ruptured tubo-ovarian abscess, and pelvic malignancy. Sometimes, a specific lesion cannot be diagnosed preoperatively and there is no other choice.

REFERENCES

Frank BW: Abdominal distension and ascites. In Friedman HH (ed): *Problem-Oriented Medical Diagnosis.* Boston, Little, Brown, 1979.

Stenchever MA: Significant symptoms and signs in different age groups. In Droegemueller W et al (eds): *Comprehensive Gynecology.* St. Louis, CV Mosby, 1987.

29. ABDOMINAL PAIN

Because abdominal pain is a frequently encountered clinical surgical on-call problem, it is given special emphasis here. Use this problem along with Problem 28, Abdominal Distention, to evaluate most cases of acute abdomen.

I. **Problem.** A 60-year-old woman presents in the emergency center with right upper quadrant tenderness and jaundice.

II. **Immediate Questions**

A. **What are the vital signs?** Fever indicates an inflammatory process. Hypotension and tachycardia may indicate shock due to sepsis or hemorrhage. Fever may be absent in the elderly and in patients receiving immunosuppressive or antipyretic medications.

B. **Where is the pain located?** This is only a general guide to the diagnosis of abdominal pain, since early in the course of the illness pain may be "shifted" away from the actual site of the pathologic process, then become generalized late in the course.

The classic example is appendicitis, in which discomfort is initially periumbilical or epigastric and later becomes localized in the right lower quadrant. If the process goes unchecked, generalized abdominal pain (peritonitis) may result. Referred pain to the groin can be seen with ureteral colic, and referred back pain with pancreatitis or a ruptured abdominal aneurysm (see Figures 1–2 and 1–3, pages 4 and 6).

C. **When did it start?** Acute, explosive pain is typical of a perforated viscus, ruptured aneurysm or abscess, or ectopic pregnancy. Pain intensifying over 1–2 hours is typical of acute cholecystitis, infarcted or torsional leiomyoma, acute pancreatitis, strangulated bowel, mesenteric thrombosis, proximal small bowel obstruction, or renal or ureteral colic. Vague pain that increases over several hours is most often seen with acute appendicitis, distal small bowel and large bowel obstructions, uncomplicated peptic ulcer disease, and various gynecologic and genitourinary conditions (see Figure 1–3, page 6).

D. **What is the quality of the pain (dull, sharp, burning, intermittent, constant, worst in life)?** Classically described patterns include "burning" (peptic ulcer disease), "searing" (ruptured aortic aneurysm), or "intermittent" (renal or ureteral colic) (see Figure 1–3). Have the patient scale the severity of the pain such as from 1 (least painful) to 10 (most painful). This gives a guide to follow the course more objectively.

E. **What makes the pain better or worse?** Pain that increases with deep inspiration is associated with diaphragmatic irritation (pleurisy, inflammatory lesions of the upper abdomen). Food often relieves the pain of peptic ulcer disease. Narcotics will relieve colic but be of little help in pain due to strangulated bowel or mesenteric thrombosis. Bending forward often relieves the pain of pancreatitis.

F. **What are the associated symptoms, if any?** Vomiting with the onset of pain is seen in peritoneal irritation or perforation of a hollow viscus and is a prominent feature of upper abdominal diseases such as Boerhaave's syndrome, acute gastritis, or pancreatitis. In distal small bowel or large bowel obstruction, nausea is usually present long before vomiting begins. **Hematemesis** suggests upper GI bleeding (ulcer disease, Mallory-Weiss syndrome). **Diarrhea**, if severe and associated with abdominal pain, suggests infectious gastroenteritis and, if bloody, may represent ischemic colitis, ulcerative colitis, Crohn's disease, or amebic dysentery. **Constipation** alternating with diarrhea may be seen with diverticular disease or irritable bowel syndrome. Although constipation is often nonspecific, **obstipation** (absence of passage of both stool and flatus) is strongly suggestive of mechanical bowel obstruction. **Hematuria** suggests a genitourinary cause such as stone or infection.

G. **What is the character of the vomitus?** (see Problem 61, page 228).

H. **When did the patient eat last?** This allows assessment of the time course of the illness and is particularly important if anesthesia is planned.

I. **What is the patient's menstrual history?** Missed or late period may suggest an ectopic pregnancy. Mittelschmerz is pain due to a ruptured ovarian follicle (see Problems 57 and 73, pages 215 and 276).

J. **What is the patient's past medical and surgical history?** Knowledge of a prior history of ulcers, gallstones, alcohol abuse, or previous operations along with a list of current medications will aid in establishing the cause. A history of blunt abdominal trauma 1–3 days prior to the onset of pain may signify subcapsular hemorrhage of the liver, spleen, or kidney.

III. **Differential Diagnosis.** Abdominal pain has intra-abdominal and extra-abdominal sources and can be associated with both medical and surgical diseases. The list is too long to reproduce in its entirety here, but some of the more frequent causes follow (also see Table 1–1, page 8).

A. **Intra-abdominal**
   1. **Hollow viscera.** Hollow viscera can perforate in the face of obstruction. Perforation represents an acute surgical emergency.
      a. **Upper abdominal.** Esophagitis, gastritis, peptic ulcer disease, cholecystitis.
      b. **Mid gut.** Small bowel obstruction or infarction. Obstruction may be due to adhesions (benign or malignant), hernias (internal or external), or volvulus.
      c. **Lower abdominal.** Inflammatory bowel disease, appendicitis, mesenteric lymphadenitis, obstruction.
      d. **Gastroenteritis, colitis.**
   2. **Solid organs**
      a. **Liver.** Hepatitis.
      b. **Pancreas.** Pancreatitis.
      c. **Spleen.** Splenic infarction.
      d. **Kidney.** Stones, pyelonephritis, abscess.
   3. **Pelvic**
      a. Pelvic inflammatory disease.
      b. Ectopic pregnancy (rupture is a surgical emergency).
      c. Degenerating fibroids.

        d. Carcinomas.

        e. Other, including fibroid torsion, cysts, endometriosis, ovarian torsion.

    4. Vascular. Vascular catastrophes are surgical emergencies.

        a. Ruptured aneurysm.

        b. Dissecting aneurysm.

        c. Mesenteric thrombosis or embolism.

        d. Splenic or hepatic rupture, usually post-traumatic.

B. Extra-abdominal. These may rarely present as referred abdominal pain. The most important to remember are sickle cell crisis, pneumonia (especially lower lobe), myocardial infarction, and rarely, diabetic ketoacidosis. These tend to be "medical" diseases, and surgery is not generally indicated.

C. Other

    1. Trauma patient. Blunt trauma may cause injuries to solid viscera (spleen, liver, kidney, pancreas) or to fixed structures such as the duodenum. Penetrating trauma may injure any intra-abdominal structure.

    2. Postoperative. Postoperative abdominal pain usually improves significantly in uncomplicated cases during the first 2–3 postoperative days. Persistent pain may indicate a problem such as obstruction or abscess formation. Uncomplicated postoperative pain is derived from both visceral fibers, due to surgical injury to peritoneal linings, and to somatic fibers innervating the abdominal wall.

    3. Critically ill patient. Patients suffering severe stress from such serious insults as multiple trauma and burns, often complicated by sepsis, may suffer from potentially life-threatening intra-abdominal events.

        a. Acute stress gastritis (usually manifested as massive upper GI bleeding).

        b. Curling's ulcer with or without perforation.

        c. A calculous cholecystitis and cholestasis from chronic use of total parenteral nutrition.

IV. Database

A. Physical examination key points (see Table 1–2, page 9)

    1. Vital signs. Writhing in agony is typical of colic, while a motionless patient is suggestive of peritoneal irritation.

    2. Heart. Look for evidence of cardiac decompensation, especially in a patient with preexisting coronary disease (distended neck veins, S3 gallop, peripheral edema), which may direct attention toward a myocardial infarction or atrial fibrillation to suggest emboli.

    3. Lungs. Listen for basilar rales or rhonchi indicating possible pneumonia. Dullness to percussion may represent pleural effusion or consolidation.

4. **Abdomen**
   a. **Inspection.** Note the presence of distention (obstruction, ileus, ascites), scaphoid (perforated ulcer), flank ecchymoses (hemorrhagic pancreatitis), caput medusae (portal hypertension), and surgical scars (adhesions, tumor).
   b. **Auscultation.** Listen for bowel sounds (absent or occasional tinkle with obstruction or ileus, hyperperistaltic with gastroenteritis, "rushes" with small bowel obstruction).
   c. **Percussion.** Tympany is associated with distended loops of bowel, dullness and a fluid wave with ascites; loss of liver dullness is associated with free air.
   d. **Palpation.** Guarding, rigidity, and rebound tenderness are hallmarks of peritonitis. Localized tenderness is often seen with cholecystitis, appendicitis, salpingitis, and diverticulitis. Costovertebral angle tenderness is common with pyelonephritis. **Murphy's sign** is inspiratory arrest while palpating the gallbladder in acute cholecystitis. Pain with active hip flexion, the **psoas sign,** can represent a retrocecal appendix or psoas abscess. The **obturator sign** (pain on internal and external rotation of the flexed thigh) can be found with a retrocecal appendix or obturator herniation. Masses may also be detected.
5. **Rectal examination.** A mass suggests a rectal carcinoma, fissures point to Crohn's disease, and unilateral tenderness is suggestive of appendicitis (usually retrocecal) or an abscess. If stool is present, evaluate for occult blood.
6. **Skin.** Look for jaundice and spider angiomas, seen with liver disease. Cool, clammy skin from peripheral vasoconstriction is an ominous sign of severe hypotension.

B. **Laboratory data**
   1. **Hemogram.** Anemia may indicate hemorrhage from an ulcer, colon cancer, leaking aneurysm, etc. Leukocytosis indicates the presence of inflammation. A low white count is more typical of viral infections such as gastroenteritis or mesenteric adenitis. Serial hematocrits should be obtained when following a patient suspected of having an ectopic pregnancy.
   2. **Serum electrolytes, BUN, creatinine.** Bowel obstruction with vomiting can cause hypokalemia or dehydration (BUN/creatinine ratio > 20 : 1).
   3. **Bilirubin, SGOT (AST), SGPT (ALT), alkaline phosphatase.** Hepatitis, cholecystitis, and other liver diseases may be diagnosed through these tests.
   4. **Amylase.** Markedly elevated levels are associated with

pancreatitis. Amylase can also be elevated with perforated ulcer and small bowel obstruction. Occasionally, a pseudocyst or hemorrhagic pancreatitis may result in a normal amylase level.

5. **Arterial blood gases.** Hypoxia is often an early sign of sepsis. Acidosis may be present with ischemic bowel.
6. **Pregnancy test.** All premenopausal women should be tested to rule out ectopic pregnancy, whether they use birth control or not. A urine or serum pregnancy test should be obtained.
7. **Urinalysis.** Hematuria may indicate nephrolithiasis; pyuria and hematuria can be present in urinary tract infections or rarely in appendicitis.
8. **Cervical culture.** Send a specimen specifically for gonorrhea, chlamydia, and aerobic and anaerobic cultures if pelvic inflammatory disease is suspected.

C. Radiologic and other studies
1. **Flat and upright abdominal films.** If the patient is debilitated, a lateral decubitus view may be substituted for the upright film. Observe for the following key elements: gas pattern, bowel dilatation, air-fluid levels, presence of air in the rectum, pancreatic calcifications, loss of psoas margin, displacement of hollow viscera, gall and renal stones, portal vein air, and aortic calcifications.
2. **Chest film.** X-ray may reveal pneumonia, widened mediastinum (dissecting aneurysm), or pleural effusion or elevation of a hemidiaphragm (subdiaphragmatic inflammatory process). Free air under the diaphragm suggests a perforation and is most often seen on the upright chest film.
3. **Ultrasound.** Echo may reveal gallstones, ectopic pregnancy, pelvic mass, or other abnormalities.
4. **Electrocardiogram.** The ECG may rule out myocardial infarction as the cause of upper abdominal distress and nausea.
5. **Other tests as clinically indicated**
   a. Intravenous pyelogram.
   b. Abdominal CT scan or magnetic resonance imaging.
   c. Biliary scintigraphy.
   d. Contrast bowel studies: upper GI swallow and enemas (barium, dilute barium, Gastrografin).
   e. Endoscopic studies: esophagogastroduodenoscopy (EGD), colonoscopy, endoscopic retrograde cholangiopancreatography (ERCP).
   f. Arteriography.
   g. Peritoneal lavage or paracentesis (see Procedure 24, page 385) or culdocentesis (Procedure 9, page 357).

V. Plan. Abdominal pain can present a diagnostic dilemma, in any patient but even more so in patients at the extremes of age or in those unable to communicate. The surgeon's goal is to determine if abdominal pain requires surgical treatment in order to prevent further morbidity. In rough terms, pain present 6 or more hours that does not improve is likely to have a cause requiring surgical intervention. Many cases of abdominal pain have no definite diagnosis before laparotomy. A brief period of observation may ultimately point to the cause, but operation is safer in most cases. The use of analgesics remains controversial, but most clinicians now believe moderate doses of pain medicine will not mask symptoms while making the patient much more comfortable. Specific types of therapy and operations for each possible diagnosis cannot be described here but can be found in surgical and medical textbooks. It is essential to recognize that certain conditions are life-threatening and usually require urgent operation (see Table 1–1, page 8).

A. Observation. With the exception of catastrophes that require urgent surgical exploration (see Table 1–1), most cases of abdominal pain require close observation, medical management, and occasionally analgesics. In the case of postoperative abdominal pain, analgesics are used most frequently.

1. Keep the patient NPO and consider nasogastric suction, especially if vomiting is present.
2. Begin intravenous hydration (see Chapter 4) with careful attention to intake and output.
3. Parenteral analgesics are used carefully to avoid masking pathologic processes.
4. Serial physical examinations by the same examiner will be very useful in determining progression of symptoms and securing the diagnosis.
5. Patients suspected of having pelvic inflammatory disease should be treated with cefoxitin 2.0 g IV q6h and doxycycline 100 mg IV q12h. Alternative therapy includes clindamycin 900 mg IV q8h and gentamicin (2.0 mg/kg IV loading dose, then 1.5 mg/kg IV q8h). If the patient is to be discharged, give ceftriaxone 250 mg IM (single dose) and doxycycline 100 mg PO bid for 14 days. Alternative therapy includes cefoxitin 2 g IM and probenecid 1 g PO concurrently with doxycycline as above. If the patient is pregnant or allergic to tetracycline, use erythromycin 500 mg qid for 7 days.

B. Surgery. Vascular catastrophes, perforated viscus, most causes of bowel obstruction, many splenic and hepatic injuries, ruptured ectopic pregnancies, and appendicitis all require emergency operation. Indications for urgent operation without a precise preoperative diagnosis are outlined in Table 1–11.

TABLE 1–11. INDICATIONS FOR URGENT OPERATION IN PATIENTS WITH ACUTE ABDOMEN.

Physical findings
  Involuntary guarding or rigidity, especially if spreading
  Increasing or severe localized tenderness
  Tense or progressive distention
  Tender abdominal or rectal mass with high fever or hypotension
  Rectal bleeding with shock or acidosis
  Equivocal abdominal findings along with—
    Septicemia (high fever, marked or rising leukocytosis, mental changes, or increasing
      glucose intolerance in a diabetic patient)
    Bleeding (unexplained shock or acidosis, falling hematocrit)
    Suspected ischemia (acidosis, fever, tachycardia)
    Deterioration on conservative treatment

Radiologic findings
  Pneumoperitoneum
  Gross or progressive bowel distention
  Free extravasation of contrast material
  Space-occupying lesion on scan, with fever
  Mesenteric occlusion or angiography

Endoscopic findings
  Perforated or uncontrollably bleeding lesion

Paracentesis findings
  Blood, bile, pus, bowel contents, or urine

From Way LW (ed): Current Surgical Diagnosis and Treatment, *8th ed. Norwalk, Connecticut, Appleton & Lange, 1988.*

REFERENCES

Boey JH: Acute abdomen. In Way L (ed): *Current Surgical Diagnosis and Treatment.* Norwalk, CT, Appleton & Lange, 1988.

Droegemueller W et al (eds): *Comprehensive Gynecology.* St. Louis, CV Mosby, 1987.

Sanford JP: *Guide to Antimicrobial Therapy 1991.* West Bethesda, MD, Antimicrobial Therapy Inc, 1991.

Silen W: *Cope's Early Diagnosis of the Acute Abdomen.* New York, Oxford University Press, 1984.

Stenchever MA: Significant symptoms and signs in different age groups. In Droegemueller W et al (eds): *Comprehensive Gynecology.* St. Louis, CV Mosby, 1987, pp 148–167.

30. ACIDOSIS

I. Problem. A patient with sepsis and accompanying adult respiratory distress syndrome (ARDS) requires intubation and mechanical ventilation. The initial arterial blood gas following intubation reveals a pH of 7.14.

II. Immediate Questions

A. Is the acidosis respiratory, metabolic, or a combination of both? Often the blood gas report will give the calculated base excess/deficit at the end (eg, $PO_2/PCO_2/pH$/bicarbonate/base excess). If the base excess is negative (or a positive deficit), the acidosis is at least partially metabolic. If the base excess is not reported with the blood gas results, the differentiation between metabolic and respiratory can still be quickly made. If PCO_2 is > 40, the acidosis is at least partially respiratory. For every 10 mm Hg that PCO_2 is > 40, the pH will be lowered by 0.08 in normal circumstances. For example, if the PCO_2 is 60, one would expect an acidosis of 7.24; any additional acidosis can be attributed to metabolic causes.

B. What is the patient's volume status? A common cause of metabolic acidosis in the acute setting is lactic acidosis due to poor tissue perfusion. Examine the patient and look at the recent urine output and cardiac filling pressures, if available, to gauge the patient's intravascular volume. Volume contraction, usually diuretic induced, is often associated with alkalosis.

C. Is there any problem with the ventilator circuitry? In a non-intubated patient with respiratory acidosis, there is usually apparent difficulty with breathing. In a patient on a ventilator, respiratory acidosis may not be clinically apparent if the patient is sedated or obtunded. Check the ventilator circuitry, the exhaled volume, and the ventilator settings to make certain there is no technical explanation for the acidosis. Verify the position of the endotracheal tube on chest x-ray, since it can slip distally into the right mainstem bronchus.

D. Are there arrhythmias or ectopy? With a profound acidosis of any cause, there may be disturbances of the cardiac rhythm or ventricular ectopy. Obtain an ECG and monitor the patient.

III. Differential Diagnosis.

As explained above, the most important initial distinction in diagnosing the cause of acidosis is between respiratory and metabolic mechanisms. In the acutely ill surgical patient, both causes may be present as in the patient in this example.

A. Respiratory acidosis. By definition, this is alveolar hypoventilation.

1. Pulmonary conditions
   a. Asthma. An asthmatic patient who has progressed to respiratory acidosis has very severe disease and usually requires prompt intubation.
   b. Mechanical upper airway obstruction. A foreign body or laryngospasm may be the cause.

  c. **Space-occupying lesions.** Pneumothorax, pleural effusion, or hemothorax may result in respiratory compromise.
  d. **Severe pulmonary edema.** Edema may occur with, eg, congestive heart failure.
  e. **Pneumonia.** This is usually associated with baseline respiratory compromise such as chronic obstructive pulmonary disease.
 2. **Drugs/toxins**
  a. **Alcohol ingestion.**
  b. **Narcotics/sedative overdose.**
  c. **Neuromuscular blocking agents,** eg, curare.
 3. **Neuromuscular conditions**
  a. **Myasthenia gravis.**
  b. **Pickwickian syndrome.**
  c. **Cerebrovascular accident.**
  d. **Guillain-Barré syndrome.**
B. **Metabolic acidosis.** This can be subdivided into conditions with a normal anion gap and those with an increased anion gap implying an elevated unmeasured anion. The anion gap is calculated by $[Na] - ([Cl] + [HCO_3])$. The normal range is 8–12 meq/L.
 1. **Normal anion gap**
  a. **Loss of bicarbonate.** Usually the loss is from the GI tract as diarrhea, small bowel fistula, pancreatic-cutaneous fistula, or a large amount of external biliary drainage.
  b. **Renal tubular acidosis.**
 2. **Elevated anion gap**
  a. **Lactic acidosis.** Poor perfusion leads to interference with normal oxidative metabolism.
  b. **Diabetic ketoacidosis.**
  c. **Alcoholic ketoacidosis.**
  d. **Chronic renal insufficiency.** Elevated unmeasured anions include sulfates and phosphates.
  e. **Drugs or poisoning.** Overdosage of aspirin or ingestion of methyl alcohol, ethylene glycol, or paraldehyde can all be factors.

IV. **Database**

 A. **Physical examination key points**
  1. **Vital signs.** Look for evidence of hypoventilation, hypotension, tachycardia, or fever. Sepsis can produce shock, a common cause of acidosis.
  2. **Lungs.** Evaluate for absent or decreased breath sounds, stridor in upper airway obstruction, wheezes, rales.

3. **Abdomen.** Peritoneal signs indicate an acute abdomen Marked distention may inhibit respiration.
4. **Skin.** Look for cool, clammy, mottled skin on the extremities as in shock with clamped-down peripheral perfusion.
5. **HEENT.** Ketosis or fruity odor on the breath suggests diabetic ketoacidosis. Look for tracheal shift from a space-occupying lesion or venous distention (congestive heart failure or tension pneumothorax).
6. **Neuromuscular examination.** Generalized weakness or focal neurologic signs, depressed level of consciousness, obtundation, or coma should be noted.

B. **Laboratory data**
1. **Hemogram.** Leukocytosis is seen with sepsis, and anemia is common with chronic renal insufficiency.
2. **Electrolytes, BUN, and creatinine.** An elevated serum chloride is found in non-anion-gap metabolic acidosis. Calculate the anion gap from the electrolytes. Renal insufficiency may be present.
3. **Arterial blood gases.** Repeat these determinations to follow therapeutic interventions.
4. **Blood glucose, ketones.** Elevations are associated with diabetic ketoacidosis.
5. **Lactate.** Elevated levels occur with sepsis and poor perfusion.

C. **Radiologic and other studies**
1. **Chest x-rays.** Chest films are used to evaluate for infiltrates, pulmonary edema, effusions, and endotracheal tube position (ideal position is approximately 2 cm above the carina).
2. **Electrocardiogram with rhythm strip.** Obtain an ECG to evaluate for arrhythmias.
3. **Electromyography.** This and other specialized neurology tests may be needed to diagnose primary neurologic conditions.

V. **Plan.** In general, for both respiratory and metabolic acidosis, treatment of the underlying cause is the primary goal. In emergent situations the two methods to reverse the acidosis acutely are to administer sodium bicarbonate intravenously and to hyperventilate the patient. Be sure to check serial pH values to monitor the progress of therapy.

A. **Metabolic acidosis**
1. **Bicarbonate therapy.** In general, administer IV bicarbonate if pH is < 7.20.
   a. Calculate the total body bicarbonate need by: patient's

weight (in kg) $\times 0.40 \times (24 - [HCO_3]) =$ total meq of HCO_3 needed.

    b. Give 50% of this amount over the first 12 hours as a mixture of bicarbonate with D_5W.

    c. Complications of bicarbonate therapy include:

        (1) Hypernatremia.

        (2) Volume overload.

        (3) Hypokalemia, caused by intracellular shifts of potassium as the pH increases.

  2. Treat underlying causes

    a. Volume resuscitate in sepsis, hemorrhagic shock, and other causes of lactic acidosis.

    b. Give insulin and saline for diabetic ketoacidosis (page 40).

    c. Perform dialysis as needed for renal failure.

 B. Respiratory acidosis. The main goal is to treat the underlying cause.

    1. If necessary, intubate the patient and treat with mechanical ventilation. If a patient is already intubated and has a significant respiratory acidosis, then increase alveolar ventilation by either raising the tidal volume (up to 10–15 mL/kg) while following peak inspiratory pressures, or increase the respiratory rate.

    2. In an emergent situation, disconnect the patient from the ventilator and hyperventilate by hand. The importance of good pulmonary toilet, ie, suctioning of secretions, cannot be overemphasized. Sedation is often a necessary adjunct to mechanical ventilation (see Chapter 6).

REFERENCES

Davenport H: *The ABC of Acid-Base Chemistry,* 6th ed. Chicago, University of Chicago Press, 1974.

Haist SA, Robbins JB, Gomella LG (eds): *Internal Medicine On Call.* Norwalk, Connecticut, Appleton & Lange, 1991.

31. ALKALOSIS

 I. Problem. One day after anterior exenteration for a recurrent cervical carcinoma, a 47-year-old woman in the ICU is on a ventilator and has a pH of 7.56.

 II. Immediate Questions

    A. What are the patient's respiratory rate and tidal volume on the ventilator? Alkalosis may be due to overventilation. The minute ventilation is what is important. Thus, rate (intermittent mandatory ventilation or assist control) as well as volume for each delivered breath (tidal volume) are important. The tidal volume should be set at 10–15 cc/kg. Minute ventilation = rate × tidal volume, so a change in either parameter will affect the minute ventilation.

B. What medications is the patient taking? Thiazide diuretics can result in a "contraction" alkalosis, and excess bicarbonate and bicarbonate precursors (such as acetate in hyperalimentation solutions) can cause a metabolic alkalosis.

C. What is the composition of IV fluids? Be sure there is no added bicarbonate (avoid Ringer's lactate) and make sure the patient is receiving sufficient chloride (80–100 meq/d as NaCl, plus losses).

D. Is an NG tube in place, or is there vomiting? Nasogastric tube drainage of HCl from the GI tract is a common cause of hypochloremic alkalosis in surgical patients.

III. Differential Diagnosis. The key differential point here is similar to that for the acidoses, that is, to determine whether the origin is metabolic or respiratory.

A. Metabolic alkalosis. This is usually seen as an elevated serum bicarbonate. The compensation is usually by hypoventilation and increased renal excretion of bicarbonate. It is diagnosed by an increased pH with normal or increased arterial PCO_2.
  1. Loss of HCl (chloride responsive)
    a. Nasogastric suction, vomiting.
    b. Villous adenoma (potassium wasting).
    c. Diuretics (especially thiazides).
    d. Posthypercapnia.
  2. Chloride resistant
    a. Bicarbonate administration (oral and parenteral).
    b. Chronic hypokalemia.
    c. Primary hyperaldosteronism.
    d. Cushing's syndrome, exogenous steroids.

B. Respiratory alkalosis. Hyperventilation results in a decreased PCO_2. The compensatory mechanism is through increased renal bicarbonate excretion.
  1. Anxiety.
  2. Hypermetabolic states (fever, early sepsis).
  3. Iatrogenic. Ventilator rate is set for too many breaths, or tidal volume is too high.
  4. Pregnancy.
  5. Cirrhosis.
  6. Cardiac disease (see Problem 36, page 141).

7. **Pulmonary disease** (see Problem 39, page 153).
8. **Brainstem lesion** (see Problem 58, page 219).
9. **Salicylate intoxication** (early, with metabolic acidosis later).

IV. Database

A. Physical examination key points

1. **Vital signs.** Pay particular attention to the respiratory rate. Tachypnea may signify a respiratory cause.
2. **Lungs.** Check for signs of pulmonary edema (rales).
3. **Skin.** Look for changes associated with alcohol abuse such as palmar erythema, spider angiomas, etc.

B. Laboratory data

1. **Serum electrolytes,** with particular attention to hypokalemia that may accompany alkalosis.
2. **Arterial blood gases,** as noted above.
3. **Serum salicylate levels,** if aspirin intoxication is suspected.
4. **Spot urine electrolytes for chloride.** This is most helpful in the diagnosis and treatment of metabolic alkalosis. If the **urine chloride is < 10 meq/L,** this represents a "chloride-responsive" alkalosis (caused by diuretics, GI tract losses, others) that can often be corrected by administration of chloride-containing IV fluids. A **urine chloride > 10 meq/L** represents a "chloride-resistant" alkalosis (caused by adrenal diseases, exogenous steroid use) and usually cannot be corrected by chloride infusion.

V. Plan. It is essential to identify the cause of alkalosis and treat it.

A. **Discontinue all exogenous bicarbonate.** Bicarbonate precursors such as the acetate salts (amino acids) found in hyperalimentation solutions should also be evaluated. If hyperalimentation is essential, attempt to increase the chloride salts in the solution; the amino acid content may need to be reduced.

B. **Begin IV replacement.** For alkalosis due to loss of HCl, give NaCl as normal saline IV. For alkalosis that is chloride resistant, give KCl IV.

C. **Give sedation.** Sedate with agents such as diazepam to decrease anxiety that may be causing respiratory alkalosis.

D. **Increase FiCO$_2$.** Use a rebreathing mask for respiratory alkalosis in the nonintubated patient, or decrease the minute ventilation by reducing the rate or tidal volume. Be sure the tidal volume is set for 10–15 cc/kg.

   E. Treat hypokalemia. Use KCl supplementation.

   F. Replace volume losses. Replace fluid volume lost through the nasogastric tube, usually using D5½NS with 20 meq KCl/L.

REFERENCE

Shapiro BA, Harrison RA, Walter JR: *Clinical Application of Blood Gases,* 4th ed. Chicago, Year Book, 1990.

32. ANAPHYLACTIC REACTION

I. Problem. A postoperative patient has developed severe dyspnea and a generalized rash after receiving intravenous penicillin.

II. Immediate Questions. The respiratory distress and hypotension can be life threatening and the patient should be seen immediately.

   A. What are the patient's vital signs? Tachycardia is a common finding and could represent the response to hypoxia, fear, hypotension, and arrhythmia. Hypotension requires immediate treatment in this setting.

   B. Can the patient communicate appropriately? Appropriate answers to simple questions indicate that cerebral oxygenation is adequate for the time being. Inability to speak points to severe respiratory deterioration or to upper airway obstruction from laryngospasm or laryngeal edema.

   C. What medication did the patient receive? Many medications can cause anaphylaxis, but the most common in this setting are penicillin, other beta-lactam antibiotics (cephalosporins), and intravenous contrast materials. Aspirin and other nonsteroidal anti-inflammatory agents may cause reactions in sensitive patients. Transfusion reactions are discussed in Problem 71 (page 270). Insect stings are another cause and are managed essentially the same way.

III. Differential Diagnosis. Anaphylaxis technically refers to the signs and symptoms caused by an antigen-mediated release of IgE-induced mediators. It can be localized (as in allergic rhinitis) or systemic and life threatening.

   A. Acute allergic reaction (anaphylaxis). In the hospital setting, anaphylaxis is most often caused by the medications noted in II-C above. Less frequently, it may be caused by food, environmental agents (dust, pollen), or insects.

   B. Upper airway obstruction. This may result from laryngeal edema caused by a foreign body and classically presents as stridor.

   C. Acute asthma attack. Wheezing with a prior history of asthma is usually present.

   D. Pulmonary embolus. Especially in the postoperative setting, this must be thought of in the patient acutely short of breath.

   E. Other. Additional causes for this constellation of symptoms are discussed in other sections: dyspnea (Problem 39, page 153), hypotension (Problem 54, page 199), pruritus and wheezing (Problem 75, page 284).

IV. Database. Knowledge of the patient's allergies and current medications is essential. The relationship of medication administration to onset of symptoms is also important, since anaphylaxis usually occurs several minutes into administration of the medication.

   A. Physical examination key points

      1. Vital signs. Hypotension must be recognized early.

      2. Lungs. Listen for sneezing (suggests bronchospasm), stridor (suggests laryngospasm), and adequacy of air movement.

      3. Skin. Generalized rash, urticaria, and pruritus often accompany an acute anaphylactic reaction.

      4. Extremities. Look for evidence of cyanosis.

      5. Mental status. Somnolence in this setting demands immediate respiratory support and is frequently indicative of severe hypercapnia.

   B. Laboratory data

      1. Arterial blood gases. Determine the level of hypoxia or hypercapnia, but usually the problem must be treated before results are available.

   C. Radiologic and other studies

      1. Chest x-ray. When time permits, a chest x-ray will rule out other causes of respiratory distress (congestive heart failure, pneumonia, etc).

      2. Electrocardiogram. Acute myocardial infarction can present as pulmonary edema with severe dyspnea. Right ventricular strain can be seen in pulmonary embolus. Myocardial infarction may result from severe hypotension in anaphylaxis.

V. Plan. Treatment should be initiated quickly based on clinical findings and before performing other studies and lab exams. Be prepared to initiate cardiopulmonary resuscitation (CPR).

A. **Oxygen.** Oxygen by face mask should be instituted for moderate to severe dyspnea. Intubation may be required if the patient is severely somnolent or unable to manage secretions, or if arterial blood gases reveal elevated PCO_2 or a low PO_2.

B. **Epinephrine.** Epinephrine 0.3–0.5 mL of 1 : 1000 solution SQ should be given immediately for laryngospasm, with dramatic improvement often seen. The epinephrine used for CPR is a 1 : 10, 000 solution given IV and should **not** be used in this situation. Use epinephrine with caution in patients over 40 years of age.

C. **Diphenhydramine (Benadryl).** Benadryl 25–50 mg IM should follow epinephrine to reduce the effects of histamine release, although its usefulness is primarily for lesser degrees of anaphylaxis such as mild urticaria. It may be given intravenously in patients with a moderate reaction, or in the elderly, in whom epinephrine should be used with caution if at all. This is an excellent drug for use during pregnancy with minimal side effects to patient and fetus.

D. **High-dose glucocorticoids.** Hydrocortisone 100 mg IV may be needed if the patient fails to respond to epinephrine and diphenhydramine.

E. **Blood pressure.** Normally the pressure responds to correction with epinephrine and diphenhydramine, but normal saline with volume repletion and occasionally pressors (dopamine) may be needed to support pressure.

F. **Monitoring.** Resolution of the respiratory distress associated with anaphylaxis is usually so dramatic that ICU monitoring after the episode is often unnecessary. Clinical judgment is needed, however. Exceptions would be the elderly or severely ill, patients with arrhythmias, or patients who appeared near to respiratory arrest prior to treatment.

REFERENCE

Wasserman SI: Anaphylaxis. In Middleton E, Reed CE, Ellis EF (eds): *Allergy: Principles and Practice,* 2nd ed. St. Louis, CV Mosby, 1983.

33. BRADYCARDIA

I. **Problem.** A patient who has undergone total vaginal hysterectomy is found to have a heart rate of 42 on a routine postoperative vital signs check.

II. **Immediate Questions**

A. **What is the patient's blood pressure, and is she alert and** oriented? The initial answers define the severity of the problem. Since the clinical relevance of a significant bradycardia is reduced perfusion pressure, the adequacy of perfusion—both blood pressure and mental status—should be rapidly assessed.

B. **What is the patient's normal resting heart rate?** The range of normal heart rates is wide, and a rate of 42 in a resting patient may not be abnormal in some people such as highly conditioned athletes.

C. **Are there any associated symptoms of chest pain or pressure, dyspnea, diaphoresis, or nausea?** A new bradyarrhythmia may be a manifestation of an acute cardiac event such as an inferior myocardial infarction. Question the patient about any concurrent symptoms.

D. **Has the patient felt dizzy or lightheaded in the recent past?** The clinical presentation of sinus node dysfunction is frequently episodic syncope or near-syncope.

E. **What medications is the patient taking, and does she have a pacemaker?** Certain medications such as beta blockers (propranolol, etc) can lead to bradycardia. A patient with a pacemaker may be suffering from pacer malfunction.

F. **Does the patient have a history of cardiovascular disease?** This may further clarify the nature of the slow heart rate.

III. **Differential Diagnosis.** Disturbances in the cardiac conduction pathway leading to bradyarrhythmias are due to dysfunction at the level of the sinus node or the atrioventricular (AV) node/Purkinje system. Within these two categories a variety of conditions exist, defined by characteristic ECG patterns and associated with particular clinical conditions.

A. **Sinus node disease**
   1. **Sinus bradycardia**
      a. **Vasovagal syncope.**
      b. **High vagal tone.** This is more common in conditioned athletes and in the elderly.
      c. **Increased intracranial pressure.** Cushing's reflex results in bradycardia.
   2. **Sinus node dysfunction.** Sick sinus syndrome and tachycardia-bradycardia syndrome are variants of sinus node disease characterized by intermittent sinus pauses.
      a. **Ischemic cardiomyopathy.**
      b. **Hypertensive cardiomyopathy.**
      c. **Hypothyroidism.**
      d. **Hypothermia.**
      e. **Infiltrative diseases** (amyloidosis, etc).

B. Atrioventricular node disease
1. **First-degree AV block.** This is defined as a PR interval > 0.2 sec.
2. **Second-degree AV block,** Mobitz type I (Wenckebach). The PR interval is successively prolonged with eventual dropped ventricular beat.
   a. **Inferior myocardial infarction.**
   b. **Drug toxicity.** Frequently implicated are digoxin, beta blockers (propranolol), and calcium channel blockers (verapamil).
3. **Second-degree AV block,** Mobitz type II. This is characterized by intermittent missed ventricular beats. Associated conditions are the same as for third-degree AV block, and the condition may progress to third-degree block.
4. **Third-degree AV block** (also called AV dissociation).
   a. **Myocardial infarction.** The most common sites are anteroseptal or inferior.
   b. **Primary degenerative disease of the conducting system.**
   c. **Infiltrative conditions** (sarcoidosis, amyloidosis, neoplasms).
   d. **Infectious disease** (viral myocarditis, acute rheumatic fever, Lyme disease).

IV. **Database.** The primary means to diagnose a bradycardia is the 12-lead ECG and rhythm strip, which should be obtained concurrent with the initial history and physical exam.

A. Physical examination key points
1. **Vital signs.** Note the heart rate, blood pressure, and respiratory rate. Hypotension < 90 mm Hg requires emergent treatment.
2. **Heart.** Note any new murmurs or gallops. Notice if the rhythm is regular or irregular.
3. **Lungs.** Listen for evidence of failure (rales).
4. **Skin.** Pallor or cool, moist skin is evidence of poor perfusion or increased vagal tone.
5. **Neurologic examination.** Look for evidence of elevated intracranial pressure (papilledema). Decreased mental status is a measure of inadequate perfusion pressure.

B. Laboratory data
1. **Electrolytes, calcium.** Hypokalemia can potentiate digoxin toxicity, and hypocalcemia can result in a prolonged QT interval and bradycardia.
2. **CPK with isoenzymes** to evaluate myocardial injury (see Chapter 2, page 305).

3. **Digoxin level,** if indicated. Toxicity is often manifest as bradycardia. Toxic levels are usually > 2.5 ng/mL.
4. **Thyroid hormone levels.** Hypothyroidism can cause bradycardia.
5. **Arterial blood gases,** if indicated by respiratory distress or dyspnea.

C. Radiologic and other studies

1. **Electrocardiogram.** The ECG should be analyzed systematically looking for atrial rate (lead II is good), ventricular rate, PR interval, relation of P waves to QRS complexes, and evidence of ischemia (inverted T waves, ST segment depression).
2. **Chest x-ray.** Changes in the cardiac silhouette and lung fields may be associated with myocardial dysfunction.
3. **Specialized tests.** Tests conducted by cardiologists include electrophysiologic mapping to define the precise location of blocks, and complete autonomic blockade (using atropine and propranolol) to determine the intrinsic heart rate and document the contribution of vagal tone to the bradycardia.

V. Plan. The treatment plan will be dictated by the type and degree of bradycardia and any underlying clinical condition. Remember that not all bradycardia is clinically significant. Use extreme caution, especially in the elderly, when treating bradycardia. In urgent situations treat with atropine IV, give oxygen, and obtain an ECG as soon as possible.

A. Drug therapy should be used in cases of acute, clinically significant bradycardia usually associated with hypotension.

1. **Atropine.** 0.5–1.0 mg IV (0.01 mg/kg); may be repeated q5–10 min to a total dose of 2 mg.
2. **Isoproterenol** (Isuprel). 1–3 µg/min IV as continuous infusion if no response to atropine. Titrate up to 10 µg/min as needed.

B. Treat the underlying condition

1. **Myocardial ischemia.** Treat with nitrates (such as sublingual nitroglycerin) and oxygen.
2. **Increased intracranial pressure.** Maneuvers to decrease pressure include mannitol diuresis, elevating the head of the bed, and intubation and mechanical hyperventilation.

C. Pacemaker therapy. If the bradyarrhythmia does not respond to medical therapy, or in certain critical situations listed below, then a temporary ventricular pacer wire should be passed to treat the bradycardia. If this option is needed, contact the cardiology consultant.

1. **Indications for temporary pacemaker.**
   a. Transient second-degree AV block with an inferior myocardial infarction.
   b. AV block due to drug toxicity.
   c. As temporizing measure prior to permanent pacemaker.
2. **Indications for permanent pacemaker.**
   a. Sinus node dysfunction: must be documented to be symptomatic.
   b. Second- or third-degree AV block associated with an acute myocardial infarction.
   c. Symptomatic Mobitz type II and third-degree AV block.

D. **Digoxin toxicity.** Check the level, hold medication, and consider digoxin antibody (Digibind) 60 mg per 1 mg digoxin IV.

REFERENCE

Zipes DP: Management of cardiac arrhythmias: pharmacological, electrical, and surgical techniques. In Braunwald E (ed): *Heart Disease: A Textbook of Cardiovascular Medicine,* 3rd ed. Philadelphia, WB Saunders, 1991.

34. BRIGHT RED BLOOD PER RECTUM (HEMATOCHEZIA)

I. **Problem.** You are called to see a 60-year-old woman who is passing red blood per rectum 3 days after undergoing wide local excision of the vulva.

II. **Immediate Questions**

A. **What are the vital signs?** Look for signs of hemodynamically significant blood loss such as tachycardia or hypotension. The initial management focuses on maintaining intravascular volume and perfusion pressure. Orthostasis is the best on-the-ward estimate of volume loss.

B. **What volume of blood has been passed, and over what time period?** The volume of blood may help to assess the significance of the bleed, since the hematocrit may not decrease until later.

C. **What was the most recent hematocrit?** A baseline value is needed to assess the amount of bleeding.

D. **What is the nature of the stool?** Coating of the stool often indicates an anal process such as hemorrhoids but may also be due to a lower GI malignancy. Bright red blood is more likely to be from the distal left colon. Melena usually signifies bleeding proximal to the right colon.

E. **What medications is the patient taking, and is there any his-**

tory of alcohol abuse? Alcoholism may suggest varices; ulcerogenic medications include aspirin and other nonsteroidal anti-inflammatory agents; excessive anticoagulation or heparinization may cause GI tract bleeding.

F. Has the patient had recent GI tract surgery? It is not unusual to have some bloody bowel movements immediately after GI tract surgery.

G. Are there any associated symptoms? Crampy abdominal pain suggests infection, inflammatory bowel disease, or diverticulitis. A change in bowel habits or decreased caliber of stools may indicate a neoplasm, whereas polyps and angiodysplasia are usually free of other symptoms.

III. Differential Diagnosis

A. Diverticular disease. Diverticula represent a common cause (up to 70%) of massive lower GI bleeding, usually from the left side.

B. Angiodysplasia. These are usually right-sided lesions and thus most often associated with melena. The natural history of bleeding from angiodysplasia generally includes rebleeding, which is usually venous or capillary as contrasted with the arterial bleeding associated with diverticula.

C. Polyps. Villous adenomas can also cause potassium loss.

D. Carcinoma. Usually bleeding represents adenocarcinoma of the large intestine, but cervical, ovarian, endometrial, vulvar, vaginal, and fallopian tube carcinoma can invade the colon.

E. Inflammatory bowel disease. Bloody diarrhea is more frequently associated with ulcerative colitis than with Crohn's disease.

F. Hemorrhoids. While their presence is not unusual, this does not preclude the presence of simultaneous malignancy or angiodysplasia.

G. Mesenteric thrombosis. This may lead to ischemic bowel.

H. Meckel's diverticulitis.

I. Anal fissures.

J. Excessive anticoagulation. Be sure to review all medications the patient is taking. Check clotting studies as needed.

K. Massive upper GI bleed. Hemorrhage results in rapid intestinal transit and resulting hematemesis (see Problem 43, page 168). Blood is an excellent cathartic. Remember that lower GI bleeding can originate anywhere in the GI tract.

L. Factitious bleeding. Bleeding from other sites, such as the cervix or postoperative incisions (eg, vulva), may be confused with rectal bleeding.

M. Area of surgical excision. The surgical field may have an active bleeder or hematoma that can present as hematochezia.

IV. Database

A. Physical examination key points

1. **Vital signs.** Look for evidence of hypovolemia (tachycardia and hypotension). Fever may represent inflammatory bowel disease or infectious gastroenteritis.

2. **Abdomen.** Palpate for masses or tenderness. A left lower quadrant mass may be associated with diverticulitis, and a right lower quadrant mass with Crohn's disease. Bowel sounds may be hyperactive since blood is a cathartic.

3. **Vulva.** Examine a vulvectomy site for possible pararectal bleeding or fistula.

4. **Rectum.** Hemorrhoids, fissures, or masses may be detected.

B. Laboratory data

1. **Hemogram.** Serial hematocrit checks are helpful since a massive bleed may not reflect itself in a change in hematocrit for some time. Microcytic/hypochromic indices are indicative of chronic blood loss.

2. **Clotting studies.** Prothrombin time, partial thromboplastin time, and platelet count may reveal a coagulation disorder. Bleeding time may reflect platelet dysfunction from aspirin or a nonsteroidal anti-inflammatory agent.

3. **Blood bank.** Obtain a type and cross-match.

4. **Stool cultures.** *Salmonella, Shigella, Clostridium difficile,* and *Campylobacter* can cause bloody diarrhea.

C. Radiologic and other studies

1. **Nasogastric tube.** Pass a nasogastric tube to rule out upper GI bleeding.

2. **Angiography.** This is indicated for the diagnosis of lower GI bleeding in any patient who requires more than 2 units of blood to maintain the hematocrit or who becomes hypotensive. Remember that angiography is impossible with barium in the gut. For it to be helpful, bleeding must usually be > 0.5–1.0 mL/min. Selective embolization or vasopressin infusion may be possible to control bleeding.

3. **Radiolabeled red cell study** (usually $^{99m}T_c$). This can sometimes localize lesions in the GI tract, especially with

slower rates of bleeding than needed for angiography (0.2 mL/min).

4. **Sigmoidoscopy.** This study will detect a low-lying source of bleeding. Colonoscopy is occasionally used and may allow fulguration from bleeding sites such as angiodysplasia.

5. **Upper GI endoscopy** (esophagogastroduodenoscopy [EDG]). While a nasogastric tube can usually rule out upper GI sources of bleeding, an inconclusive workup for lower GI bleeding necessitates a definitive look at the upper GI tract.

V. Plan. Approximately 80% of all patients with lower GI bleeding stop bleeding spontaneously. Acute, severe hemorrhage is potentially life threatening and should be treated first.

A. Acute intervention. Large-bore IVs (16 gauge) should be placed for repletion of volume. Use crystalloid unless there is a low hematocrit, in which case blood is preferred. Attempt to keep hematocrit around 30%. A Foley catheter will allow more accurate assessment of volume status. Consider a CVP line if there is any instability, and in the elderly patient. Correct coagulopathy with platelets or fresh-frozen plasma.

B. Diagnosis and treatment. A suggested algorithm for the diagnosis and treatment of acute lower GI bleeding is outlined in Figure 1–6.

1. Treatment is directed at the cause. If a bleeding diverticulum is found, initial therapy is intra-arterial infusion of vasopressin rather than resection.

2. The combined approach of angiography and colonoscopy can usually localize the bleeding site. For extreme cases in which the site cannot be identified, subtotal colectomy is usually indicated.

3. Surgery may eventually be needed to treat lesions such as gynecologic malignancies, adenocarcinomas, (colon) polyps, hemorrhoids, and the lesions of inflammatory bowel disease.

4. Local care for hemorrhoids includes sitz baths, stool softeners (Doss), and suppositories (Anusol, etc).

5. Infectious diarrhea from *C. difficile* is treated with oral Flagyl or vancomycin.

6. Radiation therapy may be indicated in advanced gynecologic malignancies invading the rectosigmoid colon.

REFERENCES

Cochio TA et al: Impact of modern diagnostic methods on the management of active rectal bleeding. *Am J Surg* 143:607, 1982.

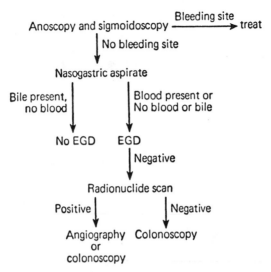

Figure 1–6. Suggested scheme for the management of lower gastrointestinal hemorrhage. (*From Schrock TR: Large Intestine. In Way LW [ed]:* Current Surgical Diagnosis and Treatment, *8th ed. San Mateo, California, Appleton & Lange, 1988.*)

Kadir S, Ernst C: Current concepts in angiographic management of gastrointestinal bleeding. *Curr Probl Surg* 20:283, 1983.

35. CARDIOPULMONARY ARREST

I. **Problem.** One week after radical vulvectomy, a patient is found unresponsive and pulseless in bed.

II. **Immediate Questions**

  A. **Is the patient responsive?** Basic cardiopulmonary resuscitation (CPR) begins with a vigorous attempt to arouse the patient. Call the patient and shake her by the shoulders.

  B. **Is the airway obstructed?** Finger sweep or suction out the patient's mouth. Listen for air movement.

  C. **Are there vital signs?** Check for carotid pulse and blood pressure. After these basic questions are asked and maneuvers performed, begin mouth-to-mouth or, preferably, ventilation with 100% oxygen by bag and mask, and chest compressions. The following questions are then asked as advanced cardiac life support (ACLS) is started.

D. What medications is the patient on? Cardiac medications are particularly important, especially antiarrhythmics and digoxin. An adverse reaction to a recently administered medication may be determined.

E. Are there any recent lab values, particularly potassium or hematocrit? Hyperkalemia (usually > 7 meq/L) or severe anemia, usually acute, may cause a cardiac arrest.

F. What are the patient's major medical problems? Ask about coronary artery disease, previous myocardial infarction, hypertension, previous pulmonary embolus, and recent surgery.

III. Differential Diagnosis. Arrest rhythms include ventricular fibrillation and tachycardia, asystole, and electromechanical dissociation (EMD). Causes of cardiopulmonary arrest may include:

A. Cardiac
1. **Myocardial infarction.**
2. **Congestive heart failure.**
3. **Ventricular arrhythmias.**
4. **Cardiac tamponade,** usually post-traumatic.

B. Pulmonary
1. **Pulmonary embolus.**
2. **Acute respiratory failure.**
3. **Aspiration.**
4. **Tension pneumothorax.**

C. Hemorrhagic. Undiagnosed severe bleeding such as from a ruptured aortic aneurysm can result in cardiac arrest.

D. Metabolic
1. **Hypokalemia, hyperkalemia.** Either may induce arrhythmias.
2. **Acidosis.** Severe acidosis may suppress myocardial function.
3. **Warming from hypothermia.** Arrhythmias may be induced.

IV. Database

A. Physical examination key points. As described, check responsiveness and vital signs. Resuscitation should always be initiated before a detailed physical exam is performed.
1. Check ventilation and perform airway opening maneuvers (jaw thrust or chin lift) as needed.
2. Look for tracheal deviation as evidence of a tension pneumothorax.

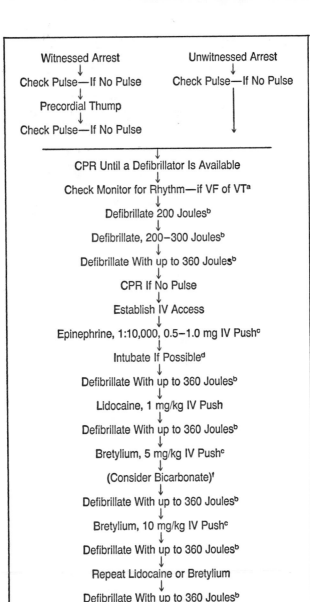

Witnessed Arrest

Check Pulse—If No Pulse

Precordial Thump

Check Pulse—If No Pulse

Unwitnessed Arrest

Check Pulse—If No Pulse

CPR Until a Defibrillator Is Available

Check Monitor for Rhythm—if VF of VT[a]

Defibrillate 200 Joules[b]

Defibrillate, 200–300 Joules[b]

Defibrillate With up to 360 Joules[b]

CPR If No Pulse

Establish IV Access

Epinephrine, 1:10,000, 0.5–1.0 mg IV Push[c]

Intubate If Possible[d]

Defibrillate With up to 360 Joules[b]

Lidocaine, 1 mg/kg IV Push

Defibrillate With up to 360 Joules[b]

Bretylium, 5 mg/kg IV Push[c]

(Consider Bicarbonate)[f]

Defibrillate With up to 360 Joules[b]

Bretylium, 10 mg/kg IV Push[c]

Defibrillate With up to 360 Joules[b]

Repeat Lidocaine or Bretylium

Defibrillate With up to 360 Joules[b]

      3. Distended neck veins may indicate pericardial tamponade or pneumothorax.

  B. Laboratory Data. These should be obtained as soon as possible, but should not delay the start of therapy.

      1. Arterial blood gases.

      2. Serum electrolytes, with special attention to potassium.

      3. Complete blood count. Especially important is the hematocrit.

  C. Radiologic and other studies

      1. Continuous cardiac monitoring, frequently checking lead placement.

      2. Other studies may be performed after the patient has been resuscitated.

V. Plan. Therapy for cardiac arrest is based on following the specific algorithms outlined by the American Heart Association (AHA). Specific AHA algorithms for ventricular fibrillation, ventricular tachycardia, asystole, and electromechanical dissociation are shown in Figures 1–7 through 1–10. Frequently used resuscitation medications are located inside the back cover. Every physician should have these memorized. In addition, successful resuscitation is based on a team approach with one leader monitoring the rhythm and ordering therapy according to the appropriate algorithm. Everyone must remain calm and must be assigned a specific job. Resuscitation be-

---

Figure 1–7. Ventricular fibrillation and pulseless tachycardia. (*From Standards for CPR and ECC. JAMA 255:21, 1986. Used with permission.*) See opposite page.

—Ventricular fibrillation (and pulseless ventricular tachycardia). This sequence was developed to assist in teaching how to treat a broad range of patients with ventricular fibrillation (VF) or pulseless ventricular tachycardia (VT). Some patients may require care not specified herein. This algorithm should not be construed as prohibiting such flexibility. Flow of algorithm presumes that VF is continuing. CPR indicates cardiopulmonary resuscitation.

[a]Pulseless VT should be treated identically to VF.

[b]Check pulse and rhythm after each shock. If VF recurs after transiently converting (rather than persists without ever converting), use whatever energy level has previously been successful for defibrillation.

[c]Epinephrine should be repeated every 5 minutes.

[d]Intubation is preferable. If it can be accomplished simultaneously with other techniques, then the earlier the better. However, defibrillation and epinephrine are more important initially if the patient can be ventilated without intubation.

[e]Some may prefer repeated doses of lidocaine, which may be given in 0.5 mg/kg boluses every 8 minutes to a total dose of 3 mg/kg.

[f]Value of sodium bicarbonate is questionable during cardiac arrest, and it is not recommended for routine cardiac arrest sequence. Consideration of its use in a dose of 1 meq/kg is appropriate at this point. Half of original dose may be repeated every 10 minutes if it is used.

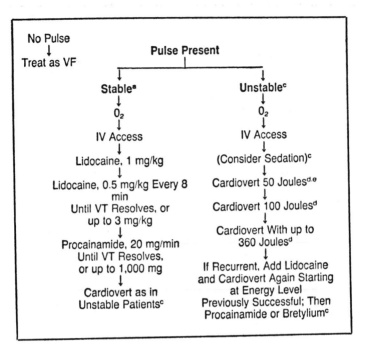

Figure 1–8. Ventricular tachycardia. (*From Standards for CPR and ECC. JAMA 255:21, 1986. Used with permission.*)

—Sustained ventricular tachycardia (VT). This sequence was developed to assist in teaching how to treat a broad range of patients with sustained VT. Some patients may require care not specified herein. This algorithm should not be construed as prohibiting such flexibility. Flow of algorithm presumes that VT is continuing. VF indicates ventricular fibrillation.

aIf patient becomes unstable (see footnote b for definition) at any time, move to "Unstable" arm of algorithm.

bUnstable indicates symptoms (eg, chest pain or dyspnea), hypotension (systolic blood pressure <90 mm Hg), congestive heart failure, ischemia, or infarction.

cSedation should be considered for all patients, including those defined in footnote b as unstable, except those who are hemodynamically unstable (eg, hypotensive, in pulmonary edema, or unconscious).

dIf hypotension, pulmonary edema, or unconsciousness is present, unsynchronized cardioversion should be done to avoid delay associated with synchronization.

eIn the absence of hypotension, pulmonary edema, or unconsciousness, a precordial thump may be employed prior to cardioversion.

fOnce VT has resolved, begin intravenous (IV) infusion of antiarrhythmic agent that has aided resolution of VT. If hypotension, pulmonary edema, or unconsciousness is present, use lidocaine if cardioversion alone is unsuccessful, followed by bretylium. In all other patients, recommended order of therapy is lidocaine, procainamide, and then bretylium.

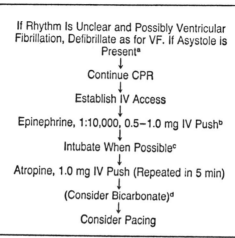

Figure 1–9. Asystole. (*From Standards for CPR and ECC. JAMA 255:21, 1986. Used with permission.*)

—Asystole (cardiac standstill). This sequence was developed to assist in teaching how to treat a broad range of patients with asystole. Some patients may require care not specified herein. This algorithm should not be construed to prohibit such flexibility. Flow of algorithm presumes asystole is continuing. VF indicates ventricular fibrillation; IV, intravenous.

[a]Asystole should be confirmed in two leads.

[b]Epinephrine should be repeated every five minutes.

[c]Intubation is preferable; if it can be accomplished simultaneously with other techniques, then the earlier the better. However, cardiopulmonary resuscitation (CPR) and use of epinephrine are more important initially if patient can be ventilated without intubation. (Endotracheal epinephrine may be used.)

[d]Value of sodium bicarbonate is questionable during cardiac arrest, and it is not recommended for the routine cardiac arrest sequence. Consideration of its use in a dose of 1 mEq/kg is appropriate at this point. Half of original dose may be repeated every ten minutes if it is used.

gins with the ABCs: *A*irway (intubate whenever possible), *B*reathing (ventilate), and *C*irculation (chest compression). For adults, the ratio of 5 compressions to 1 breath is used in two-person CPR.

A. Ventricular fibrillation and pulseless tachycardia (see Figure 1–7). Torsades de pointes, a rare ventricular arrhythmia, is treated with temporary pacemaker, rarely bretylium, but never lidocaine. Most often congenital or drug induced, it is characterized by "twisting" or direction changes of the QRS complex around the isoelectric line.

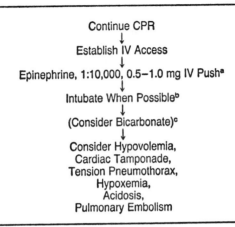

Continue CPR
↓
Establish IV Access
↓
Epinephrine, 1:10,000, 0.5–1.0 mg IV Push[a]
↓
Intubate When Possible[b]
↓
(Consider Bicarbonate)[c]
↓
Consider Hypovolemia,
Cardiac Tamponade,
Tension Pneumothorax,
Hypoxemia,
Acidosis,
Pulmonary Embolism

Figure 1–10. Electromechanical dissociation. (*From Standards for CPR and ECC. JAMA 255:21, 1986. Used with permission.*)

—Electromechanical dissociation. This sequence was developed to assist in teaching how to treat a broad range of patients with electromechanical dissociation. Some patients may require care not specified herein. This algorithm should not be construed to prohibit such flexibility. Flow of algorithm presumes that electromechanical dissociation is continuing. CPR indicates cardiopulmonary resuscitation; IV, intravenous.

[a]Epinephrine should be repeated every five minutes.

[b]Intubation is preferable. If it can be accomplished simultaneously with other techniques, then the earlier the better. However, epinephrine is more important initially if the patient can be ventilated without intubation.

[c]Value of sodium bicarbonate is questionable during cardiac arrest, and it is not recommended for routine cardiac arrest sequence. Consideration of its use in a dose of 1mEq/kg is appropriate at this point. Half of original dose may be repeated every ten minutes if it is used.

    B. Ventricular tachycardia. See the algorithm in Figure 1–8.

    C. Asystole. See the algorithm in Figure 1–9. The prognosis is very poor in cases of asystole. Defibrillate if there is any question about the rhythm being fine ventricular tachycardia.

    D. Electromechanical dissociation. See the algorithm in Figure 1–10. In surgical patients always consider pulmonary embolism, especially in high-risk patients (obese, previous embolism, certain pelvic and orthopedic cases), and hypovolemia as causes of EMD. In trauma patients, consider tension pneumothorax and cardiac tamponade. Treat hypovolemia with aggressive fluid resuscitation, tension pneumothorax with tube thoracostomy, and pericardial tamponade with pericardiocentesis.

REFERENCE

Standards and Guidelines for Cardiopulmonary Resuscitation (CPR) and Emergency Cardiac Care (ECC). *JAMA* 255:2905, 1986.

36. CHEST PAIN

I. **Problem.** Four days following total exenteration, a 50-year-old patient tells the nurse of an ongoing episode of chest pain that has lasted for 10 minutes.

II. **Immediate Questions.** The conditions that lead a patient to complain of "chest pain" range from inconsequential to life threatening. The purpose of the immediate questions is to determine the urgency of response, and in particular to ascertain whether ischemic heart disease is the cause of the pain.

A. **Does the patient have a prior history of coronary artery disease, and if so, does the current pain resemble previous episodes of angina pectoris?** In a patient with documented cardiac disease, particularly if the current episode resembles previous known anginal attacks, the pain should be treated as myocardial ischemia with sublingual nitroglycerin (0.4 mg typical initial dose) without delay.

B. **What is the location, nature, and severity of the pain?** Location of the pain (substernal, epigastric), radiation to other areas (jaw, arm, flank, abdomen), nature of the pain (burning, crushing, tearing, stabbing), and the severity can help define patterns of chest pain that fit certain diagnostic categories. However, chest pain cannot be defined by clinical criteria alone. There is considerable overlap in pain from varied causes since the thoracic viscera share common neural pathways. Classic angina is retrosternal and may radiate to the jaw or left arm. Thoracic aortic dissection is usually described as tearing or ripping, and peptic ulcer is often burning or gnawing.

C. **What was the patient doing when the pain began?** The inciting activity (or factors that alleviate pain) at the onset of an episode of chest pain is helpful in defining the diagnosis. Classic angina is brought on by exertion, pleuritic pain is exacerbated by coughing, and esophagitis is often exacerbated by recumbency.

D. **Are there any symptoms associated with the episode of chest pain?** Inquire specifically about nausea, dyspnea, diaphoresis, dizziness, syncope, abdominal pain, pleuritic pain, palpitations, and presence of acid taste in the mouth.

III. **Differential Diagnosis.** The differential diagnosis of chest pain is one of the classic points of discussion in medical school clerkships because of the frequency of the complaint, the range of diagnostic possibilities, and the importance of making the correct diagnosis.

A. **Cardiac/Vascular**
   1. **Acute myocardial infarction.** Crushing retrosternal chest pain lasting > 1 hour and unrelieved by nitroglycerin.
   2. **Angina pectoris.** The pain of angina is typically described as crushing, substernal, often with radiation to the arms or jaw. There is often associated nausea, diaphoresis, dyspnea, or palpitations, and it is usually relieved by nitroglycerin.
      a. **Coronary artery disease.**
      b. **Coronary artery spasm** (Prinzmetal's angina). This variant angina usually occurs at rest.
      c. **Aortic regurgitation or mitral valve prolapse.** A heart murmur will usually be present.
   3. **Aortic dissection.** The pain is tearing in nature and radiates to the back. It is usually associated with a history of hypertension.
   4. **Acute pericarditis.** A friction rub may be present and an effusion is typically seen on echocardiogram.
      a. **Infectious.** Most commonly this will be viral or tuberculosis.
      b. **Myocardial infarction.** There can be early pericarditis in the first few days or pericarditis 1–4 weeks post MI (Dressler's syndrome).
      c. **Uremia.**
      d. **Malignancy.** Most often this will be breast or bronchogenic.
      e. **Connective tissue diseases.**
   5. **Primary pulmonary hypertension.** The pain is mild and dyspnea on exertion is a prominent symptom.

B. **Pulmonary**
   1. **Pulmonary embolus/infarction.**
   2. **Pneumothorax.** Onset is acute, often with dyspnea. Suspect pneumothorax in young patients or those with chronic obstructive pulmonary disease.
   3. **Pleurodynia.** Also known as Bornholm's disease, this is caused by coxsackie viral illnesses.
   4. **Pneumonia/pleuritis.** This pain is typically pleuritic (made worse on deep inspiration).

C. **Gastrointestinal**

1. **Gastroesophageal reflux.** The patient often describes an acid taste in the mouth, associated with recumbency.
2. **Esophageal spasm.** This is easily confused with angina pectoris since it may cause substernal pain that is relieved by nitrates.
3. **Gastritis.** Alcoholism is commonly associated.
4. **Peptic ulcer disease.** Pain is typically epigastric and classically is relieved by eating.
5. **Biliary colic.** Pain is usually associated with eating, especially fatty foods, and is located in the epigastrium or right upper quadrant.
6. **Pancreatitis.**

D. **Musculoskeletal.** Pain can be reproduced by palpation of the chest wall.
   1. **Costochondritis.** Point tenderness is present over the costochondral junction.
   2. **Muscle strain/spasm.** There is often a history of exercise or exertion.
   3. **Rib fractures after trauma.**

IV. Database

A. **Physical examination key points**
   1. **Vital signs.** Hypotension is an ominous sign and may represent cardiovascular collapse (extensive MI, dissecting aneurysm, pulmonary embolus, or tension pneumothorax). Hypertension in the face of MI or aortic dissection requires emergency therapy to reduce the pressure. Fever may represent an embolus (usually low grade) or other inflammatory process (pneumonia, pleurisy, pericarditis). Tachycardia may also require urgent cardioversion.
   2. **Heart.** A murmur occurs with valvular disease, a friction rub with pericarditis (note: this is a "normal finding" immediately after open heart surgery), and a displaced point of maximal impulse with congestive heart failure (CHF).
   3. **Lungs.** Rales occur with CHF, dullness to percussion with fluid or pneumonic consolidation, friction rub with pleural inflammation, and decreased breath sounds with fluid or pneumothorax.
   4. **Abdomen.** Determine the presence or absence of bowel sounds, inflammation, or other evidence of an intra-abdominal lesion.
   5. **HEENT.** Thrush (especially in immunosuppressed patients) may represent *Candida* esophagitis.
   6. **Neck.** Venous distention is seen with CHF or pneumothorax.

7. **Chest.** Chest wall tenderness or contusion is present with rib fracture; sternal instability after median sternotomy may indicate infection. Point costochondral tenderness occurs with costochondritis.

8. **Neurologic examination.** Aortic dissection may cause a characteristic hemiplegia.

9. **Extremities.** There may be edema with CHF or asymmetric swelling with venous thrombosis.

B. **Laboratory data**

1. **Hemogram.** Look for leukocytosis in infectious illnesses, particularly lymphocytosis in viral conditions.

2. **CPK with isoenzymes** should be followed every 8 hours to evaluate myocardial injury.

3. **Arterial blood gases.** These should be obtained in most cases, and always if there is any dyspnea.

C. **Radiologic and other studies**

1. **Electrocardiogram.** Obtain a baseline study. Evaluate systematically and compare to prior ECGs. Document the presence and degree of pain at the time of the ECG. ECG findings of an MI may include Q waves, ST wave changes (depression or elevation), or T wave inversions. With a subendocardial infarction the Q wave may be absent. Arrhythmias may also be present.

2. **Chest x-ray.** If there is any possibility of myocardial ischemia, obtain the CXR as a portable so that the patient is not left unmonitored in the radiology department. Look for pneumothorax, effusions, infiltrates, globular heart shadow (pericardial effusion), and silhouette of the thoracic aorta and mediastinum (widened with aneurysm or dissection).

3. **Echocardiogram.** This will evaluate for pericardial effusion, cardiac wall motion, valvular disease, and aortic dissection.

4. **Aortogram/contrast CT scan.** These studies are done to diagnose aortic dissection.

5. **Venogram/ventilation.** A perfusion scan or pulmonary angiogram can diagnose pulmonary emboli. A negative V/Q scan essentially rules out embolism. However, an equivocal or "probable" scan requires confirmation with pulmonary arteriography or else the patient should be treated based on clinical grounds.

V. **Plan.** The treatment plan is dictated by establishing the correct diagnosis. Of the conditions listed above, **myocardial ischemia, aortic dissection, tension pneumothorax, and pulmonary embolism are the most immediately life threatening** but are treatable. If you have a reasonable suspicion of myocardial ischemia as the source of pain, do not hesitate to treat the patient accordingly. The most commonly confused diagnoses are esophageal spasm and musculoskeletal pain.

A. Emergency management
1. Treat with oxygen therapy by mask or cannula.
2. Obtain an ECG and leave the leads in place to serve as a monitor and for repeating the ECG if pain recurs or increases.
3. Request a STAT portable chest x-ray and a room air blood gas.
4. If myocardial ischemia is a possibility, treat with sublingual nitroglycerin as a diagnostic and therapeutic trial.

B. Myocardial ischemia
1. **Nitrates.** Use sublingual nitroglycerin; 0.4 mg (1/150 grain) is a typical starting dose. Monitor symptomatic relief and blood pressure, and repeat q5–10min for up to 3 doses if necessary. If nitroglycerin is effective but pain recurs, establish a nitroglycerin drip at 10–20 µg/min and titrate to pain relief. Keep systolic BP above 90.
2. **Morphine.** If pain is not relieved by nitroglycerin or if the patient cannot tolerate nitrates, treat with morphine 1–3 mg IV.
3. **Oxygen.** 4 L by nasal prongs (approximately equal to 35% mask).
4. **Lidocaine.** If the ECG shows clear-cut infarction or if there is prominent ectopy, treat with a 75–100 mg bolus IV, then begin continuous IV infusion at 2 mg/min.
5. **Continue monitoring** and make arrangements yourself or through Cardiology to admit the patient to CCU/ICU.
6. **Coronary thrombolysis** using streptokinase, urokinase, or tissue plasminogen activator may be indicated.

C. Aortic dissection. Initial treatment attempts to eliminate pain and reduce systolic blood pressure. Surgical correction is indicated for all symptomatic aneurysms.
1. **Nitroprusside** (Nipride). Begin a continuous infusion of 0.5–1.0 µg/kg/min and titrate up to control blood pressure.
2. **Propranolol.** Decreasing systolic blood pressure acutely may cause a rebound increase in contractility and shear force. Treat with propranolol 1–3 mg IV prior to Nipride.
3. **Morphine.** Use 1–3 mg IV prn to relieve pain.

D. Pulmonary embolus
1. Check baseline coagulation parameters (PT/PTT).
2. Give heparin in an IV bolus of either 10,000 units or 100 units/kg, then begin a continuous IV infusion of 10 units/kg/h. Check partial thromboplastin time in 3–4 hours and adjust heparin to keep it approximately twice normal.
3. If anticoagulation is contraindicated, place an intracaval fil-

ter. Filters are also indicated in patients who present with recurrent emboli despite adequate anticoagulation.

E. Pneumothorax. Treat by tube thoracostomy.

F. Pericarditis. Monitor for tamponade and give indomethacin or other anti-inflammatory agents.

G. Gastritis/esophagitis
  1. Antacids.
  2. H_2 blockers (cimetidine, ranitidine).

H. Costochondritis. Treat with nonsteroidal anti-inflammatory drugs (ibuprofen, etc).

REFERENCE

Alexander J: Chest Pain—how serious is it? *Hosp Med* 23:24, 1987.

37. CVP ABNORMALITIES

I. Problem. The central venous pressure (CVP) catheter placed in a patient who will undergo tumor debulking in the morning is not functioning.

II. Immediate Questions

  A. What is the appearance of the tracing? A CVP should have a slowly undulating waveform that varies with the patient's respirations if properly positioned in the chest. Absence of a waveform may indicate that the catheter is clotted. In the absence of a transducer, the column of fluid in the manometer should fluctuate with respirations.

  B. Can blood be aspirated from the line? Inability to aspirate blood does not imply a nonfunctioning catheter that cannot be used for fluid infusions. It may mean the tip is against the vessel, but also may indicate a kinked or clotted line.

  C. How long has the line been in place? The longer a line is in place, the higher the incidence of infection.

  D. Is the line in the correct position? This must be evaluated on chest x-ray. The tip should be in the superior vena cava. If there is any question, get a new film and compare it to the x-ray performed when the tube was placed.

III. Differential Diagnosis

  A. Clotted catheter. This happens more frequently with slowly running lines.

B. **Catheter in incorrect position.** This is evaluated by chest x-ray. Subclavian lines occasionally go up into the neck and will not fluctuate with respiration.

C. **Kinked catheter.** This includes kinking of the line at the skin entry site, or kinking under the clavicle due to the angle of placement to enter the vein. It can usually be seen as an acute bend on x-ray.

D. **Other mechanical problems.** Cracking of the catheter at the hub, or a loose connection.

E. **Flush line or transfuser malfunction.** These possibilities are easily ruled out by checking the system. The nursing staff can be very helpful in this evaluation.

F. **Infected catheter.** Any question of sepsis originating in a central venous line requires expeditious evaluation. The best technique involves drawing cultures through the catheter, removing the line, and culturing the tip.

IV. Database

A. Physical examination key points

1. **Vital signs.** Fever signifies infection, whereas tachycardia and hypotension may represent excessive bleeding, tension pneumothorax, or hemothorax.
2. **Lungs.** Diminished breath sounds may indicate a pneumothorax, hemothorax, or hydrothorax.
3. **HEENT.** Tracheal deviation may indicate an expanding hematoma or tension pneumothorax.
4. **Deep line site.** Inspect for evidence of cellulitis, bleeding, catheter kinking, or leakage from a cracked hub. Check the transducer and flush line.

B. Laboratory data

1. Draw blood cultures such as DuPont Isolator if sepsis must be evaluated. Obtain cultures from both the catheter and peripherally.
2. Obtain a complete blood count or coagulation profile if bleeding is present.

V. Plan.
Replacing the line will usually solve problems associated with the line itself. Unless the line is infected, it can be changed over a guide wire. Be sure to suture it in place carefully to avoid kinking at the hub. All line manipulations should be performed using sterile technique with the patient in Trendelenburg (head-down) position to prevent air embolus.

A. Clotted catheter. A new line thought to be clotted can often be declotted safely with a syringe. The decision to attempt to declot a catheter should be approached cautiously since the clot may act as an embolus. The catheter can be gently aspirated or flushed with a 1 cc tuberculin syringe. The smaller diameter of this syringe more closely matches the diameter of the catheter and will transmit more pressure than a larger syringe. Use heparin flush solution (100 units/mL). Streptokinase can also be used to declot a line (see Chapter 7, page 552, for dose), but side effects can limit its use.

B. Kinked catheter. Inspection of the site may reveal a kinked catheter that can be easily corrected by repositioning the skin sutures using sterile technique. A subclavian catheter that is kinked at the entry to the vein under the clavicle must be replaced. Compared with internal jugular lines, subclavian lines are the easiest to affix to the skin and prevent kinking.

C. Misdirected catheter. This usually requires removal and replacement, often to another site.

D. Bleeding. Site bleeding can usually be controlled with direct pressure.

E. Workup of the infected catheter. Draw one culture from the line, another from a peripheral site, and evaluate the colony counts at 24 hours as described by Mosca. If the colony count from the line is 5 or more times greater than the peripherally drawn culture, the line is implicated as the culprit and must be replaced at another site. If the catheter is for long-term access (ie, Hickman), antibiotics should be given through the catheter rather than removing it as initial therapy.

F. Hints for catheter insertion (see Procedure 8, page 354). There are many "tricks" to inserting a central venous catheter, most of which are personal preferences rather than proven helpful tools.
   1. The most common locations are subclavian and internal jugular (IJ). The problem with IJ lines is fixing them to the patient for long periods of time. Subclavian lines are easier to fix to the skin. Femoral lines are acceptable when there is no upper body alternative and when rapid access is needed during cardiopulmonary resuscitation.
   2. Most commonly for subclavian lines, the patient is placed in Trendelenburg position with a roll between the scapulae. This presumably makes the vein more prominent and simplifies puncture, but recent evidence in the literature contradicts this commonly held view (Jesseph et al, 1987). The needle is passed below the clavicle and aimed toward the sternal notch. After good blood return is attained, the syringe

is removed, carefully holding the needle still. Watch for spontaneous blood return. The guidewire is passed through the needle and the needle removed. The guidewire should pass easily. Remember that if the guidewire goes to the right ventricle, arrythmias may be induced. The skin is nicked with a needle and the catheter is passed over the guidewire. After removal, the guidewire should be nearly straight. Affix the catheter at the hub to the skin.

3. The internal jugular vein is approached with the patient turning her head toward the opposite side. The needle is inserted two fingerbreadths above the clavicle in the v-shaped area between the two heads of the sternocleidomastoid muscle. Aim for the ipsilateral nipple. Identifying the vein with a small needle (eg, 20-gauge) before using the large needle to pass the guidewire is highly recommended.

4. In inserting a line, there are four signs of successful placement:
   a. Blood is easily aspirated through the syringe.
   b. The guidewire passes easily.
   c. On removal, the guidewire is nearly straight.
   d. Blood is easily aspirated through the catheter after placement.

REFERENCES

Fares L, Cohn J: Improved subclavian cannulation technique. *Surg Gynecol Obstet* 162:277, 1986.

Jesseph J, Conces D, Augustyn G: Patient positioning for subclavian vein catheterization. *Arch Surg* 122:1207, 1987.

Miller J, Venus B, Mathru M: Comparison of the sterility of long term central venous catheterization using single lumen, triple lumen, and pulmonary artery catheters. *Crit Care Med* 12:634, 1984.

Mosca R et al: The benefits of isolator cultures in the management of suspected catheter sepsis. *Surgery* (in press).

38. DRAIN MANAGEMENT

I. **Problem.** A 60-year-old patient has increased output from her surgical drains.

II. **Immediate Questions**

A. **What operative procedure did the patient have and what surgical sites are being drained?** Surgical drains can be used for drainage of purulent material and necrotic debris from Bartholin or pelvic abscesses as well as prophylactically to decrease blood and lymph accumulation after major intra-abdominal surgery. Drains can be placed in the cul-de-sac and brought out through the vagina or a stab wound lateral to the abdominal incision. Exit wounds through the primary incision will result in an increased incidence of wound infections.

B. What type of drain was placed intraoperatively? Surgical drains are of two basic types: passive or active. Passive drainage is accomplished by gravity or capillary action. Drainage is further facilitated by transient increases in intra-abdominal pressure, as with coughing. Passive surgical drains include Penrose, Foley, Malecot, and Word catheters. Active drainage is accomplished by suction from a simple bulb device or a suction pump. These systems may be closed, like the Hemovac and Jackson-Pratt drains, or open to air to keep the holes in the main tube from becoming blocked, like the sump drain. Closed suction drainage will provide for removal of fluids and apposition of the tissues while preventing contamination with bacteria.

C. What is the nature of the drainage fluid? The character, odor, and amount of drainage should be noted. Body fluids include serous/serosanguineous fluids, blood, pus, lymph, bile, pancreatic juice, intestinal contents, and urine. Some of these fluids can be identified by gross visual inspection and others by laboratory analysis.

D. Are there any new symptoms concurrent with the change in drain output? Look specifically for increased pain, signs of infection, hypotension, and abdominal distention.

III. Differential Diagnosis

A. Increased drainage. Increased bloody drainage can be due to vessel leakage and may even be caused by catheter erosion into a vessel. Increased serous drainage may be from increased lymph drainage, particularly with increased activity.

B. Purulent drainage. This indicates infection.

C. Intestinal drainage. This may represent a fistula to the skin wound and is of great concern after any operation.

D. Urine drainage. This may represent fistulas anywhere along the urinary tract.

E. Sudden cessation of drainage. Tissue debris, especially in smaller catheters, is a principal source of catheter occlusion. Drains can be walled off from the general peritoneal cavity within about 6 hours. Intra-abdominal fluid can be collecting without drainage from the catheters. Therefore, regular examinations of the abdomen are necessary for early identification of intra-abdominal fluid collections.

F. Drain exit wound infection. Erythema, induration, and pain at the drain exit site are indicators of infection in the subcutaneous tract.

G. Loss of catheter. It is important to record the number, position, and types of drains used at the time of surgery and to document their removal. Drains should contain radiopaque markers for easy identification on x-rays. Drains should be sutured to the skin.

IV. Database

A. Physical examination key points

1. **Vital signs.** Look for signs of infection (tachycardia, fever) and volume loss.
2. **Abdomen.** Pain, abdominal distention, or a fluid wave may be present with accumulating fluid.
3. **Skin.** Erythema, induration, and pain around the catheter site suggest infection.
4. **Drainage fluid.** Examine the fluid for color, odor, and volume. Also examine the tube for clots or other obstructing material.

B. Laboratory data

1. **Hemogram.** Leukocytosis and left shift suggest infection. Decreasing hematocrit may suggest continued intra-abdominal blood loss.
2. **Drain hematocrit.** This will confirm continued intra-abdominal loss of blood. Drain hematocrit may be compared to central hematocrit.
3. **Drain culture and gram stain.** These are done to evaluate for infection.
4. **Chemistries.** The drain fluid can be sent for urea nitrogen or creatinine determinations to document leakage of urine. Urine urea nitrogen and creatinine are markedly elevated relative to serum values.
5. **Coagulation profile (PT/PTT, platelets).** If bleeding is excessive, a coagulopathy may be present.

C. Radiologic and other studies

1. **CT scans and ultrasound.** These studies may localize undrained fluid collections.
2. **Plain films.** Most drains are marked with a radiopaque stripe, and drain position can be verified with plain films.
3. **Angiography.** An angiogram may help to localize the bleeding site if the rate is at least 1 mL/min.
4. **Fistulography.** This contrast study is useful to identify the origin of a cutaneous fistula.

V. Plan. Note: Idiosyncrasies in management of drains are extensive. Check with a senior physician before any drain is removed.

  A. General drain care. All drains should have local care including at least daily cleansing of the skin around the exit site with an antiseptic pad. Gauze pads are placed above and below the drain and taped to the skin. Exit wounds close rapidly after drains are removed. In a diabetic or immunosuppressed patient, the sites may heal more slowly and be a source of infection. If the site becomes infected, it should be opened and cared for as an open wound. Penrose drains are usually removed gradually by advancing 2–4 cm per day until they are out. Suction drains are pulled at once after the suction is relieved. Suction drains are easier to care for than Penrose drains, and skin excoriation is minimized; in addition, more accuracy can be achieved in measuring drainage. These drains should be stripped daily to prevent catheter obstruction by tissue debris.

  B. Specific drain care
    1. Pelvic abscess. Drains from infected areas can be removed at 48–72 hours postoperatively if the drainage is serous and less than about 40 mL per day. If intraoperative cultures were positive or the patient does not become afebrile, the drain should not be removed for several days. Drainage of purulent or malodorous fluid contraindicates the removal of drains. If a patient has persistent fever and leukocytosis for over 72 hours, the presence of an abscess should be excluded by further workup (see Problem 64, page 240).
    2. Radical pelvic and groin surgery. Drains should be left in place until the drainage has decreased to 30–50 mL in 24 hours. This will prevent lymphocyst formation. Drains left in too long act as foreign bodies and channels for entry of bacteria.
    3. Word catheter. The Word catheter used to drain a Bartholin abscess should be left in place for 6 weeks. This allows a fistula tract to develop around the catheter to provide continuous drainage of the gland.
    4. Increased bloody output. Document the rate of bleeding by accurately noting output every 30–60 minutes and following serial hematocrits and coagulation parameters. Replace fluids, including blood products, as needed.

REFERENCES

Edlich RF et al: Technical factors in wound management. In Hunt TK, Dunphy JE (eds): *Fundamentals of Wound Management.* New York, Appleton-Century-Crofts, 1979, pp 440–443.

Moss JP: Historical and current perspectives on surgical drainage. *Surg Gynecol Obstet* 152:517, 1981.

39. DYSPNEA

I. **Problem.** You are covering the gynecologic service when a postoperative patient experiences difficulty in breathing.

II. **Immediate Questions**

A. **What was the patient doing when the dyspnea occurred?** Shortness of breath with exertional activity may or may not indicate an underlying problem, depending on the severity of the dyspnea. Dyspnea associated with a reclining position (ie, orthopnea) points to cardiac dysfunction.

B. **Did the dyspnea occur abruptly or did it have a gradual onset?** The differential diagnosis for acute dyspnea differs from subacute or chronic dyspnea and often points to a specific event such as a pulmonary embolus, pneumothorax, or myocardial infarction. Factors resulting in a gradual onset are chronic bronchitis, emphysema, chronic asthma, sarcoidosis, lymphangitic carcinomatosis, anemia, obesity, and congestive heart failure.

C. **What is the baseline respiratory status of the patient?** A complaint of "not getting enough air" in a well-trained athlete indicates more serious dysfunction than an equivalent complaint in a chronic smoker with emphysema. Inquire specifically about current work and recreational physical activities.

D. **What is the patient's past history?** This will help eliminate some of the causes. Shortness of breath is more ominous in a young healthy woman than in an older patient. From the history one can ascertain if there is congenital heart disease, thyroid disease, myasthenia gravis, Guillain-Barré syndrome, or a cerebrovascular accident. A smoking history is most significant. Diuretic use preoperatively could help to explain the problem. From the nursing records one could determine if there was a drug overdose.

E. **Are there other symptoms, such as chest pain, coincident with the dyspnea?** Chest pain could result from a cardiac disorder including angina pectoris or myocardial infarction, but other causes include esophageal spasm, esophagitis, herpes zoster, or anxiety with hyperventilation syndrome. Pleuritic pain suggests infection, pulmonary embolus, or pleural effusion. Abdominal pain with large incisions could cause enough discomfort to decrease respiratory effort as well as ascites. Cough would be expected with pneumonia, but pulmonary embolus and congestive heart failure could cause similar symptoms. Hives and itching point to an allergic response. Gurgling suggests inability to clear secretions, possibly from a new-onset stroke or oversedation.

F. Is there wheezing or stridor? Both acute asthma attacks and anaphylactic reactions are readily treatable but must be identified and have appropriate therapy instituted quickly.

III. Differential Diagnosis. As noted above, dyspnea may be classified as acute or subacute/chronic. Within each category, the underlying mechanism is predominantly either pulmonary or cardiac.

A. Acute
　　1. Pulmonary
　　　　a. Pneumothorax. This can be traumatic (associated with rib fractures), may progress over hours, and can be associated with a hemothorax. Pneumothorax must be considered when evaluating patients after debulking tumor from the diaphragm.
　　　　b. Pulmonary embolus. Maintain a high index of suspicion. Risk factors include immobilization, recent surgery, neoplastic disease, and estrogen use.
　　　　c. Asthma/allergic reactions. Asthma is clearly identified by wheezing. Anaphylactic reactions are recognizable by stridor, atopic history, hives, and facial edema (see Problem 32, page 124).
　　　　d. Aspirated foreign body. This is usually obvious by history, but in a young or mentally impaired patient physical exam and radiologic studies may be needed.
　　　　e. Reflux with aspiration.
　　　　f. Amniotic fluid embolism. Immediately before or during delivery, amniotic fluid can embolize in the pulmonary vasculature.
　　2. Acute myocardial infarction. This is a possibility especially if there are cardiac risk factors. An MI is usually associated with chest pain or pressure, but not always.
　　3. Anxiety attack. Anxiety is not a common cause of shortness of breath, and it is often difficult to exclude organic causes. A further complication is its association with chest pain. Often tachypnea cycles with periods of normal breathing, and tachypnea may resolve when patients are not aware of being observed.

B. Subacute/chronic
　　1. Pulmonary
　　　　a. Chronic obstructive pulmonary disease (COPD). These patients usually have a smoking history with

baseline dyspnea on exertion. In progression of baseline dyspnea look for evidence of an infectious process.
   b. **Pneumonia.** This is often associated with leukocytosis, fever, productive sputum, and chest x-ray changes (infiltrates).
   c. **Interstitial lung disease.** A chest x-ray and pulmonary function test are diagnostic.
2. **Cardiac**
   a. **Congestive heart failure.** Physical exam shows elevated jugular venous pressure, rales, peripheral edema, cardiac gallop, and displacement of the left ventricular impulse. Dyspnea is associated with lying down.

IV. Database
A. Physical examination key points
1. **Vital signs.** Fever may signify infection but can also be seen with a pulmonary embolus. Tachypnea may accompany hypoxia, embolus, or a pneumothorax.
2. **Heart.** Look for elevated jugular venous pressure, displacement of the left ventricular impulse, and a new murmur of mitral regurgitation. Check for pulsus paradoxus.
3. **Lungs.** Observe respiratory rate, work of breathing, and use of accessory muscles. Listen for wheezes, stridor, rales, evidence of consolidation, and decreased breath sounds.
4. **Extremities.** Leg swelling is evidence for deep venous thrombosis. Evaluate for evidence of cyanosis.
5. **Neurologic examination.** Confusion and drowsiness may signify severe hypoxia.

B. Laboratory data
1. **Hemogram.** Leukocytosis may be present with infection.
2. **Arterial blood gases.** They document the level of respiratory compromise and guide therapeutic decisions.
3. **Sputum gram stain/culture.** These should be obtained in patients with pneumonia or tracheobronchitis.
4. **Blood chemistries.** Results may reveal evidence of renal failure.

C. Radiologic and other studies
1. **Chest x-ray.** Of obvious importance, if the patient is in distress, obtain a stat portable CXR. Aspiration typically reveals an infiltrate in the inferior segment of the right upper lobe or apical segment of the lower lobe. Straphylococcal pneumonia may reveal cavitary lesions.
2. **Electrocardiogram.** Always obtain an ECG if there is any question of a cardiac cause.
3. **Pulmonary function tests.** These are not applicable to the

acute situation but are helpful in patients with obstructive or restrictive chronic lung disease.

4. **Ventilation/perfusion scan.** The V/Q scan will evaluate for pulmonary embolism.
5. **Pulmonary angiography.** Especially with an equivocal V/Q scan, angiography is the "gold standard" in the diagnosis of pulmonary emboli.
6. **Multiple gated acquisition (MUGA) scan.** This documents left ventricular ejection fraction and level of congestive heart failure.
7. **Exercise tolerance test.** An exercise test is useful if the episode of dyspnea is related to ischemic heart disease.

V. Plan

A. Emergency management

1. **Oxygen supplementation.** If the patient is short of breath, institute oxygen therapy. Acutely, 100% FIO_2 may be used with adjustments made to keep atrial oxygen at least 60–80 mm Hg or oxygen saturation > 90% based on blood gas measurements. Long-term oxygen therapy at this level can cause toxicity. Do not worry about suppressing the hypoxic drive (chronic lung disease) in the acute situation. Patients with a history of COPD and CO_2 retention may be at increased risk to lose their "hypoxic drive" to breath, but it is impossible to predict which patients will be affected.
2. A stat portable chest x-ray, ECG, and blood gases are usually indicated if the cause is not immediately obvious.

B. Asthma

1. In most cases, order a stat treatment of Alupent nebulizer 0.3 mL in 2–3 mL normal saline administered by a respiratory therapist.
2. In younger patients in extreme distress, give 1 : 1000 epinephrine 0.25 mL (or 0.01 mL/kg) SQ.
3. If the patient is not taking theophylline, start loading doses of aminophylline 5–6 mg/kg IV over 20–30 minutes.

C. Anaphylaxis (see Problem 32, page 124).

D. Myocardial ischemia. If immediate evaluation is consistent with myocardial ischemia, give sublingual nitroglycerin (see Problem 35, page 134).

E. Acute congestive heart failure. Treat with oxygen and diuretics (furosemide 10–40 mg IV depending upon prior exposure). Sit the patient upright if blood pressure allow this.

F. Pneumonia. Treat with antibiotics and pulmonary toilet.

1. **Pneumococcal pneumonia.** Give penicillin G aqueous 600, 000–2 million units IV q6h.

2. **Mycoplasma or Legionella pneumonia.** Administer erythromycin 500 mg IV or PO q6h.

3. **Staphylococcal pneumonia.** Treat with nafcillin or cephalothin 1.5–2.0 g IV q4h.

4. **Aspiration pneumonia.**
   a. Protect the patient from further aspiration.
   b. Give aqueous penicillin G 2 million units IV q4h.

5. **Pneumocystis pneumonia.** Treat with IV pentamidine or trimethroprim-sulfamethoxazole.

6. **Gram-negative.** Administer an aminoglycoside plus a cephalosporin IV.

G. **Pneumothorax.** Place a chest tube as outlined in Procedure 13, page 363.

H. **Pulmonary embolism.** Anticoagulate the patient as described in Problem 68, page 263.

REFERENCES

Blacklow RS (ed): *MacBryde's Signs and Symptoms: Applied Pathologic Physiology and Clinical Interpretation, 6th ed.* Philadelphia, JB Lippincott, 1983, pp 335–346.

Ginsburg AD: *Clinical Reasoning in Patient Care.* Hagerstown, MD, Harper & Row, 1980, pp 30–44.

Raffin TA: Approach to patient with dyspnea. *Hosp Med* 20:45, 1984.

40. DYSURIA

I. **Problem.** A patient complains of dysuria.

II. **Immediate Questions**

A. **How long has the symptom been present?** Knowing the time course of any illness can give an etiologic clue. If the illness is more chronic, check on any previous urinalysis available.

B. **What is the patient's urologic history? Specifically, is there a prior history of infections or stone disease?** Some patients, especially female, are prone to recurrent urinary tract infections.

C. **Are there any associated voiding symptoms?** Fever, chills, and back pain are often signs of upper urinary tract infection (pyelonephritis). Frequency, urgency, and pain on urination suggest lower urinary tract infection (cystitis, urethritis).

D. **Has the patient recently had a Foley catheter removed?** A catheter may result in infection or mild urethral irritation.

E. **Is the patient pregnant?** Urinary tract infections and pyelonephritis increase the risk of premature labor.

III. Differential Diagnosis

A. Urinary tract infection

1. **Upper.** Pyelonephritis may occasionally cause dysuria, although this is infrequent.
2. **Lower.** Cystitis is often associated with urgency and frequency. Urethritis may be gonococcal or nongonococcal, often caused by *Chlamydia*.

B. Vaginitis.
Patients may present with initial complaints of dysuria. The infection can be due to *Candida, Trichomonas,* or *Gardnerella* organisms. Atrophic vaginitis occurs in postmenopausal women.

C. Genital infections.
Infections such as herpes or those due to condylomas can cause dysuria.

D. Chemical irritants.
Allergic reactions to a variety of agents (deodorant, douches) can affect urination.

E. Post procedure.
A frequent complaint after bladder catheterization or cystoscopy, it usually resolves spontaneously if no infection intervenes.

F. Urethral syndrome.
This is a frequent syndrome in women with dysuria and voiding complaints without evidence of urinary tract infection.

G. Miscellaneous.
Urethral stricture, bladder, tumor, urolithiasis, interstitial cystitis, and radiation can account for dysuria.

IV. Database

A. Physical examination key points

1. **Abdominal examination.** Look for signs of suprapubic or costovertebral angle tenderness.
2. **Genitalia.** Do a complete pelvic examination including the uterus and urethra. Vaginal discharge suggests vaginitis.

B. Laboratory data

1. **Urinalysis and culture.** Pyuria (> 5 WBC/HPF), the presence of leukocyte esterase or nitrites, and a positive culture suggest a urinary tract infection.
2. **Hemogram.** Leukocytosis and a left shift will be seen with acute pyelonephritis. They are not normally seen in urethritis or cystitis.
3. **Culture and gram stain of urethral discharge.** Thayer-Martin media should be used if gonorrhea is suspected. *N. gonorrhoeae* can be seen as gram-negative intracellular diplococci on gram stain.
4. **Urine cytology.** Dysuria may be a subtle manifestation of transitional cell carcinoma.

C. Radiologic and other studies

     1. **A full urologic evaluation** (excretory urography, cystoscopy, etc) may be required for definitive diagnosis but is rarely performed acutely in this setting.

V. Plan

A. Uncomplicated lower urinary tract infection. A positive urinalysis (as above) is enough reason to start antibiotic therapy. If the patient is otherwise healthy and not systemically septic, then oral antibiotics (such as trimethoprim-sulfamethoxazole) may be started. All sulfa drugs are contraindicated during pregnancy.

B. Pyelonephritis. A patient with signs of systemic sepsis, ie, fever, chills, nausea, malaise, or hypotension (often associated with acute pyelonephritis) should be evaluated with appropriate cultures (blood and urine), and systemic antibiotics should be started. A third-generation cephalosporin (cefoperazone, ceftazidime, etc) or ampicillin with an aminoglycoside are good choices until culture and sensitivities are available.

C. Vaginitis. Vaginitis should be treated appropriately: nystatin vaginal cream or suppositories for *Candida,* oral metronidazole for *Trichomonas* (see Chapter 7 for prescribing during pregnancy), Premarin cream for atrophic vaginitis.

D. Urethritis/cervicitis
    1. **Gonococcal urethritis/cervicitis.** Many regimens are available: procaine penicillin G 4.8 million units IM plus probenecid 1 g PO, ceftriaxone 250 mg IM, or ampicillin 3 g PO. This is followed by a 7-day course of tetracycline, doxycycline, or erythromycin.
    2. **Nongonococcal urethritis (NGU) (Chlamydia)/cervicitis.** Give doxycycline 100 mg PO bid or tetracycline 500 mg PO qid for 7–10 days.

E. Symptomatic relief. Symptomatic relief of dysuria can usually be achieved using phenazopyridine (Pyridium) 100–200 mg PO tid (turns urine orange) while workup or treatment is in progress. A small subset of patients with dysuria are sensitive to excessively alkaline or acidic urine, which may vary with diet.

REFERENCE

Contiguglia SR, Mishell JL, Kelin MH: Renal and urinary tract disorders. In Friedman HH (ed): *Problem-Oriented Medical Diagnosis.* Boston, Little, Brown, 1979.

41. FOLEY CATHETER PROBLEMS

I. Problem. Two days after an anterior urethropexy, the patient's Foley catheter is not draining.

II. Immediate Questions

A. What has the urine output been? If the urine output has slowly tapered off, then the problem may be oliguria rather than a non-functioning Foley. A catheter that has never put out urine may not be in the bladder.

B. Is the urine grossly bloody, or are there clots in the tubing or collection bag? Clots or tissue fragments such as those present after a bladder resection can obstruct the flow of urine in a Foley catheter. Similarly, intraoperative bladder trauma in an abdominal case can lead to bleeding.

C. Is the patient complaining of any pain? Bladder distention often causes severe lower abdominal pain; bladder spasms are painful and may cause urine to leak out around the catheter rather than pass through it.

D. Was any difficulty encountered in catheter insertion? Problematic urethral catheterization should raise the possibility that the catheter is not in the bladder.

III. Differential Diagnosis

A. Low urine output. It may be due to dehydration, hemorrhage, acute renal failure, as well as a host of other causes (see Problem 62, page 232).

B. Obstructed Foley catheter
    1. Kinking of catheter or tubing.
    2. Clots and tissue fragments. These are most common after transurethral resection of the bladder. Grossly bloody urine suggests a clot has formed. Tea-colored or "rusty" urine suggests that an organized clot may be present even though the urine is no longer grossly bloody. Bleeding will often accompany "accidental" catheter removal with the balloon still inflated and can occur with any coagulopathy.
    3. Sediment/stones. Chronically indwelling catheters (usually > 1 month) can become encrusted and obstructed. Calculi can lodge in the catheter.

C. Improperly positioned Foley catheter. Patients who have undergone radical pelvic surgery are difficult to catheterize. Not uncommonly, the catheter is placed in the markedly distended vagina rather than the urethra. A very infrequent occurrence is placement of a suprapubic catheter in the peritoneal cavity and not the bladder. These complications can be prevented by observing urine in the catheter drainage system.

D. Bladder spasms. The patient may complain of severe suprapubic pain, pain radiating to the perineum, or urine loss from around the catheter. Spasms are common after bladder surgery, cystocele repair, or surgery around the bladder. Spasms may be the only catheter complaint or may be so severe as to obstruct the flow of urine.

E. Bladder disruption. This may be due to blunt abdominal trauma, or it may be an operative complication or caused by severe distention secondary to a blocked catheter.

F. Inability to deflate the Foley balloon. This problem is rare with modern catheters.

IV. Database

A. Physical examination key points

1. **Vital signs.** Check for tachycardia or hypotension characteristic of hypovolemia.
2. **Abdominal examination.** Determine if the bladder is distended (suprapubic dullness to percussion with or without tenderness), which may be indicative of an obstructed Foley catheter.
3. **Genital examination.** Bleeding at the meatus suggests urethral trauma or partial removal of the catheter with the balloon inflated.
4. **Rectal examination.** Identify vaginal or pelvic displacement of the Foley catheter.
5. **Skin.** Look for signs of hypovolemia causing low urine output, such as skin turgor, appearance of mucous membranes, etc.

B. Laboratory data.
Most problems of this nature are usually mechanical, so laboratory data are somewhat limited in this setting.

1. **BUN and serum creatinine.** Elevations may be seen in renal insufficiency.
2. **Coagulation studies.** These are indicated especially if severe bleeding is present.

C. Radiologic and other studies.
In the acute setting of a Foley catheter problem, these are usually not needed. Ultrasound may demonstrate hydronephrosis in cases of obstructive uropathy.

V. Plan

A. Verify function. A rule of thumb is that a catheter that will not irrigate is in the urethra and not in the bladder. Start by irrigating the catheter with aseptic technique using a catheter-tipped 60 mL syringe and sterile normal saline. This may dislodge any clots obstructing the catheter. If sterile saline cannot be satisfactorily instilled and aspirated, the catheter should be replaced.

Catheter irrigation or replacement in any patient who has undergone bladder surgery must be done with extreme care.

B. **Oliguria.** If the catheter irrigates freely, do a workup for anuria (see Problem 62, page 232).

C. **Spasms.** Bladder spasms can be treated with oxybutynin (Ditropan), propantheline (Pro-Banthine), or belladonna and opium (B & O) suppositories (see Chapter 7 for dosages). Be **sure** to discontinue these medications before removing the catheter, to allow normal bladder function.

D. **Faulty balloon.** There are several techniques to deflate a balloon that will not empty.
   1. Injecting 5–10 mL of mineral oil into the inflation port will cause the balloon of a latex catheter to rupture in 5–10 minutes.
   2. Threading a 16 French central venous catheter into the inflation channel (after the valve is removed) may bypass the obstruction.
   3. As a last resort, ultrasound-directed transvesical needle puncture of the balloon may be needed.

REFERENCE

Andriole UT: Care of the indwelling catheter. In Kayes D (ed): *Urinary Tract Infection and Its Management.* St. Louis, CV Mosby, 1972, pp 256–260.

42. GENITAL ULCERS

I. **Problem.** You are consulted by the Medicine Service to evaluate a 25-year-old woman with genital ulcers.

II. **Immediate Questions**

A. **Is the patient sexually active?** Most ulcerative lesions of the vulva are due to sexually transmitted diseases (STDs). If the patient has a reliable history of sexual inactivity, these possibilities are unlikely.

B. **Has the patient sustained any trauma to the genital region?** Traumatic injury to the genitalia may appear as ulcerative lesions. These may occur as a result of injury during intercourse or accidental injury from other activities (eg, straddle injuries).

C. **Is the lesion painful?** This is probably the most useful question in differentiating between the various infectious causes of genital ulcers. Unless secondarily infected, ulcers due to syphilis (*Treponema pallidum*) or lymphogranuloma venereum (*Chlamy-*

dia trachomatis serotypes L1, L2, and L3) are painless. Conversely, ulcers due to chancroid (*Haemophilus ducreyi*), herpes genitalis (herpes simplex virus), and granuloma inguinale (*Calymmatobacterium granulomatis*) are usually exquisitely painful. Neoplastic causes of vulvar ulcers (invasive squamous cell carcinoma) are generally either asymptomatic or pruritic. The rare presentation of cutaneous tuberculosis (*Mycobacterium tuberculosis*) on the vulva is usually asymptomatic.

D. How long has the ulcer been present? If the ulcer has been present for several weeks without evidence of healing, one should strongly suspect malignancy. The primary chancre of syphilis generally heals in 2–6 weeks. Primary herpetic lesions last anywhere from 2–3 weeks, whereas recurrent herpes genitalis lasts 5–10 days. The typically painful ulcers of chancroid usually heal within a week. Lymphogranuloma venereum (LGV) ulcers heal rapidly and disappear within a few days. Ulcers due to invasive carcinoma tend to progress and do not heal over.

E. Is there a recent new partner? Frequently, a careful sexual history can uncover information which is helpful in determining the cause of genital ulcers. Incubation periods are:

> Chancroid: 3–5 days
> Syphilis: 10–90 days
> LGV: 4–21 days
> Granuloma inguinale: 7 days–several months

F. Does the sexual partner have a diagnosis/symptoms? Transmission of an STD is a possibility.

G. Does the patient have a history of prior STD? What was the treatment? Certain of the infectious genital ulcers have a tendency to recur, particularly if they were inadequately treated.

H. Is she an IV drug user? Using the groin? Secondary infection of injection sites can cause ulcers.

I. What is her HIV status? Risk factors? Genital ulcers may heal slowly or disseminate in the immunocompromised host.

III. Differential Diagnosis

A. Lymphogranuloma venereum. LGV is caused by *Chlamydia trachomatis* serotypes L1, L2, and L3, and is not commonly seen in the United States. The first stage of LGV is characterized by a papular or vesicular lesion, usually on the posterior vulva, which subsequently ulcerates. It often goes unnoticed by the patient since it is painless and heals spontaneously in several days. The second stage is typified by unilateral inquinal adenopathy, often accompanied by systemic symptoms (headache, myalgias, etc). About 10–20% will demonstrate a groove between the superficial inguinal and deep femoral lymph node chains, the so-called groove sign. These nodes may then suppurate, leading to draining sinuses (third stage).

B. Granuloma inguinale. Also known as donovanosis, the disease is caused by *Calymmatobacterium granulomatis*. It is quite uncommon in the United States. The clinical presentation is subtle, characterized by the onset of a painless papule or nodule which eventually ulcerates. The lesions are most frequently found on the external genitalia but may also be seen in the perianal, oral, and inguinal regions.

C. Chancroid. Also called "soft chancre," it is caused by *Haemophilus ducreyi.* Like LGV, syphilis, and granuloma inguinale, it is sexually transmitted. Unlike syphilis, it is relatively rare in the United States, though scattered epidemics have been seen in some inner city populations. Chancroid typically presents with multiple small papules that become pustular and eventually ulcerate. The ulcerative lesion is **very tender,** shallow with a ragged edge, and sits on an erythematous base ("halo"). Large, tender inguinal lymphadenopathy lesions called **buboes** develop in about half the patients. These may suppurate, resulting in a draining inguinal ulcer.

D. Herpes genitalis. This disease is caused by the herpes simplex virus (HSV) type 1 (15%) or type 2 (85%). Primary herpes may cause constitutional symptoms (headache, high fever, malaise, myalgias) along with very painful vulvovaginal lesions and inguinal adenopathy. The lesions begin as multiple papules and progress to vesicles which rupture, leaving numerous small ulcers. These may coalesce into larger ulcers. The lesions are present in primary herpes for 2–3 weeks. Uncommonly, primary herpes can cause hepatitis, meningitis, or encephalitis. Severe vulvar pain and sacral nerve dyssynergy can cause acute urine retention. Recurrent genital HSV disease has a similar but milder presentation which lasts (on average) half as long as primary HSV. Persistent or disseminated herpes should prompt an investigation for underlying immune competence (ie, HIV status).

E. Syphilis. Syphilis is caused by the spirochete *Treponema pallidum.* The primary lesion (chancre) is painless with a raised border, central ulceration, and an indurated base. However, many syphilitic chancres are atypical. The chancre appears anytime from 10 days–3 months after exposure. Although easier to visualize on the vulva, it more commonly presents on the cervix or in the vagina where it may be missed. Other sites of chancre involvement include the mouth, anus, nipple, and oropharynx. The chancre resolves spontaneously in 2–6 weeks. If untreated, secondary syphilis develops (ie, condyloma latum) followed by a latent phase. If still untreated, about 1 in 3 patients will develop tertiary syphilis with involvement of the cardiovascular, musculoskeletal, or central nervous system. Transplacental passage of the spirochete with fetal infection can occur at any stage.

F. Carcinoma. Invasive squamous cell carcinoma of the vulva or basal cell carcinoma may present as a genital ulcer. Biopsy is the only reliable way to exclude malignancy.

G. Behçet's disease. The disorder is characterized by the triad of genital ulcerations, oropharyngeal ulcerations, and uveitis. It may also cause a vasculitis, gastrointestinal tract involvement, synovitis, and neurologic symptoms.

H. Trauma.

IV. Database

A. Physical examination key points

1. **Vital signs.** Fever may be present, particularly with primary herpes genitalis or secondarily infected genital ulcers of any cause.
2. **Oral cavity.** The mucosa should be inspected for lesions.
3. **Eyes.** Uveitis occurs in Behçet's disease. Look for inflammation of the choroid as noted by deposits of yellow or white dots on the cornea.
4. **Vulva.** The physical appearance of the lesion(s) is important to direct further diagnostic studies. Note if the lesion is tender (herpes, chancroid, granuloma inguinale, trauma, secondarily infected ulcers) or not (LGV, syphilis, most neoplasms), and whether it is secondarily infected (ie, covered with an exudate). **Syphilitic** chancres appear "punched out", ie, a smooth raised border with a clean, non-necrotic, indurated base. Contrast that with the lesion of **chancroid,** which has a "dirty" (necrotic) base without induration (hence the term "soft" chancre). In addition, chancroid usually causes multiple shallow lesions with shaggy, irregular borders. The lesion of **LGV** begins most often on the posterior portion of the vulva as a papule or vesicle and then ulcerates. The vulvar lesion of **granuloma inguinale** produces a characteristic beefy red, granulomatous, velvety ulcer. **Herpetic** lesions begin as small clusters of vesicles on an erythematous base which rupture, leaving small ulcers that crust over and heal.
5. **Inguinal lymph nodes.**
   a. **Syphilis.** There is a painless inguinal adenopathy.

b. **Herpes.** Inguinal adenopathy is seen only with primary herpes.
c. **Granuloma inguinale.** No adenopathy occurs unless the patient is secondarily infected.
d. **Chancroid.** Buboes develop 7–10 days after the lesion appears. They are unilateral in > 50% of patients and may rupture, resulting in inguinal ulcer.
e. **LGV.** A unilateral progressive adenopathy begins 1–4 weeks after the initial lesion. The "groove sign" is seen in 10–20% of patients.

B. Laboratory data

1. **Biopsy.** Unless the examiner is convinced that the lesion is nonneoplastic, a biopsy should be performed and sent for histologic analysis. The procedure can be performed simply with a local anesthetic and a dermatologic (Keyes) punch biopsy instrument. Suturing is rarely necessary.

2. **Culture.** If the lesion is not biopsied, it should be abraded at the base so that it weeps serum and then cultured. Because these ulcers are usually from STDs, other STDs should be sought (gonorrhea and *Chlamydia* cervical culture, HIV, HBsAG, and syphilis serology). The investigation of the various infectious causes is as follows.

   a. **Syphilis.** Dark-field microscopy allows visualization of the spirochetes. Serologic testing is usually negative if the primary chancre is present.
   b. **Herpes.** Unroof vesicles and collect fluid on a cotton swab for culture. The specimen must be sent in viral transport media.
   c. **LGV.** Complement fixation is probably the most frequently used test, and if > 1 : 64 is considered diagnostic. Besides serum for complement fixation, a swab of the lesion should be obtained and sent for culture and direct fluorescent antibody (FA). The specimen should only be sent in *Chlamydia* transport media (2SP). Fluctuant nodes can also be aspirated and sent for FA and culture. The Frei intradermal test cannot differentiate between acute and past infections.
   d. **Granuloma inguinale.** The granulomatous lesions are fairly characteristic and the diagnosis can be made clinically. A biopsy of the lesion can be sent for Giemsa or Wright stain to look for Donovan bodies (intracellular gram-negative rods).
   e. **Chancroid.** Gram stain and culture of the lesion or aspirated material from the bubo is the most definitive method to diagnose chancroid. However, the organism (*H. ducreyi*) is fastidious, and the microbiology lab

should be alerted that the specimen needs to be set up for isolation of this bacterium. Gram stain may reveal gram-negative rods, which tend to form chains. However the diagnosis must often be made by the appearance of the lesion because of the lack of corroborative microbiologic evidence.

V. Plan

A. General management

1. Specific treatment for each disease is given in Table 1–12.
2. All recent sexual partners should be examined and treated with a recommended regimen.
3. Treatment failures may occur with any of these regimens, and follow-up is mandatory.

B. Herpes in pregnancy.
During pregnancy, herpes genitalis poses unique problems with regard to mode of delivery. A management sequence based on current knowledge of the acquisi-

TABLE 1–12. TREATMENT OF SEXUALLY TRANSMITTED DISEASES.

Disease	Primary Treatment	Alternative
Syphilis	Benzathine PCN 2.4 million units IM × 1 dose	Tetracycline or erythromycin 500 mg qid × 15 days
Herpes		
Primary	Acyclovir 5 mg/kg q8h IV × 7–10 days (inpatient)	Acyclovir 200 mg 5 × daily PO × 7–10 days (outpatient)
Disseminated encephalitis hepatitis meningitis	Acyclovir 10 mg/kg q8h IV	
Frequent recurrence	Acyclovir 200 mg 5 × daily PO × 5 days	Acyclovir 800 mg PO bid × 5 days
Chronic suppression	Acyclovir 200 mg PO 2–5 × daily	Acyclovir 400 mg PO bid
LGV	Doxycycline 100 mg × 3 weeks and *aspirate* fluctuant nodes; do *not* I & D lymph nodes	Tetracycline or erythromycin 500 mg PO qid × 3 weeks
GI	Tetracycline 500 mg PO qid × 3 weeks or until all lesions are healed	
Chancroid	Ceftriaxone 250 mg IM qid × 7 days	Erythromycin 500 mg PO qid or Bactrim 2 tablets PO bid × 7 days

LGV = lymphogranuloma venereum; GI = granuloma inguinale.

TABLE 1-13. MODE OF DELIVERY FOR HERPES-INFECTED PATIENTS.

Perform Cesarean Section	Allow Vaginal Delivery
1. Active (visible) genital lesions in labor or with ROM, either primary or recurrent.	**1.** Recent recurrent lesion with subsequent negative culture and no active current lesion.
2. Primary herpes within 3–4 weeks of labor or ROM (unless negative cervical culture and no lesions).	**2.** History of herpes without lesions or symptoms.
3. Recurrent lesion within 2–3 weeks of labor or ROM (unless negative cervical culture and no lesions).	**3.** Recurrent lesion more than 3 weeks ago (must be reliable history) without culture.
4. Symptoms of recurrent lesion prior to development of a visible lesion.	

ROM = rupture of membranes.
There is currently no support for weekly cultures in the last month of gestation in the patient with a history of herpes.

tion of neonatal encephalitis and the duration of viral shedding is presented in Table 1–13.

REFERENCES

Centers for Disease Control: 1989 sexually transmitted diseases treatment guidelines. *MMWR* 38, No. S–8, 1989.
Holmes KK et al (eds): *Sexually Transmitted Diseases.* New York, McGraw-Hill, 1984.
Knox JM, Rudolph AH: Acquired infectious syphilis. In Holmes KK et al (eds): *Sexually Transmitted Diseases.* New York, McGraw-Hill, 1984.
Musher DM: Biology of *Treponema pallidum.* In Holmes KK et al (eds): *Sexually Transmitted Diseases.* New York, McGraw-Hill, 1984.
Perine PL, Osoba A: Lymphogranuloma venereum. In Holmes KK et al (eds): *Sexually Transmitted Diseases.* New York, McGraw-Hill, 1984.
Sarling PF: Natural history of syphilis. In Holmes KK et al (eds): *Sexually Transmitted Diseases.* New York, McGraw-Hill, 1984.

43. HEMATEMESIS

I. Problem. Ten days after undergoing a radical hysterectomy, a 65-year-old patient suddenly begins vomiting blood.

II. Immediate Questions

A. What are the blood pressure and orthostatic signs? The initial management focuses on maintaining intravascular volume and perfusion pressure. Orthostatic hypotension is the best on-the-ward estimate of volume loss.

B. Any bleeding tendencies? Review available history, physical examination, and lab data regarding any correctable coagulation deficit.

C. What medications is the patient taking? Ulcerogenic medications include aspirin and other nonsteroidal anti-inflammatory agents; excessive anticoagulation with warfarin or heparin may cause GI tract bleeding.

D. Any stigmata of alcohol abuse? Of the major causes of upper GI bleeding, only esophageal varices are associated with any physical signs. Obtain history and physical signs for cirrhosis and portal hypertension, but keep in mind that a diagnosis of cirrhosis does not equate with a diagnosis of variceal bleed.

E. Did the patient wretch or vomit nonbloody material prior to the hematemesis? A Mallory-Weiss tear is the fourth most common cause of hematemesis in most series, and the patient, nurses, or any observer should be carefully asked about the episode. "Coffee ground" emesis indicates that the blood was in the stomach long enough to be converted by gastric acid from hemoglobin to methemoglobin.

F. Does the patient have any history of aortic disease or a prior aortic vascular procedure? Although low on the list of causes of hematemesis, aortoduodenal fistula should always be included in the initial differential diagnosis of an upper gastrointestinal (UGI) bleed. The phenomenon of a sentinel bleed allows some of these patients to be salvaged, but only if the diagnosis is made quickly.

III. Differential Diagnosis. Hematemesis is virtually always associated with bleeding proximal to the ligament of Treitz. However, the converse is certainly not true. In most recent series, ulcer disease, gastritis, esophageal varices, and Mallory-Weiss tears account for 90–95% of episodes of hematemesis.

A. Esophagus

1. **Esophageal varices.** They may be associated with cirrhosis and portal hypertension.
2. **Mallory-Weiss tear.** Usually a mucosal tear at the gastroesophageal junction, it is associated with severe retching with or without vomiting.
3. **Esophagitis.** The classic history is of heartburn, "water brash" (regurgitation of gastric contents), and worsening of symptoms with recumbency.
4. **Esophageal tumors.** These include benign squamous or adenocarcinomas.

B. Stomach
1. **Gastritis.** Significant hematemesis usually indicates severe stress gastritis, most often alcohol related.
2. **Gastric ulcer.** Pain is classically exacerbated by eating, but may also be relieved with eating. Up to 42% are associated with duodenal ulcer.
3. **Gastric tumors.** These include metastatic gynecologic tumors such as ovarian carcinoma.
4. **Gastric varices.**

C. Duodenum
1. **Duodenal ulcer.**
2. **Aortoduodenal fistula.** This occurs almost exclusively in cases of aortic reconstruction.
3. **Metastatic gynecologic tumors** such as ovarian carcinoma.

D. Hemobilia. Bleeding into the biliary passages is usually secondary to trauma, infection, stone disease, or iatrogenic causes.

E. Systemic causes
1. **Coagulopathy** (disseminated intravascular coagulation, leukemia, etc).
2. **Osler-Weber-Rendu syndrome.** This is associated with multiple telangiectases.
3. **Peutz-Jeghers syndrome.** Multiple hamartomas occur in this disorder.

F. Non-GI source (nasopharyngeal bleeding).

IV. Database

A. Physical examination key points
1. **Vital signs.** Orthostatic blood pressure measurements are a sensitive guide to blood loss.
2. **Abdomen.** Look for scars from a prior ulcer or from a vascular or other procedure, pain or peritoneal signs, and evidence of portal hypertension such as splenomegaly, caput medusae, or ascites.
3. **Rectum.** Check for gross blood or melena.
4. **Skin.** Cool, moist, pale skin indicates significant volume loss. Look for evidence of alcohol abuse such as spider angiomas or palmar erythema, and for signs of systemic disease including multiple bruises, telangiectases, or hamartomas of the lips or oral mucosa.
5. **HEENT.** Search for evidence of epistaxis or other nasopharyngeal source.

B. Laboratory data

1. **Hemogram.** Obtain serial hematocrits and document the time drawn and relation to transfusions.
2. **Platelet count.** Verify there are adequate numbers.
3. **Coagulation studies.** PT and PTT help to identify a potentially correctable deficit in the coagulation cascade.
4. **Bleeding time.** Assesses platelet function in patients taking aspirin or nonsteroidal anti-inflammatory agents.
5. **Renal function.** This should be determined as a baseline.
6. **Liver function tests.** Do these to document liver disease.
7. **Blood bank specimen.** Remember with the initial blood draw to type and cross-match for up to 6–10 units of blood.

C. Radiologic and other studies

1. **Chest x-ray.** This will document aspiration.
2. **Place an NG tube.** This documents ongoing bleeding and clears the stomach for endoscopy. A Ewald or large Salem sump tube may be needed to evacuate large volumes of clot.
3. **Upper endoscopy.** In most hospitals this is the diagnostic procedure of choice (and sometimes is therapeutic). Diagnostic accuracy is 85–95%.
4. **UGI series.** This study may be used if endoscopy is unavailable and if bleeding has stopped. It interferes with endoscopy, and angiography is not usually a first-line study.
5. **Angiography.** Rarely used unless endoscopy does not identify the source. Diagnostic success requires bleeding > 0.5–1.0 mL/min.

V. Plan. Bleeding can be excessive, and up to 50% of patients with massive UGI bleed from varices will die. Treat volume loss, establish the diagnosis, and implement specific therapies. Continued bleeding in any of these conditions requires the appropriate surgical intervention. However, about 85% of cases will resolve without operative intervention.

A. Emergency management

1. Insert large-bore (16-gauge or larger) IV catheters and begin crystalloid.
2. Type and cross-match for packed red blood cells (6 units minimum). Attempt to keep hematocrit > 30%.
3. Monitor volume replacement.
   a. Always chart serial hematocrits, timing, and amount of transfusions since this measures the rate of bleeding, which is the major criterion to decide if surgery is needed in many instances.
   b. Place a Foley catheter to follow urine output as a measure of volume status.

      c. Insert a central line if needed, especially in patients with cardiac or respiratory disease.
   4. Correct coagulopathy with platelets or fresh-frozen plasma.
   5. Insert an NG tube and irrigate with iced saline or water until clear. Cold lavage causes vasoconstriction. The temperature of the irrigant may not be terribly important, however: what matters is clearing the material from the stomach.
   6. Consider endotracheal intubation to protect the airway from aspiration, especially with altered mental status.

B. Ulcer
   1. Give antacids via NG tube q1–2h.
   2. An H_2 blocker (cimetidine) may prevent rebleeding but probably does not stop ongoing bleeding.
   3. Coagulation of a bleeding site during endoscopy is often possible.
   4. During angiography, selective embolization or vasopressin infusion may control bleeding.

C. Stress gastritis
   1. Treat with antacids.
   2. H_2 blockers have no effect in active bleeding.

D. Esophageal varices
   1. Perform injection sclerotherapy by endoscopy.
   2. Start vasopressin 0.4–0.6 units/min by peripheral IV for 1 hour. Repeat q3h if successful.
   3. Attempt balloon tamponade (Sengstaken-Blakemore tube) only if experienced since complications of aspiration, respiratory arrest, and esophageal rupture are possible.

E. Mallory-Weiss tear
   1. Vasopressin is of unclear effectiveness.
   2. Do angiographic embolization.

F. Metastatic tumors
   1. Follow emergency recommendations above.
   2. Resect the involved gastric or duodenal tissue.

REFERENCE

Leavitt J, Barkin JS: Upper gastrointestinal bleeding. *Hosp Med* 18:102, 1982.

44. HYPERCALCEMIA

I. Problem. The clinical chemistry laboratory calls to tell you that one of your patients, a 45-year-old woman scheduled for surgery in the morning, has a serum calcium of 12.5 mg/dL (normal 8.5–10.5 mg/dL).

II. Immediate Questions

A. Is the patient symptomatic? Delirium, confusion, stupor and emotional lability, polydipsia, polyuria, anorexia, nausea, and vomiting are seen with symptomatic hypercalcemia.

B. Has the patient recently had surgery? In particular, adrenal surgery (hypoadrenalism) or long-term immobilization, which can cause excessive bone resorption.

C. What IV fluids and medications are currently being given? The patient may be receiving medications that cause increased calcium levels (thiazide diuretics, vitamin D) or administration of exogenous calcium.

III. Differential Diagnosis (see also Chapter 2.)

A. Hyperparathyroidism. About 20% of patients with hypercalcemia will have hyperparathyroidism. The primary disorder is usually diagnosed by elevated calcium, low phosphate, and elevated parathyroid hormone.

B. Malignancy. This can be caused by bone metastasis or by factors secreted by the tumors (multiple myeloma, lung, breast, kidney, cervix) and is the most frequent cause.

C. Thiazide diuretics. Agents such as hydrochlorothiazide cause increased renal resorption of calcium.

D. Sarcoidosis. The granulomatous tissue may produce a vitamin D metabolite.

E. Vitamin D intoxication. This history will usually reveal chronic ingestion.

F. Milk-alkali syndrome. This results from excessive alkali and calcium given in the treatment of peptic ulcer disease (less frequent today with the use of magnesium-containing antacids).

G. Hyperthyroidism.

H. Adrenal insufficiency.

I. Paget's disease.

J. Acute tubular necrosis (diuretic phase).

K. Acromegaly.

L. Excessive calcium administration.

M. Long-term immobilization.

IV. Database. The classic history is "stones, bones, moans, and abdominal groans" with weight loss.

A. Physical examination key points

1. **Vital signs.** Hypertension may accompany hypercalcemia.
2. **Heart.** Arrhythmias may include bradycardia or tachycardia.
3. **Abdomen.** Check for masses.
4. **Chest.** Breast carcinoma may be suggested by a mass lesion or prior mastectomy.
5. **Bones.** Tenderness to percussion may indicate metastatic disease.
6. **Nodes.** Lymphadenopathy occurs with cancer or sarcoidosis.
7. **Neurologic examination.** Weakness, hyperactive reflexes, and impaired mentation (stupor, delirium) may be present.

B. Laboratory data

1. **Serum calcium and albumin.** Confirm elevation on a repeat determination. **Caution:** The units of calcium measurement may differ from one institution to another (mg/dL vs meq/dL). If the albumin is not normal, a corrected calcium level must be determined (see page 300). Symptoms usually appear at levels of 13 mg/dL.
2. **Phosphorus.** Levels are usually low in hyperparathyroidism except when renal failure is present.
3. **Potassium and magnesium.** Decreases may be associated with a high serum calcium level.
4. **Arterial blood gases.** Acidosis occurs with hyperchlorhydria.
5. **Alkaline phosphatase.** The level is elevated in hyperparathyroidism with bone disease and metastasis to the bone.
6. **Renal function.** Renal insufficiency will exacerbate hypercalcemia.
7. **Parathyroid hormone (PTH).** The level is increased in primary or secondary hyperparathyroidism and is often decreased in hypercalcemia not due to hyperparathyroidism.

C. Radiologic and other studies

1. **Abdominal x-ray.** The film may show renal stones with hyperparathyroidism.
2. **Chest x-ray.** CXR may show hilar adenopathy with sarcoidosis or lymphoma.
3. **Skull films.** Typical punched-out lesions of multiple myeloma may be visualized.
4. **Barium swallow.** The esophagus can be displaced with parathyroid adenoma.
5. **Bone films.** They may show osteolytic lesions of metastatic cancer.
6. **Intravenous pyelogram.** The IVP will often reveal renal

stones with hyperparathyroidism and, occasionally, renal cell carcinoma which may have associated hypercalcemia.

7. **Electrocardiogram.** Hypercalcemia is associated with a shortened QT interval and prolonged PR interval.

8. **Cortisone suppression test.** There is no response in hyperparathyroidism, but metastatic cancer, myeloma, sarcoid, vitamin D intoxication, milk-alkali syndrome, and adrenal insufficiency will usually respond with a decrease in calcium.

V. Plan

A. **Initial management.** First lower the serum calcium if necessary, then control the underlying cause.

1. **Levels < 12 mg/dL.** Therapy is usually directed only at the underlying cause.

2. **Moderate elevation (12–15 mg/dL).** Treat with hydration and loop diuretics initially (see below).

3. **Severe hypercalcemia (> 15 mg/dL) or any symptomatic patient regardless of level.** This is a life-threatening emergency requiring more rigorous therapy.

B. **Specific plans**

1. Restrict calcium intake, encourage mobilization, and treat the underlying disorder in all cases.

2. Institute saline diuresis to restore volume and produce at least 1500–2000 mL per day of urine. Sodium increases calcium excretion by competing for resorption in the distal tubule. In the presence of renal or cardiac failure this must be done with caution. Monitor serum calcium, phosphate, potassium, magnesium, and BUN.

3. Furosemide 20–40 mg IV q2–4h can be given to bring calcium below 12 mg/dL after hydration. Carefully monitor serum potassium during diuresis, and replace as necessary.

4. Give mithramycin 15–25 µg/kg in 1 L saline over 3–6 hours. This agent is used most often for PTH-producing malignancies, osteolytic malignancies, vitamin D intoxication, and non-PTH-producing tumors such as myeloma.

5. Give magnesium sulfate 2 meq/kg IV over 8–12 hours (20% solution = 8 meq/mL) to correct hypomagnesemia.

6. Corticosteroids are used with malignancies. They are ineffective against primary hyperparathyroidism, and may take 1–2 weeks to produce an effect. Prednisone 5–15 mg PO qd is fairly typical dosing.

7. Dialysis is used as a last resort if extremely high calcium levels cannot be treated.

8. Other agents include calcitonin, indomethacin, phosphate, etidronate, and pamidronate.

REFERENCE

Zaloga G, Chernow B: Life threatening electrolyte and metabolic abnormalities. In Parillo J (ed): *Current Therapy in Critical Care Medicine.* Toronto, BC Decker, 1987, pp 245–257.

45. HYPERGLYCEMIA (See Problem 7, page 40).

46. HYPERKALEMIA

I. **Problem.** An obese 58-year-old patient with stage II-B adenocarcinoma of the endometrium has a potassium of 7.1 mmol/L on the second postoperative day (normal 3.5–5.1 mmol/L).

II. **Immediate Questions**

A. **What are the vital signs?** Check this first, as the cardiac effects of hyperkalemia can result in life-threatening arrhythmias.

B. **What is the patient's urine output?** Renal failure with inability to excrete either endogenous or exogenous potassium load is a common cause of acute hyperkalemia on a surgical service. Evaluate urine output and recent renal function chemistries.

C. **Is the patient receiving potassium in an intravenous solution?** Often a standard IV solution contains 20–40 meq/L of potassium, and hyperalimentation solutions may contain more. When beginning the initial evaluation of an abnormal potassium value, stop all exogenous potassium until the problem is resolved.

D. **Is the lab result accurate?** In the example given above, hyperkalemia is an almost expected outcome. However, abnormally elevated potassium levels are often entirely unexpected or inconsistent. If the lab does not notify you, inquire about hemolysis of the specimen, which can falsely elevate the potassium.

E. **Is the patient taking any medication that could raise her potassium level?** If the patient is receiving spironolactone, triamterene, or indomethacin, stop these medications immediately.

III. **Differential Diagnosis.** The measured laboratory value of 7.1 mmol/L for extracellular potassium concentration is a level that correlates with the harmful consequences of hyperkalemia. The extracellular level can be increased by redistribution of potassium from intracellular stores (where 98% of the total body potassium is located) or by a real increase in total body potassium.

A. Redistribution
1. Acidosis.
2. Insulin deficiency.
3. Digoxin overdose.
4. Succinylcholine.
5. Cellular breakdown.
   a. Rhabdomyolysis.
   b. Hemolysis.

B. Increased total body potassium
1. Renal causes
   a. **Acute renal failure.**
   b. **Chronic renal failure.** Potassium will not usually be elevated until end-stage disease.
   c. **Renal tubular dysfunction.** This may be associated with renal transplant, lupus erythematosus, sickle cell disease, or myeloma.
2. Mineralocorticoid deficiency
   a. **Addison's disease.**
   b. **Hypoaldosteronism** (hyporeninemic).
3. **Drug-induced.** Common causes:
   a. Spironolactone.
   b. Triamterene.
   c. Indomethacin, which is thought to interfere with renal prostaglandin levels.
   d. Chemotherapy. The effect may be secondary to emesis, diuresis, or direct action on kidney tubules (ie, cisplatin).

C. Pseudohyperkalemia
1. **Hemolysis of the specimen.**
2. **Prolonged period of tourniquet occlusion** prior to blood draw.
3. **Thrombocytosis/leukocytosis.** White blood cells and platelets release potassium as the clot forms.

IV. Database

A. Physical examination key points
1. **Heart.** Bradycardia, ventricular fibrillation, and asystole are seen with markedly elevated levels.
2. **Neurologic examination.** Neuromuscular findings include tingling, weakness, flaccid paralysis, and hyperactive deep tendon reflexes. However, cardiac arrest often precedes these symptoms.

B. Laboratory data
1. **Electrolytes, BUN, and creatinine.** Hyperkalemia is usu-

ally diagnosed by this study, and renal failure may be detected.

2. **Arterial blood gases.** Non-anion-gap acidosis is associated with hyperkalemia.
3. **Platelet count, white blood count.** Elevations may yield factitious hyperkalemia.
4. **Cortisol levels or ACTH stimulation test.**
5. **Myoglobin level in serum or urine.** This determination may be useful in crush injury.

C. **Radiologic and other studies**
   1. **Electrocardiogram.** The ECG is the second most important test besides the potassium level, and a means to separate pseudohyperkalemia from actual elevations of potassium. Changes seen as potassium increases include peaked T waves, flat P waves, prolonged PR interval, and a widened QRS complex progressing to a sine wave and arrest.

V. **Plan.** The severity of hyperkalemia as judged by the serum level and ECG dictate treatment. In general, aggressive treatment of hyperkalemia is indicated for a serum potassium > 7 mmol/L or if ECG changes are present. The methods of treatment ranked by the rapidity of the response are mechanisms which counteract membrane effects of hyperkalemia, move potassium into cells, and remove potassium from the body.

A. **Prevention of further hyperkalemia.** Remove all potassium from intravenous fluids.

B. **Calcium Administration.** Counteract membrane effects and protect the heart by giving calcium gluconate 10–20 mL of a 10% solution IV over 3–5 minutes with the patient on a cardiac monitor.

C. **Potassium shifts.** Transfer potassium to the intracellular compartment.
   1. **Sodium bicarbonate.** Give 1 ampule (44 meq) IV; may repeat 1–2 times q20–30min. Bicarbonate works best in acidotic patients but also has effects in patients with normal pH.
   2. **Insulin/glucose.** Administer 1 ampule of D50W and 10 units of regular insulin IV.
   3. **Combination therapy.** A combination of the above two methods consists of 1 L D10W mixed with 3 ampules of sodium bicarbonate given over 2–4 hours with regular insulin 10 units SQ q4–6h.

D. **Removal of potassium from the body**
   1. **Kayexalate** (exchange resin)
      a. **Oral.** Give 40 g in 25–50 mL of 70% sorbitol q2–4h.

    b. Rectal. Give 50–100 g in 200 mL water as a retention enema for 30 minutes q2–4h.
2. **Dialysis.** Peritoneal dialysis or hemodialysis may be effective.
3. **Furosemide.** Monitor urine output and volume status carefully. Administer furosemide IV.

REFERENCE

Demling RH, Wilson RF: Hyperkalemia. In *Decision Making in Surgical Intensive Care.* Toronto, BC Decker, 1988, pp 146–147.

47. HYPERNATREMIA

I. Problem. The clinical chemistry lab calls to tell you that an 85-year-old female patient has a serum sodium of 155 mmol/L (normal 136–145 mmol/L).

II. Immediate Questions

  A. Is the patient alert and oriented or is she seizing? Symptoms of hypernatremia (irritability, ataxia, anorexia, cramping) usually do not appear until the level is > 160 mmol/L. Levels > 180 mmol/L may result in confusion, stupor, or seizure. The more rapid the change in sodium level, the more likely it will be symptomatic.

  B. What medications is the patient taking? Diuretics can cause water loss leading to hypernatremia.

  C. What are the intake/output values for the past few days? An effective loss of total body water by fluid deprivation (inadequate administration of fluids) can cause hypernatremia.

  D. Are there underlying conditions? Certain diseases, most notably diabetes insipidus, are associated with hypernatremia.

  E. Is the lab value accurate? As with any lab result that is unexpected, the error could be from the lab itself. It may be of value to repeat the test.

  F. What is the composition of IV fluids administered? Check the sodium content of fluids. Is the patient receiving adequate free water (usually 35 mL/kg/24h for an adult)?

III. Differential Diagnosis. The differential diagnosis is best considered in light of the cause of hypernatremia. The disorder is due to loss of total body water and is rarely associated with increased total body sodium.

A. **Inadequate fluid intake.** Water deprivation may be the cause, particularly in postoperative patients.

B. **Increased water loss.** Most body fluids are hypotonic with respect to sodium; thus, excessive losses lead to hyponatremia.
   1. **Nonrenal losses**
      a. **Gastrointestinal losses.** The cause may be NG suction, diarrhea, or fistulas.
      b. **Pulmonary losses.** Insensible losses occur especially in intubated patients who are not receiving adequate humidification.
      c. **Cutaneous losses.** In a febrile patient, insensible losses increase 500 mL/24 hours for each degree centigrade increase above 38.3 degrees.
   2. **Renal losses**
      a. **Diuretics.**
      b. **Hypercalcemic nephropathy.**
      c. **Hypokalemic nephropathy.**
      d. **Diabetes insipidus** (true vs nephrogenic).
      e. **Acute tubular necrosis,** pyloric phase.
      f. **Postobstructive diuresis.** This effect is usually caused by the relief of longstanding bilateral renal obstruction.
      g. **Diabetes mellitus.** Diabetes can result from osmotic diuresis caused by glycosuria.
      h. **Drugs.** These include lithium, alcohol, phenytoin, colchicine, and mannitol.

C. **Administration of hypertonic saline.** There are no indications for the routine administration of hypertonic saline in surgical patients. Hypertonic saline solutions have been administered prior to chemotherapy such as with cisplatin.

D. **Increased mineralocorticoids or glucocorticoids**
   1. **Primary aldosteronism.**
   2. **Cushing's syndrome.**
   3. **Ectopic ACTH production.**

IV. **Database**
   A. **Physical examination key points**
      1. **Vital signs.** Orthostatic blood pressure changes, tachycardia, and decreased weight suggest volume loss.
      2. **Skin.** Check turgor. Mucous membranes may be dry with volume contraction.
      3. **Neurologic examination.** Look for signs of irritability, weakness, twitching, or seizures.

   B. **Laboratory data**
      1. **Serum electrolytes.** Often an electrolyte disorder involves more than one extracellular ion.

       2. Serum osmolality. Osmolality is increased with volume loss normal (280–295 mosm/L).

       3. Urine osmolality. Hypertonic urine suggests extrarenal fluid loss, while isotonic or hypotonic urine suggests renal losses (normal 500–1200 mosm/L).

       4. Spot urine sodium. A level < 20 meq/L suggests extrarenal volume losses.

  C. Radiologic and other studies. Not usually helpful.

V. Plan. The overall plan is to slowly replace free water to bring the serum sodium concentration down to normal levels. Volume repletion is especially important in patients showing orthostasis on blood pressure measurement. Correction should be gradual to prevent the development of cerebral edema, which can precipitate seizures.

  A. Determine the volume deficit. Use the actual total body water (TBW) to determine the volume of free water needed to correct serum sodium:

$$\text{Water deficit} = (0.6 \times \text{weight in kg}) - \text{TBW}$$

$$\text{TBW} = \frac{140}{\text{Serum Na}} \times (0.6 \times \text{weight in kg})$$

  B. Replace the deficit. Administer fluids over a 24-hour period as 5% dextrose in water. Alternatively, if a patient is receiving 5% dextrose in 0.45N saline, the extra free water can be given by increasing the rate of fluid and changing it to 5% dextrose in 0.2N saline.

  C. Treat the underlying cause.

       1. Replace unusually large nonrenal losses of free water, such as small bowel or pancreatic fistula drainage (see Chapter 4 on fluids and electrolytes).

       2. Treat diabetes mellitus with insulin (see Problem 7, page 40).

       3. Treat diabetes insipidus with adequate free water or with vasopressin.

REFERENCE

Demling RH, Wilson RF: Hypernatremia. In *Decision Making in Surgical Intensive Care.* Toronto, BC Decker, 1988, pp 142–143.

48. HYPERTENSION

I. Problem. After total abdominal hysterectomy and bilateral salpingo-oophorectomy, a 45-year-old woman has a blood pressure of 190/110 in the recovery room.

II. Immediate Questions

A. Is there associated tachycardia and tachypnea? Postoperative pain is often manifested by tachycardia and hypertension; the addition of tachypnea should alert you to the possibility of postoperative hypoxia, especially in the presence of agitation.

B. Is there a past history of hypertension? Mild blood pressure elevations are often seen in hypertensive patients after large intraoperative fluid infusions; this is rarely worrisome in the absence of other findings.

C. Is the patient having chest pain? Severe hypertension often places significant strain on the heart of a patient with a history of coronary artery disease; it can cause angina or infarction and requires rapid control. Aortic dissection is also an emergency and may cause back and chest pain.

D. What are the patient's usual and current medications? Sympathomimetic agents at incorrect doses can cause hypertension. Carefully check dilutions and rates of all drips. Steroids and oral contraceptives can elevate the blood pressure. To prevent postoperative hypertension, most cardiac medications and antihypertensives, with the exception of diuretics, should be given in their usual doses with a small sip of water the morning of operation.

III. Differential Diagnosis.

Classically, there are six surgically correctable causes of hypertension: coarctation of the aorta, pheochromocytoma, Cushing's syndrome, primary hyperaldosteronism, unilateral renal parenchymal disease, and renovascular hypertension. (See also Table 1–14, page 200.)

A. Postoperative
1. **Pain-induced.**
2. **Fluid overload.**
3. **Hypoxia.**
4. **Vasospasm.** Loss of body temperature frequently takes place during surgery; this often results in the patient "clamping down" to preserve body heat.

B. Essential hypertension. Among patients with chronic hypertension, there is no known cause in 90–95% of cases.

C. Secondary hypertension
1. **Renal.** The problem may be vascular or parenchymal.
2. **Endocrine.** Causes include pheochromocytoma and Cushing's syndrome.
3. **Drug-induced.** Oral contraceptives, amphetamines, ketamine, and other sympathomimetics may cause hypertension.

4. **Pregnancy.** Preeclampsia or eclampsia may be responsible (see Problems 8, 18, and 21 on pages 44, 76, and 88).
5. **Coarctation.**
6. **Increased intracranial pressure.** This is usually associated with bradycardia and may be caused by tumor, subarachnoid bleed, or other factors.
7. **Polycythemia vera.**

D. **Factitious.** Using too small a blood pressure cuff on an obese arm may falsely elevate readings.

IV. Database

A. **Physical examination key points**
1. **Vital signs.** Measure pressure in both arms. Check the core body temperature, especially in patients in the recovery room, as hypothermia may markedly raise pressure.
2. **Lungs.** Listen for rales indicating pulmonary edema and possible heart failure.
3. **Abdomen.** Look for a pulsatile mass with aneurysm or a bruit with renovascular hypertension.
4. **HEENT.** Papilledema, retinal hemorrhages, or exudates may be present. Papilledema represents increased intracranial pressure or malignant hypertension.
5. **Neurologic examination.** Focal changes may represent cerebral ischemia.

B. **Laboratory data**
1. **Arterial blood gases.** These tests should be performed if there is any question about hypoxemia.
2. **Urinalysis, BUN, and serum creatinine.** They indicate the level of renal function since hypertension can accompany renal insufficiency.
3. **Serum catecholamines, urinary vanillylmandelic acid (VMA), and metanephrines.** These are needed only if you suspect pheochromocytoma.
4. **Dexamethasone suppression test.** This can be obtained later to test for Cushing's syndrome (see page 307).

C. **Radiologic and other studies**
1. **Electrocardiogram.** Perform an ECG in most elderly patients after major cardiac, thoracic, or vascular surgery, and in patients with a history of heart disease after any major operation. In the presence of hypertension, the ECG may show ischemic changes in the absence of symptoms.
2. **Pulmonary artery catheter.** Placement of a PA catheter to determine cardiac output and pulmonary capillary wedge

pressure facilitates the evaluation of cardiac function in critically ill, hypertensive postoperative patients. Its use is not indicated in the vast majority of cases.

3. Although not typically a surgical evaluation, thorough assessment for secondary causes of hypertension should be done for new-onset hypertension in patients under 30 or over 60 and in those failing a variety of drug regimens. This often includes renal arteriography, selective renal vein renin measurements, and determination of urinary catecholamines, VMA, and serum cortisol.

V. Plan

A. Emergency management. Severe hypertension from causes including hypertensive encephalopathy, malignant hypertension, and dissecting aortic aneurysm is usually treated emergently with sodium nitroprusside (see page 528). Other agents can be used to control hypertension acutely (diazoxide, labetalol, or hydralazine) but do not offer the advantage of titration that nitroprusside does.

B. Preoperative. The goal is to obtain good control of blood pressure before performing elective procedures.

1. Check the ECG for signs of ischemia or failure.
2. All blood pressure and cardiac medications except diuretics may be given on the morning of operation.
3. Weight loss and a low-salt diet should be encouraged.
4. Typical staged therapy includes starting with a beta blocker or thiazide diuretic. Thiazides work better in black patients. If a second agent is needed, add whichever first-line agent was not used. If there are contraindications to the use of beta blockers (asthma, heart failure), central antiadrenergic agents (methyldopa, clonidine) or anti-alpha-adrenergic agents can be used. Third-line drugs include hydralazine, prazosin, and angiotensin-converting enzyme (ACE) inhibitors (captopril). Hydralazine can cause reflex tachycardia in the non-beta-blocked patient. Calcium channel blockers are now frequently used. Drug doses are listed in Chapter 7.

C. Postoperative

1. Ensure adequate oxygenation and pain relief, and warm the patient with blankets or heating blanket if necessary.
2. **Mild hypertension.** This can be treated with a variety of agents. In the immediate postoperative period, sublingual nifedipine 10–20 mg is useful and rarely causes hypotension. Hydralazine 5–10 mg IV may be used in elderly patients. Sedation and pain control are often all that are needed to control mild hypertension. Mild, persistent hyper-

tension can be further treated by temporarily adding a diuretic, such as furosemide, to the regimen to help the patient excrete mobilized fluids. Hypertension of pregnancy is treated with alpha-methyldopa, which seems to be safe for the fetus.

3. **Severe hypertension,** for example after major vascular surgery. This often requires parenteral administration of vasodilators; rarely, parenteral beta blockers are used if there is a significant history of coronary artery disease and myocardial infarction without heart failure. The vasodilator of choice is sodium nitroprusside.

REFERENCE

Gal TJ, Cooperman LH: Hypertension in the immediate postoperative period. *Br J Anaesth* 47:70, 1975.

Wish JB, Cohen JJ: Renal disease and hypertension. In Molitch ME: *Management of Medical Problems in Surgical Patients.* Philadelphia, FA Davis, 1982, pp 508–589.

49. HYPOCALCEMIA (See also Chapter 2, page 300.)

I. Problem. A gynecologic oncology patient with a history of Stage III-B squamous carcinoma of the cervix treated with definitive radiation presents with a calcium of 7.7 mg/dL (normal 8.5–10.5 mg/dL).

II. Immediate Questions

A. Are there any symptoms relevant to the low calcium? Asymptomatic hypocalcemia usually does not require emergency treatment. Signs and symptoms of hypocalcemia may include peripheral and perioral paresthesia, Trousseau's sign (carpopedal spasm), Chvostek's sign, confusion, muscle twitching, tetany, or seizures.

B. Does the low calcium level represent the true ionized calcium? Most laboratories report total serum calcium. However, a decrease of 1 g/dL in serum albumin will reduce protein-bound calcium by 0.8 mg/dL. Obtain serum albumin values and correct appropriately for the total calcium level, or determine ionized calcium (see page 300).

III. Differential Diagnosis. The causes of low ionized serum calcium can be categorized as parathyroid hormone (PTH) deficits, vitamin D deficits, magnesium deficiency, and loss or displacement of calcium.

A. Parathyroid hormone deficits

1. **Decreased PTH levels.** These may result from:
   a. **Surgical excision or injury,** including thyroid surgery.
   b. **Infiltrative diseases** such as hemochromatosis, amyloid, or metastatic cancer.
   c. **Idiopathic causes.**
   d. **Irradiation** to the thyroid or parathyroid.
2. **Decreased PTH activity**
   a. **Pseudohypoparathyroidism.** There is resistance to PTH at the tissue level. The PTH level is elevated and can be suppressed by calcium infusion.

B. **Vitamin D deficiency.** Causes include:
   1. **Malnutrition**
   2. **Malabsorption**
      a. **Pancreatitis.**
      b. **Post gastrectomy.**
      c. **Short gut syndrome.**
      d. **Laxative abuse.**
      e. **Sprue.**
      f. **Hepatobiliary disease** with bile salt.
      g. **Radiation enteritis.**
   3. **Defective metabolism**
      a. **Liver disease.** Failure to synthesize 25-hydroxyvitamin D.
      b. **Renal disease.** Failure to make 1, 25-dihydroxyvitamin D.
      c. **Anticonvulsive treatment.** Phenobarbital and phenytoin produce inactive metabolites of vitamin D.

C. **Magnesium deficiency.** This results in decreased PTH release and activity; correcting the magnesium deficit will often restore the calcium level.

D. **Calcium loss/displacement**
   1. **Hyperphosphatemia.** Bone deposition of calcium is increased in this disorder
      a. **Acute phosphate ingestion.**
      b. **Acute phosphate release by rhabdomyolysis, tumor lysis.**
      c. **Renal failure.** In chronic renal failure, decreased levels of 1, 24-dihydroxyvitamin D also contribute to hypocalcemia.
   2. **Acute pancreatitis.**
   3. **Osteoblastic metastases,** especially breast.
   4. **Medullary carcinoma of the thyroid** due to increased thyrocalcitonin.
   5. **Decreased bone resorption** caused by agents such as actinomycin, calcitonin, or mithramycin.

IV. Database

A. Physical examination key points

1. **Skin.** Look for dermatitis and eczema with chronic hypocalcemia.
2. **HEENT.** Cataracts may be present. Laryngospasm is rare but life threatening. Look for surgical scars on the neck.
3. **Neurologic examination.** Confusion, spasm, twitching, facial grimacing, and hyperactive deep tendon reflexes may be present.
4. **Specific tests for tetany of hypocalcemia**
   a. **Chvostek's sign.** This is present in 5–10% of "normal" patients. Tap on the facial nerve near the zygoma in the patient's jaw and observe for twitch.
   b. **Trousseau's sign.** Inflate a blood pressure cuff higher than systolic pressure for 3 minutes and observe for carpal spasm.

B. Laboratory data

1. **Serum electrolytes,** particularly calcium, phosphate, potassium, and magnesium. Calcium must be interpreted in terms of the serum albumin. Hypomagnesemia and hyperkalemia may potentiate the symptoms of hypocalcemia.
2. **Serum albumin.** Albumin is measured to follow correction of calcium levels, as noted on page 300. Low albumin will not affect the ionized calcium levels.
3. **Renal function tests (BUN and creatinine).** These determinations may reveal evidence of chronic renal insufficiency.
4. **Parathyroid hormone levels.**
5. **Vitamin D levels.** Obtain 25-hydroxy and 1, 25-dihydroxy vitamin D levels.
6. **Cyclic adenosine monophosphate.** Urinary cyclic AMP gives an index of parathyroid function and is increased with elevated PTH levels.
7. **Fecal fat.** This test is useful to evaluate steatorrhea.

C. Radiologic and other studies

1. **Electrocardiogram.** The ECG shows a prolonged QT interval with marked hypocalcemia.
2. **Bone films.** Bone changes are seen with renal failure or osteoblastic metastases.

V. Plan. Assess the patient for tetany, which can potentially progress to laryngeal spasm or seizures and requires acute treatment. Otherwise, establish the diagnosis by blood tests of calcium, albumin, magnesium, phosphate, and PTH level, and begin appropriate oral therapy.

A. Emergency treatment. Emergency treatment is usually needed for Ca < 1.5 mmol/L to prevent fatal laryngospasm. Give 200–300 mg of elemental calcium rapidly IV.

B. Chronic therapy. With primary PTH deficiency the goal is to give 2–4 g of oral calcium daily, then add vitamin D as necessary. In vitamin D disorder, always supplement with vitamin D.
   1. **Calcium carbonate.** There is 240 mg of calcium per 600 mg tablet.
   2. **Os-Cal 500.** A 1.25 g calcium carbonate tablet provides 500 mg of elemental calcium.
   3. **Dihydrotachysterol vitamin D$_2$.** Give 0.25–1.0 μg/gd.

C. Magnesium deficiency. Infuse 1–2 g of 10% magnesium sulfate IV over 20 minutes or add 40–80 meq MgSO$_4$ to a liter of IV fluid.

REFERENCE

Zaloga G, Chernow B: Life threatening electrolyte and metabolic abnormalities. In Parillo J (ed): *Current Therapy in Critical Care Medicine.* Toronto, BC Decker, 1987, pp 245–257.

50. HYPOGLYCEMIA (See Problem 9, page 48.)

51. HYPOKALEMIA (See also Chapter 2, page 322.)

I. Problem. A 72-year-old woman on long-term diuretic therapy for heart failure develops abdominal distention and ileus. Her serum potassium is 2.5 mmol/L (normal 3.5–5.1 mmol/L).

II. Immediate Questions

A. What medications is the patient taking? Loop diuretics, with furosemide the most typical example, are kaliuretic and cause significant renal potassium wasting. Thiazide diuretics can cause hypokalemia, but the level is rarely dangerous except when digoxin is used concomitantly. Hypokalemia will potentiate digitalis toxicity. Amphotericin causes potassium wasting by direct renal toxic effects.

B. Is there a history of vomiting, nasogastric suction, or diarrhea? Gastrointestinal losses are a common cause of hypokalemia in the surgical patient.

C. What are the vital signs? Look for irregular pulse, which in the postoperative patient could represent new premature atrial or ventricular contractions (PACs and PVCs) due to increased myocardial irritability.

D. Is the patient symptomatic? Symptoms of hypokalemia include weakness, nausea, vomiting, and abdominal tenderness.

III. Differential Diagnosis

A. Potassium losses

1. **Gastrointestinal**
   a. Prolonged NG suction without replacement can cause hypokalemia through direct losses, induced renal losses, and potassium shifts into the cells due to development of metabolic alkalosis.
   b. Intractable vomiting can cause hypokalemia through the same mechanism as NG suction.
   c. Bowel obstruction can result in hypokalemia through pooling of secretions and inefficient potassium absorption.
   d. Diarrhea, fistula, and villous adenoma are all associated with hypokalemia.

2. **Renal.** Causes include:
   a. **Diuretics,** especially loop diuretics such as furosemide.
   b. **Renal tubular acidosis.** This results in hypokalemia when K^+ is secreted and H^+ is absorbed.
   c. **Antibiotics** including carbenicillin, others. Amphotericin may also cause magnesium wasting.
   d. **Diuresis,** including postobstructive diuresis or the diuretic phase of acute tubular necrosis (ATN).

B. Potassium redistribution

1. **Alkalosis.** Cation balance requires that as H^+ moves out of cells to correct alkalosis, K^+ moves in.
2. **Insulin.** Insulin administration results in glucose and potassium transport into cells.

C. Inadequate intake.
This is most often iatrogenic (administration of potassium-free IV fluids over a prolonged time period). In the absence of other losses, normal daily potassium requirements with normal renal function are 40–60 meq/24h.

IV. Database.
Since potassium is the principal intracellular cation, hypokalemia usually represents a significant loss of body potassium. Thus, serum levels of 3.0 meq/L (mmol/L) often represent total deficits of 100–200 meq in the adult.

A. Physical examination key points

1. **Heart.** Irregular pulse may represent new arrhythmias (PAC, PVC) or digoxin toxicity.
2. **Abdomen.** Look for evidence of distention and listen for bowel sounds. Obstruction can cause hypokalemia; rarely, ileus results from hypokalemia and thus exacerbates the condition. Vomiting may cause hypokalemia or indicate digitalis toxicity.
3. **Neurologic examination.** Severe hypokalemia can cause blunting of reflexes, paresthesia, and paralysis.

B. Laboratory data

1. **Serum electrolytes.** Hypocalcemia and hypomagnesemia may coexist.
2. **Arterial blood gases.** Severe electrolyte abnormalities often have accompanying acid-base defects. Renal tubular acidosis and metabolic alkalosis often result in hypokalemia.
3. **Urine electrolytes.** These determinations are useful only in the patient off diuretics. Renal wasting can be evaluated by simple "spot" determinations of urine K^+, Na^+, and osmolality (see page 333).
4. **Digoxin.** Obtain the level if appropriate.

C. Radiologic and other studies.
An electrocardiogram with rhythm strip should be done on the patient with evidence of digitalis toxicity, new PACs, and new PVCs as manifested by a new irregular pulse.

V. Plan. More severe cases of hypokalemia, usually levels < 3.0 mmol/L, or those associated with ECG abnormalities should be treated aggressively because of the potential for life-threatening arrhythmias. Aggressive potassium replacement should be performed only after good renal function has been documented.

A. Parenteral replacement

1. **Indications.** Parenteral replacement should be considered in the following situations: digoxin toxicity or significant arrhythmia, severe hypokalemia (< 3.0 mmol/L), and patients who cannot take oral replacement (NPO, ileus, nausea and vomiting). Parenteral administration ideally should be done through a central venous catheter. Most other hypokalemia can be safely corrected in a slow, controlled fashion with oral supplementation.
2. **Replacement.** Maximum concentrations of KCl used in peripheral veins generally should not exceed 40 meq/L due to the damaging effects of high concentrations on the veins, although in an emergent situation 60 meq/L may be attempted. KCl 10–20 meq diluted in 50–100 mL D5W or NS

can be infused over 1 hour through a central line safely, and repeated as needed when severe depletion or life-threatening hypokalemia is present. Special care must be taken to ensure slow infusion of these high doses. For lesser degrees of hypokalemia that require parenteral replacement, 10–40 meq/h may be infused peripherally.

3. **Monitoring.** Check serum levels frequently (every 2–4 hours depending on clinical response) to avoid hyperkalemia. ECG or ICU monitoring is required if arrhythmias are present or for rapid infusions of KCl.

B. **Oral replacement** (see also Chapter 7, page 541). Oral treatment is generally indicated for asymptomatic, mild levels of potassium repletion (K usually > 3.0 meq/L). Oral replacements include liquids and powders. Slow-release pills typically contain < 10 meq/tablet and are thus not usually appropriate for repletion therapy. Replacement doses should be 40–120 meq qd in divided doses depending on the patient's weight and level of hypokalemia. Maintenance therapy, if needed, should be given in doses of 20–40 meq qd using the preparation best tolerated by the patient. In patients with normal renal function, it is difficult to induce hyperkalemia by oral administration of potassium. Another important exception is to avoid the use of potassium supplements in patients on potassium-sparing diuretics (triamterene, spironolactone, amiloride, others) to prevent hyperkalemia.

C. **Replacement of ongoing losses.** Large amounts of nasogastric aspirate should be replaced milliliter for milliliter with D5½NS containing 20 meq/L KCl q4–6h.

D. **Refractory cases.** Rarely, hypokalemia may not be correctable due to concomitant hypomagnesemia or hypocalcemia. Replace as described in Problem 49, page 185.

REFERENCE

Kunaw RT, Stein T: Disorders of hypo and hyper-kalemia. *Clin Nephrol* 7:173, 1977.

52. HYPOMAGNESEMIA

I. **Problem.** A 43-year-old patient being treated with cisplatin for a Stage III-C ovarian carcinoma presents with a magnesium level of 0.5 meq/L (normal 1.5–2.1 meq/L).

II. **Immediate Questions**

A. **What are the patient's vital signs?** Magnesium deficiency is associated with cardiac arrhythmias including atrial fibrillation, supraventricular tachycardia, ventricular tachycardia, and ventricular fibrillation. Determining that the patient is not in any immediate distress and does not have hypotension or a tachyarrhythmia is important.

B. Is the patient tremulous or currently having a seizure? Tremor, tetany, muscle fasciculations, and seizures are all associated with magnesium deficiency. Determining the presence of these neurologic problems will help guide the urgency of treatment.

C. Is the patient receiving chemotherapy? Chemotherapeutic agents such as cisplatin can be nephrotoxic and result in increased urinary excretion of magnesium.

III. Differential Diagnosis. The diagnosis of magnesium deficiency generally rests on a high degree of suspicion, clinical assessment, and measurement of serum magnesium. It is important to recognize that serum magnesium levels do not always correlate well with intracellular magnesium levels. Thus, it is possible to have total body or intracellular magnesium depletion with normal (or even high) serum magnesium levels. For this reason, several groups have suggested that an initial 24-hour urine collection for magnesium or a 24-hour urine magnesium retention test after parenteral administration of magnesium be done to determine whether magnesium depletion is really present. Although such tests may be useful in specific settings, the acutely ill patient is generally treated on the basis of serum level and good clinical judgment.

A. Hypocalcemia. The signs and symptoms of hypocalcemia are similar to those of hypomagnesemia, and often both problems are present in a single patient. Hypocalcemia that does not correct with intravenous supplementation suggests the presence of magnesium deficiency.

B. Hypokalemia. Potassium depletion often coexists with hypomagnesemia and can cause arrhythmias and muscle weakness, similar to the effects of hypomagnesemia. Hypokalemia that does not correct appropriately with potassium repletion also suggests magnesium depletion.

C. Lab error. Error is more likely if a colorimetric assay is used. When in doubt, ask the lab to repeat the test and controls.

D. Causes of hypomagnesemia
1. **Increased excretion**
    a. **Medications.** Medications, especially diuretics, antibiotics (ticarcillin, amphotericin B), aminoglycosides, cisplatin, and cyclosporin, often cause hypomagnesemia.

   b. Alcoholism. Decreased intake and renal magnesium wasting make alcoholism a very common cause.
   c. Diabetes mellitus. Hypomagnesemia is commonly seen in patients treated for diabetic ketoacidosis.
   d. Renal tubular disorders with magnesium wasting.
   e. Hypercalcemia/hypercalciuria.
   f. Hyperaldosteronism/Bartter's syndrome.
   g. Excessive lactation.
   h. Marked diaphoresis.
2. **Reduced intake/malabsorption**
   a. Starvation. This is a common cause.
   b. Bowel bypass or resection.
   c. Total parenteral nutrition without adequate magnesium supplementation.
   d. Chronic malabsorption syndrome, such as with pancreatic insufficiency.
   e. Chronic diarrhea.
3. **Miscellaneous**
   a. Acute pancreatitis.
   b. Hypoalbuminemia.
   c. Vitamin D therapy resulting in hypercalciuria.

IV. **Database**
   A. **Physical examination key points**
      1. **Vital signs.** Obtain blood pressure and pulse to evaluate for the presence of hypotension and tachyarrhythmias. While taking blood pressure, leave the cuff inflated for 3 minutes to check for carpal spasm (Trousseau's sign).
      2. **HEENT.** Check for Chvostek's sign (tapping over the facial nerve produces twitching of the mouth and eye). Nystagmus may be present.
      3. **Heart.** Check for regularity of rhythm.
      4. **Abdomen.** Evaluate for evidence of pancreatitis, absent bowel sounds, and tenderness. Stigmata of chronic liver disease such as hepatosplenomegaly, caput medusae, ascites, spider angiomas, and palmar erythema suggest chronic alcohol abuse.
      5. **Neurologic examination.** Hyperactive reflexes, muscle fasciculations, seizures, or tetany can result from hypomagnesemia. Hyperactive reflexes may also be seen with alcohol withdrawal.
      6. **Mental status.** Psychosis, depression, and agitation may be present.

   B. **Laboratory data**
      1. **Serum electrolytes, glucose, calcium, and phosphorus.**

Hypomagnesemia frequently accompanies other electrolyte abnormalities, especially hypocalcemia, hypokalemia, and alkalosis. If the patient is an alcoholic, then hypophosphatemia is also likely. Diabetics are prone to develop hypomagnesemia (especially in the setting of diabetic ketoacidosis).

2. **24-hour urine for magnesium.** This may be helpful if the diagnosis is in question or if there is a suspicion of renal magnesium wasting.

3. **Magnesium retention test.** This can be done using either parenteral or oral magnesium and may be helpful in certain subsets of patients in whom either the diagnosis is in question or malabsorption is suspected.

4. **Miscellaneous.** Obtain additional tests as indicated by the clinical situation: liver function studies in alcoholics, serum amylase if pancreatitis is suspected, and so forth.

C. Radiologic and other studies. Electrocardiographic findings may include prolongation of the PR, QT, and QRS intervals as well as ST depression and T waves. Rhythm disturbances include supraventricular arrhythmias as well as ventricular tachycardia and ventricular fibrillation.

V. Plan. The urgency of treatment depends on the clinical setting. The patient who is having neurologic or cardiac manifestations should be treated urgently with parenteral intravenous therapy. Asymptomatic individuals may be treated with oral magnesium. Many clinicians treat magnesium levels less than 1.0 meq/L with parenteral magnesium regardless of the fact that there is not always a good correlation between serum levels and intracellular levels, as noted earlier.

A. Intravenous magnesium sulfate. Magnesium sulfate 1 g (2 mL of a 50% solution of $MgSO_4$) equals 98 mg of elemental magnesium, which is equivalent to 8 meq $MgSO_4$ or 4 mmol Mg^{2+}. If the patient is in tetany or status epilepticus or is having significant cardiac arrhythmias, then 2 g of magnesium sulfate can be given IV over 10–20 minutes. For slightly less urgent situations, 1 g/h may be given q3–4h with close monitoring of deep tendon reflexes. In patients with renal insufficiency, magnesium should be administered only in life-threatening situations and monitoring of deep tendon reflexes is required every hour. As long as signs and symptoms of hypomagnesemia are improving, the infusion can then be slowed so that the patient receives approximately 10 g of magnesium sulfate in the first 24 hours. Selected patients may require more or less, based on clinical findings. Subsequently, 5–6 g of magnesium sulfate may be given over each 24 hours for the next 3–4 days to replenish body reserves.

    B. Intramuscular magnesium sulfate. Give 1–2 g IM q4h for 5 doses during the first 24 hours (following the patient's clinical status and serum levels as described earlier). This can then be followed by 1 g IM q6h for 2–3 days. Many patients complain about pain with the injections.

    C. Oral magnesium oxide (20 meq of magnesium per 400 mg tablet). Give 1 or 2 tablets per day for chronic maintenance therapy (may cause diarrhea, especially at higher doses).

    D. Miscellaneous. Treat other electrolyte disorders, especially hypocalcemia or hypokalemia (see Problems 49 and 51, pages 185 and 188) as well as other underlying illnesses.

REFERENCES

Elin RJ: Magnesium metabolism in health and disease. *DM* 34:161, 1988.
Massry S: Magnesium homeostasis and its clinical pathophysiology. *Res Staff Physician* 27:106, 1981.

53. HYPONATREMIA (See also Chapter 2, page 326.)

  I. Problem. An elderly woman admitted for a mastectomy has a sodium of 119 mmol/L on routine admission labs (normal 136–145 mmol/L).

  II. Immediate Questions

    A. Does the patient have any CNS symptomatology relevant to the hyponatremia? Symptomatic hyponatremia manifests primarily CNS symptoms since brain cells become edematous in a hypoosmotic state. Inquire about lethargy, agitation, disorientation, or obtundation.

    B. Are there any recent prior sodium levels to document the chronicity of the hyponatremia? The rate at which hyponatremia develops correlates directly with the severity of the symptoms it produces. Acute changes in sodium are more likely to produce severe symptoms.

    C. Does the patient take diuretics? A common cause of hyponatremia is chronic diuretic use.

    D. Is the hyponatremia real or is it a laboratory artifact? Osmotic agents and space-occupying compounds (glucose, triglycerides) at high concentrations can alter the reported laboratory value for sodium. Note the concentration of glucose and triglycerides, and adjust the measured sodium up to true levels (see III-A1).

    E. Is the patient receiving IV fluids? Overhydration with excess free water is the most common cause of hyponatremia in the surgical patient.

F. **Has the patient had recent surgery?** Surgery and anesthesia often result in a temporary syndrome of inappropriate antidiuretic hormone secretion (SIADH) and transient hyponatremia.

III. **Differential Diagnosis.** The initial differentiation is between true hyponatremia and laboratory artifact. True hyponatremia may then be classified according to the patient's volume status as **hypovolemic, euvolemic,** or **hypervolemic** (see IV-A below). Hypovolemic hyponatremia may be further classified by serum and urine chemistries.

A. **Laboratory artifact (pseudohyponatremia)**
   1. **Osmotic agents.** Hyperglycemia is most common. Adjust the serum sodium upward by 1.6 meq/L for each excess 100 mg/dL of glucose over the normal value of 100 mg/dL.
   2. **Space-occupying compounds.** Lipids are the most common. The lab can ultracentrifuge the specimen to find the correct plasma level.

B. **Hypovolemic hyponatremia**
   1. **Spot urinary Na < 10 meq/L**
      a. **GI fluid losses** (vomiting or diarrhea). In surreptitious vomiting or bulimia the urine chloride is usually < 10 meq/L.
      b. **Third space fluid loss** such as with pancreatitis or peritonitis.
      c. **Burns.**
   2. **Spot urinary Na > 10 meq/L**
      a. **Diuretic usage.** Caused by thiazide (eg, hydrochlorothiazide) and loop (furosemide) diuretics and often associated with hypokalemia and alkalosis; with surreptitious diuretic use, urinary chloride can be > 20 meq/L.
      b. **Renal disorders.** Medullary cystic disease, polycystic disease, and chronic interstitial nephritis can result in hyponatremia.
      c. **Addison's disease.** Hyperkalemia and low urinary potassium are also found.
      d. **Osmotic diuresis.** This is most commonly due to glucose, mannitol, or ketones.

C. **Euvolemic hyponatremia**
   1. **SIADH.** The diagnosis of SIADH is based on the finding of low serum osmolality, elevated urine sodium (> 20 mmol/L), and slightly concentrated urine (osmolality near that of sodium).

a. **Postoperative.** Anesthesia and surgical procedures cause increased ADH.
b. **Tumors.** Small cell lung cancer is most common, but ADH can also be elevated with cancer of the colon, esophagus, or duodenum and with lymphoma, carcinoids, and occasionally gynecologic malignancies.
c. **Pulmonary infections** such as TB and other bacterial pneumonia.
d. **CNS disorders** including trauma, tumors, and infections.
e. **Stress,** including perioperative stress.
f. **Drugs.** Oral hypoglycemic drugs, chemotherapeutic agents (cyclophosphamide, vincristine), psychiatric drugs (haloperidol, tricyclic antidepressants), and clofibrate can all raise ADH.

2. **Hypothyroidism.**
3. **Hypopituitarism.**

D. **Hypervolemic hyponatremia**
1. **Congestive heart failure.**
2. **Cirrhosis.**
3. **Renal disease.**
    a. **Chronic renal failure.**
    b. **Nephrotic syndrome.**

IV. Database

A. **Physical examination key points.** As apparent from the differential diagnosis, close attention should be paid to assessment of the volume status.
1. **Vital signs.** Evaluate for orthostatic blood pressure changes. Measure supine and standing blood pressures. A drop in blood pressure > 10 mm Hg or a pulse increase of > 10 bpm is highly suggestive of volume depletion. Tachypnea may suggest volume overload and pulmonary edema.
2. **Heart.** An S3 gallop murmur suggests volume overload.
3. **Lungs.** Rales may be heard with volume overload.
4. **Abdomen.** Look for hepatosplenomegaly and other evidence of cirrhosis or ascites. A hepatojugular reflux may be present in congestive heart failure (CHF).
5. **Skin.** Tissue turgor will be diminished and mucous membranes dry with dehydration. Edema suggests volume overload. Evidence of cirrhosis is jaundice and a caput medusae.
6. **HEENT.** Evaluate the internal jugular vein with the bed raised at 45 degrees (veins are flat with volume depletion and markedly engorged with volume overload).

7. **Neurologic examination.** Hyperactive deep tendon reflexes, altered mental status, confusion, coma, or seizures usually indicate a sodium of < 125 mmol/L.

B. **Laboratory data**
   1. **Electrolytes.** Other abnormalities may exist.
   2. **Spot urine electrolytes and creatinine.** Obtain these prior to any diuretic treatment.
   3. **Urine and serum osmolality.** Serum osmolality will be normal in cases of laboratory artifact but decreased in true hyponatremia.
   4. **Liver function tests.** These are performed to detect liver disease.
   5. **Arterial blood gases.** Acidosis or alkalosis may be present.
   6. **Thyroid function.**
   7. **Cortisol levels, ACTH stimulation test.**
   8. **Cultures** (blood and sputum).

C. **Radiologic and other studies**
   1. **Chest x-ray.** Look for evidence of CHF or a lung tumor.
   2. **Head CT scan** if indicated.
   3. **Water load test.** Bring the serum sodium to a safe level by fluid restriction, then challenge with 20 mL/kg of water PO and collect urine hourly for 5 hours. If < 75% of intake volume is excreted or if urine osmolality fails to decrease to < 200, then SIADH is present.

V. **Plan.** The cause of the hyponatremia and the presence and severity of symptoms guide therapy. Aggressive therapy for severe symptoms (eg, coma) will be discussed as well as specific therapies for certain diagnoses.

A. **Emergency therapy.** Usually for severe CNS symptoms (seizures, coma).
   1. Normal saline and furosemide 1 mg/kg IV. Use the combination of normal saline and diuretics to achieve a net negative volume balance. Carefully document volume in and volume out. Supplement fluids with potassium as needed.
   2. Hypertonic saline (3%) is rarely, if ever, needed. Some institutions have banned its use entirely because of possible serious complications.

B. **Hypovolemic hyponatremia**
   1. For almost all causes, treat by repleting volume and sodium. Normal saline is given IV.
   2. For diuretic-induced hyponatremia, repletion of lost body potassium is also needed.

C. **Euvolemic hyponatremia** (patient is not edematous).
   1. **SIADH.** Restrict water to 800–1000 mL daily. Give dem-

eclocycline (300–600 mg bid orally) for chronic SIADH, such as due to neoplasia, but onset may take up to a week.

    2. Hypothyroidism. Treat with thyroid replacement.

    3. Hypopituitarism. Treat with hormone replacement.

D. Hypervolemic hyponatremia (patient is edematous).

    1. Restrict IV and oral fluids.

        a. CHF. Treat with digoxin, diuretics (furosemide), and water restriction; captopril is also useful.

        b. Nephrotic syndrome. Steroids, water restriction, increased protein intake, and furosemide are commonly used.

        c. Cirrhosis. Treat with water restriction, diuretics, and portosystemic shunt if indicated (urine sodium > 20 meq/L).

    2. Renal failure. Treat with water restriction, loop diuretics (furosemide), and dialysis if indicated.

REFERENCE

Watson AJ: Hyponatremia. *Primary Care Emergency Decisions* 3:48, 1987.

54. HYPOTENSION (Shock)

I. Problem. A 40-year-old woman who underwent total abdominal hysterectomy for leiomyoma uteri earlier today has a blood pressure of 80/50.

II. Immediate Questions

    A. What is the pulse? Particularly in surgical patients, in whom there is often an induced hypovolemic state, the pulse can give clues to the cause of hypotension. A high pulse rate indicates a cardiovascular response to hypovolemia, while a normal pulse is less suggestive of a hypovolemic state.

    B. What have the blood pressure readings been preop? Be sure this is not the patient's resting pressure. Again, looking at the pulse helps to discern this important point. Always double-check any arterial line blood pressure readings with a careful cuff determination.

    C. When was the patient's surgery? If this is the first night postop, then hypovolemia is especially likely.

    D. What is the cardiac rhythm? Abnormal rhythms, especially atrial fibrillation or flutter, can cause hypotension.

    E. What is the patient's mental status? See if the low blood pressure is affecting the perfusion of critical organs.

    F. What are the current medications? A patient taking beta blockers can have a lower pulse, which will worsen hypotension by blunting reflex tachycardia. Narcotics and some sedatives can induce hypotension. Anaphylactic reactions may be caused by medications or intravenous contrast agents (see Problem 32, page 124).

G. What is the fluid balance? Urine output gives a clue to the patient's volume status. A decreasing urine output with hypotension suggests poor renal perfusion. Be sure the patient has been adequately hydrated and that excessive losses, such as nasogastric (NG) drainage, are being replaced.

H. Is there any obvious bleeding source? Inquire about blood on the dressings, bloody NG drainage, increased chest tube drainage, mediastinal tube output, or intraperitoneal drain output.

III. Differential Diagnosis. Table 1–14 helps to classify various causes of altered blood pressure and pulse. It is intended as a memory aid rather than a strict diagnostic tool. As a rule of thumb, a blood pressure < 90 mm Hg in an adult is considered hypotension. Hypotension may cause **shock,** a state characterized by inadequate tissue perfusion. Shock can be classified as follows.

A. Hypovolemic. This condition is often seen in surgical patients.
    1. Hemorrhagic
        a. Traumatic. Patients in shock often have significant blood loss that may not be readily apparent (chest, abdomen, retroperitoneal, or bleeding into fracture sites such as the pelvis or long bones, or into soft tissues). Alternatively, there may be obvious external bleeding.
        b. Postoperative. Internal hemorrhage may occur postoperatively or there may be direct exsanguination through surgically placed drains, etc.
        c. Others. There may be disseminated intravascular coagulation (DIC), GI tract bleeding, or ruptured aneurysms; ruptured ovarian cyst or ectopic pregnancy should be suspected.
    2. Fluid losses. Fluid can be lost through severe vomiting, di-

TABLE 1–14. DIAGNOSIS OF ALTERED BLOOD PRESSURE AND PULSE.

	Tachycardia	Bradycardia
Hypertension pain	Hypoxia	Increased intracranial pressure
Hypotension	Shock	Heart block

From Gomella LG, Lefor AT (eds): Surgery on Call. Norwalk, Connecticut, Appleton & Lange, 1990.

arrhea, sweating, extensive burns, and "third space losses" (pancreatitis, bowel obstruction). It can also be due to inadequate hydration during surgery with continued vasodilation and evaporative losses from an open abdomen.

B. Neurogenic. This is seen in patients with spinal cord trauma characterized by hypotension and a normal pulse. These patients will usually have normal urine output after fluid administration. They may require large amounts of fluid due to loss of sympathetic tone.

C. Vasogenic. Septic shock, anaphylactic reactions, or adrenocortical insufficiency may cause decreased vascular tone. In surgical patients, septic shock is the most frequent of this type; usually it is a hyperdynamic state with high cardiac output and low peripheral vascular resistance.

D. Cardiogenic. This results from "pump failure" (usually due to myocardial infarction or cardiomyopathy) or arrhythmia (atrial fibrillation, complete heart block). Tension pneumothorax or pulmonary embolus can lead to cardiogenic shock by decreasing venous return. Lesions such as pericardial tamponade, aortic valve disease (late), and septal rupture can also present with hypotension.

IV. Database

A. Physical examination key points

1. **Vital signs.** Confirm arterial line pressure readings with a cuff pressure to rule out technical errors. Tachycardia is the usual response to hypotension. Irregularity of the pulse suggests an arrhythmia. Tachypnea may indicate hypoxia or acidosis due to poor perfusion or early sepsis. Fever might suggest sepsis; however, elderly or debilitated (immunosuppressed) patients may be afebrile in the face of sepsis and occasionally hypothermia can be a sign of sepsis.

2. **Heart.** Check for new murmurs, arrhythmias, or rubs. Heart sounds may be muffled with cardiac tamponade.

3. **Lungs.** Rales suggest congestive heart failure (CHF); wheezing and stridor occur with anaphylaxis; decreased breath sounds may indicate hemothorax or pneumothorax. Rib fractures may be associated with hemothorax or pneumothorax and sternal tenderness with pericardial tamponade (such as in steering wheel trauma).

4. **Abdomen.** Distention, pulsatile mass, flank ecchymoses,

and active bleeding at drain sites or wound dressings may suggest the cause.

5. **Skin.** Good skin turgor and mucous membranes are clinical signs of hydration; cool, clammy skin may indicate shock.
6. **Neck.** Check for jugular venous distention. Bulging neck veins are compatible with congestive failure, pericardial tamponade, or tension pneumothorax.
7. **Rectum.** Gross (hematochezia) or occult blood.
8. **Pelvis.** Pelvic fractures can result in a large amount of blood loss. Pelvic examination in females may reveal a gynecologic cause (ectopic pregnancy or ruptured hemorrhagic cyst).
9. **Extremities.** Absent or "thready" pulses are consistent with shock; long bone fractures (especially of the femur) may result in significant bleeding into soft tissues. Examine IV sites for evidence of infection. Edema is often seen with CHF.

B. **Laboratory data**
1. **Hemogram.** Because the hematocrit may not drop for some time after an acute bleed, serial hematocrit determinations are essential.
2. **Serum electrolytes.** Addisonian crisis causes hyperkalemia with hyponatremia.
3. **Coagulation panel (prothrombin time, partial thromboplastin time, platelet count).** If excessive bleeding due to DIC is suspected, fibrinogen and fibrin split products should also be determined.
4. **Arterial blood gases.** Early sepsis may result in respiratory alkalosis; acidosis may indicate inadequate tissue perfusion; hypoxia may require ventilatory support.
5. **Cardiac injury panel.** Creatine phosphokinase (q8h times 4) and lactate dehydrogenase (q12h times 3) isoenzymes may reveal evidence of myocardial injury (see Chapter 2, pages 305, 316).
6. **Serum pregnancy test.** This is especially important if a ruptured ectopic pregnancy is suspected.
7. **Type and cross-match.** Blood should be set up immediately.

C. **Radiologic and other studies**
1. **Chest x-ray.** Look for evidence of CHF, cardiac enlargement, pneumothorax, or hemothorax.
2. **Electrocardiogram.** Myocardial ischemia may show flipped T waves or ST segment depression; arrhythmias may be noted.
3. **Pulmonary artery (PA) catheter.** A PA catheter is helpful in managing a patient in whom fluid overload would be particularly dangerous. By using a PA catheter, filling pressures are

directly measured so iatrogenic pulmonary edema can be avoided. It can also help to differentiate cardiogenic from hypovolemic or vasogenic causes. (See Procedure 8, page 354, for diagnostic and insertion details.)

4. **Angiogram.** This study may help to identify bleeding sites (especially with GI tract bleeding). A pulmonary angiogram may be needed to diagnose pulmonary embolus with an equivocal V/Q scan.

5. **Nuclear ventilation/perfusion scan.** The V/Q scan is used to diagnose pulmonary embolus.

6. **Echocardiogram.** Echo is used to examine valves (mitral stenosis, aortic insufficiency, etc), pericardial fluid, as well as intracardiac thrombi.

7. **Blood, sputum, and urine cultures.** These should be obtained in cases of suspected sepsis.

8. **Peritoneal tap, thoracentesis, or culdocentesis** if indicated (see procedures 9, 24, and 30, pages 357, 385, and 393).

V. **Plan.** Reestablish adequate tissue perfusion as soon as possible if the patient is in shock. In general, a blood pressure > 90 mm Hg and urine output of at least 0.5–1 mL/kg/min is acceptable.

A. **Emergency management**
   1. Control external hemorrhage with direct pressure.
   2. Establish good venous access and closely monitor the patient.
   3. Trendelenburg position (supine with feet higher than head) may acutely improve cerebral perfusion and blood pressure. A pneumatic antishock garment (PASG or MAST suit) is useful in the trauma patient with acute blood loss.
   4. Except for cardiogenic shock, replace volume acutely with IV crystalloid (lactated Ringer's, etc).
   5. Place a Foley catheter for urinary output monitoring.
   6. Provide supplemental oxygen or ventilatory support if needed. Correct severe acidosis with IV sodium bicarbonate.
   7. Insert a central venous pressure (CVP) line or PA catheter to better manage volume replacement and accurately diagnose the cause of shock.

B. **Hypovolemic shock.** Restore intravascular volume.
   1. Place two large-bore (18-gauge or greater) IV lines.
   2. Administer fluids. Use blood if the hematocrit is low or crystalloid (normal saline or lactated Ringer's) if blood is not available or if hematocrit is "acceptable" (ie, > 35%).
   3. Titrate fluids by following blood pressure and urine output.

4. A PA catheter may help to guide fluid administration. A CVP line is useful for following trends in the pressure reading.
5. Do not use pressor agents (eg, dopamine) unless there is persistent hypotension despite adequate cardiac filling pressures (a "full tank": wedge pressure > 12 mm Hg). Hypotension with low filling pressures (wedge pressure < 6 mm Hg) is initially treated with intravenous fluids. A CVP or PA catheter is necessary for monitoring when using pressor agents.
6. With good filling pressures and adequate cardiac output, the next step is peripheral vasoconstrictors such as epinephrine or levophed in a patient who is still hypotensive.

C. Neurogenic shock

1. Use moderate IV fluids to avoid volume overload.
2. Low-dose vasopressors (dopamine) may help support blood pressure.
3. A major neurologic injury may not be obvious at the time of presentation in an unconscious trauma patient.

D. Vasogenic shock

1. **Septic shock.** Treatment is directed at the underlying sepsis.
   a. Measure cardiac output and systemic vascular resistance (typically, high cardiac output with low systemic resistance) with a PA catheter.
   b. Administer IV fluids to support pressure and urine output.
   c. Culture aggressively to identify the source.
   d. Treat the underlying cause of sepsis. Initiate appropriate antibiotics, and consider laparotomy or percutaneous drainage of an abscess if indicated.
   e. Use pressors as needed. First-line therapy is often with dopamine (discussed in Chapter 7). The lowest effective dose to maintain blood pressure and urine output should be used. Physiologic effects of dopamine are as follows:

   3–5 µg/kg/min: renal and splanchnic vasodilatation via dopamine receptors

   5–10 µg/kg/min: positive inotropic effect via beta–1 receptors

   > 10 µg/kg/min: peripheral vasoconstriction via alpha receptors

2. Anaphylactic shock (see Problem 32, page 124).

E. Cardiogenic shock

1. Cardiac output is maximized by the judicious use of inotropic agents (dopamine or dobutamine). Dobutamine is the drug of choice for pump failure. The severe pulmonary edema is

treated with diuretics (eg, furosemide) and vasodilators (eg, nitrates).
2. Myocardial ischemia is treated with oxygen, morphine for pain relief, and nitrates acutely.
3. Arrhythmia is identified and treated appropriately to return the patient to normal sinus rhythm.
4. Pulmonary embolus (see Problems 39 and 68, pages 153 and 263).
5. Pneumothorax (see Problem 36, page 141).

REFERENCE

Marsciano TH: Hypotension in the surgical patient. In Cutler BS et al (eds): *Manual of Clinical Problems in Surgery.* Boston, Little Brown, 1984, pp 21–26.

55. INSOMNIA

I. **Problem.** A patient hospitalized for 14 days of intravenous antibiotics for fasciitis complains of lying awake for hours at night.

II. **Immediate Questions**

A. **Is the patient bothered by pain?** Most surgical patients experience some degree of pain, either postoperatively or related to the admission diagnosis. Painful stimuli coupled with the disruptive situation of being in the hospital (noise, interruptions, a strange bed) can understandably produce insomnia. Make sure the patient is receiving adequate pain medication in addition to sleeping pills.

B. **What is the patient's sleep pattern during the day?** Certainly, a patient who sleeps for extended periods during the day will not be able to drop off to sleep at night. Discuss this matter with the patient and, if available, with the social service/recreational therapy department.

C. **Does the patient take sleeping medications chronically?** Virtually all sleep medications show a tolerance effect and disruption of sleep patterns that can lead to less restful sleep with chronic usage. Take a detailed drug history to evaluate how withdrawal or tolerance may be contributing to the insomnia.

D. **Does the patient have difficulty lying down in a recumbent position?** Ask specifically about shortness of breath (orthopnea) and calf pain (ischemic rest pain) as causes for disrupted sleep.

E. **What is the patient's sleep pattern?** Early morning awakening is commonly associated with depression. Anxiety usually causes difficulty in getting to sleep initially.

III. Differential Diagnosis

A. Medical causes

1. **Pain.** Inadequate control is often correctable.
2. **Congestive heart failure (CHF).** Orthopnea is the hallmark.
3. **Peripheral vascular disease.** Ischemic rest pain indicates advanced disease.
4. **Hyperthyroidism.** Other symptoms include tachycardia, heat intolerance, and tremors.
5. **Sleep apnea syndrome.** This is most often seen with morbid obesity.

B. Drugs/Toxins

1. **Tolerance to sleeping medications or tranquilizers from chronic usage.**
2. **Alcohol abuse.** There may be secondary chronic disruption of appropriate sleep patterns.

C. Psychiatric causes

1. **Depressive illness,** either bipolar or unipolar.
2. **Anxiety disorders.**

D. Situational factors

1. **Noise.** The patient may be situated close to the nursing station or have a noisy roommate.
2. **Anger.** There may be unexpressed anger toward the staff or family.
3. **Anxiety.** The patient may experience either appropriate or inappropriate anxiety about her medical condition.

IV. Database.

The most important portion of the database in insomnia is the history, including evaluation of the patient's mental status. Other studies add little except in rare cases.

A. Physical examination key points

1. **Cardiopulmonary.** Look for evidence of rales, displaced point of maximum impulse, or gallop rhythm to suggest CHF.
2. **Extremities.** Decreased or absent pulses, pallor on elevation, or dependent rubor may suggest ischemic rest pain.
3. **Neurologic examination.** Evaluate the patient's mental status for anxiety or depression.

B. Laboratory data.

Most often, the cause of insomnia will be determined without the use of laboratory tests.

1. **Screening chemistries.** Include hepatic and renal function.
2. **Thyroid hormone levels.** Obtain these if clinically indicated.

C. Radiologic and other studies

1. **Chest x-ray** if indicated, such as to evaluate CHF.
2. **Ankle/brachial blood pressure** or other vascular studies, if indicated, to evaluate vascular insufficiency.

V. Plan. Most important is to determine whether medical, psychologic, or situational causes explain why the patient cannot sleep. Most cases are attributable to a situational cause or just being in the hospital. For this reason, it is wise to include a prn sleeping medication with all admission and postoperative orders unless specifically contraindicated. Any medical problem should be treated and pain should be adequately controlled.

A. Symptomatic treatment
   1. Oral sleeping medications
      a. Benzodiazepines are most frequently used for the short-term treatment of insomnia.
         (1) Triazolam (Halcion). Give 0.125–0.25 mg (0.125 in the elderly).
         (2) Temazepam (Restoril). Give 15–30 mg.
         (3) Flurazepam (Dalmane). Give 15–30 mg. Flurazepam used to be the "standard order" but was found to have prolonged and cumulative effects, and triazolam is becoming the new standard.
      b. Other oral agents
         (1) Chloral hydrate. Give 500–1000 mg (do not use in renal or hepatic failure).
         (2) Diphenhydramine (Benadryl). Give 25–50 mg PO.
   2. Nonoral sleeping medications
      a. Chloral hydrate. Give 500–1000 mg PR.
      b. Pentobarbital (Nembutal). Give 100 mg PR or IM.
   3. Nonmedical treatments. These are often as effective and may include discussing apprehensions with the patient, moving the patient to another room, or initiating psychiatric therapy for a patient who is depressed.

REFERENCE

Kaley A et al: Insomnia and other sleep disorders. *Med Clin North Am* 66:971, 1982.

56. INTRAVENOUS INFILTRATION (INCLUDING CHEMOTHERAPY)

I. Problem. The floor nurse calls to tell you that your patient, an 80-year-old diabetic female with endometrial cancer admitted for antibiotic therapy secondary to staphylococcal infection, has an apparent intravenous infiltration.

II. Immediate Questions

A. Is the patient symptomatic? Extravasation should be suspected if:
  1. The patient complains of swelling or redness at the injection site. This is not always present at the time of the extravasation, and may not be obvious for several days to months.
  2. Burning, stinging, pain, or streaking is observed at the injection site.
  3. Absent or sluggish blood return is noted.
  4. There is a change in the amount of pressure needed for the infusion.

B. What IV fluids and IV medications are currently ordered?
One hazard of intravenous drug therapy is the possible leakage of IV fluids and medications from the vein into the surrounding tissues. Prolonged administration of intravenous solutions combined with the administration of intermittent medications can lead to infiltration. The majority of these infiltrations are recognized early, remain localized, and heal spontaneously without medical intervention. However, some infiltrations cause severe tissue damage that can lead to necrosis and severe extravasation injury. The chemical and physical properties of the extravasated fluid may alter cell function by changing the osmotic fluid exchange in the interstitial tissues. This process leads to loss of capillary wall integrity, cell death, and tissue necrosis. The severity of the tissue damage is determined by a combination of many factors: the amount of drug extravasated, the tissue exposure time, vasospasticity, the amount of pressure exerted during the infusion, the anatomic site involved, the agent's osmolality, its specific tissue toxicity, and the patient's general health.

C. Does the patient have risk factors for extravasation?
  1. **Anatomic factors.** Venous integrity, vessel diameter, and local blood flow are associated with the development of infiltration. Injections into small, fragile veins or into veins with decreased circulation can result in high drug concentrations and extravasation.
  2. **Physiologic factors.** Debilitated patients with generalized vascular disease, diabetes mellitus, or Raynauld's syndrome seem more prone to local vascular and extravascular toxicity.
  3. **Mechanical factors.** Patients receiving intravenous fluids and medications via an IV infusion pump have an increased chance of tissue damage if infiltration occurs. Ischemia can result from fluid being forced by gravity or by infusion pump into a limited tissue space. Decreasing cellular pH, loss of capillary wall integrity, increased edema, and eventually cell death will follow. Intravenous infusion pumps that have a high maximum flow pressure are more likely to be associ-

ated with extravasation injury than a pump with a maximum flow pressure < 20 lb/in^2 (volumetric cassette pumps). Occlusion alarm devices are usually preset to sound only at pressures > 25 lb/in^2, by which time the damage is already done.

4. **Pharmacologic factors.** The amount of drug extravasated and the duration of drug exposure may determine the severity of tissue damage. Known vesicants should be mixed in the appropriate volume of diluent and administered over the shortest time recommended.

5. **Logistic factors.** Dorsal hand veins, which are the most accessible, are most often associated with serious extravasation injury, as are the ankle, dorsum of the foot, and wrist. Vital nerves and tendons at these sites make extravasation especially morbid. The optimal site for venipuncture when administering a known vesicant is the proximal forearm over the muscle bulk of the flexor or extensor muscles. Next in order of preference would be the dorsum of the hand, the wrist, and the antecubital fossa.

6. **Iatrogenic factors.** Repeated venipuncture attempts can lead to drug leakage. Also, delay in recognizing the infiltration and taking appropriate measures immediately after extravasation leads to more severe local reactions. It is believed that extravasation can be minimized by using a systematic technique of drug administration.

III. Differential Diagnosis

A. **Vesicant extravasation.** Morbidity from infiltration of vesicating agents may range from temporary local pain and inflammation at the site of injection to extensive tissue necrosis with loss of motor function, sensory function, or both in the affected extremity. Table 1–15 reviews the known tissue necrotizing drugs and their suggested antidotes where applicable.

1. **Hyperosmotic agents.** Solutions of dextrose and urea having an osmolality greater than that of serum (281–289 mosm/L), solutions containing high concentrations of calcium or potassium, solutions with high concentrations of dextrose and amino acids (hypertonic parenteral nutrition solutions), and radiographic contrast dyes can be corrosive to subcutaneous tissue if infiltration occurs.

2. **Ischemia-inducing agents.** Vasopressors, certain cation solutions including potassium and calcium, and alpha-adrenergic stimulators such as metaraminol, dopamine, dobutamine, epinephrine, and norepinephrine can cause smooth muscle around capillaries to constrict, leading to

TABLE 1–15. SUGGESTED ANTIDOTES FOR TISSUE NECROSING AND IRRITATING AGENTS.

Specific Agents	Local Antidote	Dosage
Aminophylline	Hyaluronidase 15 μ/mL	0.2 ml × 5 injections
Amsacrine (M-AMSA)	None known	
Bisantrene	Sodium bicarbonate 5.4%	5 mL
Calcium solutions	Hyaluronidase 15 μ/mL	0.2 mL × 5 injections
Carmustine	Sodium bicarbonate 8.4%	5 mL
Cisplatin	Sodium thiosulfate 10%	4 mL
	plus sterile H_2O	6 mL
Dacarbazine	Sodium thiosulfate 10%	4 mL
	plus sterile H_2O	6 mL
Dactinomycin	Sodium thiosulfate 10%	4 mL
	plus sterile H_2O	6 mL
	or ascorbic acid injection	50 mg
Daunorubicin	Sodium bicarbonate 8.4%	5 mL
	plus dexamethasone	4 mL
Dextrose 10%	Hyaluronidase 15 μ/mL	0.2 mL × 5 injections
Dobutamine	Phentolamine	5–10 mg
Dopamine	Phentolamine	5–10 mg
Doxorubicin	Hydrocortisone sodium succinate	50–200 mg
	plus hydrocortisone cream 1%	apply bid
	or sodium bicarbonate 8.4%	5 mL
Epinephrine	Phentolamine	5–10 mL
Estramustine phosphate	Sodium thiosulfate 10%	4 mL
	plus sterile H_2O	6 mL
Etoposide (VP-16-213)	Hyaluronidase 15 μ/mL	0.25 × 5 injections
Maytansine	None known	
Mechlorethamine	Sodium thiosulfate 10%	4 mL
	plus sterile H_2O	6 mL
Metaraminol	Phentolamine	5–10 mg
Mithramycin	Sodium edetate	150 mg
Mitoguazone (methyl-GAG)	None known	
Mitomycin C	Sodium thiosulfate 10%	4 mL
	plus sterile H_2O	6 mL
Nafcillin	Hyaluronidase 15 μ/mL	0.2 mL × 5 injections
Norepinephrine	Phentolamine	10–15 mg
Parenteral nutrition solutions	Hyaluronidase 15 μ/mL	0.2 mL × 5 injections
Potassium solutions	Hyaluronidase 15 μ/mL	0.2 mL × 5 injections
Pyrazofurin	None known	
Radiographic contrast media	Hyaluronidase 15 μ/mL	0.2 mL × 5 injections
Streptozocin	None known	
Teniposide (VM-26)	Hyaluronidase 15 μ/mL	0.2 mL × 5 injections
Vasopressin	Guanethidine	10 mg
	plus sodium chloride 0.9%	10 mL
	plus heparin	1000 U
Vinblastine	Sodium bicarbonate 8.4%	5 mL
	or hyaluronidase plus heat	150 μ
Vincristine	Hydrocortisone sodium succinate	25–50 mg/mL
	or sodium bicarbonate 8.4%	5 mL
	or hyaluronidase plus heat	150 U
Vindesine	Hyaluronidase plus heat	150 U

ischemic tissue necrosis by prolonged depolarization and contraction of smooth muscle sphincters.

3. **Direct cellular toxicity.** Chemotherapeutic agents such as doxorubicin, dactinomycin, mitomycin C, mithramycin, and daunorubicin bind with tissue deoxyribonucleic acid (DNA) and cause significant extravasation necrosis. Agents such as vincristine, vinblastine, and nitrogen mustard do not bind with DNA and are less likely to cause severe tissue damage when extravasated. Sodium bicarbonate and thiopental sodium are very alkaline and can cause severe tissue necrosis. Dilantin, digoxin, nitroglycerin, chlordiazepoxide, and diazepam are poorly water soluble and, when prepared with propylene glycol or ethyl alcohol, cause tissue damage if infiltration occurs.

B. **Intravenous infiltration of cytotoxic chemotherapy.** These patients are at high risk for extravasation because of a tendency to have fragile, thin, mobile veins that require several puncture attempts. Repeated courses of chemotherapy may increase the risk of extravasation secondary to numerous intravenous doses over a short period of time.

C. **Diabetic-related infiltration complications.** Patients with diabetes mellitus or other vascular diseases seem more prone to extravasation. Once extravasation has occurred, tissue repair is slowed, presumably because of diabetic-induced small vessel disease.

D. **Age-associated intravenous complications.** Elderly, debilitated patients have a higher incidence of extravasation. They tend to have more fragile, mobile veins and are often less likely to verbalize discomfort (especially at night, or when receiving antiemetics or sedatives).

IV. Database

A. **Physical examination key points**

1. **Inspection of the extremity.** The presentation of an extravasation injury depends on the drug used and volume of solution infiltrated. The least traumatic type of extravasation injury appears as a painful, erythematous swelling surrounding the area with blanching of the skin at the IV cannula site during the first 24–48 hours after extravasation. The pain may last several minutes to several hours but will eventually subside, and the redness and swelling will gradually diminish over several weeks without permanent damage. If part of the skin thickness is involved, blisters may appear with splotching and darkening of the skin. When the full thickness is involved, the area appears very leukoplakic

and later scabs may develop. Swelling at the IV site may be obvious at first, but evidence of tissue injury may take another 24 hours.

During the following weeks, the swelling may decrease. The affected skin becomes depressed below the surrounding skin and very obvious demarcated margins evolve, demonstrating the impending tissue necrosis. An obvious black scab will appear on the skin surface. This demarcation of the wound usually occurs by 2 weeks. Once painful necrosis is established, surgical consultation should be obtained for debridement. Multiple debridements and skin grafting may be indicated. Severe damage to the nerves and tendons can also occur. The extent of soft tissue damage should not be underestimated, and the extravasation injury should be treated aggressively. The extremity should be observed carefully for increasing swelling, diminishing pulses, and increasing pain with passive extension of the fingers as indicators of early Volkmann's ischemic contracture.

2. **Vital signs.** Fever would indicate a possible infection. Since bacterial infection could slow wound healing and potentially worsen the injury, many physicians prophylactically treat with antibiotic therapy.

B. **Laboratory data.** A complete blood count is done to evaluate for potential problems related to immunosuppression secondary to prior chemotherapy.

V. **Plan.** Treatment of extravasation varies widely between institutions. There is much controversy such as local heat versus cooling, administering a specific antidote versus steroids, leaving the IV cannula in place versus removal, etc. It is important both medically and legally, however, that an institution have an extravasation policy to deliver consistent care to these patients. The plan described here covers these controversial issues. Optimum patient care requires prompt and consistent management of an extravasation using currently recommended methods. The goals of treatment are early recognition, palliation, and prevention of severe tissue damage. Table 1–16 describes one suggested plan for managing a patient with an expected infiltration.

A. **Initial recommendations**
   1. Use careful infusion technique to prevent extravasation.
   2. Stop the infusion at the first sign of infiltration.
      a. Assess the line for patency by one of the following methods:
         (1) Gravity check. Lower the IV fluids below arm level. If

TABLE 1–16. MANAGEMENT OF EXTRAVASATION.

1. Stop the infusion immediately, leaving the needle in place.
2. Withdraw 3–5 mL of blood and solution.
3. If unable to aspirate blood, remove needle and aspirate any solution using a pincushion technique with a 27-gauge needle and syringe.
4. Consult the policy specific for the drug to establish further therapy.
5. Inject the specific antidote (optional).
6. Apply ice (heat for vinca alkaloids) and elevate the limb for 48 hours.
7. Document the occurrence of the infiltration in the medical record.
8. Evaluate the lesion daily for signs of induration, inflammation, ulceration, and tissue necrosis.
9. At the first sign of ulceration or tissue necrosis, consult a plastic surgeon.

blood returns, the needle is probably secure in the vein.
- (2) "Kink and pinch" method. Kinking the IV lines and pinching the injection bulb should result in a backflush of blood. This method also increases pressure in the vein.
- (3) Aspiration. Attempt aspiration through a three-way stopcock to assess patency.
- b. **Beware:** Good blood return is possible with an infiltrated line. Extravasation can occur without the patient experiencing any discomfort. **If in doubt, pull it out!**
- B. **Management.** Drug extravasation can be managed by leaving the cannula in place to permit aspiration of vesicant and administration of antidote, or by removing the cannula and administering antidote by multiple intradermal and subcutaneous injections.
  1. When the needle is in place, withdraw 3–5 mL of blood in order to remove some of the drug.
  2. When the needle is removed, use a 27-gauge TB syringe to aspirate the subcutaneous bleb and withdraw as much of the remaining solution as possible.
  3. Locally instill the recommended amount of antidote according to hospital policy.
     - a. Antidotes may be instilled through the existing IV line to purposely infiltrate the area. Alternatively, antidotes may be injected via a 1 mL TB syringe with 25-gauge needle. Small amounts are injected subcutaneously in a circle around the infiltrated area. The needle is changed before each injection of antidote.
     - b. Local injections of steroids are frequently used to reduce the inflammatory response, although no definitive advantage to healing has been established.

    c. Hyaluronidase has been successful in treating extravasations of vincristine, vinblastine, and vindesine. Success with hyaluronidase has been reported in the treatment of extravasated podophyllotoxins (etoposide, teniposide). Extravasation of dextrose 10%, parenteral nutrition solutions, calcium solutions, potassium solutions, aminophylline, nafcillin, and radiocontrast dye have also been treated with hyaluronidase.

    d. Extravasations of catecholamine are usually treated with phentolamine, an alpha-adrenergic blocking agent that decreases local vasoconstriction and ischemia. Phentolamine administration is standard practice for early vasopressor infiltration in many institutions.

4. Ice packs. Ice is applied with most drugs except the vinca alkaloids. Apply the ice pack to the affected area for 20–50 minutes of every hour for 24–72 hours (Oncology Nursing Society, 1984).

5. Moist heat packs. For vinca alkaloids, moist heat packs are applied for 20–50 minutes of every hour for 24–72 hours.

6. Elevate and rest the affected extremity. Use of skin traction, a stockinette dressing, and an observation window is recommended.

    a. Elevate the extremity for 48 hours.

    b. After 48 hours the patient should use the extremity normally. Physical therapy may be necessary to reduce patient discomfort and stiffness.

7. Document the incident. Records indicating venipuncture sites for chemotherapy and other vesicating agents provide valuable information for patient management and legal protection. Documentation should include:

    a. Date.

    b. Time.

    c. Needle size and type.

    d. Insertion site.

    e. Drug sequence.

    f. Drug administration technique.

    g. Approximate amount of drug extravasated.

    h. Nursing management of the extravasation.

    i. Photo documentation.

    j. Patient complaints and statements.

    k. Appearance of the site.

    l. Physician notification.

    m. Follow-up measures.

8. Photograph the suspected area when possible for documentation and follow-up.

9. Apply topical ointment (silver sulfadiazine cream) if skin breakdown occurs. Cover lightly with an occlusive sterile

dressing or wet-to-dry povidone-iodine dressings. Avoid applying pressure to the suspected infiltration site.
   10. **Plastic surgery consultation.** It is recommended that surgical consultation be obtained when ulceration appears unless the treating physician is skilled in wound healing.

REFERENCES

Cancer chemotherapy guidelines and recommendations for nursing education and practice. *J Oncol Nurs Soc* 11:19, 1984.

Dorr RT: Extravasation of vesicant antineoplastics: clinical and experimental findings. *Ariz Med* 38:271, 1981.

Hirsh JD, Conlon PF: Implementing guidelines for managing extravasation of antineoplastics. *Am J Hosp Pharm* 40:1516, 1983.

Ignoffo RJ, Friedman MA: Therapy of local toxicities caused by extravasation of cancer chemotherapeutic drugs. *Cancer Treat Rev* 7:17, 1980.

Larson DL: Treatment of tissue extravasation by antitumor agents. *Cancer* 49:1796, 1982.

Lynch DJ, Key JC, White RR: Management and prevention of infiltration and extravasation injury. *Surg Clin North Am* 59:939, 1979.

MacCara ME: Extravasation: a hazard of intravenous therapy. *Drug Intell Clin Pharm* 17:713, 1983.

Rudolph R, Larson DL: Etiology and treatment of chemotherapeutic agent extravasation injuries: a review. J Clin Oncol 5:1116, 1987.

Shelly D: Cancer chemotherapy extravasation: conservative versus aggressive medical management. Hosp Pharmacol 21:784, 1986.

Upton J, Mulliken JB, Murray JE: Major intravenous extravasation injuries. *Am J Surg* 137:497, 1979.

57. MENSES: MISSED OR CHANGED

   I. Problem. You are called to see a 19-year-old para 0 college student with a history of the last menses being different and missing the previous menses. She has mild cramps and some lower abdominal discomfort.

II. Immediate Questions

   A. What are the vital signs? Elevation of pulse and reduction in blood pressure suggest loss of hemodynamic status. An elevated temperature suggests an infectious process.

   B. What volume of blood has been passed? Have the patient describe the amount of bleeding as contrasted to her normal menstrual events. A normal menses is associated with some 25–60 mL blood loss.

   C. When was her last menstrual period and was it completely normal? Menses that are normal in time of onset, amount of bleeding, and associated symptoms almost never occur in a woman who is pregnant. Deviations from any of these criteria are of concern.

D. What is the interval between the missed period and the onset of irregular bleeding? A menses of about 4 weeks suggests a pregnancy-related problem, while a week or less is more suggestive of Halban's disease or dysfunctional uterine bleeding.

E. Obtain a brief history of her menstrual periods. A history of normal menarche and regular menses indicates a more acute event, while a history of irregular periods suggests a more chronic underlying problem.

F. Is she sexually active? Exposure to sperm is important, and most women will be forthright in answering this question.

G. What form of contraception is she using? Oral contraceptives are associated with pill-induced amenorrhea and breakthrough bleeding. Aggressive contraceptive use tends to reduce the chance of pregnancy. An IUD may also cause irregular bleeding.

H. Has the patient had any gynecologic surgery? The presence or absence of pelvic organs is important.

I. When was her last gynecologic examination? Information concerning her prior use of health care is important in planning further management.

J. Ask about exercise habits. Strenuous physical activity, particularly running or ballet dancing in a young woman, is associated with amenorrhea and irregular bleeding episodes.

K. Is there a history of psychotropic drug use? Tranquilizers and antidepressants are associated with amenorrhea and irregular periods.

L. Use of recreational drugs. Methadone and cocaine are associated with menstrual irregularities.

III. Differential Diagnosis

A. Threatened abortion. The best diagnosis in a sexually active woman with a missed period and abnormal bleeding is an ectopic pregnancy. Good contraceptive use only slightly modifies the risk.

B. Ectopic pregnancy. A missed period, irregular bleeding, and abdominal discomfort are also associated with ectopic pregnancy.

C. Stress amenorrhea. Strenuous physical activity, psychotropic drug use, or recreational drug use are all associated with irregular periods.

D. Oral contraceptive use. The more usual story for this diagnosis is one of gradually decreasing amounts of bleeding at the time of expected menses.

E. Polycystic ovary. This condition is associated with menstrual irregularity and elevations in luteinizing hormone (LH) and testosterone levels.

F. Halban's disease. A persistent corpus luteum may cause amenorrhea and then an abnormal bleeding event.

G. Early and mild pelvic inflammatory disease. Although not usually associated with amenorrhea, it does happen.

H. Factitious vaginal bleeding. Some women will confuse a heavy discharge with bleeding, or it may come from the bladder or rectum.

I. Dysfunctional uterine bleeding of unknown cause. If after careful evaluation an acceptable cause is not found, then this rather nonspecific term may be used.

IV. Database

A. Physical examination key points

1. **Vital signs.** Check pulse and blood pressure for evidence of hypovolemia. Fever may indicate an associated pelvic infection.

2. **Cardiorespiratory examination.** Evaluate in preparation for a general anesthetic.

3. **Abdominal examination.** Inspection and examination for local areas of tenderness, rebound tenderness, referred tenderness, and bowel sounds are important in assessing the potential for an extrauterine process or pelvic infection. Diffuse lower abdominal pain suggests pelvic inflammatory disease or abortion, while unilateral pain suggests an ectopic pregnancy.

4. **Pelvic examination**

   a. **Vulva and vagina.** Inspect for inflammation, irritation, and amount of blood. Also to be noted is the source of bleeding (cervical os or surface of cervix) and whether the os is open or closed.

   b. **Cervix.** Inspect with a speculum for evidence of erosion or inflammation. Evaluate for blood coming from the os and whether the cervical os is closed or dilated. Manually examine the cervix for consistency, size, and position. Is the cervix soft or hard? Softness suggests pregnancy.

   c. **Uterus.** Perform a manual examination for size, shape,

and consistency. Softness and enlargement suggest pregnancy, but a small uterus does not rule it out.
- **d. Adnexa.** Manually examine for masses or tenderness. Unilateral tenderness and enlargement suggest an ectopic pregnancy, while bilateral pain and tenderness suggest pelvic inflammatory disease. A unilateral moderately enlarged ovary suggests a persistent corpus luteum (associated with early pregnancy or Halban's disease).
- **5. Rectal examination.** Rule out this area by evaluating the cul-de-sac, adnexa, and appendiceal area for masses, tenderness, or fullness suggestive of blood or fluid in the posterior pouch.

B. Laboratory data
- **1. Hemogram.** This is useful for baseline data and to evaluate the patient's general status. A low value suggests intraperitoneal bleeding. An elevated WBC suggests infection, blood, or both in the peritoneal cavity.
- **2. Serum or urine pregnancy test.** A quantitative titer is very valuable since serial determinations of human chorionic gonadotropin (HCG) will assist in evaluating the status and location of the pregnancy. A level lower than expected by dates suggests an ectopic pregnancy or incomplete abortion. A normal level that doubles in 2 days is supportive of a normal intrauterine process, while less than this tends to occur with an abnormal pregnancy or location.
- **3. Urinalysis.** Rule out hematuria as a source of bleeding.
- **4. Hormone levels.** Obtain serum luteinizing hormone (LH), testosterone, and prolactin if HCG is negative, to evaluate hypothalamic, pituitary, and ovarian causes.

C. Radiologic and other studies
- **1. Sonography.** An echo study by abdominal or transvaginal probe is essential if the pregnancy test is positive, and more so if the quantitative HCG level is above 6000 MIU. Patients with levels above this should have evidence of an intrauterine pregnancy, while an empty uterine cavity is strongly associated with an ectopic pregnancy. A discrete ectopic pregnancy seen in the adnexal area is relatively rare. Adnexal cysts or inflammatory processes may be seen.
- **2. Culdocentesis.** With a positive pregnancy test and evidence of fluid in the cul-de-sac, a small-bore needle can be passed through the posterior fornix into the peritoneal cavity to detect blood. In cases of intraperitoneal bleeding, the blood obtained should not clot. (See Procedure 9, p. 357.)
- **3. Endometrial biopsy.** This may be carried out if the pregnancy test is negative. It provides evidence about the

patient's hormone status. A finding of proliferative tissue suggests an anovulatory event which causes irregular uterine bleeding. (See Procedures 11 and 12, pages 361 and 362.)

V. Plan. The most important step is determining if a pregnancy exists or not.

   A. Acute intervention. If the pregnancy test is positive, the location of the pregnancy must be determined. In patients with signs of an acute process, sonography indicating an empty uterine cavity, unilateral adnexal pain, and suggestive evidence of internal bleeding require surgery. Laparoscopy is the most definitive diagnostic step and should be carried out.

   B. Less acute status. If the pregnancy test is positive, the patient is in stable condition, and the status of the pregnancy is not clear, then admission with serial determination of serum HCG levels and repeat sonography provide a safe manner in which to observe the patient until the differential between a threatened abortion and an ectopic pregnancy can be made.

   C. Very stable patient. The patient may be allowed home but needs to return for serial HCG levels and repeat ultrasound studies if doubling does not occur.

   D. Negative pregnancy test. The cause of dysfunctional bleeding can be largely determined from the history, namely, drug use, pill use, tranquilizers, excessive exercise, and obesity. In addition, the LH, testosterone, and prolactin levels help to rule out polycystic ovaries.

REFERENCE

Cartwright PS: Ectopic pregnancy. In Jones HW III, Wentz AC, Burnett LS (eds): *Novak's Textbook of Gynecology,* 11th ed. Baltimore, Williams & Wilkins, 1988.

58. MENTAL STATUS CHANGES

I. Problem. A 39-year-old patient is 24 hours status post radical hysterectomy for cervical cancer. The ICU nurse reports that the patient is restless, agitated, confused, and possibly delusional.

II. Immediate Questions

   A. What happened to the patient before this occurred? Has she received a new medication? Almost any drug can cause changes in mental status. Pharmacologic agents are grouped into four main categories including antihypertensives, anticholinergics, anticonvulsants, and psychotropic medications. Family members can be helpful in eliciting the exact events leading to the patient's change in mental status. They can verify if the patient has had a mental illness in the past or if she experienced considerable anxiety associated with loss of her uterus and the diagnosis of cancer.

B. What is the patient's past medical history? Withdrawal from medications or from alcohol can cause various psychologic states as well as delirium tremens. The patient might not readily admit to a drinking problem, and a family member might be more helpful. Decreased blood flow in cardiac disease can cause enough cerebral hypoxia to produce the above symptoms. Pulmonary disease can do the same. If the patient was taking psychotropic medications preoperatively for a psychiatric diagnosis, then these need to be continued in the postoperative period.

C. What is the patient's baseline mental status? Mental retardation will make patients more prone to changes in mental status when they are placed in a foreign environment. Family members will again be helpful.

D. What are the patient's signs? Shock of any cause can result in poor cerebral perfusion and altered mental status. A changing respiratory pattern may indicate increased intracranial pressure, with initial slowing followed by a rapid respiratory rate.

E. Was the patient fully awake at any time since surgery? Get an idea of the time course for the change in neurologic status.

F. Is the patient a diabetic? Either hypoglycemia or hyperglycemia may cause altered mental status.

G. Are there any intravenous fluids? Depending on composition, these can lead to metabolic changes that cause somnolence and coma.

H. Was there a traumatic event? For example, did the patient fall out of bed?

I. Are there other symptoms? Syncope could be associated with hypotension or anemia causing decreased cerebral oxygenation. Chest pain would signify cardiac disease, and pleuritic chest pain could be from a pulmonary source. Inability to move an extremity or aphasia is a sign of stroke.

III. Differential Diagnosis

A. Trauma

1. **Subdural hematoma.** This is the most common intracranial mass lesion resulting from head injury.

    2. Epidural hematoma. An epidural hematoma is usually associated with a skull fracture and lacerated meningeal vessel.

    3. Concussion. This is a clinical diagnosis of cerebral dysfunction that clears within 24 hours.

    4. Contusion. A contusion is usually associated with neurologic deficits that persist longer than 24 hours after injury and that demonstrate small hemorrhages in the cerebral parenchyma on CT scan.

B. Metabolic causes

    1. Exogenous. These include alcohol (including withdrawal "delirium tremens"), drugs (including drug withdrawal), anesthetic agents (delayed clearance postop), or poisoning.

        a. Barbiturates, tranquilizers, anticholinergics, ethanol, opiates, antihypertensives, phenothiazines, lithium carbonate, or phenytoin.

        b. Paraldehyde is a common by-product of various chemotherapeutic agents.

        c. Street drugs.

    2. Endogenous

        a. Endocrine

            (1) **Pancreas.** Insulin, hypoglycemia, hyperglycemia.

            (2) **Pituitary.** Hyperpituitarism and hypopituitarism.

            (3) **Thyroid.** Hyperthyroidism and hypothyroidism.

            (4) **Adrenal.**

            (5) **Parathyroid.**

        b. Fluids/electrolytes

            (1) **Sodium.** Hyponatremia and hypernatremia may cause confusion.

            (2) **Hypokalemia, hyperkalemia.**

            (3) **Hypocalcemia, hypercalcemia.**

            (4) **Hypomagnesemia, hypermagnesemia.**

            (5) **Acidosis** (especially respiratory) **or alkalosis.**

            (6) **Osmolarity disturbances** (hyperosmolar coma).

        c. Organ failure, including renal, hepatic, or pulmonary: hypoxia, hypercapnia, or fat embolism syndrome (related to long bone fracture).

C. Infections

    1. Central nervous system infections (meningitis, encephalitis).

    2. Systemic sepsis.

D. Tumors

    1. Primary or metastatic to the CNS.

    2. Paraneoplastic syndromes.

E. Psychiatric causes. In psychogenic coma the neurologic and laboratory profiles are completely normal. Depression may also cause dementia, especially in the elderly. ICU psychosis and postcardiotomy delirium are occasionally seen.

F. Miscellaneous
1. **Seizures,** including postictal states.
2. **Cerebrovascular disease** including infarction or hemorrhage, arteriovenous malformation (AVM), or hypertensive encephalopathy.
3. **Syncope** (see Problem 69, page 266).
4. **Decreased cardiac output (shock)** (see Problem 54, page 199).
5. **Other CNS diseases.** These are usually more chronic. They include Alzheimer's, normal pressure hydrocephalus, and Wernicke's encephalopathy (thiamine deficiency).

IV. Database. If postop, determine the nature, onset, and duration of the event as well as anesthetic use by the patient postop, medications given, and IV fluids administered.

A. Physical examination key points
1. **Vital signs.** Hypertension, hypotension, tachycardia, bradycardia, and respiratory rate may give a clue to the diagnosis.
2. **HEENT.** Papilledema (increased intracranial pressure from a mass or hypertensive encephalopathy), meningeal signs such as nuchal rigidity (meningitis), pupillary reaction (pinpoint with narcotic; unilateral, fixed, and dilated with herniation; dilated and fixed with anoxia). Conjunctival and fundal petechiae occur with a fat embolism and fruity breath with ketoacidosis. Bruits may indicate a stroke.
3. **Skin.** Jaundice, spider angiomas, and palmer erythema are present with liver disease.
4. **Cardiopulmonary examination.** New-onset arrhythmia, congestive heart failure, as well as Stokes-Adams syndrome can cause decreased cerebral blood flow and hypoxia.
5. **Abdominal examination.** Look for enlarged liver from hepatic insufficiency or cardiac failure.
6. **Extremities.** Look for calf tenderness as well as unilateral edema, since this can be from venous thrombi. Bilateral massive edema can result from cardiac as well as renal failure.
7. **Mini-mental status examination.** Assess the level of consciousness (alert, drowsy, stupor, or coma). Check orientation to year, season, date, day, and month as well as to state, county, town, hospital, and floor. Test memory, attention span, and calculation. Test repetition, reading, writing, as well as copying.

       8. **Full neurologic examination.** Look for focal deficits, possibly from an intracranial process. Thyroid disease can cause slowing of the return portion of deep tendon reflexes. (See Appendix for the Glasgow Coma Scale including spontaneous movements and response to pain.)

  B. Laboratory data
    1. **Hemogram** to evaluate for infection, anemia.
    2. **Complete blood chemistries** (including electrolytes, BUN, creatinine, calcium, magnesium, osmolality). Glucose can be rapidly checked with a fingerstick glucometer available on most nursing units.
    3. **Arterial blood gases.** A respiratory or metabolic cause may be found.
    4. **Serum ammonia.** Elevation is indicative of hepatic failure.
    5. **Urine and serum toxicology screening** if indicated.
    6. **Other labs,** which will not be immediately available, include folate, B_{12}, free T_4, TSH, bromide, ceruloplasmin, HIV, and lead.
    7. **Cultures** if indicated for sepsis.

  C. Radiologic and other studies
    1. **Chest x-ray,** especially if an infectious or pulmonary source is possible.
    2. **CT scan of the head** if there is any indication of a CNS cause for coma, especially focal signs, papilledema.
    3. **Lumbar puncture** (see Procedure 21, page 377).
    4. **Electrocardiogram.** Evidence of myocardial infarction or artrial fibrillation (mural thrombi with emboli) may be seen.
    5. **Electroencephalogram.** Seizures and cerebral infarction alter brain wave patterns.

V. Plan. While therapy for changing neurologic status must be directed at the underlying cause, certain initial steps should be taken immediately. Start basic life support to ensure adequate airway, breathing, and circulation. Intubation may be necessary to protect the airway.

  A. Metabolic causes. Treat the defect shown on lab studies (refer to the specific abnormality in the index). A single ampule of 50% dextrose can be given IV if there is any suspicion of hypoglycemia. The effect on a patient in diabetic ketoacidosis is minimal, so it is always safer to give the dextrose.

  B. Exogenous causes. Any suspicion of narcotic-induced somnolence can be safely treated with naloxone 0.4–0.8 mg IV push. Repeat doses may be necessary (up to 4–5 ampules are commonly given in this situation).

C. **Tumor.** Somnolence in the presence of metastatic or primary CNS tumor is an emergency usually treated by radiotherapy. Give a dexamethasone bolus of 0.1–0.2 mg/kg.

D. **Infection.** Treat with high-dose antibiotics as appropriate to the organisms identified on gram stain.

E. **Cardiac syncope or low cardiac output.** Treat by approaching the underlying cardiac problem.

F. **Vascular causes.** Intracranial bleeding is usually treated like other causes of increased intracranial pressure. Contact the neurosurgical consultant. Increased intracranial pressure should be emergently treated since herniation may occur. Intubation with hyperventilation, osmotic diuresis with mannitol (1–1.5 g/kg over 20 minutes), and steroids (dexamethasone 10 mg IV) may acutely decrease intracranial pressure.

REFERENCES

Friedman HH (ed): *Problem-Oriented Medical Diagnosis.* Boston, Little, Brown, 1983.
Plum F, Posner J: *The Diagnosis of Stupor and Coma.* Philadelphia, FA Davis, 1980.
Schwartz SI, Shives GT, Spencer FC (eds): *Principles of Surgery,* 5th ed. New York, McGraw-Hill, 1989, pp. 486–490.

59. NASOGASTRIC TUBE MANAGEMENT: BLOODY DRAINAGE

I. **Problem.** Three days after total abdominal hysterectomy and small bowel resection, a 43-year-old woman has bloody output from her nasogastric (NG) tube.

II. **Immediate Questions**

A. **How long has the NG tube been in place?** A tube that has just been placed may have bloody drainage from the trauma of insertion or as a result of recent gastric surgery. An old tube may show blood from local mucosal irritation.

B. **How much bloody drainage has there been?** A tube passing large amounts of bright red blood is obviously a more critical situation than one passing a few red streaks.

C. **Is the patient status post upper gastrointestinal surgery?** There may be a marginal ulcer at an old anastomotic site or, if the surgery was recent, there may be bleeding at a newly formed anastomosis.

D. **Is the patient receiving antacids, and what is the pH of the** fluid? The presence of acidic gastric secretions increases the likelihood that gastritis will develop. Specifically, the pH should be kept greater than 4–5 for mucosal protection.

III. Differential Diagnosis

A. Insertion trauma, usually nasopharyngeal in origin.

B. Mucosal irritation, often from a tube that has been in place for some time. There is usually an associated acidic pH.

C. Suture line disruption or hemorrhage, especially in a patient recently operated upon.

D. Swallowed pharyngeal blood from an upper source of bleeding perhaps unrelated to the nasogastric tube.

E. Ulceration (Curling, Cushing, or preexisting). Look for associated conditions: burns, head injury, etc.

F. Gastric erosion/gastritis/esophagitis/varices.

G. Coagulopathy.

IV. Database

A. Physical examination key points

1. **Vital signs.** Look for tachycardia or hypotension as evidence of sepsis or excessive blood loss.
2. **HEENT.** Check for evidence of obvious pharyngeal bleeding.
3. **Abdomen.** Peritoneal signs, epigastric tenderness, or gastric distention may be present.

B. Laboratory data

1. **Hemogram.** Obtain this to check for excessive blood loss or thrombocytopenia.
2. **Coagulation studies.** Determine prothrombin time and partial thromboplastin time to rule out coagulopathy.

C. Radiologic and other studies

1. **Chest x-ray.** Order an upright film to look for free intra-abdominal air. Look at the mediastinum and both lung fields for air that may be a result of esophageal perforation after forceful vomiting (Boerhaave's syndrome).
2. **pH.** Check the pH of the gastric fluid; it must be maintained > 3.5.

V. Plan. Determine whether the cause of bleeding is serious enough to require specific aggressive therapy. Is there hypotension or hemodynamic instability? Place a large-bore IV (16-gauge or larger) and begin fluid and blood replacement. The presence of peritoneal signs or new free intra-abdominal air usually requires emergency laparotomy.

A. **NG irrigation.** Irrigate the NG tube with saline. The temperature of the saline is not important; room temperature is acceptable. This will enable diagnosis of further bleeding as well as the therapeutic maneuver of removing clots from the stomach which lead to distention and persistent bleeding.

B. **Antacid therapy.** A pH < 3.5 should be corrected with antacids and H_2 antagonists (Maalox 30 ML q2h via NG tube). Intravenous H_2 blockers (cimetidine, etc) should also be used.

C. **Endoscopy.** Perform upper GI endoscopy if bleeding persists. (See Problem 43, page 168, for a discussion of persistent bleeding.)

REFERENCE

Eastwood G: Upper GI bleeding: differential diagnosis. *Hosp Med* 23:57, 1987.

60. NASOGASTRIC TUBE MANAGEMENT: CHANGE IN AMOUNT OF OUTPUT

I. **Problem.** A 46-year-old woman has a sudden increase in the amount of nasogastric (NG) tube aspirate on the fifth hospital day after tumor debulking for ovarian cancer. Another patient, after small bowel resection, has minimal NG aspirate.

II. **Immediate Questions**

A. **Is there associated abdominal distress?** If the patient developed a generalized ileus or an obstruction, the output may increase.

B. **Is the output bilious?** Bilious NG output indicates a more distal problem with bile reflux into the stomach or a nasogastric tube placed distal to the pylorus.

C. **Is the tube functioning?** Tubes often become obstructed with mucus or antacids. Listen for a whistle on the sump tube, indicating patency, and verify that the suction is functioning.

D. **Is the patient passing flatus or stool?** Often, decreased NG output correlates with return of bowel function.

E. **Is the patient taking anything by mouth?** Ice chips and sips of liquids can often be excessive and give rise to spuriously increased tube output.

III. Differential Diagnosis. See page 400 for the average daily production of saliva and gastric, duodenal, and biliary tract fluids as a guide to the expected average daily production of GI fluids.

A. Increased output
1. **Tip of tube distal to pylorus.** The tube aspirates all biliary and pancreatic secretions as well as gastric output.
2. **Distal bowel obstruction or gastric outlet obstruction.**
3. **Return to higher secretory state.** This may occur after discontinuation of H_2 blockers such as cimetidine.
4. **Tip of tube above GE junction.** The tube may actually be coiled in back of the throat.

IV. Database. Ask the patient about any abdominal complaints, and in particular ask about the passage of flatus or stool as a guide to overall bowel function.

A. Physical examination key points
1. **HEENT.** Look for whether the tube is coiled or kinked in the mouth or throat.
2. **Abdomen.** Listen for bowel sounds and their quality. No sounds may indicate ileus or far-advanced obstruction. High-pitched, hollow sounds indicate obstruction. Distention may mean obstruction or ileus.
3. **Rectum.** Determine the presence or absence of stool.

B. Laboratory data
1. **Serum electrolytes.** Carefully monitor hydration status and potassium and bicarbonate levels during nasogastric suction.
2. **Nasogastric aspirate pH.** A pH > 6 indicates use of antacids or, more likely, that the tip of the catheter is distal to the pylorus.

C. Radiologic and other studies
1. **Upright chest x-ray.** Look for a large stomach bubble indicating poor gastric emptying. Check the position of the tube tip and verify that it is in the stomach.
2. **Upright and flat abdominal x-rays.** These studies may show distended bowel indicating ileus or obstruction.
3. **Contrast swallow.** When partial bowel obstruction or upper GI obstruction is contemplated, serial films after Gastrografin or dilute barium swallow will show normal or delayed emptying and passage of contrast. Contrast should **not** be used in the presence of ileus or complete obstruction.

V. Plan. The first priority is simply to determine that the NG tube is functioning and is in a proper position. **Manipulation of nasogastric tubes must be performed with full understanding of the nature of the surgical procedure for which the tube was placed.**

A. Verify position. This is based on x-ray confirmation. Flushing the tube with 40–60 cc of air and listening over the stomach results in a typical crackle or pop; however, this may also be heard with the tube in the distal esophagus or duodenum.

B. Verify function. Sump tubes should whistle continuously on low suction. Most tubes need to be flushed with saline (30 mL) every 3–4 hours to maintain patency.

C. Increased output
1. **Poor gastric emptying (no obstruction).** Try metoclopramide 10 mg IV q6h.
2. **Distal obstruction.** Continue NG suction; consider further workup (x-ray contrast studies as above) and possibly operation to relieve obstruction.
3. **Ileus.** Exercise patience, especially if the patient is immediately postop. Correct electrolyte abnormalities, particularly hypokalemia, with parenteral solution. Continue NG suction. Prolonged ileus may indicate intra-abdominal sepsis.

D. Decreased output
1. Most often this indicates return of bowel function. Correlate with physical examination and passage of flatus or stool. Remove the tube if appropriate.
2. Irrigate the tube to clear it, or advance the tube into the stomach if it is not positioned correctly.

REFERENCE

Ranson JHC: Complications of small intestine surgery. In Hardy JD (ed): *Complications in Surgery and Their Management.* Philadelphia, WB Saunders, 1981.

61. NAUSEA AND VOMITING

I. Problem. One week following tumor debulking for ovarian carcinoma, a patient complains of nausea and then vomits repeatedly.

II. Immediate Questions

A. Are there any associated symptoms, particularly gastrointestinal? Nausea and vomiting may accompany a wide spectrum of illnesses covering most body systems. Inquire about related concurrent symptoms to focus the differential diagnosis. Specifically, ask about abdominal pain, abdominal distention, diarrhea, or constipation/obstipation associated with the nausea and vomiting.

B. What is the appearance and odor of the vomitus? Sometimes the vomited material can give clues to the nature of the underlying dysfunction. First, look and test for blood (see Problem 43, page 168). Feculent vomitus indicates stasis or distal obstruction. Bilious vomit merely implies a patent pyloric channel. A change in the vomit from bilious to bloody may indicate a Mallory-Weiss tear.

C. How is the vomiting related to eating or to specific medications? In the postoperative setting, note if the vomiting correlates with beginning or advancing an enteral diet. Vomiting 1 or 2 hours after eating (especially if the vomit is partially digested food) points to gastric stasis or gastric outlet obstruction. Vomiting concurrent with or immediately after eating is often psychogenic. Certain medications such as narcotics or nonsteroidal anti-inflammatory drugs can cause vomiting.

D. Is the vomiting projectile? Projectile vomiting is often associated with CNS dysfunction. However, it may also occur with certain types of food poisoning.

III. Differential Diagnosis. The differential list that follows is structured around the primary system involved in the underlying cause of nausea and vomiting (Also refer to Problems 1, 28, and 29, pages 1, 104, and 110).

  A. Gastrointestinal
    1. **General**
      a. **Peritonitis.** The patient is often febrile.
      b. **Postoperative ileus.** Normal GI tract function usually returns within 48 hours after laparotomy, unless complications intervene.
      c. **Mechanical obstruction at any level.**
      d. **Gastroenteritis.** This may be related to either a virus or a toxin (food poisoning).
      e. **Tumor.** Metastatic mesenteric implants may cause an ileus through obstructive or neurogenic mechanisms.
    2. **Stomach**
      a. **Gastric outlet obstruction.**
      b. **Peptic ulcer disease.**
      c. **Gastric atony.** This may be due to diabetes.
    3. **Hepatobiliary/pancreas**
      a. **Biliary colic or acute cholecystitis.**
      b. **Pancreatitis.**
      c. **Hepatitis.**

      4. Colon
         a. Diverticulitis.
         b. **Malignant obstruction** from colorectal or ovarian can-
            cer.
         c. Appendicitis.
   B. Metabolic
      1. Uremia.
      2. Hepatic failure.
      3. Metabolic acidosis.
      4. Electrolyte abnormalities.
         a. Hypercalcemia.
         b. Hyperkalemia.
   C. Endocrine
      1. **Diabetes.** Gastroparesis may be involved.
      2. **Adrenal insufficiency.** This may follow abrupt withdrawal
         of chronic steroids.
      3. Hypothyroidism.
   D. Drugs/toxins
      1. Alcohol abuse.
      2. Botulism.
      3. **Food poisoning** (eg, staphylococcal).
      4. Food or drug allergy.
      5. **Narcotics.** Codeine is a common offender.
      6. **Nonsteroidal anti-inflammatory drugs** (eg, ibuprofen).
      7. Chemotherapeutic agents.
   E. Cardiopulmonary
      1. **Acute myocardial infarction,** particularly inferior myocar-
         dial infarction.
      2. Congestive heart failure (CHF).
   F. Genitourinary
      1. **Renal colic.** Hematuria and flank pain are usually present.
      2. Pelvic inflammatory disease.
      3. **Pregnancy,** particularly in the first trimester.
   G. Nervous system
      1. **Space-occupying CNS lesion.** Increased intracranial pres-
         sure can cause nausea and vomiting which may be projec-
         tile.
      2. Migraine headache.
      3. Labyrinthitis or motion sickness.
   H. **Acute febrile illnesses,** particularly in the pediatric age group.

IV. Database
   A. Physical examination key points

1. **Vital signs.** Orthostatic blood pressure changes suggest volume depletion; fever suggests an inflammatory component.
2. **HEENT.** Look for pharyngitis, otitis, or other evidence of acute infections; papilledema may indicate increased intracranial pressure.
3. **Skin.** Assess skin turgor and mucous membranes to estimate volume status. Yellowing of the skin may signify jaundice.
4. **Abdomen.** Evaluate for bowel sounds, abdominal distention, peritoneal signs, and areas of tenderness.
5. **Rectum.** Look for evidence of fecal impaction, rectal mass, or occult blood in the stool.
6. **Pelvic examination.** It may diagnose pelvic inflammatory disease.
7. **Neurologic examination.** Mental status changes may signify a CNS lesion or severe electrolyte abnormalities.

B. **Laboratory data**
   1. **Hemogram.** This is indicated for signs of infection.
   2. **Electrolytes.** Hypochloremia and hypokalemia may result from severe vomiting.
   3. **BUN and creatinine.** These determinations give an idea about fluid balance and may reveal unsuspected renal failure.
   4. **Liver function tests.** Hepatitis or other liver disease may be found.
   5. **Amylase.** Determine the level if pancreatitis is suspected.
   6. **Urinalysis and urine culture.** These tests may reveal infection; blood may be seen with stones or infection.
   7. **Arterial blood gases,** if indicated. Protracted vomiting may cause metabolic alkalosis; ischemic bowel and chronic renal failure may cause acidosis.
   8. **Human chorionic gonadotropin.** Urinary HCG is used to diagnose pregnancy.

C. **Radiologic and other studies**
   1. **KUB (kidneys, ureter, bladder) and upright abdominal films.** In most patients with vomiting, and always if there is abdominal distention, obtain abdominal films. Look for air-fluid levels and dilated bowel.
   2. **Chest x-ray.** A chest film can aid in the diagnosis of pneumonia or CHF and can show evidence of aspiration. Look for free abdominal air on the upright film.
   3. **Electrocardiogram.** Obtain an ECG if there is a possibility of ischemic heart disease.
   4. **Abdominal ultrasound/HIDA scan.** Perform these studies if there is a possibility of biliary colic.

    5. Upper GI series/upper endoscopy. If significant obstruction is likely, use Gastrografin instead of barium.

    6. Barium enema/colonoscopy. These studies are appropriate when there is evidence of a colonic lesion or obstruction.

    7. CT scan of the head. CT should be performed if an intracranial lesion is suspected.

V. Plan. Immediately make the patient NPO. If the patient is volume depleted, begin intravenous replacement; if not depleted, begin maintenance IV fluids (see Chapter 4). Narcotics are common offenders in the postoperative surgical patient, and switching to another agent (from Demerol to morphine, for example) may solve the problem.

  A. Abdominal cause. Place a nasogastric tube if there is persistent vomiting, mechanical obstruction, or abdominal distention. Proceed with the diagnostic workup.

  B. Nonabdominal causes. These comprise metabolic disorders, labyrinthitis, and minor infections including acute viral gastroenteritis. Assess volume status, administer intravenous fluids if indicated, treat the underlying disorder, and treat vomiting with antiemetics. Frequently used antiemetics include:

    1. Prochlorperazine (Compazine) 10 mg IM or PO q6h or 25 mg PR bid.

    2. Trimethobenzamide (Tigan) 250 mg PO or 200 mg IM or PR q6–8h.

    3. Promethazine (Phenergan) 12.5–25 mg PO or 25 mg IM q8h.

    4. Meclizine (Antivert) 25–50 mg PO q8–12h; useful for nausea in labyrinthitis or vertigo.

    5. Metochlopramide (Reglan) 10 mg IV or PO q6h; particularly useful in diabetes or other situations with poor gastric emptying.

    6. Ondansetron (Zofran) 0.15 mg/kg given over 15 minutes, 30 minutes before and 4 and 8 hours after chemotherapy; useful for patients receiving cisplatin.

REFERENCE

McGuigan JE, Wolfe MM: Anorexia, nausea and vomiting. In Blacklow RS (ed): MacBryde's *Signs and Symptoms: Applied Pathologic Physiology and Clinical Interpretation,* 6th edition. Philadelphia, JB Lippincott, 1983.

62. OLIGURIA/ANURIA

  I. Problem. One day following total pelvic exenteration and reconstruction, a patient has sequential hourly urine outputs of 22, 15, 9, and 4 mL via an indwelling Foley catheter.

II. Immediate Questions

A. What is the patient's volume status?
The most common cause of oliguria in the postoperative setting is hypovolemia. An important differential diagnosis is acute tubular necrosis (ATN), usually secondary to ischemia, which is also related to hypovolemia. Assess volume status by the means available, ie, left-sided pressures from a pulmonary artery catheter, central venous pressures, weight change, and always by physical exam. Do not let elevated weight dissuade you if other assessments point to a decreased intravascular volume. Be sure that hypovolemia is not a result of hemorrhage.

B. Did the patient suffer any periods of documented hypotension?
As mentioned, ischemic ATN is a cause of oliguria on a surgical service. Review the anesthesia record, noting any episodes of hypotension intraoperatively.

C. What is the baseline renal function?
If there is preexisting renal insufficiency, any ischemic or toxic insult to the kidneys will be amplified.

D. Is the patient taking any nephrotoxic drugs?
Aminoglycosides (gentamicin, etc) are the major offenders. Send off appropriate samples for drug levels and hold the next dose until the results are back.

E. Is the patient taking any medication that is excreted by the kidneys?
Digoxin and antibiotics are the most important medications in this category. Either modify or hold the dose until renal function improves or drug levels become available.

F. Is the patient receiving chemotherapy?
Cisplatin can be nephrotoxic.

G. Does the patient have a history of carcinoma?
Bilateral ureteral compression may result in oliguria.

H. Has the patient recently undergone surgery?
Pelvic dissections and hysterectomy may result in inadvertent ureteral ligation.

I. Is the Foley catheter patent?
Most nurses will think of this before you do, but flush the catheter at least once to make sure the oliguria is a real reflection of renal function (see Problem 41, page 159).

III. Differential Diagnosis.
Oliguria is defined as urine output < 500

mL/d and anuria as output < 100 ml/d. The differential diagnosis for acute oliguria is identical to that for acute renal failure and may be viewed as from prerenal, renal, or postrenal causes.

A. Prerenal, relating to renal hypoperfusion.
  1. **Shock/hypovolemia**
      a. **Hemorrhage,** either traumatic or as a postoperative complication.
      b. **Inadequate fluid administration.** Especially during prolonged surgery when the abdomen or retroperitoneum is open, excessive fluid can be lost by evaporation.
      c. **Sepsis** causing decreased renal perfusion due to diminished systemic vascular resistance.
  2. **Apparent intravascular hypovolemia.** This consists of a relative decrease in the effective circulating volume.
      a. **"Third space" losses.** These are very common in the initial postoperative period following major operations or with major burns.
      b. **Congestive heart failure.**
      c. **Cirrhosis.** The patient may have associated hepatorenal syndrome.
      d. **Nephrotic syndrome.**
  3. **Vascular**
      a. **Renal artery occlusion** (acute or chronic).
      b. **Aortic dissection.**
      c. **Emboli** (eg, cholesterol).

B. Renal
  1. **Acute tubular necrosis**
      a. **Ischemic,** secondary to shock or sepsis.
      b. **Toxic,** such as from medications (aminoglycosides), contrast media, or heavy metals.
  2. **Acute interstitial nephritis**
      a. **Drugs** including beta-lactamase-resistant penicillins, nonsteroidal anti-inflammatory agents (ibuprofen, etc).
      b. **Hypercalcemia.** This can cause nephrocalcinosis.
  3. **Acute glomerular disease**
      a. **Malignant hypertension.**
      b. **Immune complex disease.**
      c. **Systemic diseases** (Wegener's, thrombotic thrombocytopenic purpura, systemic lupus erythematosus, Goodpasture's).

C. Postrenal
  1. **Urethral obstruction** from carcinoma, catheter obstruction.
  2. **Bilateral ureteral obstruction** caused by carcinoma, retroperitoneal fibrosis, clots, papillary tissue, calculi, and inadvertent surgical kinking or ligation.

IV. Database

A. Physical examination key points

1. **Vital signs.** Look for weight change and orthostatic signs to document fluid loss. Fever occurs with sepsis.
2. **Skin.** Tissue turgor, mucous membranes, or edema will help to evaluate the volume status.
3. **Cardiopulmonary examination.** Check for rales, elevated venous pressure, or cardiac gallop.
4. **Abdomen.** Determine if there is ascites or a distended bladder.
5. **Extremities.** Assess perfusion by color and temperature.

B. Laboratory data

1. **Hemogram.** Perform blood studies for evidence of infection or anemia.
2. **Drug levels.** Obtain levels of any nephrotoxic drugs (eg, aminoglycosides) or drugs cleared by the kidneys (digoxin).
3. **Urinalysis.** Protein and red blood cell casts support glomerular disease. Eosinophils are associated with hypersensitivity reactions and interstitial nephritis. WBC casts may indicate glomerulonephritis. Hyaline and fine granular casts may indicate prerenal azotemia, while glomerular and epithelial casts suggest ATN. A benign sediment raises the possibility of obstruction.
4. **Urine electrolytes and creatinine.** Obtain these levels prior to giving diuretics. Urinary sodium > 20 meq/L indicates a prerenal cause; < 20 meq/L is suggestive of a renal cause. Calculate fractional excretion of sodium (FEna) as urinary sodium × plasma creatinine ÷ urine creatinine × plasma sodium. If FEna > 1 the cause is likely renal; if FEna < 1 it is likely prerenal. (See also page 333.)

C. Radiologic and other studies

1. **Ultrasound.** Echo is the test of choice to examine the collecting system for signs of chronic obstruction; it also estimates renal size.
2. **Chest x-ray.** Studies may reveal congestive failure.
3. **Kidneys, ureter, bladder.** KUB may reveal obstructing renal calculi.
4. **Intravenous pyelogram.** A combination of ultrasound, renal scan, and retrograde studies will give equivalent information without nephrotoxic contrast media. However, IVP remains the gold standard for evaluation of acute unilateral obstruction.
5. **Renal scan.** A technetium-labeled DTPA nuclear medicine study is done to assess blood flow to the kidneys; it is also useful in differentiating a parenchymal lesion from an obstructive process.

6. **Angiography.** Order if an angiogram is needed to visualize vascular anatomy, but this is rarely needed acutely.

7. **Renal biopsy.** Occasionally a biopsy is needed to determine the specific diagnosis of a renal cause of oliguria, but it is not needed acutely.

8. **Catheterization.** A central venous pressure (CVP) line or pulmonary artery (PA) catheter will give useful information about volume status.

V. Plan. As a general rule, the minimal acceptable urine output in an adult is 0.5–1 mL/kg/h. Accurate intake and output records are essential; consider inserting a Foley catheter if one is not in place. Review the patient's medications and stop or alter all nephrotoxic or renal-excreted drugs and remove potassium from the IV fluids.

A. Foley catheter drainage. Make sure the Foley catheter is working by irrigating with 50 mL normal saline using a catheter-tipped syringe. The fluid should pass easily and the entire amount should be aspirated. If a catheter problem is noted, correct it.

B. Fluid challenge. As stated above, oliguria in most surgical patients equals hypovolemia. In almost every case it is appropriate to give the patient a potassium-free volume challenge (eg, 500 mL of normal saline). In patients with fragile cardiorespiratory status, smaller boluses should be given and central venous catheters used to monitor volume status.

C. Prerenal management
1. Treat with volume boluses to increase urine output and adjust the baseline IV rate upward.
2. Monitor volume replacement with central lines and central venous pressures (eg, keep CVP > 10 mm Hg) if needed. Maintain hematocrit usually > 25–30%.
3. Give specific criteria to be notified for (eg, call house officer for urine output < 30 mL/h); a typical limit is 0.5 mL/kg/h.

D. Renal management
1. Monitor volume status with central lines. Restrict total fluid intake to insensible losses plus drainage volume and urine output.
2. Remove potassium from IV solutions unless it is abnormally low. Follow electrolytes closely, especially potassium.
3. Attempt to increase urine output once volume status is corrected.
   a. **Furosemide.** Use escalating doses to obtain the response of increased urine output. One method is to start with 80 mg IV, then 160 and 320 mg IV.

    b. Mannitol. Give 12.5–25 g (50–100 mL of a 25% solution) IV to induce osmotic diuresis.

   4. Review medications. Adjust doses or stop nephrotoxic drugs.

E. Postrenal management. A blocked Foley catheter can be treated as outlined in Problem 41 (page 159). Most other causes can be acutely managed with a Foley catheter and percutaneous nephrostomy tubes with subsequent attempt at antegrade passage of a ureteral stent or surgical correction.

REFERENCE

Palani CK, Moss GK: Oliguria, anuria: acute renal failure. In Condon RE, DeCosse JJ (eds): *Surgical Care.* Philadelphia, Lea & Febiger, 1980, pp 199–211.

63. PASSED TISSUE

I. Problem. You are called to see a 27-year-old para 1001 who reports she has passed something from her vagina that looks fleshy.

II. Immediate Questions

   A. Is there a history of fever and chills? The passage of an unrecognized tampon may be associated with toxic shock syndrome (TSS).

   B. Was any bleeding associated with the passage of tissue? Mild bleeding before and after the event strongly suggests a pregnancy-related problem. No bleeding suggests an intravaginal foreign body.

   C. When was her last menstrual period (LMP), and was it completely normal? A period that is normal in time of onset, amount of bleeding, and associated symptoms almost never occurs in a woman who is pregnant. The sequence of events after the LMP should be established.

   D. What is the interval between her LMP and the current complaint? If more than 4 weeks, a pregnancy-related problem is very possible. Under 4 weeks makes this less likely. Exactly 4 weeks suggests a menstrual-related event.

   E. Does she have any bleeding at present? Small amounts of spotting suggest an intrauterine source for the tissue.

   F. Does she have any lower abdominal pain? Cramps and discomfort suggest an intrauterine source for the tissue.

   G. Obtain a brief history of her menstrual periods. A history of normal menarche and regular periods indicates a more acute event, while irregular periods suggest a more chronic underlying problem.

H. Is she sexually active? Exposure to sperm is important information, and most women will be forthright in answering this question.

I. What form of contraception is she using? Oral contraceptives are not associated with passage of a decidual cast. An intrauterine device (IUD) may be passed at the time of a menstrual period and appear to be fleshy when covered with a blood clot.

J. Has the patient had any gynecologic surgery? The presence or absence of pelvic organs is important.

K. When was her last gynecologic examination? Information concerning her use of health care and what was noted is important in planning further management.

L. Was there a bad odor when the material was passed? Forgotten tampons and condoms are usually associated with an offensive odor.

M. Did she bring the material with her, and what does it look like? In some cases it will clearly be products of conception or foreign matter, while in other cases it is difficult to be certain exactly what the material is. If she did not bring the material, then one must assume it is pregnancy related.

III. Differential Diagnosis

A. Spontaneous abortion. The best diagnosis is a sexually active woman with a story of passing tissue is spontaneous abortion.

B. Incomplete spontaneous abortion. Although she reports passage of tissue, it may be incomplete.

C. Ectopic pregnancy. The fleshy tissue may be a decidual cast and the patient may have an ectopic pregnancy. With changes in hormone level, the decidualized endometrium may be passed and thus look fleshy.

D. Halban's disease. A persistent corpus luteum may cause a decidualized endometrium that passes upon decline of the progesterone level.

E. Foreign body. Forgotten tampons and condoms may be misinterpreted by the patient.

IV. Database

A. Physical examination key points

1. **Vital signs.** Check pulse and blood pressure for evidence of hypovolemia and shock. Fever may indicate an associated pelvic infection or TSS secondary to a retained tampon.
2. **Cardiorespiratory examination.** Evaluation is in preparation for an anesthetic.
3. **Abdominal examination.** Inspection and examination for local areas of tenderness, rebound tenderness, referred tenderness, and bowel sounds are important in assessing the potential for an extrauterine process or pelvic infection. Diffuse lower abdominal pain suggests pelvic inflammatory disease or abortion, while unilateral pain suggests ectopic pregnancy.
4. **Pelvic examination.** Inspect the vulva and vagina for inflammation, irritation, and evidence of surface irritation consistent with a retained tampon. Inspect the cervix with a speculum for signs of erosion or inflammation and amount of bleeding, if any; cervical softening is suggestive of a pregnancy state. The uterus should be evaluated for changes in size, shape, and consistency. Although a large, soft, globular uterus is indicative of pregnancy, a small uterus does not rule it out. Ectopic pregnancies present as unilateral adnexal enlargement with increased tenderness. A unilateral, moderately enlarged, nontender ovary suggests a persistent corpus luteum (associated with early pregnancy or Halban's disease).
5. **Rectal examination.** To rule out this area as a source of the bleeding, evaluate the cul-de-sac, adnexa, and appendiceal area for masses, tenderness, or fullness suggestive of blood or fluid in the posterior pouch.

B. Laboratory data

1. **Hemogram.** This is useful for baseline data and to evaluate the patient's general status. A low value suggests blood loss. An elevated WBC suggests infection.
2. **Serum or urine pregnancy test.** A quantitative value is very valuable since serial determinations of human chorionic gonadotropin will assist in evaluating the status and location of the pregnancy. A level lower than expected by dates suggests an ectopic pregnancy or abortion. A normal level that doubles in 2 days is supportive of a normal intrauterine process, while less than this tends to occur with an abnormal pregnancy or location.

C. Radiologic and other studies

1. **Sonography.** An echo study using an abdominal or transvaginal probe is essential if the pregnancy test is positive and the material passed has features of a decidual cast.

Negative adnexa and evidence of blood in the uterine cavity suggest a complete abortion.

2. **Endometrial biopsy.** This may be carried out if the pregnancy test is negative. It provides evidence about the patient's hormone status. A finding of proliferative tissue suggests an anovulatory event which causes irregular uterine bleeding (see Procedure 12, page 362).

V. Plan. The most important step is determining if a pregnancy exists or not.

A. **Acute intervention.** If the tissue passed is suggestive of products of conception and the os is slightly open, then a therapeutic dilation and curettage must be carried out with reasonable dispatch. If the adnexa are negative for masses while the patient is under anesthesia, no further procedures are necessary. The tissue must be sent for rush examination. If evidence of pregnancy is not found, careful evaluation including laparoscopy for a possible ectopic pregnancy must be carried out.

B. **Conservative care.** If the tissue appears to be a complete pregnancy, the cervical os is closed, no bleeding is present, and the hematocrit is stable, the patient may be sent home and the tissue sent for rush pathologic assessment. If products of conception are not found, then the patient must return for further evaluation to rule out the presence of an ectopic pregnancy.

C. **The pregnancy test is negative.** The patient may be reassured she is not pregnant and that subsequent menstrual events will be evaluated.

D. **The material is clearly a foreign body.** Most patients are acutely embarrassed and will leave promptly. Simple douching for a day or so will help to reduce the odor and promote healing. An antibiotic is not necessary as a prophylactic for TSS.

REFERENCE

Wentz AC: Abnormal uterine bleeding. In Jones HW III, Wentz AC, Burnett LS (eds): *Novak's Textbook of Gynecology,* 11th ed., Baltimore, Williams & Wilkins, 1988.

64. POSTOPERATIVE FEVER

I. **Problem.** A 42-year-old woman develops a temperature of 38.6 °C (101.5°F) 4 days following hysterectomy.

II. **Immediate Questions**

A. **Is the patient experiencing pain?** The presence and location of pain often cues the examiner and focuses the remainder of the examination. Deep pelvic pain or fullness suggests a pelvic hematoma, pelvic abscess, or cuff abscess. More superficial abdominal pain may be due to abdominal wall hematomas/abscesses or simple wound infections. Intense incisional pain out of proportion to the wound's appearance may be the first clue to a serious wound infection (eg, necrotizing fasciitis).

B. Has the patient been taking antibiotics perioperatively or postoperatively? If the patient is already being treated for an infection without response (ie, 48–72 hours after the first dose), several considerations must be entertained. Inappropriate antibiotics or dosage, resistant organisms, inaccurate diagnosis, an unresponsive abscess (pelvic or abdominal wall), or drug fever are all reasonable possibilities in this scenario.

C. Does the patient have respiratory symptoms (dyspnea, cough, tachypnea)? Involvement of the respiratory tract is a significant cause of postoperative infectious morbidity, particularly following upper abdominal procedures.

D. When was the onset of fever? The onset of fever relative to the operative procedure is particularly helpful in determining the cause. Early fever (< 48 hours) may be due to unrecognized ureteral injury, unrecognized established infections, "early" wound infections (due to group A strep), aspiration pneumonia, or contaminated intravenous solutions. Most diagnoses of atelectasis are tenuous at best, and should have objective findings to support the diagnosis (x-ray). Most febrile morbidity results from fevers that develop 3–8 days following surgery. These are often due to "routine" abdominal wound infections, urinary tract infections, or cellulitis or abscess of the cuff. Late-onset fever (> 8 days) may be due to transfusion-related infections (eg, cytomegalovirus, hepatitis), late pelvic abscesses or pelvic cellulitis, or osteomyelitis (after MMK-type urethropexy).

E. Does the patient have GI complaints (nausea and vomiting or diarrhea)? Nausea and vomiting may suggest bowel obstruction or hypomotility (ie, adynamic ileus). Adynamic ileus is a frequent complication of pelvic floor peritonitis as the small bowel which sits in the basin of the pelvic floor becomes inflamed, suspending normal peristalsis. Diarrhea in the face of fever may be nonspecific but should arouse suspicion of pseudomembranous colitis, particularly if the patient has received antibiotics (even a single dose for prophylaxis).

F. What procedure was performed? Postoperative febrile morbidity (defined as temperature > 38.0 °C or 100.4 °F on two readings at least 6 hours apart beyond the first 24 hours after surgery) occurs more frequently following vaginal than abdominal hysterectomy. Also, following abdominal hysterectomy, both incision sites (abdominal and vaginal) should be considered possible sources of infection. Alternatively, "clean cases" in which the vaginal cuff is not opened (eg, ovarian cystectomy) result in lower postoperative febrile morbidity and wound infection rates when compared to "clean-contaminated" cases (ie, where the cuff is opened).

G. Does the patient have urinary complaints or flank pain? The urinary tract is a common site of postoperative infection. The complaint of dysuria is not specific for infection since irritation from an indwelling catheter can produce this symptom without infection. High fever as a result of simple cystitis is uncommon, and if the urinary tract is implicated, a temperature > 38.0 °C suggests upper tract disease (ie, pyelonephritis). The triad of flank pain, fever, and tachycardia should raise concern about ureteral injury (ligation, laceration, or kinking resulting in obstruction). This will usually present in the first 3 postoperative days. Oliguria may be a sign of hypovolemia (hemorrhage or inadequate fluid intake) or septic shock. Anuria may be due to an obstructed indwelling catheter (associated with bladder distention) or bilateral ureteral ligation.

H. Is the patient receiving a blood product transfusion? Fever during blood transfusion is common and disappears after the transfusion is stopped.

III. Differential Diagnosis

A. Pelvic cuff cellulitis or abscess. Postoperative pelvic infections are fairly common following hysterectomy because the procedure is "clean-contaminated" (ie, the peritoneum is exposed to vaginal flora). The advent of routine use of prophylactic antibiotics has substantially reduced postoperative infectious morbidity following vaginal hysterectomy. The most frequent complaint associated with pelvic cuff cellulitis is a sense of fullness in the lower abdomen associated with fever, most frequently 3–6 days following surgery.

B. Urinary tract infection or injury. Indwelling urinary catheters are almost universally used during and following hysterectomy. The longer the catheter remains in place, the more likely the urinary tract is to be colonized with bacteria. Fever associated with significant flank tenderness indicates either upper tract infection (pyelonephritis) or ureteral injury (ligation, crush injury, laceration).

C. Pelvic hematoma. Significant bleeding into the abdomen or retroperitoneal space is often accompanied by fever and a drop in hematocrit. Persistent fever, particularly if it is not responsive to appropriate antibiotics, suggests secondary infection. A hematoma of the abdominal wound or in the space of Retzius (eg, during retropubic urethropexy) can also cause fever without definite infection.

D. Abdominal wound infection. Most wound infections are seen 4–8 days following surgery. Abnormal appearance of the wound (erythema, induration, and drainage) is the initial clue. A wound cannot definitely be considered infected without purulent drainage. Frequently, pressure on the wound edges is helpful to force the underlying fluid collection to surface.

E. Pulmonary disorders.

1. **Pneumonia.** Pneumonia that presents early in the postoperative period (during the first 24 hours) is most likely due to aspiration. Later in the postoperative course, pneumonia complicating atelectasis may develop, particularly in patients with preexisting pulmonary disease. Findings of respiratory distress, abnormalities on auscultation, arterial hypoxia, tachypnea, and a pulmonary infiltrate on x-ray are all supportive of this diagnosis.

2. **Embolism.** Bed rest and vascular damage from surgery both are thrombogenic and may cause lower extremity thrombophlebitis, which can result in pulmonary embolism. Pulmonary embolism can cause fever if it is associated with septic pelvic vein thrombosis or pulmonary infarction. Pulmonary embolism occurs more frequently following extensive procedures (eg, radical vulvectomy) and in the morbidly obese. Tachypnea, tachycardia, arterial hypoxia, and pleuritic chest pain all suggest the diagnosis (see Problems 36 and 39, pages 141 and 153).

F. Intravenous catheter infections. Catheter infections and urinary tract infections are the two most frequent nosocomial infections in all hospitalized patients.

G. Drug fever. Persistent fever without an obvious source may be due to a drug reaction. Occasionally in drug fever, eosinophilia is present and strongly supports the diagnosis. However, eosinophilia is not sensitive enough to be a reliable indicator of drug fever. Discontinuing the drug is usually followed by defervescence within 48 hours.

IV. Database

A. Physical examination key points

1. **Vital signs.** Hypotension and tachycardia are both signs of impending septic shock. A rapid respiratory rate may also be

a clue to the cause of fever (ie, aspiration pneumonia, septic pulmonary embolism).

2. **Chest.** Carefully percuss and auscultate all lung fields. Abnormal findings or respiratory difficulties should be followed by chest x-ray and arterial blood gases.

3. **Abdomen.** The absence of bowel sounds (ileus) may be due to pelvic peritonitis, bowel ischemia, or prolonged intraoperative handling. The incision should be carefully inspected and palpated for abnormalities: erythema, induration, or abnormal discharge (culture) or underlying flatulence (incise and drain). The site and severity of abdominal tenderness should be noted. Flank tenderness is present with ureteral injury and pyelonephritis. Any drain sites should be inspected and the character of the drainage noted.

4. **Speculum examination.** This is mandatory in the febrile patient following hysterectomy. The integrity of the suture lines and status of the cuff are particularly important. Cuff abscess can often be revealed just by applying pressure from a cotton swab. Palpate carefully, noting tenderness and the presence of any pelvic masses. Rectal exam is also mandatory, and is helpful to evaluate the posterior portion of the pelvic basin.

5. **Extremities.** Intravenous sites must be inspected. In a febrile patient, any of the following is an indication for line change:
   a. Central lines older than 7 days.
   b. Peripheral lines older than 3 days.
   c. Any sign of phlebitis.
   d. Severe pain at the site.

B. **Laboratory data.** The following tests should be ordered for a febrile patient when the clinical circumstances dictate.

1. **Hemogram.** Elevated WBC count is compatible with, but not diagnostic of, an infectious process. The so-called left shift, which consists of numerous immature polymorphonuclear leukocytes (band forms), suggests an acute inflammatory process. The finding of eosinophilia in the proper clinical scenario (no other fever source on exam and the patient is taking antibiotics) is compatible with drug fever. A low hemoglobin may be due to blood loss at surgery or hematoma formation, but is also seen with intra-abdominal abscess.

2. **Arterial blood gases,** particularly if the patient is acutely ill. Respiratory alkalosis is the initial finding in sepsis, followed by metabolic acidosis. Hypoxia occurs with pneumonia and pulmonary embolism.

3. **Cultures**
   a. Vaginal cuff site.

    b. Incision, if drainage is present.
    c. Blood.
    d. Sputum, if there are respiratory symptoms and an infiltrate is seen on x-ray.
    e. Urine.
    f. Central intravenous lines. Send the catheter tip.

C. Radiologic and other studies
    1. Chest x-ray. Order chest films if there are pulmonary signs or symptoms (increased respiratory rate, productive cough, rales on examination, shortness of breath).
    2. Abdominal ultrasound. An echo study is useful if pelvic abscess, ureteral obstruction, or underlying wound fluid collections are suspected.
    3. CT scan. If pelvis ultrasound is negative and a pelvic abscess is still being considered, CT scan is more sensitive. Also, come centers have success with diagnosing septic pelvic thrombophlebitis with a pelvic CT scan.
    4. Intravenous pyelogram. Order an IVP if there is any question of ureteral injury. It can diagnose either obstructive lesions, ureteral injury, or suggest a bladder laceration.

V. Plan

    A. Acute treatment. Management of septic shock is beyond the scope of this manual; however, if the patient is febrile, tachycardiac, and hypotensive, the following should be done.
        1. Transfer the patient to the ICU.
        2. Maintain adequate oxygenation.
        3. Perform rapid intravenous volume expansion (1–2 L of normal saline), preferably with hemodynamic monitoring.
        4. Obtain appropriate lab tests.

    B. Persistent fever. (see Table 1–17 for treatment of persistent fever.)

REFERENCES

Faro S: Other soft tissue infections. In Faro S, Gilstrap L (eds): *Infections and Pregnancy.* New York, Alan R. Liss, 1989.
Ledger WJ: Hospital acquired gynecologic infections. In *Infection in the Female,* 2nd edition. Philadelphia, Lea & Febiger, 1986.

65. POSTOPERATIVE HEMORRHAGE

    I. Problem. You are called to see a 52-year-old patient with tachycardia and a falling hematocrit 6 hours postoperatively.

TABLE 1–17. TREATMENT OF PERSISTENT FEVERS.

Cause of Persistent Fever	Action
Inappropriate diagnosis	Repeat physical exam and studies
Inappropriate antibiotics	Change antibiotics
Not appropriate for site	Change antibiotics based on expected bacteriology
Unexpected resistant organism	Change antibiotic based on susceptibility testing
Wrong dose	Change dose
Second infection site	Diagnose and treat appropriately
Drug fever	Discontinue putative agent
Septic pelvic thrombophlebitis	Begin heparin
Unresponsive abscess	Drain abscess

II. Immediate Questions

A. What type of surgical procedure was performed? Postoperative hemorrhage can occur after almost any surgical procedure. Patients who have undergone a radical operation with dissection in the retroperitoneal space may experience retroperitoneal bleeding, while those who have undergone a simple hysterectomy will likely have bleeding from the vaginal cuff or vascular pedicles. Cervical conizations often are complicated by postoperative bleeding, which is severe enough to require transfusion in 5–10% of cases.

B. What intraoperative fluid losses and replacements occurred? The intraoperative estimate of blood loss, insensible fluid loss, and blood and fluid replacement should be determined. This, along with knowledge of the preoperative hematocrit, will allow calculation of the present fluid status.

C. Are there signs of active bleeding? Intra-abdominal bleeding in patients with closed system abdominal drains may be quantitated by measuring the drain output. It should be noted that the intra-abdominal blood may not all be evacuated by the drains.

D. What is the patient's clinical status? Hemodynamically significant blood loss may cause tachycardia, hypotension, postural changes in blood pressure, and decreased urine output. The patient should be assessed for confusion, obtundation, and cyanosis. Hypoxia may result from severe anemia and hypovolemia.

E. What medications is the patient receiving? Aspirin or perioperative heparin prophylaxis may cause clotting abnormalities. Other drugs may reversibly affect platelet function for several hours. These include nonsteroidal anti-inflammatory agents, steroids, tricyclic antidepressants, phenothiazines, calcium channel blocking agents, and xanthine derivatives. High-dose penicillin and carbenicillin may cause thrombocytopenia.

F. Has the patient received a massive blood transfusion?
When large volumes of blood are given over a short interval, pathologic bleeding can occur. Fresh-frozen plasma should be administered to replace labile coagulation factors (V and VIII) at a ratio of 1 unit fresh-frozen plasma for every 5 units of transfused blood.

III. Differential Diagnosis

A. Bleeding due to failed surgical hemostasis. Bleeding resulting from faulty surgical technique with failure to secure vascular pedicles adequately occurs infrequently. It is more common after vaginal than abdominal hysterectomy. Postoperative vaginal hemorrhage is most often caused by failure to secure the vaginal angles. Intra-abdominal bleeding after hysterectomy is most commonly due to difficulties in ligation of the vessels of the broad ligament. When tumor debulking is performed, bleeding may occur from denuded surfaces throughout the abdominal cavity or from the retroperitoneal space. Failure to ligate omental vessels will result in continued bleeding with hemoperitoneum formation, while bleeding in the retroperitoneal space often results in tamponade with hematoma formation. Overly vigorous "stripping" of drains either in the retroperitoneal space or in the groin may traumatize small vessels with resultant hemorrhage. Delayed postoperative hemorrhage at 7–14 days can occur due to weakening and loosening of suture material after cervical conization.

B. Bleeding due to coagulopathy. All patients with postoperative hemorrhage should be assessed for an underlying coagulopathy, either congenital or acquired. Congenital coagulopathy such as von Willebrand's disease may go undetected until the postoperative period. Acquired coagulopathies are more common and may be due to drugs, massive blood transfusion, disseminated intravascular coagulation (DIC), uremia, vitamin K deficiency, or liver disease.

IV. Database

A. Physical examination key points
1. **Vital signs.** Hypovolemia may cause tachycardia and hypotension. Postural changes should be assessed. Fever may suggest sepsis with resultant DIC.
2. **Appearance of the patient.** Hypoxia can result from severe anemia and may be manifest as confusion, somnolence, change in mental status, and cyanosis. Peripheral vasoconstriction with cool, clammy skin and diaphoresis may herald the onset of shock.

3. **Heart.** Severe blood loss with hypovolemia will result in tachycardia and possibly hypoxia. Patients with underlying coronary artery disease may experience angina.
4. **Kidneys.** Hypovolemia will result in diminished urine output. Hypotension and vasoconstriction decrease renal perfusion and can cause oliguria or anuria.
5. **Abdomen.** Intra-abdominal bleeding may be manifest by increasing abdominal girth. Bowel sounds are hypoactive. Intraperitoneal infection or abscess formation may cause severe abdominal tenderness and be the source of DIC from sepsis.
6. **Incision.** The surgical incision should be examined, especially when hemorrhage is occurring from the vagina, for possible identification of bleeding sites.
7. **Pelvic examination.** Hematomas at the vaginal cuff or elsewhere within the pelvis may be identified by pelvic exam. Intra-abdominal hemorrhage with hemoperitoneum formation will not be detected. Active bleeding from a vessel at the vaginal cuff may be identified.
8. **Skin.** Petechiae or bleeding from intravenous access sites or gums indicates the presence of a coagulopathy.

B. **Laboratory data**
   1. **Hemogram.** A stat hemogram should be obtained. The drop in hematocrit in conjunction with calculations of fluid loss and replacement perioperatively can be used to estimate the amount of excess blood loss. The initial hematocrit, however, is not useful in the patient with a massive acute bleed. Hematocrit should be measured serially since it may not reflect the true intravascular status for several hours. Leukocytosis may indicate an infectious process. Thrombocytopenia, if found, may be the cause of the coagulopathy and continued bleeding.
   2. **Coagulation parameters.** The prothrombin time (PT), partial thromboplastin time (PTT), and bleeding time should be obtained. The serum concentration of fibrinogen and fibrin degradation products should be measured if DIC is suspected.
   3. **Serum chemistries.** Elevated liver function tests may indicate liver disease. Elevated BUN and creatinine can indicate the degree of renal compromise or hypovolemia.
   4. **Blood bank.** Immediately send blood for typing and cross-matching. The number of units of packed cells to request is determined by the patient's hematocrit, or by the estimate of blood loss in the case of massive acute hemorrhage.
   5. **Arterial blood gases.** An arterial blood gas study should be obtained in a patient with mental status changes that may be secondary to hypoxia.

C. Radiologic and other studies

1. **Abdominal ultrasound.** When intra-abdominal bleeding is suspected but cannot be definitively documented, abdominal ultrasound can be used to confirm the presence of fluid accumulation within the abdominal cavity. It may also demonstrate accumulations consistent with hematomas.

2. **Abdominal-pelvic CT scan.** The CT scan can also be used to demonstrate free fluid within the abdominal cavity or the presence of hematomas. It may provide a better indication than ultrasound of the exact location and amount of fluid present.

3. **Chest x-ray.** If hypovolemic shock is present, obtain a chest x-ray.

4. **Angiography.** If severe hemorrhage is present in a patient who is not a surgical candidate or if surgical intervention fails to control the hemorrhage, angiography or a technetium 99 radiolabeled red cell study may be useful to localize the site of bleeding. Angiography can localize bleeding at a rate of 0.5–1.0 mL/min, while radiolabeled red cell studies can localize slower rates of 0.2 mL/min.

V. Plan. Fluid resuscitation with crystalloid should begin immediately. Blood should then be cross-matched. If the bleeding site is obvious and accessible, try to control the bleeding. The urgency of the situation is dictated by the volume and rate of blood loss and by the patient's clinical status. Patients in hypovolemic shock may require invasive hemodynamic monitoring and transfer to an intensive care setting.

A. Acute intervention. Large-bore (14- to 18-gauge) intravenous cannulas should be inserted and fluid resuscitation initiated. Blood may be drawn for laboratory analysis and cross-matching at the time of IV insertion. Fluid replacement may be with saline, lactated Ringer's solution, or Hespan until blood is available; the rate and volume of replacement will depend on the patient's status. Blood should be replaced as soon as possible and the hematocrit maintained at 30%. In extreme situations, O-negative blood can be utilized and pressors may be necessary if shock is present. Obvious, accessible acute bleeding should be stopped. A Foley catheter should be inserted for accurate assessment of urine output, which can be an indicator of the patient's intravascular volume status. Oxygen should be administered to patients who are hypoxic. In extremely ill patients, a central venous catheter and intensive care monitoring may be necessary to evaluate and replace intravascular volume accurately.

B. Location of the bleeding site. Once the patient is stabilized, the bleeding site should be localized. Vaginal bleeding usually originates from the vaginal cuff, which is readily accessible by pelvic examination. Intra-abdominal bleeding sites are more difficult to localize and assess. Rapidly increasing abdominal girth in a patient with a falling hematocrit indicates intra-abdominal hemorrhage, which can be assessed by ultrasound or CT scan. Bleeding from wounds is usually readily apparent during examination of the incision site.

C. Cause of hemorrhage. Examination of the patient may reveal petechiae and bleeding from intravenous sites, indicating a generalized coagulopathy. If these findings are not present, diagnosis must await return of the coagulation parameters. If the PT, PTT, or bleeding time is prolonged, a coagulopathy is present that may be contributing to the hemorrhage. If these parameters are normal, the bleeding is most probably due to failed surgical hemostasis.

D. Treatment. Therapy for postoperative hemorrhage depends on the cause, site, and volume of bleeding.

  1. Any identified coagulopathies should be corrected. Drugs that interfere with clotting should be stopped if possible. Platelets should be replaced when thrombocytopenia is found. Protamine sulfate can be administered to reverse the anticoagulant effects of heparin. If a massive blood transfusion has been given, fresh-frozen plasma should be administered. If DIC is the result of an infectious process, antibiotic therapy should be initiated.

  2. Vaginal cuff bleeding after hysterectomy can usually be localized during pelvic examination. A carefully placed suture can be utilized to ligate the bleeding point. Cauterization by electrocautery or chemical cautery can also be employed if available. Most commonly, bleeding will be located at the vaginal angles. Care should be taken not to inadvertently ligate the ureters or place a suture into the bladder. If at pelvic examination the bleeding is seen to originate from generalized venous oozing and a specific vessel cannot be identified, a vaginal pack can be utilized to obtain hemostasis. This should be left in place for 24–48 hours, during which time a Foley catheter for urinary drainage is necessary.

  3. Bleeding after cervical conization is common and can be problematic. At pelvic examination, the bleeding site from the cone bed can usually be identified and cauterized or surgically ligated. If the bleeding is originating in the endocervical canal, packing with a hemostatic agent such as Surgicel or Gelfoam may be required. Occasionally bleeding is severe enough to require repeat ligation of the paracervical vessels by placing sutures laterally at 3 and 9 o'clock.

4. Bleeding into a wound can often be controlled by application of pressure. A sandbag is useful for this purpose. If a drain is present, it should be left in place to provide drainage and prevent hematoma formation. Reopening of the wound is rarely necessary and, when performed, rarely allows identification of a specific bleeding site.

5. Intra-abdominal bleeding is the most difficult to manage. Once it is identified, try to quantitate the blood loss by measuring the output into drains, following abdominal girth measurements, obtaining serial hematocrits, or performing ultrasound or a CT scan. Blood and fluids should be replaced as needed. Often the bleeding will gradually stop without active intervention, especially if a coagulopathy has been corrected. If bleeding stops, the intra-abdominal blood will gradually be absorbed and does not require drainage as long as there are no signs of infection. If infection does occur, drainage can usually be accomplished percutaneously with ultrasound guidance.

6. Surgical intervention to control intra-abdominal bleeding is reserved for extreme cases. When 2500–3000 mL of blood loss has occurred without spontaneous resolution, surgical intervention is indicated. The exact site of bleeding can be difficult to identify at laparotomy due to distortion of the anatomy and retraction of vessels. Ligation of the anterior division of the hypogastric artery may be necessary when diffuse bleeding is occurring from the pelvis. Specific points of bleeding in the retroperitoneal space can likewise be difficult to identify. When surgical intervention is contemplated, angiography or a labeled red cell study to localize the bleeding site preoperatively may be useful. Arterial embolization can be performed and may successfully produce hemostasis.

7. Patients with severe, persistent bleeding who are not surgical candidates or who have failed conservative and surgical management should be considered for angiography and arterial embolization of the vascular supply to the area of bleeding.

REFERENCES

Fink MP: Shock: an overview. In Rippe JM et al (eds): *Intensive Care Medicine,* 2nd edition. Boston, Little, Brown, 1991, pp 1417–34.

Henry DH: Clotting abnormalities in the surgical patient. In Goldman DR et al (eds): *Medical Care of the Surgical Patient.* Philadelphia, JB Lippincott, 1982, pp 442–56.

Rosen B et al: Hemorrhage and resuscitation. In Rippe JM et al (eds): *Intensive Care Medicine,* 2nd edition. Boston, Little, Brown, 1991, pp 1435–43.

Thompson JD, Rock JA. Wiskind A: Control of pelvic hemorrhage: blood component therapy and hemorrhagic shock. In Thompson JD, Rock JA (eds): *TeLinde's Operative Gynecology*, 7th edition. Philadelphia, JB Lippincott, 1992, pp 151–94.

66. RAPE

I. Problem. A 30-year-old woman is brought to the emergency room by a friend and states she has been raped.

II. Immediate Questions. Questions are aimed at eliciting important medical as well as forensic information.

   A. When did the assault occur? Since then has the patient bathed, douched, defecated, urinated, changed clothes, or brushed her teeth? Time elapsed since the assault or intervening activities may affect the recovery of evidence.

   B. Where did the assault occur? This information is frequently used by law enforcement when the patient recovers.

   C. Was the assailant known? If not, get a description. From 20–40% of all sexual assault victims know their assailant; this increases to > 80% in those under the age of 18.

   D. Was there oral, anal, or vaginal penetration? Did ejaculation occur? Was a condom used? Oral and anal penetration, in addition to or instead of vaginal penetration, is not an infrequent occurrence and affects the gathering of forensic specimens. Sexual dysfunction involving inadequate erection or lack of ejaculation affects a surprisingly large portion of male assailants.

   E. When was the most recent consensual sexual activity prior to or after the reported assault? Describe the type of sexual activity.

   F. When was the patient's last menstrual period, and does she use anything for contraception? The risk of rape-related pregnancy is 1–2%. Consider the possibility that the patient may already be pregnant.

   G. Was a weapon used? In 30–40% of cases a gun, knife, or blunt instrument is used to threaten or injure the victim.

   H. Was there any drug or alcohol use by the patient or assailant prior to or during the assault? Information which might be used in prosecution or defense should be anticipated and appropriate laboratory studies ordered.

   I. Does the patient have a history of previous sexual assaults or psychiatric problems? Victims are at increased risk for serious psychologic sequelae.

   J. In cases of suspected childhood sexual abuse:

        1. Remember that the abuse is often chronic and try to find out when it first occurred.
        2. Avoid yes and no questions.
        3. Communicate on the patient's level.
        4. Drawing pictures or use of anatomically correct dolls may be helpful.
        5. Reassure the child that he/she has not done anything wrong.

III. Differential Diagnosis. It is not up to the physician to decide whether or not a sexual assault has occurred. In documentation, use nonjudgmental and unbiased terminology such as "reported" or "suspected" sexual assault. Avoid terms such as "alleged rape" since this may seem to imply that the physician did not believe the patient. Consider the possibility of preexisting or transmitted infection from sexual assault. Also, the possibility of preexisting pregnancy or pregnancy occurring from an act of sexual violence must not be overlooked.

IV. Database

    A. Physical examination key points
        1. Observe the patient's mental status and emotional state, and describe in a nonjudgmental manner. Many women present with a flat or seemingly inappropriate affect after sexual assault.
        2. Describe any disturbances in attire, ie, torn or stained clothing, etc. Any clothing which is potential evidence of force should be submitted to the police for more detailed forensic evaluation.
        3. Look for evidence of extragenital trauma. Ask the woman to demonstrate where she was grabbed or struck. Describe the location and appearance of scratches, bruises, lacerations, bites, etc. Consider taking photographs.
        4. Pelvic examination. General anesthesia may be required if the patient is a child. Use of colposcopy and application of toluidine blue have been reported to enhance detection of subtle abrasions or other evidence of trauma.
        5. External genitalia. Examine the mons, vulva, and thighs for matted hairs, dried secretions, foreign material, or trauma. Describe the location and appearance of any lacerations, swelling, abrasions, tenderness, or erythema. In a child, the size of the hymenal opening is somewhat variable, but visibility of vaginal rugae through a patulous introitus in a girl under the age of 10 is indicative of coitus.

    6. **Speculum examination.** Describe the presence of any vaginal secretions, blood, foreign materials, or lacerations.

    7. **Bimanual/rectovaginal examination.** Note uterine size, any adnexal enlargements, tenderness, or unassociated pelvic abnormalities. A tender adnexal mass effect may represent a hematoma in the broad ligament. A statement about the anal sphincter, especially if anal penetration is reported, is important. Look for skin tears, hyperpigmentation, and thickening of the perianal skin in cases of chronic sexual abuse of children.

B. Laboratory data. Hospitals in most larger cities now have available sexual assault kits for organized collection of forensic evidence. Critical to the collection of evidence is maintenance of a "chain of custody." A method should be established to ensure that all persons responsible for handling or storing evidentiary material can be easily traced. A written record showing the date, time, and signatures of persons involved in the transfer should be kept for each item. Meticulously label all specimens with the patient's name, identification number, and the source of the item. Avoid cross-contamination of specimens. Use the same type or brand of swab throughout the exam and provide control swabs for each specimen obtained. Collect samples even if the patient has douched, bathed, etc, since positive findings can often still be identified.

    1. **Fingernail scrapings, if suggested by history or examination.** Skin, blood, or clothing fragments under the fingernails may be useful in identification of an assailant.

    2. **Pubic hair combings.** There is the possibility that this may contain specimens from the assailant.

    3. **Head and pubic hair pluckings.** There is the possibility that a suspect may have the victim's hair on him or vice versa. Because the root of a hair shaft possesses several characteristics helpful in determining the source of the hair, it is recommended that the hairs be plucked rather than cut.

    4. **Dried secretions or blood on skin.** Swab the area with a saline-moistened swab, let it dry, and submit, noting the site. This may allow evaluation for the presence of acid phosphatase and ABO (H) antigens.

    5. **Drug and alcohol screening,** if indicated.

    6. **Wet mount of material from the posterior vaginal fornix to examine for the presence of sperm.** Morphologically identifiable sperm are rarely detected later than 72 hours after intercourse. In evaluating data from suspected sexual assault cases, keep the following facts in mind: approximately 10% of adult males in the United States have azospermia or oligospermia; about ⅓ of rapists experience

sexual dysfunction resulting in no deposition of sperm; hundreds of thousands of vasectomies are performed in the United States each year; 1/3 of victims report douching prior to examination.

7. **Fixed smear from the posterior fornix, vulva or both for sperm** (Pap, Gram, or Giemsa stain).

8. **Endocervical culture for gonococcus and Chlamydia.** Obtain oral and rectal cultures if indicated by history.

9. **Swab from the vaginal pool and any suspicious areas about the vulva and rectum.** This can be examined for:
   a. **Acid phosphatase (ACP).** Seminal fluid is rich in ACP, while normal vaginal fluid is not. In various studies, this assay identified the presence of semen in 1.4 to 22% additional cases in which no sperm were identified.
   b. **ABO (H) antigen.** Certain individuals secrete ABO (H) antigens into body fluids such as saliva, seminal fluid, and vaginal secretions. The identification of foreign ABO (H) antigens in the vagina may be further evidence supporting the presence of semen and may exclude certain suspects.
   c. **Sperm precipitins.** Additional material may be obtained with 5–10 mL of saline vaginal irrigation.

10. **Saliva sample** to determine the patient's secretor status.

11. **Urine** to detect the presence of sperm or evidence of trauma.

12. **Human chorionic gonadotropin (HCG).** Perform a serum or urine pregnancy test if indicated.

13. **Blood type and Rh status** of the patient.

14. **Rapid plasma reagin (RPR)**—baseline.

15. **Serology.** Consider serologic testing (baseline) for hepatitis B.

16. **HIV screening.** Consider baseline HIV screening only with full informed consent.

V. Plan

A. **Obtain informed consent** prior to history, examination, and collection of evidence. Any suspected child abuse must be reported to the appropriate authorities.

B. **Treat genital and extragenital injuries** with appropriate consultation as indicated. Consider tetanus prophylaxis.

C. **Consider presumptive treatment of sexually transmitted diseases (STDs),** particularly gonorrhea, *Chlamydia,* and syphilis. In addition, treat any specific infection found in the patient and presumptively treat, if possible, for any STD found in the assailant. Recommended empiric regimens include ceftriaxone

250 mg IM followed by doxycycline 100 mg PO bid for 7 days or tetracycline 500 mg PO qid for 7 days.

D. Prophylaxis against pregnancy should be discussed and offered to patients who are at risk for pregnancy and who are HCG negative. This decision should be made in light of the patient's menstrual and contraceptive history and after full discussion of potential risks and side effects. Prophylaxis should be initiated within 72 hours after intercourse. Regimens that have been used for this purpose include:

1. Diethylstilbestrol 25 mg PO bid for 5 days.
2. Ethinyl estradiol 5 mg PO qd for 5 days.
3. Ethinyl estradiol 50 μg with norgestrel 0.5 mg (Ovral) 2 tablets PO, with repeat dose in 12 hours.
4. Conjugated estrogen (Premarin) 25 mg IV qd for 3 days.
5. Antiemetics should be offered to treat the nausea frequently associated with high-dose estrogen administration.

E. Acute crisis intervention. Early emotional support and counseling should be given, utilizing all appropriate available resources including social workers, rape crisis centers, etc. The psychologic and emotional trauma from sexual assault is often profound and prolonged.

F. Follow-up in 4–6 weeks with repeat endocervical cultures, RPR, and HCG. A second follow-up visit may be required at 8–12 weeks for repeat serologic studies as indicated (syphilis, HIV, hepatitis B). Counseling may need to be ongoing.

REFERENCES

American College of Obstetricians and Gynecologists: Sexual Assault. Tech Bull No. 101. Washington, DC, ACOG, 1987.

Centers for Disease Control: 1989 sexually transmitted diseases treatment guidelines. *MMWR* 38, No. 5–8, 1989.

Glaser J, Hammerschlag M, McCormack W: Sexually transmitted diseases in victims of sexual assault. *N Engl J Med* 315:625, 1986.

Solola A et al: Rape: management in a non-institutional setting. *Obstet Gynecol* 61:373, 1983.

Soules M et al: The spectrum of alleged rape. *J Reprod Med* 20:33, 1978.

67. SEXUALLY TRANSMITTED DISEASE EXPOSURE

I. Problem. A 17-year-old female states that her boyfriend told her he has an infection and she needs to be "checked out."

II. Immediate Questions

A. What kind of symptoms does her boyfriend have, and how

was he treated? The types of symptoms and the specific treatment may be a clue to the kind of infection involved. Transmission of infection may also occur if the sexual partner is asymptomatic.

B. **Does the patient have any symptoms?** Abnormal vaginal bleeding, dysuria, vaginal discharge, pelvic or abdominal pain, and genital sores or ulcerations may represent symptoms of an already established genital infection.

C. **When was the patient's last menstrual period, and have menses been normal?** The possibility of pregnancy must also be considered in the evaluation and treatment of any woman of reproductive age. Certain infections may adversely affect pregnancy or neonatal outcome, and treatment may need modification in the presence of pregnancy.

D. **What kind of contraception do the patient and her boyfriend use?** This question also addresses the issue of potential pregnancy at the time of evaluation or occurring during the course of treatment. Barrier types of contraception, particularly condoms, protect against the acquisition and transmission of infection. Oral contraceptives appear to protect against the development of pelvic inflammatory disease as a sequela of infectious cervicitis, whereas IUDs may promote development of upper tract infection in the presence of lower tract infection.

E. **Do either the patient or her boyfriend have other sexual partners?** To prevent the spread of infection, all potentially exposed persons should be evaluated and treated.

F. **Do either the patient or her boyfriend have a history of sexually transmitted diseases (STDs)?** In the presence of a history of STDs, a current infection may represent inadequate prior treatment or relapse. Most commonly, however, it signifies continued high-risk behavior and the need for intensive counseling.

G. **In what types of sexual practices do the couple engage?** Oral, genital, or anal/genital sex dictates the evaluation of these areas for infection. Treatment may be influenced by the anatomic site exposed or infected.

III. Differential Diagnosis

A. **Chlamydia trachomatis.** *Chlamydia* is the most common sexually transmitted organism in the United States with approximately 4.5 million genital infections per year. *Chlamydia* infections may be asymptomatic in both sexes. The most common symptoms in males are urethritis with urethral discharge and burning. Mucopurulent cervicitis is usually the initial clinical symptom in women with cervical edema, erythema, friability, and mucopurulent discharge.

B. Neisseria gonorrhoeae. Frequently symptomatic in males, urethral discharge and irritation are prominent features. In women, gonococcus (GC) is also a common cause of mucopurulent cervicitis. GC and *Chlamydia* are considered to be the most likely sexually transmitted organisms initiating upper tract infection (pelvic inflammatory disease) by ascending spread.

C. Syphilis. This is increasing in incidence. Transmission requires exposure to moist mucosal or cutaneous lesions or perinatal exposure. Transmission usually occurs only during the first few years of infection, when there is susceptibility to spontaneous mucocutaneous relapses. Clinical manifestations are highly variable and generally depend on length of infection.

D. Human papillomavirus. HPV is the most common viral sexually transmitted disease in the United States. Patients may be asymptomatically infected or develop genital warts. In women, HPV has been linked to the development of lower genital tract neoplasia. Immunosuppressed individuals may experience more severe and widespread disease with more rapid progression to invasive cancer.

E. Herpes simplex virus. Herpes transmission requires close contact with a person shedding virus at a peripheral site, mucosal surface, or secretion; the virus is then inoculated on a mucosal surface or crack in the skin. At the time of initial infection, HSV ascends the peripheral sensory nerves and establishes latency in nerve root ganglia. Up to ¾ of infected individuals are asymptomatic, but this does not prevent transmission of infection. When lesions are present, they are initially papular or vesicular, then ulcerative, and are quite tender. Over 50% of individuals experiencing a primary episode have variable systemic symptoms (fever, headache, malaise, myalgia) that begin prior to the onset of lesions. Immunosuppressed individuals may experience more frequent and severe recurrences. Recurrent episodes are usually of shorter duration, are more localized, and have milder symptoms compared with primary episodes. They are often preceded by prodromal symptoms (burning, itching, shooting pains) in the genital region.

F. Trichomonas vaginalis. Males are usually asymptomatic. Females may also be asymptomatic but have a high likelihood of developing acute symptoms with classically profuse, often frothy, greenish or yellowish vaginal discharge and highly irritative symptoms including puritus, dysuria, and dyspareunia. Predisposing factors include menses, cervical or vaginal lesions, cervical mucorrhea, or other vaginal conditions with increased pH. Mature squamous vaginal epithelium is essential for growth of trichomonads.

G. Human immunodeficiency virus. An increasing proportion of HIV infections are acquired via heterosexual transmission. Asymptomatic infection generally lasts for several years until increasing immunocompromise results in the development of opportunistic infections, malignancies, and other HIV-associated symptoms.

H. Mycoplasma/ureaplasma. Pathologic significance is controversial. Asymptomatic colonization is common, though there may be a link with infertility, poor obstetric outcome, and development of pelvic inflammatory disease.

I. Hepatitis B virus. Sexual contact is the most frequently reported mode of HBV transmission in the United States. Homosexual men, heterosexual men and women with multiple partners, and sexual partners of IV drug users are at high risk for sexual transmission of HBV.

J. Ectoparasites. Pediculosis pubis and scabies are transmitted by close, not necessarily sexual, bodily contact. Infestation results in a hypersensitivity reaction with pruritic papular or eczematous eruption.

K. Miscellaneous. Additional STDs include molluscum contagiosum, granuloma inguinale, lymphogranuloma venereum, and chancroid. These infections are seen more commonly in tropical countries, though they are increasing in the United States as well. Molluscum contagiosum exhibits umbilicated papular lesions which are nontender. The other three infections are included in the genitoulcerative lesions (see Problem 42, page 162).

IV. Database

A. Physical examination key points

1. **Vital signs.** Fever suggests an inflammatory or infectious process.
2. **Skin and mucosal surfaces.** If oral or genital contact has occurred, look for sores, fever blisters, or evidence of pharyngitis. Skin rash involving the trunk and extremities may be indicative of disseminated gonococcal infection or secondary syphilis.
3. **Abdomen.** Perform auscultation, percussion, inspection, and palpation. Look for diffuse abdominal tenderness with or without signs of peritoneal irritation which may represent pelvic inflammatory disease. Right upper quadrant tenderness may suggest the presence of perihepatitis of gonor-

rheal or chlamydial origin. Give special attention to tenderness or enlargement of inguinal lymph nodes, commonly seen with genitoulcerative disorders.

4. **Pelvic examination**
   a. Examine the external genitalia for erythema, edema, ulcers, papules or vesicles, warts, lice, nits, or other lesions. Are lesions single or multiple, tender or nontender?
   b. Perform a speculum examination looking for abnormal vaginal discharge, mucopurulent cervical discharge, and erythema or edema of the vagina and cervix.
   c. Perform bimanual examination to look for an adnexal mass and uterine or adnexal tenderness. Uterine enlargement should suggest the possibility of pregnancy and requires further evaluation.
   d. The perianal region should be examined for lesions, erythema, edema, or discharge. Rectovaginal examination will allow better assessment of the posterior pelvis for masses and tenderness.

B. **Laboratory data**
   1. **Hemogram.** Left shift and leukocytosis suggest an infectious process.
   2. **Wet mount** (normal saline/10% KOH mount of vaginal secretions). The presence of white cells without other organisms present suggests cervicitis or upper tract infection. Increased white cells are also usually seen with *Trichomonas* infections but less commonly with vaginal candidiasis and infrequently with pure bacterial vaginosis.
   3. **Vaginal pH.** Normal vaginal pH is approximately 3.5–4.5. pH is elevated with *Trichomonas* or bacterial vaginosis, and potentially elevated in the increased cervical discharge seen with cervical gonorrhea, chlamydia, or herpes infections.
   4. **Gram stain of endocervical secretions.** An increased number of white cells is indicative of cervicitis; the presence of gram-negative intracellular diplococci has high specificity for the diagnosis of gonorrhea.
   5. **Rapid plasma reagin (RPR).** If positive, represents evidence of preexisting syphilis. Biologic false positives—usually in low titer—may be seen with acute febrile illnesses, immunizations, autoimmune disorders, and IV drug use.
   6. **Urinalysis and culture.** The presence of pyuria without bacteria suggests chlamydial urethritis.
   7. **Human chorionic gonadotropin (HCG).** Perform a serum or urine pregnancy test if indicated.
   8. **HIV antibody testing.** This should be routinely offered to those with sexually transmitted diseases.

9. **Cultures.** Obtain specimens to test for GC and *Chlamydia;* include HSV if indicated.
10. **Hepatitis B antigen/antibody testing,** if indicated.
11. Burrows suggestive of scabies should be scraped vigorously and scrapings suspended in a drop of 10% KOH. Examine microscopically for adults, larvae, and eggs.

V. Plan

A. Diagnosis. The first step is to try to establish the type of exposure that has occurred. Appropriate cultures should be obtained as well as the sexual partner's records, if available. Remember that different STDs commonly coexist, and assess for the presence of other infections even if the particular type of infectious exposure is known.

B. Treatment. Specifically treat the presumed infection to which the patient has been exposed, as well as other infections found to be present. There is no current evidence that prophylactic treatment of HSV or HPV prevents establishment of infection after inoculation has taken place (see Problem 42, page 162). Specific treatment recommendations are summarized below.

1. **Chlamydia trachomatis**
   a. Doxycycline 100 mg PO bid for 7 days **or** tetracycline 500 mg PO qid for 7 days.
   b. Alternative regimen: erythromycin base 500 mg PO qid for 7 days **or** erythromycin ethylsuccinate 500 mg PO qid for 7 days.

2. **Neisseria gonorrhoeae**
   a. Ceftriaxone 250 mg IM **plus** doxycycline 100 mg PO bid for 7 days (also effective for incubating syphilis).
   b. Alternative regimens
      (1) Spectinomycin 2 g IM **plus** doxycycline.
      (2) If infection was acquired from a source proven *not* to have penicillin-resistant gonorrhea, give a penicillin such as amoxicillin 3 PO, ampicillin 3.5 g PO, or aqueous penicillin G 4.8 million units IM **with** 1 g probenecid PO **followed by** doxycycline 100 mg PO bid for 7 days.

3. **Syphilis**
   a. **Early syphilis.** Primary and secondary syphilis and early latent syphilis of < 1 year's duration.
      (1) Benzathine penicillin G 2.4 million units IM.
      (2) Alternative regimen (PCN allergy): doxycycline 100 mg PO bid for 2 weeks **or** tetracycline 500 mg PO qid for 2 weeks.
   b. **Late latent syphilis, tertiary syphilis**

        (1) Benzathine penicillin G 2.4 million units IM weekly for 3 weeks.

        (2) Alternative regimen (PCN allergy): doxycycline 100 mg PO bid for 4 weeks **or** tetracycline 500 mg PO qid for 4 weeks. Lumbar puncture may be indicated.

4. Trichomonas vaginalis
    a. Metronidazole 2 g PO.

    b. Alternative regimen: metronidazole 250 mg PO TID for 7 days.

5. Ectoparasites
    a. Treat all sexual contacts and household members.

    b. Pediculosis pubis

        (1) Permethrin 1% creme rinse applied to the affected area and washed off after 10 minutes.

        (2) Pyrethrums and piperonyl butoxide applied and washed off at 10 minutes.

        (3) Lindane 1% shampoo applied for 4 minutes and then thoroughly washed off (not recommended for pregnant or lactating women).

    c. Scabies

        (1) Lindane (1%) 1 oz of lotion or 30 g of cream applied thinly to all areas of the body from the neck down and washed off thoroughly after 8 hours (not recommended for pregnant or lactating women).

        (2) Crotamiton 10% applied to the entire body from the neck down for 2 nights and washed off thoroughly 24 hours after the second application.

6. Hepatitis B
    a. Indications for postexposure prophylaxis include:

        (1) Sexual contact with a partner who has active hepatitis B or who contracts hepatitis B.

        (2) Sexual contact with a partner positive for hepatitis B surface antigen.

    b. Hepatitis B immune globulin 0.06 mL/kg IM followed by initiation of hepatitis B vaccine series.

C. Counseling. Each patient exposed to an STD should be counseled concerning its cause, possible sequelae, and prevention. Mutually monogamous relationships or the use of condoms with a spermicide provide the best means of protection.

REFERENCES

Centers for Disease Control: 1989 sexually transmitted diseases treatment guidelines. *MMWR* 38, No. S–8, 1989.

Holmes K et al: *Sexually Transmitted Diseases,* 2nd ed. New York, McGraw-Hill, 1990.

68. SWOLLEN AND TENDER EXTREMITY

I. **Problem:** An oncology patient presents with unilateral lower extremity edema and pain.

II. Immediate Questions

A. **What are the vital signs?** Tachycardia and fever may represent infection. Tachycardia and tachypnea may be manifestations of pulmonary embolus.

B. **Is the patient short of breath?** Complaints of not getting enough air should be sought in a patient with a swollen extremity to help evaluate for pulmonary embolus.

C. **Does the patient have dorsal pedal, posterior tibial, and popliteal pulses?** Trousseau's syndrome manifests itself in oncology patients as a migratory thrombosis of the venous and arterial vessels. Patients with decreased or absent pulses require immediate attention.

III. Differential Diagnosis

A. **Venous obstruction.** In this situation it is pertinent to recall **Virchow's triad** of venous stasis, hypercoagulability, and endothelial damage.
1. **Hypercoagulability** secondary to plasminogens produced by the tumor can result in both venous and arterial thrombosis.
2. **Venous stasis** can be present in the postoperative patient who is not ambulating, as well as in the oncology patient with compression of venous vessels from tumor extension or nodal metastasis.
3. **Endothelial injury** may be secondary to tumor extension or intraoperative manipulation of pelvic and abdominal vessels. The preceding mechanisms account for thrombosis in the postoperative period and pregnancy, the latter being complicated by aortocaval compression caused by the enlarged pregnant uterus.

B. **Arterial emboli**
1. **Trousseau's syndrome.** Venous and arterial emboli are secondary to plasminogen production in tumors.
2. **Arterial stasis.** This results from tumor obstruction or ligation of the external iliac artery during a pelvic procedure.

C. **Pulmonary embolism.** Emboli may be secondary to venous obstruction, arterial embolism, or both.

D. **Lymphatic problems.** These include:

1. Lymph node metastasis secondary to pelvic tumor, the majority being vulvar carcinoma with metastasis to the inguinal nodes.
2. Lymphatic obstruction secondary to radiation teletherapy or inguinal femoral lymph node dissection.

E. **Fluid collection.** Lymphocyst formation is common after lymph node dissection. Obstruction of lymphatics secondary to fluid collections can occur in the pelvic sidewall or the groin.

F. **Infection**
   1. Cellulitis will usually occur within 7 days of performing an inguinal femoral lymph node dissection.
   2. Abscess formation can occur in any operative wound.

IV. **Database**
   A. **Physical examination key points**
      1. **Vital signs.** Tachypnea can be a sign of pulmonary embolus. Fever may be seen with cellulitis.
      2. **Lungs.** Decreased breath sounds, rales, and pleural rubs are suggestive of a pulmonary embolus or congestive heart failure.
      3. **Heart.** Note new rubs, gallops, or murmurs. An S3 gallop, loud P2, and tachycardia are suggestive of pulmonary embolism.
      4. **Extremities.** Palpate pulses and evaluate color, temperature, calf tenderness, and palpable cords. Establish a baseline circumference of the extremities and follow with serial examinations at the same site.
      5. **Pelvic examination.** Look for evidence of pelvic tumor enlargement and evaluate the inguinal region for nodal enlargement, fluid collection, or cellulitis.

   B. **Laboratory data**
      1. **Hemogram.** Evaluate platelet number as well as WBC count for possible infection.
      2. **Prothrombin time (PT) and partial thromboplastin time (PTT).** Baseline PT and PTT prior to anticoagulant therapy may be elevated in disseminated intravascular coagulation (DIC).
      3. **Fibrin degradation products (FDP) and/or fibrinopeptide A.** Oncology patients with Trousseau's syndrome present with a chronic DIC and will have elevated FDP.
      4. **Tumor markers** when appropriate, to evaluate recurrent disease.
      5. **Arterial blood gases** if suspicion of pulmonary embolism exists. Arterial oxygen saturation will not markedly improve

with oxygen administration in patients with a pulmonary embolus.

C. **Radiologic and other studies**
   1. **Chest x-ray.** Pleural effusion or a wedge-shaped infarction may be present with pulmonary embolism.
   2. **Duplex Doppler study.** When available, duplex Doppler permits diagnosis of a venous or arterial thrombus without the morbidity of intravenous radiographic contrast media. This is the most acceptable method for pregnant patients or those with allergies to iodine.
   3. **Venogram.** If duplex Doppler is not available, venography is an alternative. It should be avoided during pregnancy since it requires IV contrast plus radiation to the fetus.
   4. **Ventilation/perfusion scan.** When attempting to rule out pulmonary embolism, the V/Q scan is a very useful test.
   5. **Computerized tomography or magnetic resonance imaging.** CT and MRI are used to evaluate tumor spread in the abdomen and pelvis. Iliac, femoral, and inferior vena cava thrombus can also be diagnosed with CT or MRI.
   6. **Electrocardiogram.** Right axis deviation, sinus tachycardia (> 100 bpm), and ST segment depression may occur in patients with a pulmonary embolus. Needless to say, one must also rule out the presence of a myocardial infarction with these findings as well.

V. **Plan**

A. **Deep venous thrombosis (DVT), arterial emboli, and pulmonary embolism**
   1. **Heparinization.** Treatment consists of anticoagulation with intravenous heparin 5000–10,000 USP units as an IV bolus followed by 1000 units/h for the typical adult. Heparin is titrated until the PTT is 2 times control.
   2. **Coumadinization.** After anticoagulation with heparin for 72 hours, the patient is switched to warfarin 10 mg qd for 2 doses followed by 5 mg qd until PT is 1.5–2 times control. (The dose is titrated to maintain this level.) Anticoagulation is maintained for at least 3–6 months.
   3. Heparin is discontinued when coumadinization is achieved.
   4. Patients unable to take warfarin (ie, pregnant women) can be anticoagulated with subcutaneous heparin by dividing the parenteral dose into tid–qid subcutaneous injections.
   5. Patients with Trousseau's syndrome should be reheparinized if the thrombus enlarges during warfarin therapy.
   6. **Prevention**
      a. **Minidose heparin.** This is useful in preventing DVT

when started preoperatively in high-risk patients such as those undergoing pelvic procedures, obese patients, or patients with a past history of DVT. Give 5000 units SQ q 8–12 h.

   b. **Pneumatic compression devices.** These devices intermittently inflate around the legs, presumably reproducing muscle contractions which are very effective in preventing DVT. Early ambulation also helps to prevent DVT. Antiembolic stockings should be used with pneumatic compression devices.

B. Symptomatic lymphocyst. Prep the skin overlying the inguinal region and drain the cyst with a 20-gauge needle after anesthetizing with 1% lidocaine. Pelvic fluid can be drained percutaneously under ultrasound guidance.

C. Lymphedema. Recommend thromboembolic stockings.

D. Recurrence of tumor. Refer the patient to a gynecologic oncologist for additional therapy.

E. Cellulitis. Treat with parenteral antibiotics with sensitivity for staphylococcal, streptococcal, and gram-negative organisms (ie, nafcillin plus gentamicin or vancomycin plus gentamicin). Mild cases of inguinal cellulitis can be treated with oral dicloxacillin (see Chapter 7 for doses).

REFERENCES

Becker DM. Venous thromboembolism. Epidemiology, diagnosis, prevention. *J Gen Intern Med* 1:402, 1986.
Mohr DN et al: Recent advances in the management of venous thromboembolism. *Mayo Clin Proc* 63:281, 1988.
Sach GH, Levin J, Bell WR: Trousseau's syndrome and other manifestations of chronic disseminated coagulopathy in patients with neoplasms. Clinical, pathophysiologic and therapeutic features. *Medicine* 56:1, 1977.

69. SYNCOPE

I. Problem. A patient undergoing preoperative evaluation for pelvic pain has a syncopal episode in the radiology department.

II. Immediate Questions

A. What was the patient doing when the episode occurred? Vasovagal syncope or fainting due to orthostatic hypotension can only occur in a sitting or standing position. Syncope while lying flat is almost always cardiac in origin. Vasovagal attacks have associated factors of heat, anxiety, pain, or closed space. Syncope with exertion is often from a cardiac cause. Ask also about coughing, turning or twisting of the head, or getting up quickly.

B. Was the syncope observed, and was there any seizure activity? In determining the cause of loss of consciousness, a seizure is always in the initial differential diagnosis. Ask observers about seizure activity, examine for bites to the tongue, and evaluate rate of return to baseline consciousness. Syncopal patients recover quickly, while seizure patients have a postictal period. Incontinence is more suggestive of a seizure.

C. How did the patient feel immediately prior to the loss of consciousness? Vasovagal syncope is usually preceded by an aura, a presyncopal complex consisting of sweating, light-headedness, and abdominal queasiness. Cardiac syncope and orthostatic hypotension are usually sudden in onset. Seizure episodes may have a preceding aura.

D. Did anyone take her pulse during the episode? Vasovagal attacks are associated with bradycardia, orthostatic hypotension with tachycardia, and cardiac syncope with variable heart rates ranging from severe bradycardia in heart block to tachycardias as the cause for the syncope.

E. Is the patient diabetic or does she have any major medical conditions? Hypoglycemic spells are an infrequent but readily treatable cause of syncope. Cardiac problems may suggest the cause.

F. When was the patient's last menses? If the patient is late for her menses (> 28 days), she should be evaluated for an ectopic pregnancy.

III. Differential Diagnosis

A. Vasovagal. The simple faint is associated with the aura described above.

B. Cardiac
  1. Arrhythmias
    a. Heart block (rate usually < 40 bpm). Fainting may occur in Stokes-Adams attacks.
    b. Tachyarrhythmias (rate usually > 160 bpm with reduced cardiac output). Syncope is associated with paroxysmal atrial tachycardia, atrial fibrillation and flutter, ventricular tachycardia or fibrillation.
    c. Sick sinus syndrome.
    d. Asystole. Fainting occurs with cardiac arrest.
  2. Myocardial disease
    a. Aortic stenosis with left ventricular outflow obstruction.

       b. Idiopathic hypertrophic subaortic stenosis (IHSS) from the same mechanism as aortic stenosis.

       c. Primary pulmonary hypertension, which causes reduced pulmonary flow.

       d. Acute myocardial infarction with cardiogenic shock.

       e. Atrial myxoma.

    3. Orthostatic hypotension

       a. Hypovolemia of any cause. Consider ruptured ectopic pregnancy.

       b. Sudden posture change. Fainting in this situation may be associated with certain medications (prazosin, etc.).

       c. Neurologic and endocrine. Syncope occurs with Shy-Drager syndrome, diabetes.

C. Cerebrovascular

    1. Basilar artery insufficiency.

    2. Carotid sinus syndrome typically presents as syncope caused by turning the head to one side.

    3. Subclavian steal syndrome.

D. Miscellaneous

    1. Micturition syncope or cough syncope usually involves decreased venous return.

    2. Hypoglycemia.

    3. Hyperventilation.

    4. Hypoxia.

E. Nonsyncopal

    1. Seizure (see Problem 21, page 88).

    2. Coma.

IV. Database

A. Physical examination key points

    1. Vital signs. Check for orthostatic changes, heart rate, and rhythm. A > 20 mm Hg discrepancy in blood pressure between the two arms suggests subclavian steal.

    2. Neck. Look for carotid bruits and carotid upstroke.

    3. Heart. There may be murmurs of aortic stenosis, IHSS, or rhythm abnormalities.

    4. Rectum. Heme-positive stools or other evidence of an acute GI bleed should be sought.

    5. Pelvic examination. Evaluate for pelvic mass (ie, ectopic pregnancy). A bulging cul-de-sac may be suggestive of a hemoperitoneum.

    6. Neurologic examination. Look for dysarthria, focal signs, and mental status changes.

   7. Reproduce syncope with maneuvers such as coughing, turning the head, hyperventilation, or carotid massage.
   B. Laboratory data
   1. Hemogram. Pay close attention to the hematocrit. Decreased hematocrit may be suggestive of ectopic pregnancy or a ruptured spleen.
   2. Electrolytes and glucose. Test especially for hypoglycemia.
   3. Blood gases. Hypoxia or hyperventilation (decreased CO_2, decreased pH) may be present.
   4. Pregnancy test. Obtain a urine or serum pregnancy test to rule out pregnancy.
   C. Radiologic and other studies
   1. Chest x-ray. Especially note the cardiac silhouette for evidence of heart failure effusion.
   2. ECG with rhythm strip. Short PR intervals, delta waves, or any more obvious signs of rhythm disturbance may be present.
   3. Echocardiogram. The study may reveal myxoma, valvular lesions, or thrombi.
   4. Holter monitor. This is useful for evaluation of dysrhythmias.
   5. Pelvic ultrasound. Intrauterine pregnancy can be identified in utero with serum human chorionic gonadotropin (HCG) > 6000 mIU. An adnexal mass that presents without an intrauterine pregnancy is suggestive of an ectopic pregnancy.

V. Plan. Etiologic causes for syncope range from an inconsequential vasovagal attack to ectopic pregnancy. Therefore, treatment is dictated by the correct diagnosis. Always assess the patient for injury from a fall during syncope.

   A. Vasovagal syncope. Instruct the patient to put her head down at the onset of presyncopal symptoms.

   B. Orthostatic hypotension
   1. Assess for volume loss using orthostatic blood pressure measurements (paying close attention to possible GI bleed), and treat accordingly (see Problem 54, page 199).
   2. Instruct the patient to change positions slowly.

   C. Cardiac cause
   1. Treat the arrhythmia. If tachyarrhythmia is causing hypotension, treat as outlined in Problem 54, page 199. Cardiac arrest rhythms are treated as in Problem 35, page 134.
   2. If the initial ECG does not reveal a rhythm disturbance,

closely monitor the patient and consider a 24-hour Holter monitor.

D. Hemoperitoneum. This is a surgical emergency. The patient should undergo an exploratory laparotomy as soon as possible.

REFERENCE

Moss AJ: Diagnosis: syncope. *Hosp Med* 17:59, 1981.

70. TACHYCARDIA (SEE PROBLEM 13, PAGE 59.)

71. TRANSFUSION REACTION

I. Problem. During a transfusion of packed red blood cells, a patient's temperature rises to 39.5 °C (103.1 °F). (Blood bank products are discussed in Chapter 5.)

II. Immediate Questions

A. What are the vital signs? Hypotension should be ruled out. Tachypnea is a sign of a significant reaction. Fever is the most common manifestation of a transfusion reaction.

B. Does the patient have back or chest pain? Acute coagulopathy can develop from a major transfusion reaction. Chest pain may develop during hemodynamic stress. Other symptoms may include chills, diaphoresis, hypersensitivity reactions (hives, wheezing, pruritus), or exacerbation of congestive heart failure.

C. Has the transfusion been stopped? If not, do so and maintain an open IV line with normal saline.

III. Differential Diagnosis.
Differentiating a fever due to a transfusion reaction from other causes of postoperative fever is often difficult. Assuming no other fever source, the following transfusion reactions are possible, in order of decreasing likelihood and increasing severity.

A. White cell antigens. Unlike washed red cells, packed cells contain relatively large numbers of leukocytes. Febrile responses to these cells are usually accompanied by urticaria.

B. Minor protein reactions. Allergic reactions to transfused serum proteins can cause fever. Sometimes, anaphylaxis or acute pulmonary edema can occur.

C. ABO incompatibility. This represents a potentially life-threatening problem and fortunately is rare. Signs are seen after transfusion of relatively small quantities of blood.

   D. Contaminated blood. Bacterial contamination is rare but should be suspected when high fever and hypotension develop early during a transfusion. It is often fatal.

IV. Database

A. Physical examination key points

1. **Heart.** Examine for tachycardia and new flow murmur.
2. **Lungs.** Listen for rales and wheezing.
3. **Abdomen.** Pain, especially in the flanks, should be looked for.
4. **Skin.** Examine for rash or hives.

B. Laboratory data

1. **Blood bank specimen.** Two freshly drawn clot tubes (redtop tubes) should be returned to the blood bank with the remaining untransfused blood. A repeat cross-match will be performed. In addition, most blood banks require a heparinized specimen to perform an indirect Coombs' test looking for previous sensitization.
2. **Urinalysis.** Hematuria after a transfusion reaction represents hemoglobinuria after hemolysis from a major ABO incompatibility.
3. **Hemogram.** Schistocytes may be present in a transfusion reaction; a worsening anemia may develop in the face of massive red cell destruction.
4. **Serum for free hemoglobin and haptoglobin.** Free hemoglobin will be present with a reaction and haptoglobin will be decreased.
5. **Other lab tests** as clinically indicated. Coagulation studies can help to diagnose thrombocytopenia and disseminated intravascular coagulation (DIC). Monitor renal function by obtaining BUN and creatinine along with serum electrolytes. Arterial blood gases are rarely indicated (cardiovascular collapse).

C. Radiologic and other studies. These are not routinely needed, but are ordered as clinically indicated.

V. Plan

A. Immediately stop the transfusion. Consultation with the blood bank pathologist is usually indicated to evaluate the reaction as well as to discuss any further transfusions.

B. **Maintain IV access.** Monitor urine output and vital signs closely, and keep open a normal saline IV.

C. **Send the blood bank appropriate specimens** (see B-1 above). Make sure the bag is returned to the blood bank immediately.

D. **Mild reactions.** Usually these consist of fever without any evidence of more severe symptoms or hemolysis.
   1. Antihistamines (diphenhydramine 25–50 mg IM or IV) and acetaminophen may reverse mild allergic and febrile reactions.
   2. Transfusion can usually be restarted.

E. **Severe reactions.** A severe reaction usually signifies that acute hemolysis has taken place. One of the major goals is to prevent renal failure.
   1. **Circulatory support.** Maintain adequate blood pressure with volume or pressors. Diuresis with furosemide or mannitol, usually with D5W, should be started to prevent renal injury in the setting of marked hemolysis. Also consider alkalinization of the urine with bicarbonate to further protect the kidney.
   2. **Antibiotics.** These will be needed if examination of the remaining untransfused unit reveals evidence of bacterial contamination. The organisms are usually gram-negative bacilli.

F. **Known reactions.** Patients with known febrile reactions to blood products can be pretreated with antihistamines (diphenhydramine), antipyretics, or steroids to avoid the reaction. Special blood bank products (leukocyte-poor red cell packs) may occasionally be used in this setting.

REFERENCE

Greenwalt TJ: Pathogenesis and management of hemolytic transfusion reactions. *Semin Hematol* 18:84, 1981.

72. URINE IN THE VAGINA

I. **Problem.** A 56-year-old woman is complaining of urine leaking from her vagina.

II. **Immediate Questions**

A. **Has the patient had recent pelvic surgery?** The most important etiologic factor for urinary vaginal fistulas is gynecologic surgery, chiefly a hysterectomy. Other causes include urologic procedures, obstetric injury, pelvic cancers, extensive pelvic trauma, and radiation complications.

B. What medical problems does the patient have? Other predisposing factors for fistula formation are arteriosclerosis, hypertension, diabetes mellitus, obesity, and pelvic inflammatory disease.

C. Has the patient had previous pelvic irradiation? Urinary tract complications resulting from radiation therapy for carcinoma of the cervix can occur as long as 30 years after treatment.

D. When did the patient start losing urine, and how much? Depending on the pathogenesis, fistulas caused by trauma manifest themselves immediately after surgery, while fistulas caused by tissue necrosis take 5–14 days to appear. The amount of urine lost is directly related to the size and location of the fistula.

E. Are there any associated symptoms? Vesicovaginal fistulas are usually painless. Enterovaginal fistulas and vaginitis are usually irritating to the skin of the vulva.

III. Differential Diagnosis

A. Vesicovaginal fistula. Vesicovaginal fistulas usually present as a painless, watery discharge. With a small fistula, patients may void normally and leak only small amounts of urine. The flow may increase when the patient changes to certain positions. However, large fistulas usually leak constantly and urine does not collect in the bladder to allow normal voiding.

B. Ureterovaginal fistula. These fistulas can be associated with hydroureter and hydronephrosis. Occasionally urine can also extravasate intraperitoneally with accompanying fever, flank pain, and paralytic ileus. This complication may be present in patients who have undergone radical hysterectomy.

C. Urethrovaginal fistula. These fistulas may occur following surgical repair of a cystocele or urethral diverticulum, or with obstetric trauma. A high urethrovaginal fistula is often associated with damage to the internal urethral sphincter and accompanied by urinary incontinence. When the fistula is in the middle or lower third of the urethra, the patient may have no symptoms except spraying of the urinary stream.

D. Severe stress or urge incontinence. When loss of urine is due to weakness of the sphincter, urine usually can be seen to spurt from the urethral meatus with straining.

E. Vaginitis. The large amount of vaginal drainage may not be urine but a heavy vaginal discharge. The patient may also complain of burning on urination and a foul odor to the vaginal drainage.

F. Enterovaginal fistula. Small bowel drainage from the vagina is extremely irritating to the skin of the vulva and perineum.

IV. Database

A. Physical examination key points

1. **Vital signs.** Fever may suggest infection or fistula formation
2. **Abdomen.** Perform percussion and palpation to detect an overdistended bladder leading to stress incontinence.
3. **Pelvic examination.** On vaginal exam, look and palpate for urethrovaginal and vesicovaginal fistulas. Frequently, with small fistulas, a small reddened area in the upper vagina can be seen where urine escapes. A small wire probe may help in identifying the area.
4. **Skin.** Extensive irritation of the vulva from drainage may suggest an enterovaginal fistula or vaginitis.

B. Laboratory data

1. **Hemogram.** Leukocytosis and left shift may suggest an infectious process or fistula formation.
2. **Serum electrolytes.** An elevated serum creatinine indicates impairment of renal function.
3. **Urinalysis.** Evaluate the urinary sediment for leukocytes, erythrocytes, and bacteria.

C. Radiologic and other studies

1. **Dye tests**
   a. If the fistula cannot be visualized, the bladder may be filled with 200–300 mL of a dilute solution of methylene blue and the vagina inspected. If no leakage is demonstrated, place a tampon in the vagina and instruct the patient to drink fluids and to walk. After several hours, remove the tampon and look for staining.
   b. If no methylene blue staining is found, the dye test should be repeated by giving the patient 10 mL of 0.4% indigo carmine intravenously or 200 mg of phenazopyridine orally. Staining of the tampon at this point indicates a ureterovaginal fistula.
   c. A test is also available for the diagnosis of enterovaginal fistula. After the patient takes Congo red or a charcoal solution by mouth, red coloration or charcoal particles appear in the vagina.
2. **Intravenous pyelogram.** An IVP can identify ureterovaginal fistula or ureteral obstruction with concurrent hydronephrosis and hydroureter.
3. **Retrograde pyelogram.** This study gives the exact localization of the obstruction when its position is not clear from the IVP.

4. **Cystogram.** This x-ray can be used to show the fistula channel in vesicovaginal fistulas. The x-ray should be taken from an oblique side angle and again after evacuation of the bladder.

5. **Small bowel series.** An enterovaginal fistula can be identified by contrast study of the small bowel.

6. **Nuclear medicine studies.** These are noninvasive techniques used to assess renal function in patients with ureteral obstruction.

7. **Cystoscopy and urethroscopy.** Cystoscopy can determine the size and location of the vesicovaginal fistula and its proximity to the ureters. If the ureteral orifices are close to the fistula tract, a ureteral catheter should be placed prior to surgery. It is also necessary to identify causes of fistula formation such as sutures or neoplasms.

V. Plan

A. Acute intervention. Placement of a large Foley catheter may reduce the amount of urinary leakage. Continued Foley catheter drainage with bladder decompression can be attempted for 1–2 months to encourage spontaneous closure of the fistula.

B. Specific treatment plans. The optimal time for repair has long been debated. However, the best guide is the condition of the fistula itself. When the area is clean, pliable, uninflamed, and free of edema, repair can be attempted. In postmenopausal women, 2–4 weeks of estrogen therapy will decrease the friability and increase the vascularity of the vaginal mucosa so that healing is improved.

1. **Ureteral fistula.** Therapy requires elimination of incontinence in addition to maintaining renal function. Placement of a nephrostomy tube serves as a palliative or temporary measure to prevent kidney failure in obstruction and to decrease the intraperitoneal leakage of urine. The catheter is inserted percutaneously under fluoroscopic guidance and can be left in place for weeks to years. The ureter should be splinted by inserting a stent in either the retrograde direction through the bladder or via a percutaneous nephrostomy in the antegrade direction. Ureterovaginal fistulas heal spontaneously in 5–7% of cases.

2. **Vesicovaginal fistula.** Spontaneous recovery occurs in 1–6% of cases and can be expected only in nonirradiated patients. If spontaneous healing has not taken place after 1–2 months, surgical measures are necessary.

3. **Urethrovaginal fistula.** Distal urethral fistulas are usually asymptomatic and surgical intervention is unnecessary.

With these fistulas, a simple marsupialization between the fistula and the external meatus of the urethra can be done. If incontinence is occurring because urethral closure is insufficient, surgical intervention is necessary.

REFERENCES

Kunz J: Gynecologic complications in gynecologic surgery and radiotherapy. New York, S Karger, 1984.
Thompson D: Vesicovaginal fistulas. In Thompson JD, Rock JA (eds): *TeLinde's Operative Gynecology,* 7th ed. Philadelphia, JB Lippincott, 1992, pp 785–810.

73. VAGINAL BLEEDING (Missed or changed menses is discussed in Problem 57, page 215.)

I. **Problem.** You are called to see a 58-year-old multiparous postmenopausal woman who complains of moderate vaginal bleeding for 2 days.

II. **Immediate Questions**

A. **What are the vital signs?** Elevation of pulse and reduction in blood pressure suggest loss of hemodynamic status.

B. **What volume of blood has been passed?** Has the patient given her answer in relation to her memory of normal menstrual events? A normal menstrual period is associated with 25–60 mL blood loss.

C. **When was her last normal menstrual period?** This provides information about the duration of amenorrhea.

D. **Is this the first episode of postmenopausal bleeding?** Recurrent episodes are more significant than a single event.

E. **If there were previous episodes, what diagnostic studies were done?** Knowledge of the results of past diagnostic studies helps to plan current management.

F. **Has the patient had any gynecologic surgery?** The presence or absence of pelvic organs is important.

G. **Has the patient been taking hormones, and if so, which ones and how much?** Unopposed estrogen causes proliferation, while a combination of estrogen and progesterone results in an almost inactive endometrium.

H. **When was her last gynecologic examination?** Information concerning her use of health care and what she was told may be helpful in planning further management.

   I. Has the patient had intercourse recently? Local trauma is a frequent cause of bleeding in a postmenopausal patient.

   J. Is there any history of diabetes mellitus or hypertension? Both conditions are associated with an increased likelihood of cancer of the endometrium.

III. Differential Diagnosis

   A. Vulvovaginitis. Local irritation or inflammation more often causes minimal bleeding, but it can be persistent at times.

   B. Cancer of the vulva. This is usually associated with a lesion noted by the patient before the onset of bleeding.

   C. Cancer of the cervix. Cervical cancer is less common in the postmenopausal patient, and this presentation is very rare in a patient who has had annual cancer detection smears.

   D. Cancer of the endometrium. A likely cause of her bleeding, endometrial cancer is even more likely if she is using estrogen alone but much less likely if she is taking a combination of estrogen and progesterone. There may be an associated pyometra.

   E. Endometrial hyperplasia or polyp. This is the most likely cause of her bleeding.

   F. Rectal bleeding. Patients will often be uncertain from where the bleeding originates (see Problem 34, page 130).

   G. Bloody urine. Patients will on occasion confuse urethral bleeding with vaginal bleeding.

IV. Database

   A. Physical examination key points

      1. Vital signs. Increased pulse and decreased blood pressure are indicative of hypovolemia. Fever may indicate an associated pyometra.

      2. Abdominal examination. Abdominal masses such as ovarian and uterine tumors as well as fibroids may be palpated.

      3. Pelvic examination. Inspect the vulva and vagina for inflammation, irritation, or a local lesion which may be carcinoma. A hard, fixed cervix is suggestive of cervical cancer. Fibroids usually present as an irregular enlarged uterus, whereas endometrial carcinoma is usually symmetric.

      4. Rectal examination. To rule out this area as a source of the bleeding, evaluate the cul-de-sac area for masses or tenderness.

B. Laboratory data

1. **Hemogram.** This is useful for baseline data and to evaluate the general status of the patient. If values are very low, defer biopsies until the patient's total status is evaluated.

2. **Cancer detection smear.** Obtain this only if the amount of bleeding is minimal. A bloody Pap smear is of no value and may mislead, since false negative smears are a bit higher in the presence of significant cancer.

3. **Direct biopsy.** Any suspicious lesion of the vulva or cervix should be biopsied to rule out cancer.

4. **Endometrial biopsy.** This can rule out hyperplasia or cancer of the endometrium.

5. **Cultures.** A slide using 10% KOH and normal saline is made and examined to rule out yeast, *Trichomonas,* or bacterial vaginosis. Yeast infections occur in postmenopausal women and may cause significant irritation and tissue breakdown.

C. Radiologic and other studies. Sonography would be of value only if the pelvic examination was unsatisfactory because of obesity.

V. Plan. The vast majority of postmenopausal patients stop bleeding very quickly and the amount of loss is small. These cases are rarely emergencies and the fear of cancer, not the amount of bleeding, has brought the patient to the emergency room.

A. Acute intervention. Only if there is evidence of significant blood loss will active intervention be necessary (see Problem 54, page 199).

B. Cancer. The primary concern is to rule out cancer at any site as a cause of bleeding. This requires careful assessment of the cervix, endometrium, and adnexal areas by biopsy and, if needed, laparoscopy.

C. Other causes. One malignancy is ruled out as a cause, local management of the irritation or atrophy is required. A local estrogen cream is useful for atrophic vaginitis. Basic hygiene of the external genitalia area with simple solutions or antifungal or anti-trichomonas medication. Most important is educating the patient about the value and importance of ongoing annual evaluation and screening.

REFERENCES

Goldfarb JM, Little AB: Abnormal uterine bleeding. *N Engl J Med* 302:666, 1980.

Mishell DR Jr (ed): *Menopause: Physiology and Pharmacology.* Chicago, Year Book, 1986.

74. VAGINAL DISCHARGE

I. **Problem.** A 24-year-old woman complains of a 3-day history of heavy vaginal discharge.

II. **Immediate Questions**

A. **What are the characteristics of the discharge?** Normal vaginal secretions are whitish to slightly gray in appearance, of moderate consistency, and without odor. The amount varies somewhat throughout the menstrual cycle. Consistency, color, and odor of abnormal vaginal secretions may be a clue to their specific cause.

B. **Are there associated symptoms?** Lower abdominal or pelvic pain, fever, or both may indicate the presence of upper genital tract infection. Irritative symptoms such as burning or itching are most consistent with *Candida, Trichomonas,* allergic or irritative phenomena, or atrophic vaginitis.

C. **How recent has the patient been sexually active?** Patients who are currently or recently sexually active, particularly in non-monogamous relationships, are at increased risk for sexually transmitted diseases (STDs). If the sexual partner also has genital symptoms, an STD is more likely.

D. **If she is sexually active, is any form of contraception being used?** Barrier forms of contraception offer varying degrees of protection against STDs. The presence of an IUD, particularly with multiple sexual partners, predisposes to acquisition of pelvic inflammatory disease (PID), whereas oral contraceptives are protective against PID.

E. **When was the last menstrual period and was it normal?** The presence of pregnancy must always be considered and may influence the acquisition or significance of certain infections which might result in vaginal discharge. In an older woman, the possibility of vaginal discharge related to estrogen deficiency must be considered.

F. **Is there a prior history of STDs?** Sexually transmitted diseases not infrequently recur because of inadequate treatment of the patient or her partner, relapse, or reinfection secondary to continued unsafe sexual practices.

G. **When was the most recent Pap smear obtained, and have there been any abnormal Pap smears in the past?** A heavy yellowish or blood stained, often malodorous discharge may be the first sign of an invasive cervical cancer.

H. Is the patient taking any medications? Women taking antibiotics or steroids are at higher risk for vaginal candidiasis.

I. Has the patient been using or inserting any substances into her vagina? Douches, lubricants, vaginal contraceptives, or other vaginal medications may cause an allergic or irritative reaction.

J. Is there a history of any significant medical illnesses? Diabetes mellitus or immunosuppression from a variety of causes may predispose to the development of vaginal candidiasis.

III. Differential Diagnosis

A. Bacterial vaginosis. Currently considered to be the most common vaginal infection, this appears to be a disequilibrium syndrome with an overgrowth of certain organisms including *Gardnerella vaginalis,* various anaerobes, and *Mycoplasma.* It is unclear whether a particular organism initiates overgrowth, sexual inoculation is required, or host factors are responsible.

B. Candida vaginitis. Most infections are caused by *Candida albicans;* predisposing factors include an estrogen-rich environment (oral contraceptive pills, estrogen replacement, pregnancy), the administration of antibiotics which decrease the number of protective resident bacteria, and immunosuppression. Most infections are the result of self-inoculation from the GI tract, although sexual transmission may occur.

C. Trichomonas vaginalis. Infections with *Trichomonas* are almost always sexually transmitted; predisposing factors include the presence of cervical or vaginal lesions, mature squamous epithelium, and menses or other conditions which increase vaginal pH.

D. Cervicitis. This is most commonly caused by gonorrhea or *Chlamydia* but may also be seen with herpes simplex virus. Women with cervicitis are more likely to have abnormal vaginal bleeding.

E. Pelvic inflammatory disease. The diagnosis of PID should always be called into question if there are no abnormal cervical or vaginal secretions.

F. Allergic/irritative vaginitis.

G. Vaginal or cervical lesions. Invasive cervical or vaginal cancer, usually in a more advanced stage, may present with abnormal vaginal discharge.

H. **Foreign body.** Retained tampons, and in children a variety of items, may present with an abnormal discharge which is often malodorous and may contain blood.

I. **Atrophic vaginitis.** Postmenopausal patients not receiving estrogen replacement therapy may develop an abnormal and irritative vaginal discharge. The role of bacterial organisms in the development of symptoms is not well understood.

J. **Pediatric vaginitis.** Symptomatic vaginitis may be caused by a variety of bacteria including enteric organisms, hemolytic streptococci, and staphylococci. The total quantitative bacterial load appears to be important. Other common causes of vaginitis in children include pinworms, the presence of a foreign body, and, in children who have been sexually abused, gonorrhea or *Chlamydia*. Some children experiencing chronic sexual abuse develop recurrent vaginal infections that are believed to be secondary to removal of the hymen as a normal anatomic barrier.

IV. Database

A. Physical examination key points

1. **Vital signs.** Fever may suggest the presence of an upper genital tract infection.
2. **Skin.** Rash on the trunk and extremities may suggest disseminated gonococcal infection. Erythematous, thickened, pruritic areas under the arms or breasts or on the medial thighs may suggest candidal infection.
3. **Abdomen.** Look especially for tenderness in the lower abdomen, with or without signs of peritoneal irritation, which might suggest pelvic inflammatory disease. Enlarged, firm or fixed inguinal lymph nodes may indicate a neoplastic process.
4. **Pelvic examination**
   a. **External genitalia.** Look for signs of vulvar irritation including erythema, edema, or skin changes suggestive of fungal infection or allergic/irritative reaction. Signs of perianal irritation in a child may suggest the presence of pinworms. Urethral discharge and erythema may indicate the presence of urethritis secondary to gonorrhea or *Chlamydia*. The size of the hymenal opening and the presence of skin tags and hyperpigmentation may be clues to chronic sexual abuse in children.
   b. **Speculum examination.** Look for any cervical or vaginal lesions. Erythema and edema of the vaginal mucosa suggest an infectious or allergic phenomenon. Characteristics of the discharge should be noted including its consistency, color, and odor. Is the cervix friable, edem-

atous, and erythematous, suggesting cervicitis? Prominent vaginal papillae secondary to an intense inflammatory response are considered pathognomonic of *Trichomonas* infections. Thin, flattened, easily traumatized mucosal surfaces are consistent with estrogen deficiency.

c. **Bimanual/rectovaginal examination.** Cervical motion with uterine or adnexal tenderness is suggestive of an upper genital tract infection. Always change gloves before the rectovaginal exam to avoid contaminating the rectum with potentially infectious cervical or vaginal secretions.

B. **Laboratory data**
1. **Hemogram.** Left shift and leukocytosis are suggestive of a systemic process.
2. **Rapid plasma reagin or serologic test for syphilis.** In the presence of a sexually transmitted disease, these tests can rule out coexisting syphilis.
3. **Human chorionic gonadotropin.** A serum or urine pregnancy test may be indicated to rule out pregnancy.
4. **Cultures.** Obtain specimens for gonococcus, *Chlamydia,* and herpes simplex virus, if indicated.
5. **Pap smears.** Depending on the results, biopsies may be indicated.

C. **Radiologic and other studies**
1. **Wet mount (normal saline) of vaginal secretions.** The presence of trichomonads, clue cells, or budding yeast and hyphal forms may help to establish the diagnosis. Remember that more than one process may be going on at the same time. The presence of excess white cells without other findings suggests cervicitis, upper genital tract infection, or possibly a severely irritative reaction. Bacterial vaginosis does not elicit much of an inflammatory response; therefore, many white cells on wet mount, even in the presence of numerous clue cells, probably indicate a coexisting process.
2. **10% KOH mount.** Look for the presence of fungal forms.
3. **Vaginal pH.** Both *Trichomonas* and bacterial vaginosis are high pH states, generally above the normal vaginal pH of 3.5–4.5. The presence of blood, semen, excess cervical secretions, or amniotic fluid artificially raises the pH.
4. **Endocervical gram stain.** The presence of gram-negative intracellular diplococci has a high specificity for the diagnosis of gonorrheal cervicitis; > 30 WBC/HPF is consistent with cervicitis or upper genital tract infection.

V. **Plan**
A. **Identify and treat the underlying cause.** Current CDC-recom-

mended treatment regimens for common vaginal infections include:

1. **Trichomonas vaginalis.** Metronidazole 2 g PO in a single dose **or** 500 mg PO bid for 7 days. **Note:** Metronidazole has been associated with a disulfiram-like reaction. Patients should be warned not to drink alcohol while taking this medication.
2. **Candidiasis.** There are several effective regimens, including the following.
   a. Miconazole nitrate 200 mg vaginal suppository intravaginally qhs for 3 days.
   b. Clotrimazole 200 mg vaginal tablets intravaginally qhs for 3 days.
   c. Butaconazole 5 g of 2% cream intravaginally qhs for 3 days.
   d. Terconazole 80 mg suppository **or** 0.4% cream intravaginally qhs for 3 days.
   e. Miconazole nitrate 100 mg vaginal suppository **or** 5 g 2% cream intravaginally qhs for 7 days.
   f. Clotrimazole 100 mg vaginal tablets **or** 5 g of 1% cream intravaginally qhs for 7 days.
3. **Bacterial vaginosis**
   a. Metronidazole 500 mg PO bid for 7 days.
   b. Alternative regimen: clindamycin 300 mg PO bid for 7 days.

B. **Sexually transmitted diseases**
   1. See Problem 67, page 256, for appropriate treatment of gonorrheal or chlamydial cervicitis.
   2. Allergic or irritative vaginitis responds to removal of the inciting stimulus, but sometimes requires topical steroids for symptomatic relief.
   3. Atrophic vaginitis generally responds to estrogen orally, intravaginally, or by transdermal administration.

C. If an STD is diagnosed or suspected, the partner should be treated or referred for treatment.

D. The presence of an STD requires counseling the patient concerning cause and prevention of recurrent infections. Barrier methods of contraception, particularly condoms and spermicide, should be emphasized. Patients who present with recurrent or chronic vaginal candidiasis deserve further evaluation to rule out predisposing factors, such as immunosuppression. Patients with suspected STDs should be advised to avoid intercourse until treatment of both partners is completed.

E. The presence of gonococcus or *Chlamydia* requires follow-up evaluation and culture to ensure eradication of infection.

F. Any suspected child abuse must be reported to the appropriate authorities.

REFERENCES

Friedrich EG Jr: Vaginitis. *Am J Obstet Gyneol* 152:247, 1985.
Holmes KK et al (eds): *Sexually Transmitted Diseases,* 2nd ed. New York, Mc-Graw-Hill, 1990.
Jones HJ, Wentz AC, Burnett LS (eds): *Novak's Textbook of Gynecology,* 11th ed, Baltimore, Williams & Wilkins, 1988.
Sweet RL: Importance of differential diagnosis in acute vaginitis. *Am J Obstet Gyneol* 152:921, 1985.

75. WHEEZING

I. Problem. You are asked to see a ventilator-dependent postoperative patient in the ICU for new onset of wheezing.

II. Immediate Questions

　　A. Are the patient's vital signs stable? Extremes of blood pressure and pulse indicate the level of hypoxia or hypercapnia, if any. Fever could represent pulmonary infection.

　　B. Were medications given recently? Consider the possibility of an allergic reaction.

　　C. When was the last chest x-ray? Evidence of pneumonitis and endotracheal tube position can be evaluated quickly.

　　D. Is there a history of asthma or allergy? If so, has the patient been taking a medication such as theophylline and was this medication continued postoperatively in a parenteral form (aminophylline)?

III. Differential Diagnosis

　　A. Acute bronchospasm. There is usually a prior history of asthma. A subtherapeutic drug level of an antiasthmatic agent may be the cause.

　　B. Pneumonia. Fever and cough may also be present.

　　C. Allergic reaction. An allergic reaction can be due to systemically administered medication or inhalation of an allergen and may progress to anaphylaxis (see Problem 32, page 124).

　　D. Fluid overload. So-called cardiac asthma is due to pulmonary edema.

IV. Database. Obtain a list of medications and allergies.

　　A. Physical examination key points
　　　　1. Vital signs. Hypotension may accompany an anaphylactic reaction.

2. **HEENT.** Stridor may be present, suggesting laryngospasm.
3. **Lungs.** Determine the presence of breath sounds bilaterally, relative air movement, and inspiratory and expiratory wheezing.
4. **Skin.** Look for rash or other evidence of allergic reaction.
5. **Extremities.** Evaluate for edema (suggesting congestive heart failure) or cyanosis.

B. **Laboratory data**
1. **Arterial blood gases.** These tests determine the adequacy of ventilation and oxygenation.
2. **Hemogram.** Elevated WBCs could indicate pulmonary infection.
3. **Sputum gram stain and culture,** if indicated.
4. **Theophylline level,** if the patient is taking theophylline (see page 441, 557).

C. **Radiologic and other studies**
1. **Chest x-ray.** Evidence of pneumonia, pulmonary edema, or atelectasis should be sought; endotracheal tube position should be rechecked.
2. **Peak airway pressure.** This important parameter can be readily discerned from the ventilator. Values above 20–30 cm H_2O are abnormal and, in the setting of new wheezing, represent bronchospasm or fluid overload.

V. Plan

A. **Aggressive endotracheal tube suctioning with saline lavage.** Aggressive suctioning is important to the intubated patient for several reasons. First, it prevents atelectasis by removing mucus plugs and stimulating coughing; second, "pulmonary toilet" probably helps prevent microbial colonization from progressing to full-blown infection; third, it aids in diagnosis of infections.

B. **Nebulized metaproterenol (Alupent).** Give 0.3 cc in 2.5 mL saline. This is a selective beta-2 agonist used to treat acute asthma. Effects are seen within 5 minutes, and doses may be repeated q4h.

C. **Aminophylline.** Refractory bronchospasm should be treated with intravenous aminophylline.
1. Instill a 6 mg/kg loading dose over 20–30 minutes; the dose should be reduced 50% if the patient has received aminophylline in the previous 24 hours.
2. A continuous drip of 0.5 mg/kg/h should be used as maintenance, adjusted according to serum theophylline levels (10–20 μg/mL therapeutic level) and to side effects such as tachycardia.

D. Antibiotics. Bronchospasm induced by pneumonia or acute bronchitis should be treated with appropriate antibiotics as determined from culture results.

E. Nonintubated patients. These patients should likewise be treated with nebulized metaproterenol, and aminophylline as necessary.

F. Diuretics. If there is evidence of fluid overload, use agents such as furosemide.

G. Anaphylaxis (see Problem 32, page 124).

REFERENCES

Ahmad M, Lindquist C: Bronchial asthma: aspects of pathogenesis and therapy. *Postgrad Med* 62:111, 1977.
Demling RH, Wilson RF: Bronchospasm and bronchodilators. In *Decision Making in Surgical Intensive Care.* Philadelphia, BC Decker, 1988, pp 17–18.

76. WOUND DEHISCENCE

I. Problem. A nurse notifies you that the laparotomy wound in a patient who underwent total abdominal hysterectomy has opened and there is a piece of fat poking out of the wound.

II. Immediate Questions

A. Is there a wound dehiscence, and if so, to what extent? Always evaluate the wound yourself as soon as possible. Do not trust a nurse's observations, since they may overcall or undercall wound problems, and do not wait until morning to look at the wound. See how much of the wound has opened, how deeply, and if there is an evisceration. An "open wound" is not a dehiscence unless the fascia opens.

B. Did any fluid leak from the wound? Look at the dressing and ask the nurse and patient about the nature and amount of fluid. Serous or serosanguineous fluid is more ominous for a true fascial dehiscence. Grossly bloody or purulent fluid is indicative of a superficial wound infection, a liquefying hematoma, or active bleeding in the superficial tissues.

C. Are there any factors predisposing to dehiscence? Factors such as sepsis, poor nutrition, diabetes, and steroids predispose to poor wound healing and increase the likelihood of dehiscence.

III. Differential Diagnosis. A wound dehiscence is usually the result of a combination of factors including technical problems, local wound problems, poor wound healing, and increased stress on the wound.

The following list is not so much a differential diagnosis as a list of those contributing factors.

A. Technical problems
   1. **Poorly placed sutures,** either failure to take a full-thickness bite or reapproximating muscle instead of fascia.
   2. **Inappropriate suture material** such as not using a heavy enough gauge suture for an abdominal closure.
   3. **Sutures tied too tightly** usually induces tissue ischemia, causing the suture to pull out.

B. Local wound problems
   1. **Infection.**
   2. **Hematoma.**

C. Poor wound healing
   1. **Poor nutrition.**
   2. **Diabetes.**
   3. **Steroids,** either endogenous (Cushing's) or exogenous.
   4. **Uremia.**
   5. **Chemotherapy.**
   6. **Advanced malignancy.**

D. Increased tension on the wound
   1. **Abdominal distention.**
      a. **Ascites.**
      b. **Dilated bowel.**
   2. **Vomiting or coughing.**
   3. **Chronic obstructive pulmonary disease.**

IV. Database

   A. Physical examination key points. Using sterile gloves, take off all the dressings and examine the entire wound. Look for leakage of fluid when the wound is palpated, and look for signs of infection. Examine for opening of the fascia using a finger or sterile cotton swab.

   B. Laboratory data. Wound culture and gram stain are usually indicated.

V. Plan

   A. Initial management. Determine by wound examination if there is an evisceration, fascial disruption without evisceration, or a superficial wound separation. In all cases, it is safe to make the patient NPO and start antibiotics (cephalosporins are frequently used) to cover at least skin organisms until a final plan is formulated.

B. Evisceration/fascial dehiscence. Cover the wound with saline-soaked sterile gauze, then cover with a large sterile dressing. Notify the senior staff and the operating room since evisceration requires operative repair.

C. Fascial dehiscence without evisceration
1. If the overlying skin and subcutaneous tissues are intact but there is clearly a fascial defect, it may be treated by operative repair or observation. Without treatment, a ventral hernia will develop.
2. Use an abdominal binder if senior staff opts for observation. Note, however, that a binder often compromises respiratory function, especially in the immediate postoperative period.

D. Superficial wound separation
1. Healing by secondary intention is mandatory when there is an associated superficial wound infection, and is the safest management in any case. Treat with 2–4 wet-to-dry dressing changes per day (depending on the size of the defect, saline-soaked 4 × 4s are often used).
2. Some surgeons may attempt to reclose a superficial wound separation either immediately or following a period of wet-to-dry dressing changes. If this approach is used, realize that there is a substantial risk of developing a superficial infection.

REFERENCES

Greenburg AG, Saik RP, Peskin GW: Wound dehiscence. *Arch Surg* 114:143, 1979.
Hunt TK: Wound complications. In Hardy JD (ed): *Complications in Surgery and Their Management.* Philadelphia, WB Saunders, 1981, pp 24–27.

77. WOUND DRAINAGE

I. Problem. You are called to see a patient who has new drainage from a midline laparotomy incision 5 days after tumor cytoreduction and small bowel resection for ovarian cancer.

II. Immediate Questions

A. How old is the wound and what was the operative procedure? The diagnosis can be made partly on the basis of timing of the drainage as well as the type of surgery. Patients at increased risk for wound infection include those undergoing lengthy surgery, surgery for pelvic abscess, or operations on bacteria-containing organs such as bowel.

B. Was there any prior drainage and are drains present? Increased drainage from a wound may indicate that the suction or other drain is not working.

C. How was the wound closed? Wounds packed open may be expected to drain small amounts of fluid.

D. What is the character of the drainage? Bloody, serosanguineous, purulent, or intestinal contents aid in the diagnosis.

E. How much drainage is there? Quantitation is essential, especially to replace gastrointestinal tract losses in the presence of a fistula. Consider saving and weighing the dressings if volume determination is critical.

III. Differential Diagnosis

A. Wound infection. Most wound infections become clinically apparent at 5–6 days postoperatively. Usually the patient is febrile and the skin is reddened with fluctuation and induration of the subcutaneous tissue. These infections are usually caused by coliform bacilli, *Staphylococcus,* and *Streptococcus.* A rare infection due to hemolytic streptococci and staphylococci leads to the fulminating course of **necrotizing fasciitis.** This wound is painful and contains dark vesicles and widespread ecchymoses. There is rapid progression of subcutaneous and fascial necrosis and septicemia, and death occurs in 20–30% of the patients. Another rare infection is gas gangrene caused by *Clostridium* or a mixed gram-negative and microaerophilic gram-positive infection. This is manifest by severe pain and crepitation of the wound.

B. Impending dehiscence. Serosanguineous drainage from the wound after the first 24 postoperative hours suggests the possibility of an impending evisceration. When this drainage is associated with discomfort around the incision, disruption should be strongly suspected.

C. Enterocutaneous fistula. Intestinal contents draining from the wound can result from a high-output or low-output fistula. These fistulas are often caused by inadvertent suturing of a segment of intestine to the abdominal wall during fascial closure. Development of the fistula usually follows several days of abdominal pain and fever.

D. Hemorrhage. Excessive bleeding will usually exit through a fresh postoperative wound. Disseminated intravascular coagulation (DIC) may manifest as bleeding through the wound as well as at other locations (IV sites, etc).

E. Urinary fistula.

F. Ascitic leak. This usually occurs in the immediate postoperative period in a patient with known ascites.

G. **Drain malfunction.** If a surgically placed drain is occluded, the intended fluid may exit through the wound.

IV. Database

A. Physical examination key points

1. **Vital signs.** Fever, tachycardia, and signs of sepsis may suggest a wound infection.
2. **Abdomen.** Look for signs of peritonitis, distention, or fluid collection.
3. **Wound.** Examine the wound and surrounding tissues for inflammation or crepitation to suggest wound infection (see III-A).

B. Laboratory data

1. **Hemogram.** Leukocytosis with a left shift may reveal infection. A falling hematocrit may indicate severe anemia from bleeding. Platelets may be decreased in DIC or in other causes of thrombocytopenia.
2. **Coagulation profile.** Prothrombin time, partial thromboplastin time, and fibrin split products should be ordered if DIC is suspected.
3. **Culture and gram stain of drain fluid.** This is necessary to identify the cause and to direct treatment for infections.
4. **Creatinine or urea nitrogen of drain fluid.** If the drainage is thought to be urine, the creatinine and urea nitrogen will be much higher than the serum level.

C. Radiologic and other studies.

A fistulogram may be helpful if there is no clue to the origin of the drainage.

V. Plan

A. Initial management

1. Immediately treat a life-threatening complication such as evisceration (see Problem 76, page 286). Perform a diagnostic workup in less acute situations.
2. Send effluent from a wound for gram stain and culture. Chemistry determinations on clear fluid for urea nitrogen or creatinine may aid in diagnosis.

B. Wound infection

1. The wound must be opened, which can usually be done at the bedside, and packed with saline-moistened gauze after evacuating the pus from the wound.
2. Remove enough skin closure staples or sutures to fully drain the area.
3. In the presence of advancing local cellulitis, crepitation typi-

cal of a gas-forming infection, or systemic signs of infection, aggressive therapy is needed.
   a. Clostridia infection is treated by early debridement along with high-dose IV penicillin.
   b. Gas-forming nonclostridial infections are treated with broad-spectrum antibiotics.

C. Dehiscence (see Problem 76, page 286).

D. Enterocutaneous fistula. Low-output fistulas will often close spontaneously, while fistulas that remain high output will probably require surgical intervention.
   1. Place a bag over the wound to capture the effluent, protect the skin, and quantitate the drainage.
   2. Oral administration of charcoal or dye may be used to confirm the diagnosis.
   3. Sump drains may be useful to help collect the material. Nasogastric suction and keeping the patient NPO are essential.
   4. Institute early nutritional support by the parenteral route.

E. Hemorrhage
   1. Evaluate the patient's volume status. Remember that a drop in hematocrit can occur late. Replete volume with crystalloid, blood, or both.
   2. The decision whether or not to reoperate for bleeding will depend on the clinical situation. The bleeding may be from a vessel in the skin or subcutaneous fat. If such a vessel is seen, it can be cauterized at the bedside with a battery-powered cautery.
   3. Treatment for DIC should be directed at the underlying cause (eg, antibiotics for infection). Significant bleeding should be corrected with fresh-frozen plasma and platelets.

REFERENCES

Hunt TK: Disorders of repair and their management. In Hunt TK, Dunphy JE (eds): *Fundamentals of Wound Management.* New York, Appleton-Century-Crofts, 1979, pp 133–138.

Mattingly RF, Thompson JD: Opening and closing the abdomen. In *TeLinde's Operative Gynecology,* 6th ed. Philadelphia, JB Lippincott, 1985, pp 170–178.

Laboratory Tests and Their Interpretation

The range for some common normal values is given in parentheses. Check the ranges for each facility before interpreting results of any lab test. Unless specified, values reflect normal adult levels.

Acid-Fast Stain

Normal = negative.

Positive. *Mycobacterium* species *(M. tuberculosis* and atypical mycobacteria such as *M. avium-intracellulare, scrofulaceum),* Nocardia, Actinomyces.

ACTH (Adrenocorticotropic Hormone)

8 AM: 20–100 pg/mL or 20–100 ng/L; midnight value: approximately 50% of AM value.

Increased. Addison's disease, ectopic ACTH production (oat cell carcinoma, pancreatic islet cell tumors, thymic tumors, renal cell carcinoma).

Decreased. Adrenal adenoma or carcinoma, nodular adrenal hyperplasia, pituitary insufficiency.

ACTH Stimulation Test

Used to help diagnose adrenal insufficiency. Cortrosyn (an ACTH analog) is given at a dose of 0.25 mg IM or IV. Collect blood at time 0 and at 30 and 60 minutes for cortisol and aldosterone.

Normal Response:
Basal cortisol level of at least 5 µg/dL, an increase of at least 7 µg/dL, and a final cortisol of 16 µg/dL at 30 minutes or 18 µg/dL at 60 minutes.

Addison's Disease (Primary Adrenal Insufficiency):
Neither cortisol nor aldosterone increases over baseline.

Secondary Adrenal Insufficiency:
Caused by pituitary insufficiency or suppression by exogenous steroids; cortisol is unchanged but aldosterone increases. An ACTH level and pituitary stimulation tests can be used to differentiate primary from secondary adrenal insufficiency.

21-Hydroxylase Deficiency:
The 1-hour value of 12-hydroxyprogesterone can be plotted on a nomogram to predict the genotype of 21-hydroxylase deficiency.

Albumin

3.5–5.0 g/dL or 35–50 g/L.

Decreased. Malnutrition, nephrotic syndrome, cystic fibrosis, multiple myeloma, Hodgkin's disease, leukemia, protein-losing enteropathies, chronic glomerulonephritis, cirrhosis, inflammatory bowel disease, collagen vascular diseases, hyperthyroidism, last two trimesters of pregnancy.

Aldosterone

Serum, supine: 3–10 ng/dL or 0.083–0.28 nmol/L early AM, normal sodium intake; serum, upright: 5–30 ng/dL or 0.138–0.83 nmol/L; urinary: 2–16 μg/24h or 5.4–44.3 nmol/d.

Increased. Hyperaldosteronism (primary or secondary). Should be confirmed after oral or intravenous salt loading.

Decreased. Adrenal insufficiency, panhypopituitarism.

Alkaline Phosphatase

20–70 U/L.
A fractionated alkaline phosphatase is often useful to differentiate between bone or liver origin of the enzyme. The heat-stable fraction comes from liver, the heat-labile fraction from bone ("bone burns"). On a fractionated sample, if the heat-stable fraction is < 20% suspect bone origin; if 25–55%, suspect liver origin. Levels are increased in pregnancy and toxemia.

Increased. Increased calcium deposition in bone (hyperparathyroidism), Paget's disease, osteoblastic bone tumors (metastatic or osteogenic sarcoma), osteomalacia, rickets, pregnancy, childhood, liver disease such as biliary obstruction (masses, drug therapy), hyperthyroidism.

Decreased. Malnutrition, excess vitamin D ingestion, pregnancy, pregnancy-induced hypertension.

Alpha-Fetoprotein (AFP)

< 30 ng/mL or < 30 μg/L.

Increased. Hepatoma, ovarian tumors (embryonal carcinoma, malignant teratoma, endodermal sinus tumors), spina bifida (in mother's serum).

ALT (Alanine Aminotransferase) (SGPT: Serum Glutamic-Pyruvic Transaminase)

8–20 U/L.

Increased. Liver disease, liver metastasis, biliary obstruction, pancreatitis, liver congestion, hepatitis (**ALT** is more elevated than **AST** in viral hepatitis; **AST** is more elevated than **ALT** in alcoholic hepatitis).

Ammonia

Arterial: 15–45 μg N/dL or 11–32 μmol N/L.

Increased. Hepatic encephalopathy, Reye's syndrome.

Amylase

25–125 U/L.

Increased. Acute pancreatitis, pancreatic duct obstruction (stones, stricture, tumor, sphincter spasm secondary to drugs), alcohol ingestion, mumps, parotiditis, renal disease, macroamylasemia, cholecystitis, peptic ulcers, intestinal obstruction, mesenteric thrombosis, after surgery (upper abdominal), ovarian cancer, ruptured ectopic pregnancy, diabetic ketoacidosis.

Decreased. Pancreatic destruction (pancreatitis, cystic fibrosis), liver damage (hepatitis, cirrhosis).

Amylase/Creatinine Clearance Ratio

Normal < 5%.

Order urine and serum amylase and creatinine levels. The urine can be either a "spot urine" or a 2-hour collection.

$$\text{Ratio} = \frac{\text{Urine amylase} \times \text{Serum creatinine}}{\text{Urine creatinine} \times \text{Serum amylase}} \times 100$$

Increased. A ratio > 5% is virtually diagnostic of acute pancreatitis.

Androstenedione

82–338 μg/dL.

Increased. Anovulation and hirsutism.

Anion Gap

8–12 mmol/L.

The anion gap is a calculated estimate of unmeasured anions. It is used to help differentiate the cause of metabolic acidosis.

$$\text{Anion gap} = (Na^+) - (Cl^- + HCO_3^-)$$

Increased (high). (>12 mmol/L.) Lactic acidosis, ketoacidosis (diabetic, alcoholic, starvation), uremia toxins (salicylates, methanol, ethylene glycol, paraldehyde), hyperalimentation.

Decreased (low). (< 8 mmol/L.) Seen with bromide ingestion, hypernatremia, multiple myeloma, dilutional states, hypoalbuminemia.

Anticardiolipin Antibody

Normal = negative titer.

Elevated. Spontaneous abortion, intrauterine fetal death.

Antinuclear Antibodies (ANA)

Normal = negative titer.

A useful screening test in patients with symptoms suggesting collagen vascular disease, especially if titer is ≥ 1 : 160.

Positive. Systemic lupus erythematosus (SLE), drug-induced lupus-like syndromes (procainamide, hydralazine, isoniazid, etc), scleroderma, mixed connective tissue disease (MCTD), rheumatoid arthritis, polymyositis, juvenile rheumatoid arthritis (5–20%). Low titers are also seen in disorders other than collagen vascular disease.

AST (Aspartate aminotranferase) (SGOT: Serum Glutamic-Oxaloacetic Transaminase)

8–20 U/L.

Generally parallels changes in **ALT** in liver disease.

Increased. Liver disease, acute myocardial infarction, Reye's syndrome, muscle trauma and injection, pancreatitis, intestinal injury or surgery, factitious increase (erythromycin, opiates), brain damage.
Decreased. Beriberi, severe diabetes with ketoacidosis, liver disease.

B$_{12}$ (Vitamin B$_{12}$)

140–700 pg/mL or 189–516 pmol/L.

Increased. Leukemia, polycythemia vera.

Decreased. Pernicious anemia, bacterial overgrowth, dietary deficiency (rare: normally the body has 2–3 years of stores), malabsorption, pregnancy.

TABLE 2–1. NORMAL BLOOD GAS VALUES.

Measurement	Arterial Blood	Mixed Venous Blood[a]	Venous Blood
pH	7.40	7.36	7.36
(range)	(7.36–7.44)	(7.31–7.41)	(7.31–7.41)
pO_2	80–100 mm Hg	35–40 mm Hg	30–50 mm Hg
(decreases with age)			
pCO_2	35–45 mm Hg	41–51 mm Hg	40–52 mm Hg
O_2 saturation	> 95%	60–80%	60–85%
(decreases with age)			
$[HCO_3^-]$	22–26 mEq/L (mmol/L)	22–26 mEq/L (mmol/L)	22–28 mEq/L (mmol/L)
Base difference (deficit/excess)	–2 to +2	–2 to +2	–2 to +2

[a]Obtained from the right atrium, usually through a pulmonary artery catheter.
From Gomella LG (ed): Clinician's Pocket Reference, *7th ed. Norwalk, Connecticut, Appleton & Lange, 1992.*

Base Excess/Deficit

Normal blood gas values are given in Table 2–1. A decrease in base (bicarbonate) is termed **base deficit** and an increase is termed **base excess.** To determine the dose of sodium bicarbonate needed to fully correct a metabolic acidosis, use the following formula:

$$\text{meq Sodium bicarbonate} = \frac{\text{Deficit} \times \text{Patient weight (kg)}}{4}$$

Excess. Metabolic alkalosis (see Problem 31, Alkalosis, page 121), respiratory acidosis (see Problem 30, Acidosis, page 117).

Deficit. Metabolic acidosis (see Problem 30, Acidosis, page 117), respiratory alkalosis (see Problem 31, Alkalosis, page 121).

Bicarbonate (or "total CO_2")

22–29 mmol/L.

See **Carbon Dioxide.** See also Tables 2–1 and 2–2.

Increased. Metabolic alkalosis, compensation for respiratory acidosis. (See problem 30, Acidosis, page 117).

Decreased. Metabolic acidosis, compensation for respiratory alkalosis. (See problem 31, Alkalosis, page 121).

TABLE 2–2. SIMPLE ACID-BASE DISTURBANCES.

Acid-Base Disorder	Primary Abnormality	Secondary Abnormality	Expected Degree of Compensatory Response
Metabolic acidosis	$\downarrow\downarrow\downarrow[HCO_3^-]$	$\downarrow\downarrow pCO_2$	$pCO_2 = (1.5 \times [HCO_3^-]) + 8$
Metabolic alkalosis	$\uparrow\uparrow\uparrow[HCO_3^-]$	$\uparrow\uparrow pCO_2$	$\uparrow$ in $pCO_2 = \Delta HCO_3^- \times 0.6$
Acute respiratory acidosis	$\uparrow\uparrow\uparrow pCO_2$	$\uparrow[HCO_3^-]$	$\uparrow$ in $HCO_3^- = \Delta pCO_2/10$
Chronic respiratory acidosis	$\uparrow\uparrow\uparrow pCO_2$	$\uparrow\uparrow[HCO_3^-]$	$\uparrow$ in $HCO_3^- = 4 \times \Delta pCO_2/10$
Acute respiratory alkalosis	$\downarrow\downarrow\downarrow pCO_2$	$\downarrow[HCO_3^-]$	$\downarrow$ in $HCO_3^- = 2 \times \Delta pCO_2/10$
Chronic respiratory alkalosis	$\downarrow\downarrow\downarrow pCO_2$	$\downarrow\downarrow[HCO_3^-]$	$\downarrow$ in $HCO_3^- = 5 \times \Delta pCO_2/10$

From Gomella LG (ed): Clinician's Pocket Reference, *7th ed. Norwalk, Connecticut, Appleton & Lange, 1992.*

Urine Chloride < 10 meq/L (Chloride Responsive):
Diuretics, GI tract losses (NG suction, vomiting, diarrhea [villous adenoma, congenital chloride wasting diarrhea in children]), iatrogenic (inadequate chloride intake).

Urine Chloride > 10 meq/L (Chloride Resistant):
Adrenal diseases (Cushing's syndrome, hyperaldosteronism), exogenous steroid use, Bartter's syndrome, licorice ingestion.

Bilirubin

Total: < 0.2–1.0 mg/dL or 3.4–17.1 μmol/L; direct: < 0.2 mg/dL or < 3.4 μmol/L; indirect: < 0.8 mg/dL or 13.7 μmol/L.

Increased Total. Hepatic damage (hepatitis, toxins, cirrhosis), biliary obstruction (stone or tumor), hemolysis, fasting.

Increased Direct (Conjugated). Biliary obstruction (gallstone, tumor, stricture), drug-induced cholestasis, Dubin-Johnson and Rotor's syndromes.

Increased Indirect (Unconjugated). So-called hemolytic jaundice caused by any type of hemolytic anemia (transfusion reaction, sickle cell, etc), Gilbert's disease, physiologic jaundice of the newborn, Crigler-Najjar syndrome.

Bleeding Time

Duke, Ivy < 6 min; template < 10 min.

Increased. Thrombocytopenia, thrombocytopenic purpura, von Willebrand's disease, defective platelet function (aspirin, nonsteroidal anti-inflammatory drugs, uremia).

Blood Gas, Arterial

See Tables 2–1 and 2–2.

See individual components for differential diagnosis. For acid-base disorders, see the section below and Problems 30 and 31 (pages 117 and 121).

Blood Gas, Capillary

When interpreting a capillary blood gas, apply the following rules to the diagnosis of **Blood Gases, Arterial:**

pH: Same as arterial or slightly lower (normal = 7.35–7.40).
pCO_2: Same as arterial or slightly higher (normal = 40–45).
pO_2: Lower than arterial (normal = 45–60).
O_2 saturation: > 70% is acceptable. Saturation is probably more useful than pO_2 when interpreting capillary blood gas values.

Blood Gas, Venous

See Table 2–1. There is little difference between arterial and venous pH and bicarbonate (except with congestive heart failure and shock); therefore, the venous blood gas may occasionally be used to assess acid-base status, but venous oxygen levels are significantly less than arterial levels.

Blood Urea Nitrogen (BUN)

7–18 mg/dL or 1.2–3.0 mmol urea/L.

Increased. Renal failure, prerenal azotemia (decreased renal perfusion secondary to congestive heart failure, shock, volume depletion), postrenal obstruction, GI bleeding, hypercatabolic states, stress, drugs (especially aminoglycosides).

Decreased. Starvation, liver failure (hepatitis, drugs), pregnancy, infancy, nephrotic syndrome, overhydration

C-Peptide

Fasting: ≤ 4.0 ng/mL or ≤ 4.0 µg/L; 60 years: 1.4–5.5 ng/mL or 1.4–5.5 µg/L.

Decreased. Diabetes (insulin-dependent diabetes mellitus), factitious insulin administration, hypoglycemia.

CA-125

≤ 35 units/mL.

Increased. Ovarian, endometrial, and colon carcinoma, endometriosis, inflammatory bowel disease, pelvic inflammatory disease, pregnancy, hepatitis, breast lesions, benign abdominal masses.

Note: Many gynecologists utilize CA-125, ultrasound, and physical examination as a screening tool for ovarian carcinoma. Their sensitivity in detecting ovarian carcinoma is low.

Calcitonin

< 100 pg/mL or < 100 ng/L.

Increased. Medullary carcinoma of the thyroid, newborns, pregnancy, chronic renal insufficiency, Zollinger-Ellison syndrome, pernicious anemia.

Calcium, Serum

8.4–10.2 mg/dL (4.2–5.1 meq/L) or 2.5–2.55 mmol/L; ionized: 4.5–4.9 mg/dL (2.2–2.5 meq/L) or 1.1–1.2 mmol/L.

When interpreting a total calcium value, the total protein and albumin must be known. If these are not within normal limits, a corrected calcium can be roughly calculated by the following formula. Values for ionized calcium need no special corrections.

$$\text{Corrected total Ca} = 0.8 \,(\text{Normal albumin} - \text{Measured albumin}) + \text{Reported Ca}$$

Increased. Primary hyperthyroidism, parathyroid hormone (PTH) secreting tumors, vitamin D excess, metastatic bone tumors, osteoporosis, immobilization, milk-alkali syndrome, Paget's disease, idiopathic hypercalcemia of infants, infantile hypophosphatasia, thiazide drugs, chronic renal failure, sarcoidosis, multiple myeloma.

Decreased. Hypoparathyroidism (surgical, idiopathic), pseudohypoparathyroidism, insufficient vitamin D, calcium and phosphorus ingestion (pregnancy, osteomalacia, rickets), hypomagnesemia, renal tubular acidosis, hypoalbuminemia (cachexia, nephrotic syndrome, cystic fibrosis), chronic renal failure (phosphate retention), acute pancreatitis, factitious decrease because of low protein and albumin.

Calcium, Urine

Calcium-free diet; < 540 mg or 0.13–1.00 mmol per 24-hour urine; average-calcium diet: 100–300 mg per 24-hour urine.

Increased. Hyperparathyroidism, hyperthyroidism, hypervitaminosis D, distal renal tubular acidosis (type I), sarcoidosis, immobilization, osteolytic lesions (bony metastasis, multiple myeloma), Paget's disease, glucocorticoid excess (either endogenous or exogenous), furosemide.

Decreased. Thiazide diuretics, hypothyroidism, renal failure, steatorrhea, rickets, osteomalacia.

Carbon Dioxide ("Total CO_2" or Bicarbonate)

23–29 mmol/L.

See **Carbon Dioxide, Arterial,** for pCO_2 values.

Increased. Metabolic alkalosis, respiratory acidosis, emphysema, severe vomiting, primary aldosteronism, volume contraction, Bartter's syndrome.

Decreased. Metabolic acidosis, respiratory alkalosis, starvation, diabetic ketoacidosis, lactic acidosis, alcoholic ketoacidosis, toxins (methanol, ethylene glycol, paraldehyde), severe diarrhea, renal failure, drugs (salicylates, acetazolamide), dehydration, adrenal insufficiency.

Carbon Dioxide, Arterial (pCO_2)

35–45 mm Hg.
See Tables 2–1 and 2–2, pages 297 and 298.

Increased. Respiratory acidosis, compensatory increase in metabolic alkalosis (see Problem 30, page 117).

Decreased. Respiratory alkalosis, compensatory increase in metabolic acidosis (see Problem 31, page 121).

Carboxyhemoglobin

Nonsmoker < 2%; smoker < 6%; toxic > 15%.

Increased. Smokers, smoke inhalation, automobile exhaust inhalation, inadequate ventilation with faulty heating units.

Carcinoembryonic Antigen (CEA)

Nonsmoker < 3.0 ng/mL or < 3.0 μg/L; smoker < 5.0 ng/mL or < 5.0 μg/L.

Used predominantly in monitoring patients for recurrence of carcinoma, especially status post resection for ovarian or colon carcinoma.

Increased. Carcinoma (ovarian, colon, pancreas, lung, stomach, cirrhosis, chronic pulmonary disease, inflammatory bowel disease), smokers, nonneoplastic liver disease, Crohn's disease, ulcerative colitis.

Catecholamines, Fractionated

Values are variable and depend on the lab and method of assay used. Normal levels below are based on high-performance liquid chromatography (HPLC) technique.

	Plasma (supine)	Urine
Norepinephrine	70–750 pg/mL	14–80 µg/24h
	414–4435 pmol/L	82.7–473 nmol/d
Epinephrine	0–100 pg/mL	0.5–20 µg/24h
	0–546 pmol/L	2.73–109 nmol/d
Dopamine	< 30 pg/mL	65–400 µg/24h
	< 196 pmol/L	424–2612 nmol/d

Increased. Pheochromocytoma, neural crest tumors (neuroblastoma). With extra-adrenal pheochromocytoma, norepinephrine may be markedly elevated compared with epinephrine.

Cathecholamines, Urinary, Unconjugated

> 15 years old: < 100 µg/24h.

Measures free (unconjugated) epinephrine, norepinephrine, and dopamine.

Increased. Pheochromocytoma, neural crest tumors (neuroblastoma).

CBC (Complete Blood Count, Hemogram)

Normal values are given in Table 2–3. For differential diagnosis, see specific tests.

TABLE 2–3. NORMAL COMPLETE BLOOD COUNT FOR SELECTED AGE RANGES.

Determination	Adult Female	24 h–1 wk	First Day
WBC count (cells/mm²)	4500–11,000	5000–21,000	9400–34,000
[SI: 10⁹/L]	[4.5–11.0]		
RBC count (10⁶/µL)	4.15–4.87	5.1	5.1 ± 1.0
[SI: 10¹²/L]	[4.15–5.49]		
Hemoglobin (g/dL)	12.2–14.7	18.3 ± 4.0	19.5 ± 5.0
[SI: g/L]	[122–147]		
Hematocrit (%)	37.9–43.9	52.5	54.0 ± 10.0
MCH (pg)	27–31	36	38
[SI: pg]			
MCHC (g/dL)	33–37	35	36
[SI: g/L]ᵃ			
MCV (µm²)	76–100	103	106
[SI: fL]			
RDW	11.5–14.5		

ᵃTo convert from standard reference value to SI units, multiply by 10.
WBC = white blood cells; RBC = red blood cells; MCH = mean corpuscular hemogloblin; MCHC = mean corpuscular hemogloblin concentration; MCV = mean corpuscular volume; RDW = red cell distribution width.
From Gomella LG (ed): Clinician's Pocket Reference, 7th ed. Norwalk, Connecticut, Appleton & Lange, 1992.

Chloride, Serum

98–106 mEq/L.

Increased. Diarrhea, renal tubular acidosis, mineralocorticoid deficiency, hyperalimentation, medications (acetazolamide, ammonium chloride).

Decreased. Vomiting, diabetes mellitus with ketoacidosis, mineralocorticoid excess, renal disease with sodium loss.

Chloride, Urine

110–250 mmol per 24-hour urine.

See **Urinary Electrolytes.**

Cholesterol (Total)

140–200 mg/dL or 3.63–6.22 mmol/L; desired level: < 200 mg/dL or 5.18 mmol/L. Blood lipid values are given in Table 2–4.

Increased. Primary hypercholesterolemia (types IIa, IIb, III), elevated triglycerides (types I, IV, V), biliary obstruction, nephrosis, hypothyroidism, pancreatic disease (diabetes), pregnancy, hyperlipoproteinemia.

Decreased. Liver disease (hepatitis, etc), hyperthyroidism, malnutrition (cancer, starvation), chronic anemias, steroid therapy, lipoproteinemias.

High-Density Lipoprotein (HDL) Cholesterol
Fasting 30–80 mg/dL or 0.78–2.07 mmol/L.

HDL has the best correlation with the development of coronary artery disease.

Increased. Estrogen, exercise, ethanol.

Low-Density Lipoprotein (LDL) Cholesterol
Desired < 130–160 mg/dL or 3.36–4.14 mmol/L.

Increased. Excess dietary saturated fats, myocardial infarction, hyper-

TABLE 2–4. NORMAL TOTAL CHOLESTEROL LEVELS BY AGE.

Age	Standard Units	SI Units
< 29	< 200 mg/dL	< 5.20 mmol/L
30–39	< 225mg/dL	< 5.85 mmol/L
40–49	< 245mg/dL	< 6.35 mmol/L

From Gomella LG (ed): Clinician's Pocket Reference, *7th ed. Norwalk, Connecticut, Appleton & Lange, 1992.*

lipoproteinemia, biliary cirrhosis, endocrine disease (diabetes, hypothyroidism).

Decreased. Malabsorption, severe liver disease, abetalipoproteinemia.

Triglycerides
See **Triglycerides.**

Cold Agglutinins

< 1.32.

Increased. *Mycoplasma* pneumonia, viral infections (especially mononucleosis, measles, mumps), cirrhosis, some parasitic infections.

Complement C3

80–155 mg/dL or 800–1550 ng/L; > 60 years: 80–170 mg/dL or 80–1700 ng/L. Normal values may vary greatly depending on the assay used.

Increased. Rheumatoid arthritis, rheumatic fever, various neoplasms (GI, others).

Decreased. Systemic lupus erythematosus, glomerulonephritis (poststreptococcal and membranoproliferative), sepsis, subacute bacterial endocarditis (SBE), chronic active hepatitis, severe hepatic failure.

Variable. Rheumatoid arthritis.

Complement C4

20–50 mg/dL or 200–500 ng/L.

Increased. Rheumatoid arthritis (juvenile), neoplasm (GI, lung, others).

Decreased. Systemic lupus erythematosus, chronic active hepatitis, cirrhosis, glomerulonephritis, hereditary angioedema.

Complement CH50 (Total)

33–61 mg/mL or 330–610 ng/L.
Tests for complement deficiency in the classic pathway.

Increased. Acute phase reactants (tissue injury, infections, etc).

Decreased. Hereditary complement deficiencies, any cause of deficiency of individual complement components.

Coombs' Test, Direct

Normal = negative.
Uses the patient's erythrocytes; tests for the presence of antibody or complement in the patient's red blood cells.

Positive. Autoimmune hemolytic anemia (leukemia, lymphoma, collagen vascular diseases, systemic lupus erythematosus), hemolytic transfusion reaction, some drug sensitizations (methyldopa, levodopa, cephalothin), hemolytic disease of the newborn (erythroblastosis fetalis).

Coombs' Test, Indirect

Normal = negative.

Uses serum that contains antibody, usually from the patient. Useful for red cell typing.

Positive. Isoimmunization from previous transfusion, incompatible blood due to improper cross-matching.

Cortisol

Serum, 8 AM: 5.0–23.0 µg/dL or 138–635 nmol/L; serum, 4 PM: 3.0–15.0 µg/dL or 83–414 nmol/L; urine (24-hour): 10–100 µg/d or 27.6–276 nmol/d. Diurnal variation should be present.

Increased. Adrenal adenoma, adrenal carcinoma, Cushing's disease, nonpituitary ACTH-producing tumor, steroid therapy, oral contraceptives.

Decreased. Primary adrenal insufficiency (Addison's disease, congenital adrenal hyperplasia), Waterhouse-Friderichsen syndrome, adrenocorticotropic hormone (ACTH) deficiency.

Counterimmunoelectrophoresis (CIEP, CIE)

Normal = negative.

An immunologic technique that allows rapid identification of infecting organisms from serum, urine, CSF, and other body fluids. Organisms identified include *Neisseria meningitidis, Streptococcus pneumoniae, Haemophilus influenzae,* and group B streptococcus.

Creatine Phosphokinase (CPK)

25–145 mU/mL or 25–145 U/L.

Increased. Cardiac muscle damage (acute myocardial infarction, myocarditis, defibrillation), skeletal muscle damage (intramuscular injection, hypothyroidism, rhabdomyolysis, polymyositis, muscular dystrophy), brain infarction.

CPK Isoenzymes MM, MB, BB:
MB (normal < 6%) increased in acute myocardial infarction (begins in 4–8 hours, peaks at 24 hours), muscular dystrophy, and cardiac surgery; BB not frequently seen or useful.

Creatinine Clearance

85–125 mL/min or 0.819–1.204 mL/s/m^2.

A concurrent serum creatinine and 24-hour urine creatinine are needed. A shorter time interval can be used and corrected for in the formula. A quick formula is also found on page 567 under **Aminoglycoside Dosing.**

$$\text{Creatinine clearance} = \frac{\text{Urine creatinine} \times \text{Total urine volume}}{\text{Plasma creatinine} \times \text{Time}}$$

where time = 1440 minutes for 24 hours. To verify if the urine sample is a complete 24-hour collection, determine if the sample contains at least 12–20 mg/kg/24h or 106–177 µmol/kg/d of creatinine for adult females. This test is not a requirement. If the patient is an adult (150 lb = body surface area of 1.73 m$_2$), adjustment of the clearance for body size is not routinely done. Adjustment for pediatric patients is a necessity. See the Appendix for the body surface conversion. To correct for body surface area, multiply the calculated creatinine clearance by 1.73 and divide by the patient's body surface area.

Increased. Pregnancy.

Decreased. A decreased creatinine clearance results in an increase in serum creatinine, usually secondary to renal insufficiency. Clearance normally decreases with age. See **Creatinine, Serum, Increased** immediately below.

Creatinine, Serum

0.6–1.1 mg/dL.

Increased. Renal failure (prerenal, renal, or postrenal obstruction), gigantism, acromegaly, ingestion of roasted meat, aminoglycosides. Falsely elevated with ketones and certain cephalosporins, depending on assay.

Decreased. Pregnancy.

Creatinine, Urine

11–20 mg/kg/24h or 97–177 µmol/kg/d.
See **Creatinine Clearance.**

Dehydroepiandrosterone (DHEA)

Increased. Anovulation, polycystic ovaries, adrenal hyperplasia, adrenal tumors.

Decreased. Menopause.

Dehydroepiandrosterone Sulfate (DHEAS)

0.5–2.5 µg/mL.

Increased. Hyperprolactinemia, adrenal hyperplasia, adrenal tumor, polycystic ovaries, lipoid ovarian tumors.

Decreased. Menopause.

Dexamethasone Suppression Test

Used in the differential diagnosis of Cushing's syndrome.

Overnight Dexamethasone Suppression Test:
In the rapid version of this test, a patient takes 1 mg PO of dexamethasone at 11 PM and a fasting 8 AM plasma cortisol is obtained. Normally the cortisol level should be < 5 µg/dL or < 138 nmol/L. A value > 5 µg/dL or 138 nmol/L suggests the diagnosis of Cushing's syndrome; however, suppression may not occur with obesity, alcoholism, or depression. In these patients, the best screening test is a 24-hour urine for free cortisol.

Low-Dose Dexamethasone Suppression Test:
After collection of baseline serum cortisol and 24-hour urine free cortisol levels, dexamethasone 0.5 mg PO is administered q6h for 8 doses. Serum cortisol and 24-hour urine for free cortisol are repeated on the second day. Failure to suppress to a serum cortisol of < 5 µg/dL (138 nmol/L) and a urine free cortisol < 30 µg/dL (82 nmol/L) confirms Cushing's syndrome.

High-Dose Dexamethasone Suppression Test:
After the low-dose test, dexamethasone 2 mg PO q6h for 8 doses is administered. A fall in urinary free cortisol to 50% of the baseline value occurs in patients with Cushing's disease, but not in patients with adrenal tumors or ectopic ACTH production.

Estradiol, Serum

Estradiol	Normal Values
Follicular phase	25–75 pg/mL
Midcycle peak	200–600 pg/mL
Luteal phase	100–300 pg/mL
Pregnancy	
1st trimester	1–15 ng/ml
2nd trimester	5–15 ng/mL
3rd trimester	10–40 ng/mL
Postmenopause	5–25 pg/mL

Estrogen Receptors

These are determined on fresh surgical specimens. The presence of the receptors is associated with longer disease-free interval and survival from breast cancer, and greater likelihood of response to endocrine therapy.

Ethanol Level

0–trace.

Increased. 100–200 mg/100 mL (legally drunk, labile behavior); 150–300 mg/100 mL (confusion); 250–400 mg/100 mL (stupor); 350–500 mg/100 mL (coma); > 450 mg/100 mL (death).

Fecal Fat

< 6 gm/24h on a fat-free diet.

Increased. Steatorrhea (pancreatic insufficiency).

Ferritin

12–150 ng/mL or 12–150 µg/L.

Increased. Hemochromatosis, hemosiderosis, sideroblastic anemia.

Decreased. Iron deficiency (earliest and most sensitive sign before red cells show any change), severe liver disease.

Fibrin Degradation Products (FDP)

< 10 µg/mL.

Increased. Any thromboembolic condition (deep venous thrombosis, myocardial infarction, pulmonary embolus), disseminated intravascular coagulation, hepatic dysfunction.

Fibrinogen

150–450 mg/dL or 150–450 g/L.

Increased. Inflammatory processes (acute phase reactant), during the second and third trimesters of pregnancy.

Decreased. Congenital fibrinogen deficiency, disseminated intravascular coagulation (sepsis, amniotic fluid embolism, abruptio placentae, cardiac surgery), burns, neoplastic and hematologic malignancies, acute severe bleeding, snake bite.

Fibrinopeptide A

0–trace.

Increased. Disseminated intravascular coagulation, Trousseau's syndrome.

Decreased. Dysfibrinogenemia.

Folic Acid (Serum Folate)

2–14 ng/mL or 4.5–31.7 nmol/L.

Increased. Folic acid administration.

Decreased. Malnutrition, malabsorption, massive cellular growth (cancer), hemolytic anemia, megaloblastic anemia, malabsorption, pregnancy.

Follicle-Stimulating Hormone (FSH)

5–20 mIU/mL midcycle peak increases 2-fold.

Increased. (Hypergonadotropic: > 40 mIU/mL.) Postmenopausal, surgical castration and ovarian failure, gonadotropin-secreting pituitary adenoma.

Decreased. (Hypogonadotropic: < 5 mIU/mL.) Prepubertal, hypothalamic and pituitary dysfunction, pregnancy.

FTA-ABS (Fluorescent Treponemal Antibody Absorbed)

Normal = nonreactive.

Positive. Syphilis (test of choice to confirm the diagnosis). May be negative in early primary syphilis and can remain positive after adequate treatment.

Fungal Serologies

Normal = negative (< 1 : 8).

This is a complement-fixation fungal antibody screen that usually detects antibodies to *Histoplasma, Blastomyces, Aspergillus,* and *Coccidioides.*

Gastrin

< 75 pg/mL.

Increased. Zollinger-Ellison syndrome, pyloric stenosis, pernicious anemia, atrophic gastritis, ulcerative colitis, renal insufficiency, steroid or calcium administration.

Glucose

Fasting: 70–105 mg/dL or 3.89–5.83 nmol/L; 2 hours postprandial: 70–120 mg/dL or 3.89–6.67 mmol/L.

Increased. (See Problem 7, Hyperglycemia in Pregnancy, page 40.) Diabetes mellitus, Cushing's syndrome, acromegaly, increased epinephrine (injection, pheochromocytoma, stress, burns, etc), acute pancreatitis, adrenocorticotropic hormone (ACTH) administration, spurious increase caused by drawing blood from a site above an IV line containing dextrose, elderly patients, pancreatic glucagonoma.

Decreased. (See Problem 9, Hypoglycemia in Pregnancy, page 48.) Pancreatic disorders (pancreatitis, islet cell tumors), extrapancreatic tumors (carcinoma of the adrenals, stomach), hepatic disease (hepatitis, cirrhosis, tumors), endocrine disorders (early diabetes, hypothyroidism, hypopituitarism), functional disorders (after gastrectomy), pediatric problems (prematurity, infant of a diabetic mother, ketotic hypoglycemia, enzyme diseases), exogenous insulin, oral hypoglycemics, malnutrition, sepsis, and occasionally pregnancy.

Glycohemoglobin (Hemoglobin A₁C)

4.6–7.1%

Increased. Diabetes mellitus (uncontrolled; reflects levels over the preceding 3–4 months).

Decreased. Chronic renal failure.

Gram Stain

Rapid Technique
Spread a thin layer of specimen onto a glass slide and allow it to dry (air or quick gentle heat). Apply gentian violet (15–20 sec); follow with iodine (15–20 sec), then alcohol (just a few seconds until the effluent is barely decolorized). Rinse with water and counterstain with Safranin (15–20 sec). Examine under an oil immersion lens: gram positives are dark blue and gram negatives are red.

Gram-Positive Cocci:
Staphylococcus, Streptococcus, Diplococcus, Micrococcus, Peptococcus (anaerobic), and *Peptostreptococcus* (anaerobic) species.

Gram-Positive Rods:
Clostridium (anaerobic), *Corynebacterium, Listeria, Bacillus,* and *Bacteroides* (anaerobic) species.

Gram-Negative Cocci:
Neisseria (Branhamella) species.

Gram-Negative Coccoid Rods:
Haemophilus, Pasteurella, Brucella, Francisella, Yersinia, and *Bordatella* species.

Gram-Negative Straight Rods:
Acinetobacter (Mima, Herellea), Aeromonas, Bacteroides (anaerobic), *Campylobacter* (comma-shaped) species, *Eikenella, Enterobacter, Escherichia, Fusobacterium* (anaerobic), *Klebsiella, Legionella, Proteus, Providencia, Pseudomonas, Salmonella, Serratia, Shigella, Vibrio, Yersinia.*

Haptoglobin

26–185 mg/mL.

Increased. Obstructive liver disease, any inflammatory process.

Decreased. Any type of hemolysis (transfusion reaction, etc), liver disease.

Hematocrit

See Table 2–3, page 302, for normal values.

Increased. Polycythemia vera, secondary polycythemia, high altitudes, vigorous exercise, smoking, hemoconcentration (burns, shock, severe dehydration).

Decreased. Microcytic anemia (iron deficiency, severe protein deficiency, defects in porphyrin synthesis); normocytic anemia (sudden massive hemorrhage, hemolytic anemias [immune, disseminated intravascular coagulation, congenital hemoglobinopathies], poor red cell production (leukemia, medications, renal disease, chronic infections and diseases, liver disease); macrocytic anemia (megaloblastic anemia [B_{12} or folate deficiency], macrocytosis).

Hemoglobin

See Table 2–3, page 302, for normal values.

Increased. Polycythemia vera, secondary polycythemia, high altitude, vigorous exercise.

Decreased. (See **Hematocrit, Decreased.**)

Hepatitis Testing

Recommended hepatitis panel tests based on the clinical setting are shown in Table 2–5 and interpretation of testing patterns in Table 2–6.

Hepatitis Tests

HBsAg:
Hepatitis B surface antigen (formerly Australia antigen, HAA). Indicates

TABLE 2–5. HEPATITIS PANEL TESTING TO GUIDE IN THE ORDERING OF HEPATITIS PROFILES FOR GIVEN CLINICAL SETTINGS.

Medical Setting	Test	Purpose
Screening tests		
Pregnancy	HBsAg	All expectant mothers should be screened during 3rd trimester
High-risk patients on admission (homo-sexuals, dialysis patients)	HBsAg	To screen for chronic or active infection
Percutaneous inoculation		
Donor	HBsAg Anti-HBc IgM Anti-Hep C	To test patient's blood (esp. dialysis and HIV patients) for infectivity with hepatitis B and C if a health care worker is exposed
Victim	HBsAg Anti-HBc Anti-Hep C	To test an exposed health care worker for immunity or chronic infection
Pre-HBV vaccine	Anti-HBc Anti-HBs	To determine if an individual is infected or has antibodies to HBV
Screening blood donors	HBsAg Anti-HBc Anti-Hep C	Used by blood banks to screen donors for hepatitis B and C
Diagnostic Tests		
Differential diagnosis of acute jaundice, hepatitis, or fulminant liver failure	HBsAg Anti-HBc IgM Anti-HAV IgM Anti-Hep C	To differentiate between HBV, HAV, and hepatitis C in an acutely jaundiced patient with hepatitis or fulminant liver failure
Chronic hepatitis	HBsAg HBeAg Anti-HBe Anti-HDV (total + IgM)	To diagnose HBV infection If positive for HBsAg, to determine infectivity If HBsAg patient worsens or is very ill, to diagnose concomitant infection with hepatitis delta virus
Monitor		
Infant follow-up	HBsAg Anti-HBc Anti-HBs	To monitor the success of vaccination and passive immunization for perinatal transmission of HBV 12–15 months after birth
Postvaccination screening	Anti-HBs	To ensure immunity has been achieved after vaccination (CDC recommends "titer" determination, but usually qualitative assay is adequate)
Sexual contact	HBsAg Anti-HBc Anti-Hep C	To monitor sexual partners of a patient with chronic HBV or hepatitis C

From Gomella LG (ed): Clinician's Pocket Reference, *7th ed. Norwalk, Connecticut, Appleton & Lange, 1992.*

TABLE 2–6. INTERPRETATION OF VIRAL HEPATITIS SEROLOGIC TESTING PATTERNS.

Anti-HAV (IgM)	HBsAg	Anti-HBc (IgM)	Anti-HBc (Total)	Anti-C (ELISA)	Interpretation
+	–	–	–	–	Acute hepatitis A
+	+	–	+	–	Acute hepatitis A in a hepatitis B carrier
–	+	–	+	–	Chronic hepatitis B[a]
–	–	+	+	–	Acute hepatitis B
–	+	+	+	–	Acute hepatitis B
–	–	–	+	–	Past hepatitis B infection
–	–	–	–	+	Hepatitis C[b]
–	–	–	–	–	Early hepatitis C or other cause (other virus, toxin, etc)

[a]Patients with chronic hepatitis B (either active hepatitis or carrier state) should have HBeAg and anti-HBe checked to determine activity of infection and relative infectivity. Anti-HBs is used to determine the response to hepatitis B vaccination.
[b]Anti-C often takes 3–6 months before being positive. Will soon be replaced by more sensitive tests, eg, polymerase chain reaction (PCR).
From Gomella LG (ed): Clinician's Pocket Reference, 7th ed. Norwalk, Connecticut, Appleton & Lange, 1992.

either chronic or acute infection with hepatitis B. Used by blood banks to screen donors.

Total Anti-HBc:
IgG and IgM antibody to hepatitis B core antigen; confirms either previous exposure to hepatitis B virus (HBV) or ongoing infection. Used by blood banks to screen donors.

Anti-HBc IgM:
IgM antibody to hepatitis B core antigen. Early and best indicator of acute infection with hepatitis B.

HBeAg:
Hepatitis Be antigen; when present, indicates high degree of infectivity. Order only when evaluating a patient with chronic HBV infection.

Anti-HBe:
Antibody to hepatitis Be antigen; presence is associated with resolution of active inflammation, but often signifies that virus is integrated into host DNA, especially if the host remains HBsAg positive.

Anti-HBs:
Antibody to hepatitis B surface antigen; when present, typically indicates immunity associated with clinical recovery from HBV infection or previous immunization with hepatitis B vaccine. Order only to assess effectiveness of vaccine and request titer levels.

Anti-HAV:
Total antibody to hepatitis A virus; confirms previous exposure to hepatitis A virus.

Anti-HAV IgM:
IgM antibody to hepatitis A virus; indicative of recent infection with hepatitis A virus.

Anti-HDV:
Total antibody to delta hepatitis; confirms previous exposure. Order only in patients with known acute or chronic HBV infection.

Anti-HDV IgM:
IgM antibody to delta hepatitis; indicates recent infection. Order only in patients with known acute or chronic HBV infection.

Anti-HCV:
Antibody against hepatitis C (formerly known as non-A, non-B hepatitis), the major cause of posttransfusion hepatitis. Used by blood banks to screen donors. Many false positives.

HIV Antibody (HTLV-III Antibody)

Normal = negative.

Used to diagnose AIDS and to screen blood for transfusion. Detects HIV antibody by an ELISA method, and positive tests are confirmed by Western blot.

Positive. AIDS, AIDS-related complex.

5-HIAA (5-Hydroxyindoleacetic Acid)

2–8 mg or 10.4–41.6 µmol/per 24-hour urine collection.
    5-HIAA is a serotonin metabolite.

Increased. Carcinoid tumors, certain foods (banana, pineapple, tomato).

Human Chorionic Gonadotropin (HCG Beta Subunit)

Normal: < 3.0 mIU/mL; 10 days postconception: > 3 mIU/mL; 30 days: 100–5000 mIU/mL; 10 weeks: 50, 000–140, 000 mIU/mL; > 16 weeks: 10, 000–50, 000 mIU/mL; thereafter, levels slowly decline (Figure 2–1).

Increased. Pregnancy, trophoblastic disease (hydatidiform mole, choriocarcinoma [levels usually > 100, 000 mIU/mL]), ovarian tumors.

17-Hydroxycorticosteroids, Urine (17-OHCS)

2.0–9.0 mg/24h urine.

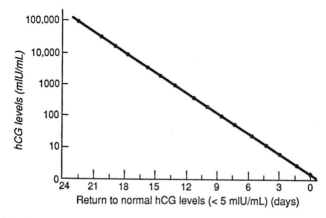

Figure 2–1. Regression of hCG. (*From Pernoll ML, Benson RC [eds]:* Current Obstetric and Gynecologic Diagnosis and Treatment, *6th ed. Norwalk, Connecticut, Appleton & Lange, 1987.*)

Increased. Administration of steroids or adrenocorticotropic hormone (ACTH), Cushing's syndrome, stress, hyperthyroidism, 11-hydroxylase deficiency, obesity, pregnancy.

Decreased. Addison's disease, decreased ACTH production (panhypopituitarism), estrogens, oral contraceptives.

17-Hydroxyprogesterone (17-OHP)

Follicular phase 15–70 ng/dL; luteal phase 35–290 ng/dL.

Increased. Congenital adrenal hyperplasia (> 8 ng/mL). If < 3 ng/mL increased ACTH stimulation test, consider 11β-hydroxylase or 21-hydroxylase deficiency.

Iron

50–170 µg/dL or 8.95–30.43 µmol/L.

Increased. Hemochromatosis, hemosiderosis caused by excessive iron intake, excess destruction or decreased production of erythrocytes, liver necrosis.

Decreased. Iron deficiency anemia, nephrosis (loss of iron-binding proteins), normochromic anemia of chronic diseases, infections, pregnancy.

Iron Binding Capacity, Total (TIBC)

250–450 µg/dL or 44.75–80.55 µmol/L.

The normal iron/TIBC ratio is 20–50%; < 15% is characteristic of iron deficiency anemia. An increased ratio is seen with hemochromatosis.

Increased. Acute and chronic blood loss, iron deficiency anemia, hepatitis, oral contraceptives, pregnancy.

Decreased. Anemia of infection and chronic diseases, cirrhosis, nephrosis, hemochromatosis.

17-Ketogenic Steroids (17-KGS)

3–15 mg or 10–52 µmol/per 24-hour urine.

Increased. Adrenal hyperplasia, Cushing's syndrome, 11- and 21-hydroxylase deficiency.

Decreased. Addison's disease, acute steroid withdrawal, anorexia nervosa, panhypopituitarism.

17-Ketosteroids (17-KS)

6–15 mg or 21–52 µmol per 24-hour urine.

Increased. Cushing's syndrome, 11- and 21-hydroxylase deficiency, severe stress, exogenous steroids, excess adrenocorticotropic hormone or androgens.

Decreased. Addison's disease, anorexia nervosa, panhypopituitarism.

KOH Prep

Normal = negative.

Positive. Superficial mycoses (Candida, Trichophyton, Microsporum, Epidermophyton, Keratinomyces).

Lactate Dehydrogenase (LDH)

45–100 U/L.

Increased. Acute myocardial infarction, cardiac surgery, prosthetic, hepatitis, pernicious anemia, malignant tumors, pulmonary embolus, hemolysis (anemias or factitious), renal infarction.

LDH Isoenzymes (LDH 1 to LDH 5):
Normally, the ratio LDH 1/LDH 2 is < 0.6–0.7. If the ratio approaches or exceeds 1, suspect a recent myocardial infarction. With an acute infarc-

tion, LDH begins to rise at 10–12 hours, peaks at 48–72 hours, and remains elevated for 7–10 days. LDH 5 is increased in hepatitis.

Lactic Acid (Lactate)

4.5–19.8 mg/dL or 0.5–2.2 mmol/L.

Increased. Lactic acidosis due to hypoxia, hemorrhage, circulatory collapse, sepsis, cirrhosis, exercise.

LE (Lupus Erythematosus) Preparation

Normal = "no cells seen".

Positive. Systemic lupus erythematosus (SLE), scleroderma, rheumatoid arthritis, drug-induced lupus (procainamide, others). ANA is more sensitive.

Lee-White Clotting Time

6–7 minutes.

Increased. Heparin therapy, plasma clotting factor deficiency (except Factors VII and XIII).

Leukocyte Alkaline Phosphatase Score (LAP Score)

70–140.

Increased. Leukemoid reaction, Hodgkin's disease, polycythemia vera, myeloproliferative disorders, pregnancy, liver disease, acute inflammation.

Decreased. Chronic myelogenous leukemia, pernicious anemia, paroxysmal nocturnal hemoglobinuria, nephrotic syndrome.

Lipase

Variable depending on the method; 10–150 U/L by turbidimetric method.

Increased. Acute pancreatitis, pancreatic duct obstruction (stone, stricture, tumor, drug-induced spasm), fat embolus syndrome (increase usually normal in mumps).

Luteinizing Hormone (LH)

5–20 mIU/mL midcycle peak increases 2- 3-fold.

Increased. (Hypergonadotropic: > 40 mIU/mL.) Postmenopausal, surgical or radiation castration, ovarian failure, polycystic ovaries.

Decreased. (Hypogonodotropic: < 5 mIU/mL.) Prepubertal, hypothalamic and pituitary dysfunction.

Magnesium, Serum

1.6–2.6 mg/dL or 0.80–1.20 mmol/L.

Increased. Renal failure, hypothyroidism, magnesium-containing antacids, Addison's disease, diabetic coma, severe dehydration, exogenous administration for premature labor or pregnancy-induced hypertension.

Decreased. Malabsorption, steatorrhea, alcoholism and cirrhosis, hyperthyroidism, aldosteronism, diuretics, acute pancreatitis, hypoparathyroidism or hyperparathyroidism, hyperalimentation, nasogastric suctioning, chronic dialysis, renal tubular acidosis, chemotherapeutic and other drugs (cisplatin, aminoglycosides).

Magnesium, Urine

6.0–10.0 meq/d or 3.00–5.00 mmol/d.

Increased. Hypermagnesemia, diuretics, hypercalcemia, metabolic acidosis, hypophosphatemia.

Decreased. Hypomagnesemia, hypocalcemia, hypoparathyroidism, metabolic alkalosis.

Metabolic Acidosis, Diagnosis of

See **Blood Gas, Arterial** and **Venous** and Problem 30, Acidosis, page 120.

Metabolic Alkalosis, Diagnosis of

See **Blood Gas, Arterial** and **Venous** and Problem 31, Alkalosis, page 121.

Metanephrines, Urine

Total: < 1.0 mg or 0.574 mmol per 24-hour urine; fractionated metanephrines-normetanephrines: < 0.9 mg or 0.517 mmol per 24-hour urine; fractionated metanephrines: < 0.4 mg or 0.230 mg per 24-hour urine.

Increased. Pheochromocytoma, neural crest tumors (neuroblastoma), false positives with drugs (phenobarbital, hydrocortisone, others).

Monospot

Normal = negative.

Positive. Mononucleosis.

Myoglobin, Urine

Normal = qualitative negative.

Positive. Conditions affecting skeletal muscle (crush injury, rhabdomyolysis, electrical burns, delirium tremens, surgical procedures), acute myocardial infarction.

Nitrogen Balance

+4 to +20 g/d or +275–1400 mmol/d; urinary nitrogen: 12–24 g or 850–1700 mmol per 24-hour urine.

Most often used in the assessment of patients on hyperalimentation. A positive nitrogen balance is usually the goal. Formula:

$$\frac{\text{Nitrogen}}{\text{balance}} = \frac{24 \text{ hour protein intake (g)}}{6.25} - 24 \text{ hour urine nitrogen} + 4)$$

5′-Nucleotidase

2–15 U/L.

Increased. Obstructive liver disease.

Osmolality, Serum

275–295 mOsm/kg.

A rough estimation of osmolality is [2 (sodium) + BUN/2.8 + glucose/18]. Will not be accurate if foreign substances that increase osmolality are present, such as mannitol.

Increased. Hyperglycemia, alcohol ingestion, increased sodium because of water loss (diabetes, hypercalcemia, diuresis), ethylene glycol ingestion, mannitol.

Decreased. Low serum sodium, diuretics, Addison's disease, hypothyroidism, inappropriate antidiuretic hormone (ADH), syndrome of inappropriate ADH (SIADH).

Osmolality, Urine

Spot 50–1400 mosm/kg; > 850 mosm/kg after 12 hours of fluid restriction.

Loss of the ability to concentrate urine, especially during fluid restriction, is an early indicator of impaired renal function.

Oxygen, Arterial (pO_2)

See Table 2–1, page 297, and chapter 6.

Decreased. Ventilation-perfusion (V/Q) abnormalities (chronic obstructive pulmonary disease, asthma, emphysema, atelectasis, pneumonia, pulmonary embolus, respiratory distress syndrome, pneumothorax, tuberculosis, cystic fibrosis, obstructed airway), alveolar hypoventilation (skeletal abnormalities, neuromuscular disorders, pickwickian syndrome), decreased pulmonary diffusing capacity (pneumoconiosis, pulmonary edema, pulmonary fibrosis [Bleomycin]), right-to-left shunt (congenital heart disease [tetralogy of Fallot, transposition, etc]).

Parathyroid Hormone (PTH)

Normal is based on its relationship to serum calcium, usually provided on the lab report. Also, reference values will vary depending on the laboratory and whether N-terminal, C-terminal, or midmolecule is measured. PTH midmolecule: 0.29–0.85 ng/mL or 29–85 pmol/L with calcium 8.4–10.2 mg/dL or 2.1–2.55 mmol/L.

Increased. Primary hyperparathyroidism, secondary hyperparathyroidism (hypocalcemic states such as chronic renal failure, others).

Decreased. Hypoparathyroidism and hypercalcemia not resulting from hyperparathyroidism, hypoparathyroidism.

Partial Thromboplastin Time (PTT)

27–38 seconds.

Prolonged. Heparin and any defect in the intrinsic clotting mechanism such as severe liver disease or disseminated intravascular coagulation (includes Factors I, II, V, VIII, IX, X, XI, and XII), prolonged use of a tourniquet before drawing a blood sample, hemophilia A and B, lupus coagulant, liver disease.

pH, Arterial

See Table 2–1, page 297.

Increased. Metabolic and respiratory alkalosis (see problem 31, Alkalosis, page 121).

Decreased. Metabolic and respiratory acidosis (see Problem 30, Acidosis, page 117).

Phosphorus

2.7–4.5 mg/dL or 0.87–1.45 mmol/L.

Increased. Hypoparathyroidism, pseudohypoparathroidism, excess vitamin D, secondary hypoparathyroidism, acute and chronic renal failure, acromegaly, tumor lysis (lymphoma or leukemia treated with chemotherapy), alkalosis, glucose, factitious increase (hemolysis of specimen), bone disease (healing fractures), Addison's disease, childhood.

Decreased. Hyperparathyroidism, alcoholism, diabetes, hyperalimentation, acidosis, alkalosis, gout, salicylate poisoning, IV administration of steroid, glucose, or insulin, hyperparathyroidism, hypokalemia, hypomagnesemia, diuretics, vitamin D deficiency, phosphate-binding antacids.

Placental Alkaline Phosphatase

150–400 mg/mL in the third trimester (values correlate with serum estriols and placental growth).

Unreliable in predicting complications of pregnancy because of its wide range.

Decreased. Fetal compromise and death.

Platelets

See Table 2–3, page 302.

Platelets may be normal in number but abnormal in function, as occurs in aspirin therapy; assess platelet function with a bleeding time.

Increased. Primary thrombocytosis (idiopathic myelofibrosis, agnogenic myeloid metaplasia, polycythemia vera, primary thrombocythemia, chronic myelogenous leukemia). Secondary thrombocytosis (collagen vascular diseases, chronic infection [osteomyelitis, tuberculosis], hepatic cirrhosis, sarcoidosis, hemolytic anemia, iron deficiency anemia, recovery from B$_{12}$ deficiency or iron deficiency, solid tumors, and lymphomas; after surgery, especially splenectomy; response to drugs such as epinephrine or withdrawal of myelosuppressive drugs). Sudden exercise, after trauma, bone fracture, after asphyxia, acute hemorrhage, after childbirth, carcinoma, myeloproliferative disorders.

Decreased. Idiopathic thrombocytopenic purpura, congenital disease, marrow suppressants (chemotherapy, thiazide diuretics, alcohol, estrogens, x-rays), burns, snake and insect bites, leukemias, aplastic anemias, hypersplenism, thrombotic thrombocytopenic purpura, infectious mononucleosis, viral infections, cirrhosis, massive transfusions, eclampsia and preeclampsia, more than 30 different drugs.

Potassium, Serum

3.5–5.1 mmol/L.

Increased. (See also Problem 46, Hyperkalemia, page 176.) Factitious increase (hemolysis of the specimen, thrombocytosis), renal failure, Addison's disease, acidosis, spironolactone, triamterene, dehydration, hemolysis, massive tissue damage, excess intake (oral or IV), potassium-containing medications, acidosis.

Decreased. (See also Problem 51, Hypokalemia, page 188.) Diuretics, decreased intake, vomiting, nasogastric suctioning, villous adenoma, diarrhea, Zollinger-Ellison syndrome, chronic pyelonephritis, renal tubular acidosis, metabolic alkalosis (primary aldosteronism, Cushing's syndrome).

Potassium, Urine

25–125 mmol per 24-hour urine; varies with diet.

See **Urinary Electrolytes.**

Progesterone, Serum

Progesterone	Normal Values
Follicular phase	< 1 ng/mL
Luteal phase	5–20 ng/mL
Pregnancy	
1st trimester	10–30 ng/ml
2nd trimester	50–100 ng/mL
3rd trimester	100–400 ng/mL
Postmenopause	< 1 ng/mL

Protein, Serum

6.0–7.8 g/dL or 60–78 g/L.

Increased. Multiple myeloma, Waldenström's macroglobulinemia, benign monoclonal gammopathy, lymphoma, sarcoidosis, chronic inflammatory disease.

Decreased. Any cause of decreased albumin, any cause of hypogammaglobulinemia such as common variable hypogammaglobulinemia, malnutrition, inflammatory bowel disease, Hodgkin's disease, leukemias.

Protein, Urine

< 100 mg per 24-hour urine; spot < 10 mg/dL (< 20 mg/dL if early morning collection); dipstick negative.

Increased. Nephrotic syndrome, glomerulonephritis, lupus nephritis, amyloidosis, venous congestion of kidney (renal vein thrombosis, severe congestive heart failure), multiple myeloma, preeclampsia, postural proteinuria, polycystic kidney disease, diabetic nephropathy, radiation nephritis, malignant hypertension.

False Positive: Gross hematuria, very concentrated urine, Pyridium, very alkaline urine.

Prothrombin Time (PT)

11.5–13.5 seconds.

PT evaluates the extrinsic clotting mechanism which includes Factors I, II, V, VII, and X.

Prolonged. Drugs such as warfarin sodium (Coumadin), decreased vitamin K, fat malabsorption, liver disease, prolonged use of a tourniquet before drawing a blood sample, disseminated intravascular coagulation (DIC), lupus anticoagulant (usually selectively increases the partial thromboplastin time).

Red Blood Cell Count

See Table 2–3, page 302. Also see **Hematocrit.**

Red Blood Cell Indices

See Table 2–3, page 302.

MCV (Mean Cell Volume)

Increased. Megaloblastic anemia (B_{12}, folate deficiency), macrocytic (normoblastic) anemia, reticulocytosis, Down's syndrome, chronic liver disease, alcoholism, hypothyroidism, aplastic anemia.

Decreased. Iron deficiency, sideroblastic anemia, thalassemia, some cases of lead poisoning, hereditary spherocytosis.

MCH (Mean Cellular Hemoglobin)

Increased. Macrocytosis (megaloblastic anemias, high reticulocyte counts).

Decreased. Microcytosis (iron deficiency).

MCHC (Mean Cellular Hemoglobin Concentration)

Increased. Very severe, prolonged dehydration; spherocytosis.

Decreased. Iron deficiency anemia, overhydration, thalassemia, sideroblastic anemia.

RDW (Red Cell Distribution Width)
Measure of the degree of anisocytosis.

Increased. Combination of macrocytic and microcytic anemia or recovery from iron deficiency anemia.

Red Blood Cell Morphology

Poikilocytosis:
Irregular RBC shape (sickle, burr, etc).

Anisocytosis:
Irregular RBC size (microcytes, macrocytes).

Basophilic Stippling:
Lead, heavy metal poisoning, thalassemia.

Howell-Jolly Bodies:
After splenectomy, some severe anemias.

Sickling:
Sickle cell disease and trait.

Nucleated RBCs:
Severe bone marrow stress (hemorrhage, hemolysis, etc), marrow replacement by tumor extramedullary hematopoiesis.

Target Cells (Leptocytes):
Thalassemia, hemoglobinopathies (sickle cell disease), obstructive jaundice, any hypochromic anemia, after splenectomy.

Spherocytes:
Hereditary spherocytosis, immune or microangiopathic hemolysis.

Helmet Cells (Schistocytes):
Microangiopathic hemolysis, hemolytic transfusion reaction, other hemolytic anemias.

Burr Cells (Acanthocytes):
Severe liver disease; high levels of bile, fatty acids, or toxins.

Polychromasia:
The appearance of a bluish-gray red cell on routine Wright's stain suggests reticulocytes.

Respiratory Acidosis, Diagnosis of

See **Blood Gas, Arterial** and **Venous** and Problem 30, Acidosis, page 117.

Respiratory Alkalosis, Diagnosis of

See **Blood Gas, Arterial** and **Venous** and Problem 31, Alkalosis, page 121.

Reticulocyte Count

0.5–1.5%.

If the patient's hematocrit is abnormal, a corrected reticulocyte count should be calculated as follows:

$$\text{Corrected reticulocyte count} = (\%)\ \text{Reticulocyte} \times \frac{\text{Patient's hematocrit}}{45\%}$$

Increased. Hemolysis, acute hemorrhage; therapeutic response to treatment of iron, vitamin B_{12} or folate deficiency.

Decreased. Infiltration of bone marrow by carcinoma, lymphoma, or leukemia; marrow aplasia, chronic infections such as osteomyelitis, toxins or drugs (> 100 reported), many anemias.

Retinol Binding Protein (RBP)

3–6 mg/dL.

Decreased. Malnutrition states, vitamin A deficiency, intestinal malabsorption of fats, chronic liver disease.

Rheumatoid Factor (RA Latex Test)

< 15 IU by microscan kit or < 1 : 40.

Increased. Rheumatoid arthritis, systemic lupus erythematosus, Sjögren's syndrome, scleroderma, dermatomyositis, polymyositis, syphilis, chronic inflammation, subacute bacterial endocarditis, hepatitis, sarcoidosis, interstitial pulmonary fibrosis.

Saline Prep

For (1) *Trichomonas,* (2) clue cell (bacterial vaginosis).

Schlicter Test

Bactericidal ≥ 1 : 8 dilution.

Used most frequently to ensure adequate antimicrobial levels in patients with osteomyelitis or bacterial endocarditis.

Sedimentation Rate (ESR)

Wintrobe Scale:
0–20 mm/h.

Zeta Scale:
40–54% normal, 55–59% mildly elevated, 60–64% moderately elevated, > 65% markedly elevated.

Westergren Scale:
< 50 years: 25 mm/h; > 50 years: 30 mm/h.

This is a very nonspecific test. The zeta method is not affected by anemia. The Westergren scale remains the preferred method.

Increased. Any type of infection, inflammation, rheumatic fever, endocarditis, neoplasm, acute myocardial infarction, pregnancy.

SGGT (Serum Gamma-Glutamyl Transpeptidase)

8–40 U/L.

Generally parallels changes in serum alkaline phosphatase and 5'-nucleotidase in liver disease.

Increased. Liver disease (hepatitis, cirrhosis, obstructive jaundice), pancreatitis, myocardial infarction.

SGOT (Serum Glutamic-Oxaloacetic Transaminase) or AST (Serum Aspartate Aminotransaminase)

8–20 U/L.

Generally parallels changes in SGPT (ALT) in liver disease.

Increased. Acute myocardial infarction, liver disease, Reye's syndrome, muscle trauma and injection, pancreatitis, intestinal injury or surgery, factitious increase (erythromycin, opiates), burns, cardiac catheterization, brain damage, severe pregnancy-induced hypertension.

Decreased. Beriberi, severe diabetes with ketoacidosis, liver disease.

SGPT (Serum Glutamic-Pyruvic Transaminase) or ALT (Serum Alanine Aminotransferase)

8–20 U/L.

Increased. Liver disease, liver metastasis, biliary obstruction, pancreatitis, liver congestion (SGPT [ALT] is more elevated than SGOT [AST] in viral hepatitis; SGOT [AST] is elevated more than SGPT [ALT] in alcoholic hepatitis), severe pregnancy-induced hypertension.

Sodium, Serum

136–145 mmol/L.

Increased. (See Problem 47, Hypernatremia, page 179.) Excess water loss (sweating, vomiting), diuresis (diabetes mellitus and insipidus, postobstructive diuresis, diuretic drugs), iatrogenic increase (improper fluid management).

Decreased. (See Problem 53, Hyponatremia, page 195.) Congestive heart failure, nephrosis, cirrhosis, sodium depletion (vomiting, diarrhea, diuretics), adrenocortical insufficiency, inappropriate secretion of antidiuretic hormone (with chronic obstructive pulmonary disease, tumors, etc), factitious (hyperlipidemia, hyperglycemia), hypokalemia.

Sodium, Urine

40–210 mmol per 24-hour urine.

See **Urinary Electrolytes.**

Stool for Fat

See **Fecal Fat.**

Stool for Occult Blood (Hemoccult Test)

Normal = negative.

Positive. (See Problem 34, Bright Red Blood per Rectum, page 000.) Swallowed blood, ingestion of red meat, any ulcerated lesion of the GI tract (ulcer, carcinoma, polyp), large doses of vitamin C (> 500 mg/d).

Stool for WBC

Normal = occasional WBC.

Increased. (Usually polys) *Shigella, Salmonella,* enteropathogenic *Escherichia coli,* ulcerative colitis, pseudomembranous colitis.

T_3 (Tri-iodothyronine) Radioimmunoassay

120–195 ng/dL or 1.85–3.00 nmol/L.

Increased. Hyperthyroidism, T^3 thyrotoxicosis, oral estrogen, pregnancy, exogenous T^4, any cause of increased thyroid-binding globulin.

Decreased. Hypothyroidism, euthyroid sick state, any cause of decreased thyroid-binding globulin.

T^3 RU (Resin Uptake)

24–34%.

Increased. Hyperthyroidism, medications (phenytoin [Dilantin], steroids, heparin, aspirin, others), nephrotic syndrome.

Decreased. Hypothyroidism, pregnancy, medications (estrogens, iodine, propylthiouracil, others).

T^4, Total (Thyroxine)

5.5–10.5 µg/dL or 71–135 nmol/L.

A good screening test for hyperthyroidism.

Increased. Hyperthyroidism, exogenous thyroid hormone, estrogens, pregnancy, severe illness, any cause of increased thyroid-binding globulin.

Decreased. Hypothyroidism, euthyroid sick state, any cause of decreased thyroid-binding globulin.

Testosterone, Serum

Testosterone	Normal Values
Follicular phase	20–80 ng/dL
Midcycle peak	20–80 ng/dL
Luteal phase	20–80 ng/dL
Postmenopause	10–40 ng/dL

Increased. Adrenogenital syndrome, ovarian stromal hyperthecosis, polycystic ovaries, menopause, ovarian tumors.

Thrombin Time

10–14 seconds.

Increased. Systemic heparin, disseminated intravascular coagulation, elevated fibrin degradation products, fibrinogen deficiency, congenitally abnormal fibrinogen molecules.

Thyroglobulin

0–60 ng/mL or < 60 µg/L.

Used primarily to detect recurrence in patients who undergo surgical resection for nonmedullary thyroid carcinoma.

Increased. Differentiated thyroid carcinomas (papillary, follicular), thyroid adenoma, Graves' disease, toxic goiter, nontoxic goiter, thyroiditis.

Decreased. Hypothyroidism, testosterone, steroids, phenytoin.

Thyroid-Binding Globulin (TBG)

1.5–3.4 mg/dL or 15–34 mg/L.

Increased. Hypothyroidism, pregnancy, oral contraceptives, estrogens, hepatic disease, acute porphyria, familial.

Decreased. Hyperthyroidism, thyrotoxicosis, androgens, anabolic steroids, corticosteroids, prednisone, nephrotic syndrome, severe illness, surgical stress, phenytoin, hepatic disease.

Thyroid-Stimulating Hormone (TSH)

0.7–5.3 mU/mL.

Newer sensitive assay that is an excellent screening test for hyperthyroidism as well as hypothyroidism. Distinguishes between low normal and decreased TSH.

Increased. Hypothyroidism.

Decreased. Hyperthyroidism. Less than 1% of hypothyroidism is from pituitary or hypothalamic disease that results in decreased TSH.

TORCH Battery

Normal = negative.

Test is based on serologic evidence of exposure to toxoplasmosis, rubella, cytomegalovirus, or herpes virus.

Transferrin

220–400 mg/dL or 2.20–4.00 g/L.

Increased. Acute and chronic blood loss, iron deficiency anemia, hepatitis, oral contraceptives.

Decreased. Anemia of chronic disease, cirrhosis, nephrosis, hemochromatosis. Poor nutritional status, chronic and acute inflammation.

Triglycerides

35–135 mg/dL or 0.40–1.53 mmol/L. Can vary with age.

Increased. Hyperlipoproteinemias (types I, IIb, III, IV, V), hypothyroidism, liver diseases, alcoholism, pancreatitis, acute myocardial infarction, nephrotic syndrome, familial increase.

Decreased. Malnutrition, congenital abetalipoproteinemia.

Uric Acid

3.0–6.5 mg/dL or 0.18–0.38 mmol/L.

Increased. Gout, renal failure, destruction of massive amounts of nucleoproteins (tumor lysis after chemotherapy, leukemia or lymphoma, anemia, chemotherapy), toxemia of pregnancy, drugs (especially diuretics), hypothyroidism, polycystic kidney disease, parathyroid diseases.

Decreased. Uricosuric drugs (salicylates, probenecid, allopurinol), Wilson's disease, Fanconi's syndrome, pregnancy.

Urinalysis, Routine

Appearance

Normal	Yellow, clear, straw colored
Pink/red	Blood, hemoglobin, myoglobin, food coloring, beets
Orange	Pyridium, bile pigments
Brown/black	Myoglobin, bile pigments, melanin, cascara bark, iron, Macrodantin, Flagyl, sickle cell crisis
Blue	Methylene blue, *Pseudomonas* urinary tract infection (rare), hereditary tryptophan metabolic disorders
Cloudy	Urinary tract infection (pyuria), blood, myoglobin, chyluria, mucus (normal in ileal loop specimens), phosphate salts (normal in alkaline urine), urates (normal in acidic urine), hyperoxaluria
Foamy	Proteinuria, bile salts

pH
4.6–8.0; newborn 5–7.

Acidic. High-protein diet, Mandelamine, acidosis, ketoacidosis (starvation, diabetic), chronic obstructive pulmonary disease, diarrhea, dehydration.

Basic. Urinary tract infection, renal tubular acidosis, diet (high-vegetable, milk, immediately after meals), sodium bicarbonate or Diamox therapy, vomiting, metabolic alkalosis, chronic renal failure.

Specific Gravity
1.001–1.035; newborn 1.012.

Increased. Volume depletion, congestive heart failure, adrenal insufficiency, diabetes mellitus, syndrome of inappropriate antidiuretic hormone, increased proteins (nephrosis). If markedly increased (1.040–1.050), suspect artifact or excretion of radiographic contrast medium or some other osmotic agent.

Decreased. Diabetes insipidus, pyelonephritis, glomerulonephritis, water load with normal renal function.

Bilirubin
Normal = negative dipstick.

Positive. Obstructive jaundice, hepatitis, cirrhosis, congestive heart failure with hepatic congestion, congenital hyperbilirubinemia (Dubin-Johnson syndrome).

Blood (Hemoglobin)
Normal = negative dipstick.

Positive. Stones, trauma, tumors, coagulopathy, infection, menses (contamination), polycystic kidneys, interstitial nephritis, hemolytic anemia.

Note: If the dipstick is positive for blood but no red cells are seen, there may be free hemoglobin (from trauma, transfusion reaction, or lysis of red cells), or myoglobin is present because of a crush injury, burn, or tissue ischemia.

Glucose
Normal = negative dipstick.

Positive. Diabetes mellitus, other endocrine disorders (pheochromocytoma, hyperthyroidism, Cushing's syndrome, hyperadrenalism), stress states (sepsis, burns), pancreatitis, renal tubular disease, iatrogenic causes (steroids, thiazides, birth control pills), false positive with vitamin C ingestion.

Ketones
Normal = negative dipstick.

Positive. Starvation, high-fat diet, alcoholic and diabetic ketoacidosis, vomiting, diarrhea, hyperthyroidism, pregnancy, febrile states.

Nitrite
Normal = negative dipstick.

Positive. Infection (a negative test does not rule out infection).

Protein
Normal = negative dipstick.

Positive. See **Protein, Urine.**

Leukocyte Esterase
Normal = negative dipstick.

Positive. Infection (test detects ≥ 5 WBC/HPF or lysed WBCs).

Reducing Substance
Normal = negative dipstick.

Positive. Glucose, fructose, galactose.

False Positives. Vitamin C, antibiotics.

Urobilinogen
Normal = negative dipstick.

Positive. Bile duct obstruction, suppression of gut flora with antibiotics.

Microscopy
Note: If the dipstick is negative and the gross appearance is normal, many laboratories are no longer performing microscopy on a routine basis.

RBCs
0–3/HPF.

Trauma, urinary tract infection, genitourinary tuberculosis, stones, urinary tract tumors (malignant and benign), glomerulonephritis, any cause of blood on dipstick (see above).

WBCs
0–4/HPF.

Increased. Infection anywhere in the urinary tract, strictures, genitourinary tuberculosis, renal tumors, acute glomerulonephritis, radiation damage, interstitial nephritis (analgesic abuse). (Glitter cells represent WBCs lysed in hypotonic solution.)

Epithelial Cells
Normal = occasional.

Increased. Acute tubular necrosis, necrotizing papillitis.

Parasites
Normal = none.

Positive. Trichomonas vaginalis, Schistosoma Haematobium.

Yeast
Normal = none.

Positive. Candida albicans (especially in diabetics, immunosuppressed patients, or if a vaginal infection is present).

Spermatozoa
(normal if after intercourse).

Crystals

Normal in Acid Urine. Calcium oxalate (small square crystals with a central cross), uric acid.

Normal in Alkaline Urine. Calcium carbonate, triple phosphate (resembles coffin lids).

Abnormal. Cystine, sulfonamide, leucine, tyrosine, cholesterol, or excessive amounts of the crystals noted above.

Contaminants:
Cotton threads, hair, wood fibers, amorphous substances (all usually unimportant).

Mucus:
(Small amounts are normal.) Large amounts suggest urethral disease. Ileal loop urine normally has large amounts.

Hyaline Cast:
(Normal = occasional.) Benign hypertension, nephrotic syndrome.

RBC Cast:
(Normal = none.) Acute glomerulonephritis, lupus nephritis, subacute bacterial endocarditis, Goodpasture's syndrome, vasculitis, malignant hypertension.

WBC Cast:
(Normal = none.) Pyelonephritis.

Epithelial Cast:
(Normal = occasional.) Tubular damage, nephrotoxin, viral infections.

Granular Cast:
(Normal = none.) Breakdown of cellular casts, leads to waxy casts.

Waxy Cast:
(Normal = none.) End stage of a granular cast, severe chronic renal disease, amyloidosis.

Fatty Cast:
(Normal = none.) Nephrotic syndrome, diabetes mellitus, damaged renal tubular epithelial cells.

Broad Cast:
(Normal = none.) Chronic renal disease.

Urinary Electrolytes

These "spot urines" are of limited value because of large variations in daily fluid and salt intake. Results are usually indeterminate if a diuretic has been given. Sodium is most useful in the differentiation of volume depletion, oliguria, or hyponatremia. Chloride is useful in the diagnosis and treatment of metabolic alkalosis. Urinary potassium levels are often used in the evaluation of hypokalemia.

Chloride < 10 mmol/L:
Chloride-sensitive metabolic alkalosis (GI losses, diuretic induced).

Chloride > 20 mmol/L:
Chloride-resistant metabolic alkalosis (Cushing's syndrome, hyperaldosteronism, exogenous steroids, alkali ingestion).

Potassium < 10 mmol/L:
Hypokalemia, potassium depletion, extrarenal loss.

Potassium > 10 mmol/L:
Renal potassium wasting (diuretics, brisk urinary output).

Sodium < 20 mmol/L:
Volume depletion, hyponatremic states, prerenal azotemia (congestive heart failure, shock, etc), hepatorenal syndrome, edematous states.

Sodium > 40 mmol/L:
Acute tubular necrosis, adrenal insufficiency, renal salt wasting, syndrome of inappropriate antidiuretic hormone (SIADH).

Sodium > 20–40 mmol/L:
Indeterminate.

Sodium > dietary intake:
SIADH, salt-wasting nephropathy, adrenal insufficiency.

Urinary Indices

Urinary indices used in determining the cause of oliguria are given in Table 2–7. Also see Problem 62, Oliguria/Anuria, page 232.

Urine Chloride

"Chloride Resistant":
(> 10 meq/L.) Adrenal diseases (Cushing's syndrome, hyperaldosteronism), exogenous steroid use, Bartter's syndrome, licorice ingestion.

"Chloride Responsive":
(< 10 mEq/L.) Diuretics, GI tract losses (nasogastric suction, vomiting,

TABLE 2–7. URINARY INDICES USEFUL IN THE DIFFERENTIAL DIAGNOSIS OF OLIGURIA.

Index	Prerenal	Renal (ATN)[a]
Urine osmolality	> 500	< 350
Urinary sodium	< 20	> 40
Urine/serum creatinine	> 40	< 20
Urine/serum osmolarity	> 1.2	< 1.2
Fractional excreted sodium[b]	< 1	> 1
Renal failure index (RFI)[c]	< 1	> 1

[a] Acute tubular necrosis (intrinsic renal failure).

[b] Fractional excreted sodium = $\dfrac{\text{Urine/Serum sodium}}{\text{Urine/Serum creatinine}} \times 100$

[c] Renal failure index = $\dfrac{\text{Urine sodium} \times \text{serum creatinine}}{\text{Urine creatinine}}$

Modified from Gomella LG (ed): Clinician's Pocket Reference, 7th ed. Norwalk, Connecticut, Appleton & Lange, 1992.

diarrhea [villous adenoma, congenital chloride-wasting diarrhea in children]), iatrogenic (inadequate chloride intake).

Vanillymandelic Acid (VMA), Urine

2.7 mg/dL or 10.1–35.4 µmol/d.

VMA is a urinary metabolite of both epinephrine and norepinephrine.

Increased. Pheochromocytoma, neural crest tumors (neuroblastoma, ganglioneuroma).

False positives. Methyldopa, chocolate, vanilla, others.

VDRL Test (RPR) (Venereal Disease Research Laboratory)

Normal = nonreactive.

Good for routine syphilis screening. Almost always positive in secondary syphilis but frequently becomes negative in late syphilis. Also, in some patients with HIV infection, the VDRL can be negative in primary and secondary syphilis.

Positive (Reactive). Syphilis (transient false positives occur with bacterial or viral illnesses, long-term systemic lupus erythematosus, pregnancy, and drug addiction). If reactive, confirm with FTA-ABS.

Western Blot for AIDS

Normal = negative.

The technique used as the reference procedure for confirming the presence or absence of HIV antibody, usually after a positive HIV antibody by ELISA determination. The HIV antigen is purified using gel electrophoresis, then attached to a nitrocellulose filter against which the serum suspected of antibody positivity is reacted. An enzyme-labeled anti-human immunoglobulin is reacted with the complex, followed by a chromogenic substrate to visualize the reaction.

White Blood Cell Count

See Table 2–3, page 302.

Increased. Infections (especially bacterial), leukemia, leukemoid reactions, tissue necrosis, after splenectomy, exercise, fever, pain, anesthesia, labor.

Decreased. Sepsis, overwhelming bacterial infections, certain nonbacterial infections (influenza, hepatitis, mononucleosis), aplastic anemia, pernicious anemia, hypersplenism, cachexia, chemotherapeutic agents, ionizing radiation.

White Blood Cell Differential

See Table 2–3, page 302.

Many hospitals are now performing the "3 Cell Differential Count" on automated machines. **Small cells** correlate with lymphocytes; **middle-sized cells** are monocytes, eosinophils, and basophils; and **large cells** are related to neutrophils (both segs and bands).

Basophils
0–1%.

Increased. Chronic myeloid leukemia, rarely in recovery from infection and from hypothyroidism.

Decreased. Acute rheumatic fever, lobar pneumonia, after steroid therapy, thyrotoxicosis, stress.

Eosinophils
0–3%.

Increased. Allergy, parasites, skin diseases, malignancy, drugs, asthma, Addison's disease, collagen vascular diseases. (A handy mnemonic is NAACP: *N*eoplasm, *A*llergy, *A*ddison's disease, *C*ollagen vascular diseases, *P*arasites.)

Decreased. After steroids or adrenocorticotropic hormone, after stress (infection, trauma, burns), Cushing's syndrome.

Lymphocytes
24–44%.

Increased. Measles, German measles, mumps, whooping cough, smallpox, chickenpox, influenza, hepatitis, infectious mononucleosis, acute infectious lymphocytosis in children, virtually any viral infection, acute and chronic lymphocytic leukemias.

Decreased. After stress, burns, trauma, normal finding in 22% of the population, uremia, some viral infections.

Lymphocytes, Atypical
0–3%.

> 20%. Infectious mononucleosis, cytomegalovirus (CMV) infection, infectious hepatitis, toxoplasmosis.

< 20%. Viral infections (mumps, rubeola, varicella), rickettsial infections, tuberculosis.

Lymphocytes, Total
< 900: severe nutritional deficit; 900–1400: moderate deficiency; 1400–1800: minimal deficiency.

Used to assess nutritional status. Calculated by multiplying the white cell count by the percentage of lymphocytes.

White Blood Cell Morphology

Auer Rods:
Acute myelogenous leukemias.

Dohle Bodies:
Severe infection, burns, malignancy, pregnancy.

Hypersegmentation:
Megaloblastic anemias, iron deficiency, myeloproliferative disorders, drug induced.

Toxic Granulation:
Severe illness (sepsis, burns, high temperature).

3 Procedures

Table 3–1 lists the supplies and instruments needed to perform the procedures presented in this chapter.

1. AMNIOCENTESIS

Indications:
1. Prenatal diagnosis (cytogenetic and biochemical analysis).
2. Evaluation of elevated maternal serum alpha-fetoprotein.

TABLE 3–1. INSTRUMENTS AND SUPPLIES USED IN THE COMPLETION OF PROCEDURES LISTED IN THIS CHAPTER.

MINOR PROCEDURE TRAY
Sterile gloves
Sterile towels/drapes
4 × 4 gauze sponges
Povidone-iodine (Betadine) prep solution
Syringes 5, 10, 20 mL
Needles 18-, 20-, 22-, 25-gauge
1 % lidocaine (with or without epinephrine)
Adhesive tape

INSTRUMENT TRAY
Scissors
Needle holder
Hemostat
Scalpel and blade (No. 10; No. 15 for delicate work)
Suture of choice (2–0 or 3–0 silk on cutting needle)

From Gomella LG (ed): Clinician's Pocket Reference, *7th ed. Norwalk, Connecticut, Appleton & Lange, 1992.*

3. Management of isoimmunized pregnancies (amniotic fluid bilirubin index).
4. Determination of fetal lung maturity (lecithin/sphingomyelin [L/S] ratio, phosphatidylglycerol [PG].
5. Management of preterm labor and premature rupture of the membranes (evaluation for chorioamnionitis, fetal lung maturity).
6. Evaluation of oligohydramnios in the absence of documented rupture of the membranes (indigo carmine infusion for documentation of amniotic fluid leakage, amnioinfusion for improved sonographic visualization of fetal anatomy).

Materials:
1. Ultrasound machine.
2. Ultrasound gel.
3. 22-gauge spinal needle of appropriate length to reach the amniotic fluid pocket (distance determined sonographically prior to procedure).
4. Three skin prep brushes or sponges with ring forceps.
5. Povidone-iodine or other antiseptic suitable for sterile skin prep.
6. Sterile drapes, sterile gloves.
7. Syringe(s) of size appropriate for the volume of amniotic fluid to be removed.
8. Needle cap.
9. 1% lidocaine plain with 5 mL syringe and 25-gauge needle (for local anesthesia, optional).
10. Specific transport and culture media (if indicated). Prepackaged

sterile amniocentesis trays are also available; however, many of these contain 20-gauge spinal needles, which may be associated with an increased risk of complications.

11. 1–2 mL of indigo carmine dye for twin studies.

Procedure:

1. Inform the patient of the indication for and nature of the procedure, expected discomfort, and risk of complications, and obtain written consent.

2. A preprocedure sonogram should be performed in all cases by qualified, experienced personnel. At a minimum, the operator should document fetal viability, fetal heart motion, placental location, and amniotic fluid volume, and evaluate the location and depth of amniotic fluid pockets. If indicated, a level II scan documenting fetal anatomy and estimated gestational age may be performed at this time.

3. Identify and mark an appropriate puncture site. This should be done sonographically using a linear-array transducer with the beam directed in the vertical plane (perpendicular to the floor) in order to accurately document the position and depth of the amniotic fluid pocket. Select a pocket away from the fetal head and trunk as close to the midline as possible, so as to avoid the large uterine vessels which are more lateral. If possible, avoid the placenta. If the placenta must be traversed, avoid the cord insertion site, placental lakes, and large placental surface vessels, which can be visualized sonographically. Visualize the selected fluid pocket in both the transverse and sagittal orientations, and localize the skin puncture site in both orientations using a finger or cotton-tipped swab placed between the transducer and the skin. Mark the puncture site on the maternal abdomen using a needle cap. After marking, reconfirm the site sonographically and measure the depth to the middle of the selected pocket.

4. Prep the maternal abdomen in a sterile fashion using povidone-iodine or another suitable antiseptic. Drape the abdomen using sterile drapes.

5. If desired, local anesthesia may be given using 1% lidocaine plain. Using a 25-gauge needle and 5 mL syringe, create a subcutaneous skin wheal, then inject the subcutaneous tissues down to the peritoneum but not to the level of the uterus. Myometrial contractions can be rapidly stimulated with the use of a local anesthetic.

6. Two techniques for needle placement may be utilized.

    a. **Needle placement without direct ultrasound guidance**

       (1) Using a ruler, measure out the distance required to reach the center of the selected fluid pocket on the needle shaft, starting from the tip of the needle.

       (2) Introduce the needle vertically through the abdominal wall and into the uterus to the measured depth, using a single

smooth motion. This should be done fairly rapidly to avoid "tenting" of the fetal membranes, which will yield a dry tap. A brief increase in resistance will be felt as the needle tip passes through the rectus fascia. An abrupt decrease in resistance may be felt as the amniotic fluid pocket is entered. Once the desired depth has been attained, remove the stylet. In many cases, amniotic fluid will begin to flow spontaneously from the needle hub.

(3) If fluid does not fill the needle hub spontaneously, attach a small syringe and aspirate gently. If no material can be aspirated (a "dry tap"), which may result from membrane "tenting," the needle may be withdrawn slightly and rapidly readvanced as long as undue resistance is not encountered.

(4) If the tap remains dry, or if blood is aspirated at any time, the location of the needle should be determined sonographically before proceeding, as described below. Alternatively, the needle may be removed, the fluid pocket and puncture site reassessed sonographically, and the procedure repeated.

b. Needle placement with direct ultrasound guidance: This method is superior to needle placement without sonographic guidance, and has been shown to reduce the incidence of bloody taps and multiple punctures. Biopsy guides are available for both linear-array and sector transducers. Many clinicians have had excellent results using a sector transducer for direct visualization without the need for additional equipment.

(1) The amniotic fluid pocket is identified and a puncture site selected using the linear-array transducer as described above.

(2) The abdomen is prepped and draped and anesthesia administered (if desired).

(3) The sector transducer is placed under the drapes approximately 3–5 cm lateral to the puncture site, oriented transversely and angled toward the site, as shown in Figure 3.1.

(4) Prior to needle insertion, reassess transducer positioning and access to the fluid pocket by pressing with a fingertip on the maternal abdomen at the proposed puncture site.

(5) Introduce the needle vertically into the subcutaneous tissues. Adjust the ultrasound beam so that the tip and entire shaft of the needle are seen sonographically, as shown in Figure 3–2, then advance the needle into the amniotic fluid pocket under direct sonographic visualization. With this method, small adjustments in needle orientation may be made at any time to avoid fetal parts which may have entered the selected fluid pocket, umbilical cord, or placenta.

(6) The ultrasound transducer may be held under the drapes

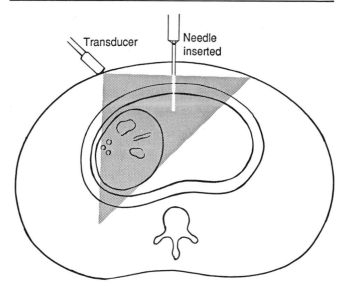

Figure 3–1. Technique for needle placement with direct ultrasound guidance.

by a sonographer or assistant, or may be draped or bagged in a sterile fashion and held by the same individual performing the amniocentesis.
  (7) If the needle tip appears to be within the amniotic fluid pocket but no amniotic fluid can be aspirated, this may be due to membrane "tenting" as described above. Withdraw the needle to the periphery of the amniotic fluid pocket and readvance rapidly.
 7. Withdraw the appropriate volume of amniotic fluid using the syringe(s). Replace the stylet prior to withdrawing the needle to prevent needle tracks from occurring.
 8. Perform a sonogram to document fetal heart motion after amniocentesis. "Streaming" of blood from the uterine puncture site may also be evaluated at this time.
 9. If the gestational age is > 24 weeks, monitor fetal heart rate and uterine activity for 30–60 minutes after the procedure to document the absence of fetal distress and/or labor.
10. If the patient is Rh negative, and the father of the baby is known to be Rh positive or his blood type is unknown, administer 300 µg of human anti-D immune globulin intramuscularly.

Complications:
 1. Rupture of the membranes (1–1.5%).

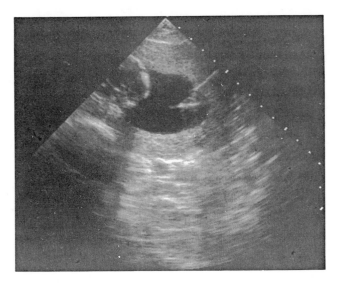

Figure 3–2. Sonogram showing needle inserted into amniotic fluid pocket under direct ultrasound guidance.

2. Fetal loss (0.5%).
3. Infection (chorioamnionitis, 0.1%).
4. Trauma to the fetus, placenta (placental or subchorionic hematoma, abruption), or umbilical cord.
5. Preterm labor.
6. Maternal or fetal hemorrhage.
7. Maternal rectus hematoma.
8. Rh sensitization.
9. Failure to obtain an adequate specimen.
10. Failure of cell growth.

Amniotic Fluid Volume and Proper Handling

The volume of amniotic fluid that should be obtained and the proper receptacle for specimen transport vary according to the indication for amniocentesis.

Prenatal Diagnosis at ≥ 15 Weeks
1. For cytogenetic analysis only, remove 20–25 mL of fluid. Discard the first 1–3 mL, which may be contaminated with maternal cells.

2. If biochemical analysis is to be performed as well, remove 30 mL, again discarding the first 1–3 mL. The specimen may be transported at room temperature in the same syringe(s) in which it was obtained, or may be transferred to another sterile container.

Prenatal Diagnosis at < 15 Weeks. Amniocentesis performed between 11 and 14 weeks is considered "early amniocentesis." The safety and efficacy of this procedure is currently under evaluation.

1. After fully counseling the patient, obtain specific written consent for early amniocentesis.
2. Remove 1 mL of amniotic fluid per week of gestation.
3. Discard the first 0.5 mL, which may be contaminated with maternal cells.
4. The specimen should be handled and transported in the same manner as amniotic fluid obtained for prenatal diagnosis at 16 weeks or greater.

Evaluation of Elevated Maternal Serum Alpha-fetoprotein. Determination of the amniotic fluid alpha-fetoprotein concentration and presence of acetylcholinesterase is indicated in some cases of elevated maternal serum alpha-fetoprotein after a complete Level II sonogram has been performed.

1. Approximately 3 mL of amniotic fluid is required for these tests.
2. Cytogenetic analysis is usually performed at the same time, in which case a total of 20–25 mL of fluid should be removed as described above under "Prenatal Diagnosis at ≥ 15 Weeks." Contamination of the amniotic fluid specimen with fetal blood will result in a falsely elevated amniotic fluid alpha-fetoprotein concentration.
3. Allow an initially blood-tinged specimen to clear prior to collecting the sample for alpha-fetoprotein.
4. Transport the specimen at room temperature in a sterile container.

Management of the Isoimmunized Pregnancy (amniotic fluid bilirubin studies, Delta OD 450)

1. Remove approximately 10 mL of amniotic fluid.
2. Place the specimen into a container in which it is shielded from light, to prevent photo-oxidation of the bilirubin which would result in underestimation of the degree of fetal hemolysis.

Fetal Lung Maturity Studies (L/S ratio, PG). Remove approximately 10 mL of amniotic fluid and transport it in a clean container. Some laboratories require that the specimen container be placed in ice until it arrives in the laboratory.

Management of Preterm Labor and Preterm Premature Rupture of the Membranes

1. Approximately 3 mL of amniotic fluid is usually required for these

cultures. The amniotic fluid should be sent for gram stain and aerobic, anaerobic, *Chlamydia, Mycoplasma,* and *Ureaplasma* cultures.

   a. Using sterile swabs, immediately place a small amount of fluid into specific transport media for *Chlamydia, Mycoplasma,* and *Ureaplasma* cultures, and into anaerobic culture media or an anaerobic culture tube prior to transport.

   b. Transport the remainder of the specimen to the laboratory in a sterile container at room temperature for gram stain and aerobic culturing.

2. Send approximately 10 mL of fluid for a fetal lung maturity profile as described above, unless the gestational age is well documented to be severely preterm.

Management of Multiple Gestations. For prenatal diagnosis in a multiple gestation in which the fetuses are in separate sacs, it is of paramount importance to obtain amniotic fluid from each separate sac.

1. The sac separation(s) should be clearly identified sonographically prior to the procedure, and puncture sites carefully selected on opposite sides of the membrane(s). Visualization of the placental cord insertion sites for each fetus may be helpful in determining which fetus belongs to each sac.

2. Following successful removal of fluid from a given sac, instill 0.5 mL of indigo carmine dye into that sac. The uterus may be gently moved about in order to disperse the dye prior to tapping the next sac. Methylene blue dye has been shown to cause hemolysis in the fetus or newborn and should not be used for this purpose.

3. Clear fluid from the next sac indicates a successful puncture. If dye is identified, the previous sac has been punctured.

4. Most clinicians believe that amniocentesis of the most accessible sac in **concordant** twins is usually sufficient to obtain information regarding the risk of respiratory distress syndrome in each infant. In **discordant** twins, however, the sac of the larger fetus should be tapped.

5. In monoamniotic twins, the absence of a visible membrane or sac separation by careful high-resolution ultrasound is usually sufficient to make the diagnosis of monoamnionicity.

   a. If the diagnosis remains in doubt (eg, in the case of inadequate ultrasound due to maternal body habitus), amnionography may be helpful.

   (1) After successful needle placement, instill 5–10 mL of water-soluble iodinated radiocontrast material, such as Urografin or Hypaque, into the amniotic sac.

   (2) After allowing the patient to move about for several minutes, obtain a flat plate abdominal x-ray film to evaluate the distribution pattern of the dye.

2. AMNIOINFUSION

Indications:
This technique is useful in the evaluation of oligohydramnios in the absence of evidence diagnostic for ruptured membranes.

Materials:
1. See Procedure 1, Amniocentesis.
2. 5 mL of $D_{10}W$.
3. 1 L of lactated Ringer's solution.
4. One tampon.

Procedure:
1. A solution similar in composition to midtrimester amniotic fluid is made by adding 5 mL of D10W to 1000 mL of lactated Ringer's.
2. Add 1–2 of indigo carmine dye to this solution to allow positive identification if the fluid leaks into the vagina following amnioinfusion.
3. Place a tampon into the vagina before starting the procedure to absorb any fluid that may leak through the cervix.
4. Insert the needle under direct ultrasound guidance, as described in Procedure 1, to avoid fetal injury, since there is little room for error in the presence of oligohydramnios.
5. After successful needle placement, obtain an amniotic fluid specimen for fetal lung maturity studies, cytogenetic analysis, or both if indicated. (See Procedure 1, Amniotic Fluid Volume and Proper Handling.)
6. Using a large syringe and maintaining sterile technique, infuse a sufficient volume of solution to visualize the fetal anatomy adequately. Depending upon the gestational age and maternal body habitus, 250–750 mL of fluid may be required, and may be infused over 5–10 minutes.
7. Unless otherwise contraindicated, the patient may sit up and move about after the infusion until the presence or absence of fluid leakage has been determined.
8. Replace the tampon 4–6 hours after the infusion, and then at 6- to 12-hour intervals for 1–2 days or until blue staining of the upper portion of the tampon is seen, confirming the diagnosis of ruptured membranes.
9. The dye begins to appear in maternal urine several hours after the infusion; therefore, it is important to distinguish staining of the lower portion of the tampon with maternal urine from staining of the upper portion due to amniotic fluid leakage.

Complications:
Rupture of the membranes (1–1.5%); fetal loss (0.5%); infection (chorioamnionitis, 0.1%); trauma to the fetus, placenta (placental or sub-

chorionic hematoma, abruption), or umbilical cord; preterm labor; maternal or fetal hemorrhage; maternal rectus hematoma; Rh sensitization; failure to obtain an adequate specimen; failure of cell growth.

3. AMNIOTIC FLUID FERN TEST

Indication:
Assessment of rupture of membranes.

Materials:
1. Sterile speculum.
2. Sterile swab.
3. Glass slide and microscope.
4. Nitrazine paper (optional).

Procedure:
1. After a sterile speculum is placed in the vagina, a sample of fluid which has "pooled" in the vault is swabbed on a glass slide and allowed to air dry.
2. Amniotic fluid produces a microscopic arborization or "fern" pattern which may be visualized with 10× magnification. False positive results may occur if cervical mucus is collected; however, the ferning pattern of mucus is more coarse. This test is unaffected by meconium, vaginal pH, and blood to amniotic fluid ratios of ≤ 1 : 10. Samples heavily contaminated with blood may not fern.
3. An additional test used to detect ruptured membranes entails the use of nitrazine paper, which has a turning point of 6.0. Normal vaginal pH in the pregnant woman ranges from 4.5–6.0; the pH of amniotic fluid is 7.0–7.5. A positive nitrazine test consists of the paper changing color from yellow to blue. False positive results are more common with the nitrazine paper test since blood, meconium, semen, alkalotic urine, cervical mucus, and vaginal infections can all raise the pH.

Complication:
Bacteria may be introduced if sterile technique is not used.

4. ARTERIAL LINE PLACEMENT

Indications:
1. When continuous blood pressure readings are needed (patient on pressors, unstable pressures, etc).
2. When frequent arterial blood gases are needed. Arterial lines decrease arterial trauma and patient discomfort.

Materials:
1. Minor procedure and instrument tray.
2. Heparin flush solution (1 : 100 dilution).
3. Pressure infusion bag with heparin flush (1 : 100).

4. Connecting tubing.
5. Transducer.
6. Monitor (per ICU protocol).
7. Arterial line catheter kit **or** 20-gauge catheter-over-needle assembly with 1 ½- to 2-inch needle (Angiocath) and 0.025-inch guidewire (optional).

Procedure:

1. The most common approach is via the **radial** artery.
2. Perform the Allen test to verify the safety of radial artery catheterization.
3. Use sterile technique (gloves, gown, and mask if possible). Sterile prep (povidone-iodine) and drape the wrist with the hand in anatomic position and a roll under the dorsum of the wrist. Tape the hand to the table before draping. Have the nurse prepare the flush bag, tubing, and transducer with particular attention to removing air bubbles.
4. Use a 20-gauge intravenous catheter flushed with heparinized saline.
5. Anesthetize the puncture site with a small amount of plain lidocaine.
6. Insert the catheter at a 45-degree angle directly over the palpable radial pulse just proximal to the wrist.
7. Continue to advance the catheter until a flashback of blood is seen in the chamber.
8. Now push the entire assembly in, going through the back wall of the artery to transfix the vessel.
9. Remove the needle portion of the IV catheter, leaving just the plastic catheter in place.
10. Slowly withdraw the catheter until blood is squirting out.
11. Insert a 0.025-inch guidewire, which should advance easily.
12. Advance the catheter over the guidewire and connect the flush bag and transducer. Be **sure** to suture the catheter in place (use 3-0 silk on a cutting needle).
13. Alternatively, some physicians attempt to pass the catheter without the aid of a guidewire.
14. Dress the catheter with gauze and tape. Tape the tubing around the patient's thumb.

Technical Tips:

1. The dorsalis pedis artery can be cannulated in a similar fashion.
2. The femoral or brachial arteries are also sometimes used.
3. With some practice, a guidewire may not always be needed. Insert the catheter into the vessel and, after getting a flashback of bright red blood, advance the catheter over the needle without transfixion of the posterior wall.
4. Any amount of heparin can make the results of a prothrombin

time (PT) or activated partial thromboplastin time (APTT) inaccurate. If blood is drawn from the arterial line and unexpectedly high results are obtained, always repeat the test. Despite removal of the first 10 mL from the line, some of the flush solution can still get into the sample tube and produce unreliable results.

5. Always compare the arterial line pressure with a cuff pressure. A difference is sometimes seen normally (10–20 mm Hg) and should be incorporated when following the blood pressure.

Complications:
Infection, hemorrhage, thrombosis of the artery, emboli, pseudo-aneurysm formation.

5. ARTERIAL PUNCTURE

Indications:
1. Blood gas determinations.
2. When arterial blood is needed for chemistry determinations (eg, ammonia levels).

Materials:
1. Blood gas sampling kit or 3–5 mL syringe (glass preferred).
2. 23 to 25-gauge needle.
3. Heparin (1000 U/mL) 1 mL.
4. Alcohol or povidine-iodine swabs.
5. Cup of ice.

Procedure:
1. For blood gas determinations, a heparinized syringe must be used. Other arterial studies do not require heparin. If a blood gas kit is not available, a 3–5 mL syringe can be "heparinized" by drawing up 1 mL of 1 : 1000 heparin solution through a small-gauge needle (23 to 25-gauge) into the syringe, pulling the plunger all the way back. The heparin is then expelled, leaving only a small amount which effectively coats the syringe.
2. Arteries in order of preference are the radial, femoral, and brachial. If using the radial artery, an **Allen test** must be performed first to verify the patency of the ulnar artery: you do not want to damage the radial artery if there is no flow in the ulnar artery. To perform the Allen test, have the patient make a tight fist. Occlude both the radial and ulnar arteries at the wrist and have the patient open her hand. While maintaining pressure on the radial artery, release the ulnar artery. If the ulnar artery is patent, the hand should flush red within 6 seconds. A radial puncture can then be safely performed. If return of color is delayed or the hand remains pale, do **not** perform the puncture because inadequate collateral flow is present. Choose an alternate site.
3. If using the femoral artery, use the mnemonic **NAVEL** to aid in

locating the important structures in the groin. Palpate the femoral artery just below the inguinal ligament. From lateral to medial, the structures are *N*erve, *A*rtery, *V*ein, *E*mtpy space, *L*ymphatic.

4. Palpate the chosen artery carefully. You may wish to inject lidocaine subcutaneously for anesthesia (use a small needle such as 26- or 27-gauge), but this often turns a "one-stick procedure" into a "two-stick procedure." Palpate the artery proximally and distally with two fingers or trap the artery between two fingers placed on either side of the vessel. Hyperextension of the joint will often bring the radial and brachial arteries closer to the surface.

5. Prep the area with either a povidone-iodine solution or alcohol swab.

6. Hold the syringe like a pencil with the needle bevel up and enter the skin at a 60- to 90-degree angle. Often you can feel the arterial pulsations as you approach the artery.

7. Maintaining a slight negative pressure on the syringe, obtain blood on the downstroke or upon slow withdrawal (after both sides of the artery have been punctured). Aspirate very slowly. A good arterial sample, because of pressure in the vessel, should require only minimal back-pressure. If a glass syringe or special blood gas syringe is used, the barrel will usually fill spontaneously and it is not necessary to withdraw on the barrel.

8. If the vessel is not encountered, withdraw the needle without coming out of the skin, and redirect it to the pulsation.

9. After obtaining the sample, withdraw the needle quickly and apply **firm** pressure at the site for at least 5 minutes, or longer if the patient is receiving anticoagulants. Even if a sample was not obtained, pressure should be applied to prevent a compartment syndrome from extravasated blood.

10. If the sample is for a blood gas determination, expel any air from the syringe, mix the contents thoroughly by twirling the syringe between your fingers (if **any** blood clots in the syringe, the blood gas cannot be run on the machine!), remove and dispose of the needle, and make the syringe airtight with a cap. Place the syringe in an ice bath if more than a few minutes will elapse before the sample is processed. The inspired oxygen concentration and time of day should be noted on the lab slip.

Complications:
Bleeding, infection, hematoma.

6. BIOPHYSICAL PROFILE

Indications:
To evaluate fetal status.

Materials:
1. Ultrasound machine.

2. Fetal monitor.

Procedure:
1. Perform a non stress test.
2. Use ultrasound to evaluate fetal breathing, limb movement, fetal tone, and amniotic fluid volume (Table 3–2) and score each factor.
3. Risk of perinatal mortality is estimated by the outcome on the biophysical profile (Tables 3–3, 3–4).

Complications:
None.

7. BLOOD CULTURES

Indications:
1. Routine workup of a fever.
2. When a subclinical bacteremia, such as subacute bacterial endocarditis (SBE), is suspected.

Materials:
1. Tourniquet.
2. Povidone-iodine solution.
3. Two 10–20 mL syringes.
4. Four 4 × 4 gauze pads.
5. Six 18- to 22-gauge needles.
6. Two sets of aerobic and anaerobic culture bottles (antibiotic retrieval devices, if available).

Procedure:
1. Apply a tourniquet above the chosen vein.
2. Paint the area chosen for puncture with povidone-iodine solution (preferably a 4 × 4 gauze soaked in the solution). This should be

TABLE 3–2. SCORING OF THE BIOPHYSICAL PROFILE.

	Normal (2)	Abnormal (1)
Amniotic fluid volume	Fluid pocket of 1 cm^2 or more	Oligohydramnios
Non stress test	Reactive	Nonreactive
Breathing	At least one episode of breathing lasting at least 30 seconds	No episode of breathing
Limb movement	Three discrete movements	Two or fewer movements
Fetal tone	At least one episode of limb or trunk extension followed by return to flexion	No episode of movement

From Pernoll ML, Benson RC (eds): Current Obstetric and Gynecologic Diagnosis and Treatment, 6th ed. Norwalk, Connecticut, Appleton & Lange, 1987.

TABLE 3–3. PERINATAL MORTALITY RATES FOLLOWING VARIOUS TEST RESULTS.[a]

Test Outcome	Perinatal Mortality Rate (per 1000 deliveries)
Biophysical profile 8–10	< 10
Contraction stress test negative	< 10
Non stress test reactive	< 10
Biophysical profile 6	?
Contraction stress test reactive positive	51
Biophysical profile 4	90
Biophysical profile 2	120
Contraction stress test nonreactive positive	211
Biophysical profile 0	600

[a]Data adapted from Freeman (1982) and from Manning (1982)
From Pernoll ML, Benson RC (eds): Current Obstetric and Gynecologic Diagnosis and Treatment, 6th ed. Norwalk, Connecticut, Appleton & Lange, 1987

repeated three times with a different gauze pad. Then wipe the area around the vein with alcohol and allow the alcohol to dry.
3. Clean the tops of the culture tubes or bottles with iodine solution.
4. Use an 18- to 22-gauge needle (or smaller if needed) and a 10–20 mL syringe. Enter the skin over the prepped vein. **Be careful not to touch the needle or the prepped skin site.** Enter the vein and draw off about 10 mL of blood. Remove the tourniquet and compress the venipuncture site.
5. Discard the needle used in the puncture and replace it with a **new, sterile** 20- to 22-gauge needle. Place a few milliliters of blood in each of the culture tubes or bottles by allowing the vacuum to draw in the appropriate volume, usually specified on the collection device. Submit the samples to the lab promptly with the appropriate lab slips completed, including the antibiotics the patient is taking. Results are usually available in 12–48 hours.

TABLE 3–4. COMPARISON OF SOME TESTS OF FETAL WELL-BEING.

Test	Cost	Risk	Time	False Positive Rate	False Negative Rate
Fetal movement counting	0	0	(0)	30–60%	? (< 5%)
Non stress test	+	0	30 minutes–2 hours	Depends on duration	0.2–0.3%
Contraction stress test	+++	+	1–2 hours	25–50%	0.1%
Biophysical profile	+++	0	1–2 hours	< 30%	0.1%

From Pernoll ML, Benson RC (eds): Current Obstetric and Gynecologic Diagnosis and Treament, 6th ed. Norwalk, Connecticut, Appleton & Lange, 1987.

Complications:
Bleeding, hematoma, infection, contaminated cultures.

8. CENTRAL VENOUS CATHETERIZATION

A central venous catheter (also known as a "deep line") is a catheter introduced into the superior vena cava, inferior vena cava, or one of their main branches.

Indications:
1. Administration of fluids and medications, especially when there is no peripheral access.
2. Administration of hyperalimentation solutions or other fluids (eg, amphotericin B) that are hypertonic and damage peripheral veins.
3. Measurement of central venous pressure (CVP).
4. Insertion of a pulmonary artery catheter or transvenous pacemaker.

Materials:
1. Minor procedure tray and instrument tray or prepackaged central venous catheter insertion kit.
2. Hat, mask, gown, sterile gloves (especially for hyperalimentation lines).
3. Central venous catheter of choice (Intracath, subclavian line).
4. IV fluid and tubing.

Procedures:
The two most common approaches employed are via the internal jugular vein and subclavian vein. The safest method is a modification of the Seldinger technique which utilizes initial placement of a guidewire into the vessel.

Subclavian Vein Technique with Prepackaged Kit and Multilumen Catheter
1. Use sterile technique (povidone-iodine prep, gloves, and a sterile field) whenever possible.
2. Place the patient head down in the **Trendelenburg position** (this helps to engorge the veins and prevent air embolism) with her head turned to the opposite side. The right side is preferred for central line placement since the dome of the pleura is lower and there is a more direct path to the right atrium. It may be helpful to place a towel roll between the patient's shoulder blades along the axis of the spine. Prep a wide area (include the neck and chest to nipples) with povidone-iodine solution and drape with sterile towels.
3. Identify the area two fingerbreadths lateral and inferior to the point where the clavicle and first rib cross, and make a skin wheal

with a 25-gauge needle and lidocaine solution. Use a 22-gauge needle to anesthetize the subcutaneous tissue.

4. Attach a thin-walled 18-gauge needle/cannula or 16-gauge Jelco needle to a 10 mL syringe and introduce it into the site of the skin wheal. Keeping the needle parallel to the skin (in the horizontal plane), advance the needle just underneath the clavicle to a point halfway between the sternal notch and thyroid cartilage (Figure 3–3). The likelihood of puncturing the pleura is increased if the needle is angled posteriorly as it is advanced under the clavicle.

5. Apply constant back-pressure on the syringe while the needle is

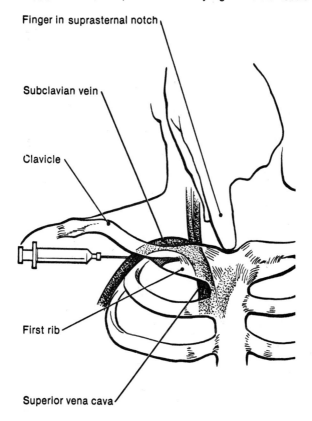

Finger in suprasternal notch

Subclavian vein

Clavicle

First rib

Superior vena cava

Figure 3–3. Technique for catheterization of the subclavian vein. (*From Gomella LG [ed]: Clinician's Pocket Reference, 7th ed. Norwalk, Connecticut, Appleton & Lange, 1992.*)

being advanced. Free return of blood indicates entry into the subclavian vein. Bright red blood that forcibly enters the syringe indicates that the subclavian artery has been entered. If this occurs, remove the needle and apply firm pressure for 10 minutes.

6. After the vein is entered, advance the cannula into the vein and remove the needle. Advance the guidewire approximately 10 cm through the cannula. Use the flexible end of the wire and do not force it. If any resistance is met, withdraw the guidewire and cannula. **Never** reinsert the needle through the cannula since this may result in shearing of the catheter tip and embolization. With the guidewire in place, remove the cannula and pass the tunnel dilator over the wire. A small nick in the skin using a No. 11 scalpel blade is often required before the dilator will pass. After the tunnel is dilated, remove the dilator and advance the central venous catheter approximately 10–12 cm into the vein. The guidewire should then be removed. If the catheter is in position, there should be good backflow of blood. If there is no backflow, the catheter may not be in the proper position or is kinked.

7. Securely suture the assembly in place with 2-0 or 3-0 silk. Apply an occlusive dressing with povidone-iodine ointment.

8. Obtain a chest film to verify placement of the catheter tip and to rule out pneumothorax. The catheter tip should lie in the superior vena cava in the vicinity of the right atrium, at about the fifth thoracic vertebra.

Subclavian Vein Technique with "Needle-Over-Cannula" (eg, Intracath)

1. Position and prepare the patient as in steps 1–3 above.
2. Attach a 10 mL syringe to the 14- or 16-gauge needle supplied with the catheter.
3. Enter the vein as in steps 4 and 5 above.
4. When venous blood is aspirated, carefully remove the syringe from the needle and advance the catheter through the needle and into the vein. It should advance easily. If resistance is met, **do not** withdraw the catheter since it can be sheared by the needle and result in a catheter embolus. **Always** remove both the needle and catheter as a unit and hold pressure over the site.
5. Lock the hub of the catheter to the needle hub and withdraw the assembly until the needle is outside the skin. Attach the needle guard securely and suture the assembly to the skin with 3-0 silk suture and a sterile dressing.
6. Obtain a chest x-ray as above.

Internal Jugular Technique (Central Approach)

1. Follow steps 1 and 2 as for the subclavian technique.
2. Locate the triangle formed by the clavicle and the two heads of the sternocleidomastoid muscle. Use a 25-gauge needle and lidocaine to raise a small skin wheal in the center of this triangle.

Change to a 22-gauge needle to anesthetize the deeper layers, and then use gentle aspiration with the same needle to initially locate the internal jugular vein.

3. Attach a thin-walled 18-gauge cannula-over-needle (supplied with most internal jugular insertion kits) or 16-gauge Intracath needle to a 10–20 mL syringe. Insert the needle through the skin wheal caudally, directed toward the ipsilateral nipple and at a 30-degree angle to the frontal plane. If the vein is not entered, withdraw the needle slightly and redirect it 5–10 degrees more laterally. Apply constant back-pressure.

4. If bright red blood forcibly fills the syringe, the carotid artery has been punctured. Remove the needle and apply firm pressure for 10 minutes.

5. Follow steps 6–8 as described for the subclavian technique.

Central Venous Catheter Removal
   1. Turn off the IV flow.
   2. Cut the retention sutures and gently withdraw the catheter.
   3. Apply pressure for at least 2–3 minutes and apply a sterile dressing.

Complications:
   1. Pneumothorax, hemothorax, hydrothorax: Listen to the chest and check a chest x-ray taken after insertion of the deep line.
   2. Arterial puncture with hematoma: Withdraw the needle and apply firm pressure. **Be very cautious in attempting an internal jugular puncture on the opposite side after entering the artery. Life-threatening tracheal and carotid compression can occur if there are bilateral carotid hematomas.**
   3. Catheter tip embolus: **Never** withdraw the catheter through the needle. It can shear off the tip.
   4. Air embolus: Make sure that the open end of a deep line is **always** covered with a finger. As little as 50–100 cc of air in a vein can be fatal. If you suspect that air embolization has occurred, place the patient's head down and turn her onto her left side to keep the air in the right atrium. Obtain a **STAT** portable chest film to see if air is present in the heart.

Interpretation:
See Tables 3–5 through 3–7 for CVP and pulmonary artery determinations and their interpretation.

9. CULDOCENTESIS

Indications:
   1. Diagnostic technique for problems of acute abdominal pain.
   2. Evaluation of a patient with signs of hypovolemia and possible intra-abdominal bleeding.
   3. Evaluation of ascites, especially in possible cases of gynecologic malignancy.

TABLE 3–5. INTERPRETATION OF CENTRAL VENOUS PRESSURE READINGS.

Reading (cm H$_2$O)	Description	Implications
< 4	Low	Fluids may be pushed
4–10	Midrange	Not clinically useful
> 10	High	Suspect congestive heart failure, cor pulmonale, or chronic obstructive pulmonary disease

From Gomella LG (ed): Clinician's Pocket Reference, *7th ed. Norwalk, Connecticut, Appleton & Lange, 1992.*

Materials:
1. Speculum.
2. Antiseptic sachas.
3. Iodine or chlorhexidine.
4. 1% lidocaine.
5. 18- to 21-gauge spinal needle.
6. Two 10 mL syringes and tenaculum.

Procedure:
1. Culdocentesis should be preceded with a careful pelvic exam to document the uterine position and rule out a pelvic mass at risk of perforation by the procedure.

TABLE 3–6. NORMAL PULMONARY ARTERY MEASUREMENTS.

Parameter	Range
Right atrial pressure	1–7 mm Hg
Right ventricular pressure	
Systolic	15–25 mm Hg
Diastolic	0–8 mm Hg
Pulmonary artery pressure	
Systolic	15–25 mm Hg
Diastolic	8–15 mm Hg
Mean	10–20 mm Hg
PCWP ("wedge pressure")	6–12 mm Hg
Cardiac output	3.5–5.5 L/min
Cardiac index	2.8–3.2 L/min/m^2
Mixed venous O$_2$ saturation	> 60%

From Gomella LG (ed): Clinician's Pocket Reference, *7th ed. Norwalk, Connecticut, Appleton & Lange, 1992.*

TABLE 3–7. DIFFERENTIAL DIAGNOSIS BASED ON PULMONARY ARTERY CATHETER READINGS.

PCWP Measurement	Implications
6–12 mm Hg	Normal
Low	Left ventricular end diastolic pressure (LVEDP) is low, and cardiac output can be increased by expanding circulating volume
High	In the absence of severe underlying cardiac disease, signifies relative pulmonary congestion due to fluid overload or congestive failure
RAP = PCWP	Biventricular compromise (cardiac tamponade, pericarditis)

From Gomella LG (ed): Clinician's Pocket Reference, 7th ed. Norwalk, Connecticut, Appleton & Lange, 1992.

2. Obtain informed consent, then prep the vagina with antiseptic such as iodine or chlorhexidine.
3. Inject 1% lidocaine submucosally in the posterior cervical fornix, then apply the tenaculum.
4. Traction is improved by applying the tenaculum to the posterior cervical lip.
5. Attach an 18- to 21-gauge spinal needle to a 10 mL syringe and fill the syringe with 1 cc of air.
6. Move the needle forward through the posterior cervical fornix, applying light pressure to the syringe until the air passes. Maintain traction on the tenaculum during advance of the spinal needle in order to maximize the surface area of the cul-de-sac for needle entry (Figure 3–4).
7. After intra-abdominal entry, ask the patient to raise herself onto her elbows to permit gravity drainage into the area of needle entry. Apply negative pressure to the syringe. Slow rotation of the needle followed by slow removal may enable a pocket of fluid to be found and aspirated.
8. If the first culdocentesis is not successful, the procedure can be repeated with a different angle of approach.
9. Although perforation of a viscus is a possibility, the complication rate has been very low. Fresh blood that clots rapidly is probably secondary to a traumatic tap, and the procedure can be repeated.
10. If blood is aspirated, spin it for hematocrit and place it into an empty glass test tube to demonstrate the presence or absence of clot.
11. If pus is aspirated, send it for gonococcus, aerobic and anaerobic, *Chlamydia, Mycoplasma,* and *Ureplasma* cultures.
12. If the patient is suspected of having a malignancy, send aspirated fluid for cytologic evaluation.

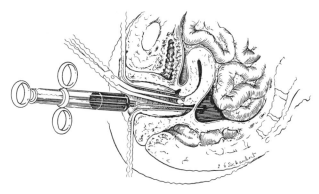

Figure 3–4. Culdocentesis. (*From Pernoll ML, Benson RC [eds]: Current Obstetric and Gynecologic Diagnosis and Treatment, 6th ed. Norwalk, Connecticut, Appleton & Lange, 1987.*)

Complications:
Infection, hemorrhage, air embolus, perforated viscus.

10. DOPPLER PRESSURES

Indications:
1. Evaluation of peripheral vascular disease.
2. Routine blood pressure measurement in infants or critically ill adults.

Materials:
1. Doppler flow monitor.
2. Conductive gel (lubricant jelly can also be used).
3. Blood pressure cuff.

Procedure:
1. Determine the blood pressure in each arm.
2. Measure the pressures in the popliteal arteries by placing a blood pressure cuff on the thigh. The pressures in the dorsalis pedis arteries (on the top of the foot) and the posterior tibial arteries (behind the medial malleolus) are determined with a blood pressure cuff on the calf.
3. Apply conductive jelly and place the Doppler probe over the artery. Inflate the blood pressure cuff until pulsatile flow is no longer heard. Deflate the cuff until flow returns. This is the systolic, or Doppler, pressure. Note that the Doppler cannot routinely deter-

mine diastolic pressure and that a palpable pulse need not be present to use the Doppler.

4. The **ankle-brachial (A/B) index** is often computed from Doppler pressure. It is equal to pressure in the ankle (usually the posterior tibial artery) divided by systolic pressure in the arm. An A/B index > 0.9 is usually normal, while an index < 0.5 is usually associated with significant peripheral vascular disease.

Complications:
None.

11. ENDOCERVICAL BIOPSY

Indications:
1. Evaluation of cervical intraepithelial neoplasia.
2. Evaluation of irregular uterine bleeding.
3. Evaluation of postmenopausal bleeding.

Note: Indications 2 and 3 usually are assessed with an endometrial biopsy.

Materials (see Figure 3–5):
1. Speculum.
2. Antiseptic sachas.
3. Iodine or chlorhexidine.
4. Tenaculum.
5. Kevorkian or Novak curet.
6. 1% lidocaine, 10 mL syringe.

Procedure:
1. Antiseptic preparation is not done because of the risk of losing a friable portion of abnormal cervix and the very low rate of curet-induced infection without preparation.
2. Move a Kevorkian forceps or Novak curet in an oscillating motion around the endocervical canal, taking care to sample the area maximally.
3. Patient discomfort can be reduced by paracervical block anesthesia with 1% lidocaine.
4. After completion, swirl the curet in buffered formalin to remove adherent endocervical fragments. Aspirate the residual blood within the endocervix with a 10 mL syringe or grasp the endocervix with a Kelly clamp and squirt blood into the container of buffered formalin. Send the formalin containing blood and tissue to the pathology lab.
5. Advise the patient that spotting can occur for 24 hours after the procedure. Intercourse is best delayed until bleeding stops. Heavy bleeding can be treated with application of silver nitrate.

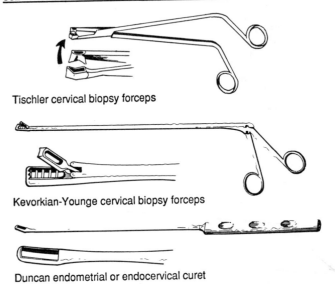

Tischler cervical biopsy forceps

Kevorkian-Younge cervical biopsy forceps

Duncan endometrial or endocervical curet

Figure 3–5. Biopsy instruments. (*From Pernoll ML, Benson RC [eds]:* Current Obstetric and Gynecologic Diagnosis and Treatment, *6th ed. Norwalk, Connecticut, Appleton & Lange, 1987.*)

Complications:
Bleeding, infection, uterine or cervical perforation with injury to the bladder or bowel.

12. ENDOMETRIAL BIOPSY

Indications:
1. Evaluation for luteal phase defects, a diagnostic technique in the evaluation of infertility or habitual abortion.
2. Evaluation of uterine bleeding in "low-risk" patients.
3. Obtaining endometrial cultures for *Chlamydia,* diagnosis of chronic endometritis of varied causes.
4. Evaluation of postmenopausal bleeding.
5. Preceding postmenopausal hormone replacement therapy.

Materials:
1. Speculum.
2. Antiseptic such as iodine or chlorhexidine.
3. Tenaculum.
4. Uterine sound.
5. Uterine curet/Pippell, Z-Sampler.

    6. 10 mL syringe and formalin.

Procedure:
    1. Careful pelvic exam should precede endometrial biopsy. In patients at risk of pregnancy, appropriate testing should precede biopsy.
    2. Obtain informed consent, then prep the vagina with antiseptic such as iodine or chlorhexidine.
    3. Application of a tenaculum to the cervix is optional but should be done if any difficulty is encountered when inserting the sampler.
    4. Several newer disposable plastic biopsy instruments are available along with the older Novak and Kevorkian samplers. The physician should refer to instructions supplied with the newer samplers. Adequacy of specimens with the newer disposable instruments has been variable.
    5. Older instruments such as the Novak or Kevorkian curet (see Figure 3–5) generally provide an adequate specimen but are uniformly more uncomfortable than the newer instruments because of their larger diameter.
    6. Once the curet passes the endocervix, advance the instrument along the natural contours of the uterus. **Never** apply undue force to the advancing curet. All quadrants of the endometrial cavity should be sampled.
    7. Insert a syringe on the free end of the Novak curet in order to apply negative pressure during biopsy.
    8. After completion, submit the specimen to the pathology lab in buffered formalin. In special circumstances, when receptor or other special studies are to be performed, the specimen can be divided and a portion fast-frozen for fresh tissue studies.
    9. Advise the patient that a small amount of spotting may occur. She should watch out for fever during the subsequent 48 hours. Intercourse should be delayed until bleeding subsides.

Complications:
Infection, bleeding, uterine perforation with injury to the bladder or bowel.

13. ENDOTRACHEAL INTUBATION

Indications:
    1. Airway management during cardiopulmonary resuscitation.
    2. Any indication for using mechanical ventilation (coma, general anesthesia, etc).

Contraindications:
    1. Massive maxillofacial trauma (relative).
    2. Fractured larynx.
    3. Suspected cervical spinal cord injury (relative).

Materials:
1. Endotracheal tube (Table 3–8).
2. Laryngoscope handle and blade (straight or curved, No. 3).
3. 10 mL syringe, adhesive tape, benzoin.
4. Suction equipment (Yankauer suction).
5. Malleable stylet (optional).
6. Oropharyngeal airway.

Procedure:
1. Orotracheal intubation is most commonly used and is described here. In the case of suspected cervical spine injury, nasotracheal intubation is preferred and orotracheal intubation should be strongly discouraged.
2. Any patient who is hypoxic or apneic must be ventilated (bag mask or mouth to mask) prior to attempting endotracheal intubation. Remember to avoid prolonged periods of no ventilation if the intubation is difficult. A rule of thumb is to hold your breath while attempting intubation. When you need to take a breath, so must the patient, and you should resume ventilation and reattempt intubation in a minute or so.
3. Extend the laryngoscope blade to 90 degrees to verify that the light is working. If there is a balloon on the tube, check it for leaks.
4. Position the patient's airway by extending the neck anteriorly while simultaneously extending the head posteriorly.
5. Hold the laryngoscope in your left hand, hold the patient's mouth open with your right hand, and use the blade to push the tongue to the patient's left while keeping it anterior to the blade. Advance the blade carefully toward the midline until the epiglottis is visualized. Use suction to clear the airway if needed.
6. If a **straight laryngoscope blade** is used, it is passed under the epiglottis and **lifted** upward to visualize the vocal cords. If a **curved blade** is used, it is placed anterior to the epiglottis (into the vallecula) and gently lifted anteriorly (Figure 3–6). In either case, **the handle should not be used to pry the epiglottis open, but rather gently lifted to expose the vocal cords.**
7. While maintaining visualization of the cords, grasp the tube in

TABLE 3–8. RECOMMENDED ENDOTRACHEAL TUBE SIZES.

Patient	Internal Diameter (mm)	
Premature infant	2.5–3.0	(uncuffed)
Newborn infant	3.5	(uncuffed)
Adult	7.0–9.0	(cuffed)

From Gomella LG (ed): Clinician's Pocket Reference, 7th ed. Norwalk, Connecticut, Appleton & Lange, 1992.

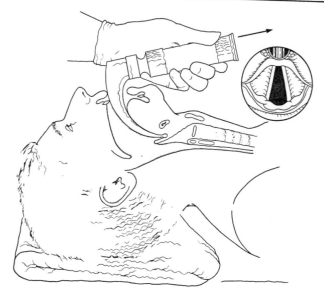

Figure 3–6. Endotracheal intubation using a curved laryngoscope blade. (*From Chesnutt M, DeWar T:* Clinical Manual of Office and Bedside Procedures, *Norwalk, Connecticut, Appleton & Lange, 1992.*)

    your right hand and pass it through the cords. With more difficult intubations, the malleable stylet can be used to direct the tube.

8. When using a cuffed tube, gently inflate air with a 10 mL syringe until there is an adequate seal (about 5 cc). Ventilate the patient while auscultating and visualizing both sides of the chest to verify positioning. If the left side does not seem to be ventilating, it may signify that the tube has been advanced down the right mainstem bronchus. Withdraw the tube 1–2 cm and recheck the breath sounds. Also auscultate over the stomach to make sure the tube is not mistakenly in the esophagus. Confirm positioning with a chest x-ray. The tip of the endotracheal tube should be a few centimeters above the carina.

9. Tape the tube in position and insert an oropharyngeal airway to prevent the patient from biting the tube.

Complications:
Bleeding, oral or pharyngeal trauma, improper tube positioning (esophageal intubation, right mainstem bronchus), aspiration, tube obstruction or kinking.

14. FEVER WORKUP

Although not a "procedure" in the true sense of the word, a fever workup involves judicious use of invasive procedures. The true definition of a "fever" can vary from service to service. General guidelines to follow are a temperature of > 101.6 °F (38.6 °C) orally on a medicine or surgery service, or ≥ 101 °F (38.3 °C) rectally or 100 °F (37.7 °C) orally in an immunocompromised patient.

When evaluating a patient for "fever," consider whether the temperature is an oral, rectal, or axillary reading (rectal temperatures are about 1 degree higher and axillary temperatures about 1 degree lower than oral); whether she has drunk any hot or cold liquids or smoked around the time of the determination; and whether she is taking any antipyretics.

General Fever Workup

1. Quickly review the chart and medication record if the patient is not familiar to you.
2. Question and examine the patient to locate any obvious sources of fever. Do all of the following before you begin to investigate the less common or less obvious causes of a fever.
   a. **Ears, nose, and throat.**
   b. **Neck:** Is there any tenderness or stiffness?
   c. **Nodes:** Any adenopathy?
   d. **Lungs:** Note the presence of rales (crackles), rhonchi (wheezes), decreased breath sounds, or dullness to percussion. Can the patient generate an effective cough?
   e. **Heart:** Determine if a heart murmur is present that may suggest subacute bacterial endocarditis (SBE).
   f. **Abdomen:** Check for the presence or absence of bowel sounds, guarding, rigidity, tenderness, bladder fullness, or costovertebral angle (CVA) tenderness.
   g. **Genitourinary:** Is there a Foley catheter in place? What does the urine look like grossly and microscopically?
   h. **Rectal examination:** Is there tenderness or fluctuance to suggest an abscess?
   i. **Pelvic examination:** This is especially important in the postpartum patient.
   j. **Wounds:** Is there any erythema, tenderness, swelling, or drainage from surgical sites?
   k. **Extremities:** Check IV sites for signs of inflammation. Look for thigh or calf tenderness and swelling.
   l. **Miscellaneous:** Consider the possibility of drug fever (the eosinophil count on the complete blood count [CBC] may be elevated) or nasogastric tube fever.
3. **Laboratory studies**

a. **Basic:** CBC with differential, urinalysis, cultures of urine, blood, sputum, wound, or spinal fluid as indicated.
b. **Other:** Studies based on your evaluation:
   (1) **Radiographic:** Such as chest or abdominal films or ultrasound exams.
   (2) **Invasive:** Lumbar puncture, thoracentesis, and paracentesis are more aggressive procedures that may be indicated.

Miscellaneous Fever Facts

1. When reviewing causes of fever in the postop patient, think of the "six Ws":
   a. **Wind:** Atelectasis secondary to intubation and anesthesia is the most common cause of a fever immediately postop. To treat, have the patient up and ambulating and getting incentive spirometry, percussion and postural drainage (P&PD), nasotracheal (NT) suctioning, etc.
   b. **Water:** Urinary tract infection; may be secondary to a bladder catheter.
   c. **Wound:** Infection.
   d. **Walking:** Phlebitis.
   e. **Wonder drugs:** Drug fever (especially with some cephalosporins).
   f. **Woman:** Endometritis or mastitis (these are common only in postpartum patients).
2. **Elevated white cell counts:** The WBC is commonly elevated secondary to catecholamine discharge after a stress such as surgery or childbirth.
3. **Temperatures of 103–105 °F (39.4–40.5 °C):** Think of lung or kidney infections or bacteremia.
4. **Lethargy, combativeness, inappropriate behavior:** Strongly consider doing a lumbar puncture to rule out meningitis.
5. **Elderly patients:** They can be extremely ill without many of the typical manifestations; they may be hypothermic or deny any tenderness. You must be very aggressive to identify the cause.

15. FOAM TEST

Indications:
To evaluate fetal lung maturity.

Materials:
1. 1 mL of amniotic fluid.
2. Two 3 mL test tubes.
3. 1 mL of normal saline.
4. 2 mL of 95% ETOH.

Procedure:
1. Fill tube A with 0.5 mL of amniotic fluid and 0.5 mL of normal saline.
2. Fill tube B with 0.25 mL of amniotic fluid and 0.75 mL of normal saline.
3. Add 1 mL of 95% ETOH to both tubes.
4. Cover the tubes and shake for 30 seconds.
5. Record the presence or absence of bubbles along the meniscus of both tubes in 15 minutes.

Complications:
None.

Interpretation:
1. A positive test is bubbles in both A and B.
2. An intermediate result is bubbles in A but not B.
3. A negative test is absence of bubbles in both tubes.

16. GASTROINTESTINAL TUBES

Indications:
1. Gastrointestinal decompression: ileus, obstruction, pancreatitis, postoperatively.
2. Lavage of the stomach with gastrointestinal bleeding or drug overdose.
3. Prevention of aspiration in an obtunded patient.
4. Feeding a patient who is unable to swallow.

Materials:
1. Gastrointestinal tube of choice (see below).
2. Lubricant jelly.
3. Catheter-tipped syringe.
4. Glass of water with a straw, stethoscope.

Types of Gastrointestinal Tubes

Nasogastric (NG) Tubes. Both the Salem sump and Levin tubes have radiopaque markings.

1. **Levin:** A tube with a single lumen, a perforated tip, and side holes for the aspiration of gastric contents. Should be connected to an intermittent suction device to prevent the stomach lining from obstructing the lumen. Sometimes it is necessary to cut off the tip to allow for the aspiration of larger pills or tablets. The size varies from 10–18 French (**1 French unit = ⅓ mm**).
2. **Salem sump:** A double-lumen tube with the smaller tube acting as an air intake vent so that continuous suction can be applied. This is the best tube for irrigation and lavage since it will not collapse upon itself. If a Salem sump tube stops working even after

it is repositioned, often a "shot" of air from a catheter-tipped syringe into the air vent will clear the tube.

Intestinal Decompression Tubes. **Do not** tape these intestinal tubes to the patient's nose or the tube will not descend. The progress of the tube can be followed on x-ray.

1. **Cantor tube:** A long single-lumen tube with a rubber balloon at the tip. The balloon is partially filled with mercury (5–7 mL using a tangentially directed 21-gauge needle, then the air is aspirated), which allows it to gravitate into the small bowel with the aid of peristalsis. Used for decompression when the bowel is obstructed distally.

2. **Miller-Abbott tube:** A long double-lumen tube with a rubber balloon at the tip. One lumen is used for aspiration; the other connects to the balloon. After the tube is in the stomach, inflate the balloon with 5–10 cc of air, inject 2–3 mL of mercury into the balloon, then aspirate the air. Functioning and indications are essentially the same as for the Cantor tube.

Feeding Tubes. Virtually any NG tube can be used as a feeding tube, but it is preferable to place a specially designed nasoduodenal "feeding tube." These are of smaller diameter (usually 8 French) and are more pliable and comfortable for the patient. Weighted tips tend to travel into the duodenum, which helps to prevent regurgitation. Most are supplied with stylets that facilitate positioning, especially if fluoroscopic guidance is needed. Always verify the position of the nasoduodenal tube with an x-ray prior to starting tube feeding. Commonly used tubes include the mercury-weighted varieties (**Keogh tube, Duo-Tube, Dobhoff**), the tungsten-weighted (**Vivonex tube**), and the unweighted pediatric feeding tubes.

Miscellaneous

1. **Sengstaken-Blakemore tube:** A triple-lumen tube used exclusively for the control of bleeding esophageal varices by tamponade. One lumen is for gastric aspiration, one is for the gastric balloon, and the third is for the esophageal balloon. Other types of tubes used to control esophageal bleeding include the **Linton** and **Minnesota** tubes.

2. **Ewald tube:** An orogastric tube used almost exclusively for gastric evacuation of blood or drug overdose. The tube is usually double lumen and larger diameter (18–36 French).

Procedure (for NG and Feeding Tubes):

1. Inform the patient of the nature of the procedure and encourage cooperation if she is able. Choose the nasal passage that appears most open. Have the patient sitting up if she is able.

2. Lubricate the distal 3–4 inches of the tube with a water-soluble jelly (K-Y Jelly or viscous lidocaine) and insert the tube gently

along the floor of the nasal passageway. Maintain gentle pressure that will allow the tube to pass into the nasopharynx.

3. When the patient can feel the tube in the back of the throat, ask her to swallow small amounts of water through a straw as you advance the tube 2–3 inches at a time.

4. To be sure the tube is in the stomach, aspirate gastric contents or blow air into the tube and listen over the stomach with your stethoscope for a "pop" or "gurgle." The position of feeding tubes **must** be verified by a chest x-ray prior to institution of feedings to prevent accidental instillation into the bronchi.

5. NG tubes are usually attached either to low wall suction (Salem sump type tubes with a vent) or to intermittent suction (Levin type tubes). The latter allows the tube to fall away from the gastric wall between suction cycles.

6. Feeding and pediatric feeding tubes in adults are more difficult to insert because they are more flexible. Many are provided with stylets that make their passage easier.

7. Tape the tube securely in place but do not allow it to apply pressure to the ala of the nose. Patients have been disfigured because of ischemic necrosis of the nose caused by a poorly positioned NG tube.

Complications:

1. Inadvertent passage into the trachea may provoke coughing or gagging.
2. If the patient is unable to cooperate, the tube often becomes coiled in the oral cavity.
3. The tube is irritating and may cause a small amount of bleeding in the mucosa of the nose, pharynx, or stomach. The drying and irritation can be lessened by throat lozenges or antiseptic spray.
4. Intracranial passage is a possibility in a patient with a basilar skull fracture.
5. Esophageal reflux may be caused by tube-induced incompetence of the distal esophageal sphincter.

17. HEELSTICK

Indication:
Frequently used to collect blood samples from infants.

Materials:

1. Alcohol swabs.
2. Lancet.
3. Capillary or caraway collection tubes.
4. Clay tube sealer.

Procedure:

1. Although the procedure is called a "heelstick," any highly vas-

cularized capillary bed can be used (finger, earlobe, or great toe). The heel can be warmed for 5–10 minutes by wrapping it in a warm washcloth.

2. Wipe the area with an alcohol swab.

3. Use a 4 mm lancet and make a quick, deep puncture so that there is free flow of blood. Wipe off the first drop, then gently squeeze the heel and touch a collection tube to the next drop of blood. The tube should fill by capillary action. Seal the end of the tube in clay.

4. Most labs can usually do laboratory determinations on small samples from the pediatric age group. A caraway tube can hold 0.3 mL of blood. One to three caraway tubes can be used for most routine tests. For a capillary blood gas, the blood is usually transferred to a 1 mL heparinized syringe and placed on ice.

5. Wrap the foot with 4 × 4 gauze squares or apply a Band-Aid.

Complications:
Bleeding, hematoma, infections.

18. INTERNAL FETAL SCALP MONITORING

Indication:
Accurate assessment of fetal heart rate (FHR) patterns during labor to screen for possible fetal distress.

Contraindications:
1. Presence of placenta previa.
2. When it is not possible to identify the portion of the fetal body where application is contemplated.

Materials:
1. Electrode (should not be applied to the fetal face, fontanels, or genitalia).
2. Sterile vaginal lubricant or povidone-iodine spray.
3. Spiral electrode.
4. Leg plate/fetal monitor.

Procedure:
1. Position the patient in the dorsal lithotomy position (knees flexed and abducted), and perform an aseptic perineal prep with sterile vaginal lubricant or povidone-iodine spray.
2. Perform a manual vaginal exam and clearly identify the fetal presenting part. The membranes **must** be ruptured prior to attachment of the spiral electrode.
3. Remove the spiral electrode from the sterile package and place the guide tube firmly against the fetal presenting part.
4. Advance the drive tube and electrode until the electrode contacts the presenting part. Maintaining pressure on the guide tube and

    drive tube, rotate the drive tube clockwise until mild resistance is
    met (usually one turn).

5. Press the arms on the drive tube grip together, which releases the
   locking device. Carefully slide the drive and guide tubes off the
   electrode wires while holding the locking device open.
6. Attach the spiral electrode wires to the color-coded leg plate and
   connect the plate to the electronic fetal monitor.

Complications:
Fetal or maternal hemorrhage, fetal infection (usually scalp abscess at
the site of insertion).

Interpretation:
Normal FHR is 120–160 beats per minute (bpm). **Accelerations** are increases in the FHR. Although they can accompany fetal distress (usually
in association with late decelerations), they are almost always a sign of
fetal well-being. **Decelerations** are transient falls in FHR related to a
uterine contraction and are of three types:

1. **Early decelerations:** This pattern is seen in normal labor. Slowing of the FHR is clearly associated with the onset of the contraction, and the FHR promptly returns to normal after the contraction
   is over. Early decelerations are usually caused by head compression, occasionally by cord compression.
2. **Late deceleration:** Slowing of the FHR occurs after the uterine
   contraction starts, and the rate does not return to normal until well
   after the contraction is over. This type of pattern is often associated with uteroplacental insufficiency (fetal acidosis or hypoxia).
3. **Variable decelerations:** This is an irregular pattern of decelerations, unassociated with contractions, caused by cord compression. If bradycardia persists, evaluate with scalp pH.

Other patterns seen include **beat-to-beat variability** (small fluctuations
in FHR, 5–15 bpm over the baseline rate, usually associated with fetal
well-being); **tachycardia** (often an early sign of fetal distress; seen with
febrile illnesses, hypoxia, and fetal thyrotoxicosis); and **bradycardia** (associated with maternal and fetal hypoxia and with fetal heart lesions,
including heart block). A **sinusoidal** pattern can be drug-induced and is
seen occasionally with severe fetal anemia.

19. INTRAUTERINE PRESSURE CATHETER PLACEMENT

Indications:
Accurate assessment of uterine contraction during labor.

Contraindication:
Presence of placenta previa.

Materials:
1. Pressure catheter and introducer.
2. Transducer connected to fetal monitor.

    3. Sterile gloves, vaginal lubricant or povidone-iodine spray.
    4. 10 mL syringe.
    5. 30 mL of sterile water.

Procedure:
    1. Prime the transducer with sterile water.
    2. Place the patient in the dorsal lithotomy position (knees flexed and abducted), and perform an aseptic perineal prep with sterile vaginal lubricant or povidine-iodine spray.
    3. Perform a manual vaginal exam and clearly identify the fetal presenting part. The membranes must be ruptured prior to insertion of the catheter.
    4. Remove the catheter from the sterile package and place the guide tube into the uterine cavity through your fingers encircling the presenting part.
    5. Prime the catheter with sterile water and thread it through the guide tube.
    6. Attach the distal catheter to the transducer and zero to air (Figure 3–7).

Complications:
Infection, placental perforation if low lying.

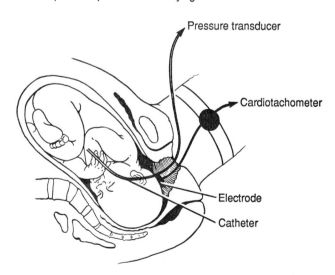

Figure 3–7. Internal fetal heart rate monitoring. (*Redrawn, with permission, from Hon EH:* Hosp Pract *[Sept] 1970;5:91.*)

20. IV TECHNIQUES

Indications:
To establish an intravenous access for administration of fluids, blood, or medications.

Materials:
1. IV fluid.
2. Connecting tubing.
3. Tourniquet.
4. Alcohol swab.
5. Intravenous cannulas (a catheter-over-needle assembly such as an Angiocath, a Jelco, or a butterfly needle).
6. Antiseptic ointment, dressing, and tape.

Procedure:
1. It helps to rip the tape into strips, attach the IV tubing to the solution, and flush the air out of the tubing before you begin. If a catheter/needle assembly is used (Angiocath, etc), it often helps to break the seal between the needle and catheter before the catheter is in the vein so that dislodging the catheter is less likely.
2. The upper, nondominant extremity is the site of choice for an IV. Choose a distal vein (dorsum of the hand) so that if the vein is lost, you can reposition the IV more proximally. Figure 3–8 demonstrates some common upper extremity veins; however, avoid veins that cross a joint space. Also avoid the leg since there is a high incidence of thrombophlebitis with IVs placed there. If no extremity vein can be found, try the external jugular. If all these fail, the next alternative is a central venous line insertion.
3. Apply a tourniquet above the proposed IV site. Carefully clean the site with an alcohol or povidine-iodine swab. If a large-bore IV (16 or 14) is to be used, local anesthesia (lidocaine injected with a 25-gauge needle) is helpful.
4. Stabilize the vein distally with the thumb of your free hand. Using the catheter-over-needle assembly (Intracath or Angiocath), either enter the vein directly or enter the skin alongside the vein first and then stick the vein along the side at about a 20-degree angle. (Direct entry and side entry techniques are illustrated in Figure 3–10.) Once the vein is punctured, blood should appear in the "flash chamber." Advance a few more millimeters to be sure that **both** the needle **and** the tip of the catheter have entered the vein. Carefully withdraw the needle as you advance the catheter into the vein (Figure 3–9). **Never withdraw the catheter over the needle since this procedure can shear off the plastic tip and cause a catheter embolus.** Remove the tourniquet and connect the IV line to the catheter. Blood loss can be minimized by compressing the vein with the thumb just proximal to the catheter.
5. Observe the site with the IV fluid running for signs of induration or swelling that indicate improper placement or damage to the vein.

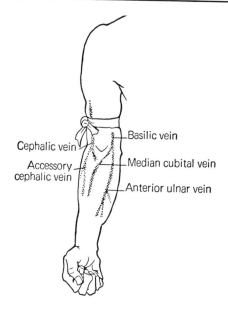

Figure 3–8. Principal veins of the arm used in venipuncture. The pattern can be highly variable. (*From Krupp MA [ed]:* The Physician's Handbook, *21st ed. Los Altos, California, Lange Medical Publications, 1985.*)

See Chapter 4 for choosing IV fluids and how to determine infusion rates.

6. Tape the IV securely in place, and apply a drop of povidone-iodine or antibiotic ointment and a sterile dressing. Ideally, the dressing should be changed every 24–48 hours to help reduce infections. Armboards are also useful to help maintain an IV site.

7. If the veins are deep and difficult to locate, a small 3–5 mL syringe can be mounted on the catheter assembly. Proper position inside the vein is determined by aspiration of blood. If blood specimens are needed from a patient who also needs an IV, this technique can be used to start the IV and collect samples at the same time.

8. If venous access is limited, a "**butterfly**" or "**scalp vein**" needle can sometimes be used (Figure 3–10). This is a small metal needle with plastic "wings" on the side. It is very useful in infants, who often have poor peripheral veins but prominent scalp veins, children, and in adults who have small, fragile veins.

Complications:
Bleeding, hematoma, infections.

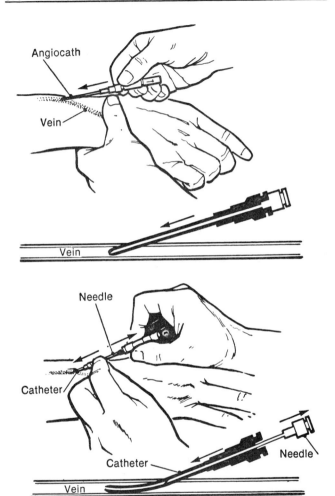

Figure 3–9. To insert a catheter-over-needle assembly into a vein, stabilize the skin and vein with gentle traction. Enter the vein and advance the catheter while removing the needle. (*From Gomella LG [ed]: Clinician's Pocket Reference, 7th ed. Norwalk, Connecticut, Appleton & Lange, 1992.*)

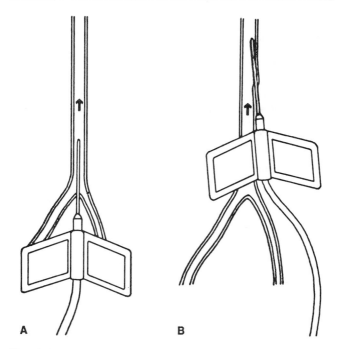

A   **B**

Figure 3–10. Example of a "butterfly" needle assembly and the two techniques of entering a vein for intravenous access: (A) direct puncture and (B) side entry. (*From Gomella TL [ed]:* Neonatology: Basic Management, On-Call Problems, Diseases, Drugs, *2nd ed. Norwalk, Connecticut, Appleton & Lange, 1992.*)

21. LUMBAR PUNCTURE

Indications:
1. Diagnostic purposes (analysis of cerebrospinal fluid [CSF].
2. Measurement of CSF pressure or its changes with various maneuvers (Valsalva, etc).
3. Injection of various agents: contrast media for myelography, antitumor drugs, analgesics, antibiotics.

Contraindications:
1. Increased intracranial pressure (papilledema, mass lesion).
2. Infection near the puncture site.
3. Planned myelography or pneumoencephalography.
4. Coagulation disorders.

Materials:
1. A sterile, disposable lumbar puncture (LP) kit or minor procedure tray.
2. Spinal needles (21-gauge for adults, 22-gauge for children).

Anatomic Considerations:
1. The objective of a lumbar puncture is to obtain a sample of CSF from the subarachnoid space. Specifically, during LP the fluid is obtained from the **lumbar cistern,** the volume of CSF located between the termination of the spinal cord (the conus medullaris) and the termination of the dura mater at the coccygeal ligament. The cistern is surrounded by the subarachnoid membrane and the overlying dura. Located within the cistern are the filum terminale and the nerve roots of the cauda equina. When an LP is done, the main body of the spinal cord is avoided and the nerve roots of the cauda are simply pushed out of the way by the needle.
2. The termination of the spinal cord in an adult is usually between L1 and L2. The safest site for an LP is the interspace between L4 and L5. An imaginary line drawn between the iliac crests (the supracristal plane) intersects the spine at either the L4 spinous process or the L4–L5 interspace exactly. A spinal needle introduced between the spinous processes of L4 and L5 penetrates the layers in the following order: skin, supraspinous ligament, interspinous ligament, ligamentum flavum, epidural space (contains loose areolar tissue, fat, and blood vessels), dura, "potential space," subarachnoid membrane, subarachnoid space (lumbar cistern).

Procedure:
1. Examine the visual fields for evidence of papilledema and review the CT scan of the head if available. Discuss the relative safety and lack of discomfort with the patient to dispel any myths about LP. Some prefer to call the procedure a "subarachnoid analysis" rather than a spinal tap. As long as the procedure and the risks are outlined, most patients will agree to LP. Have the patient sign an informed consent form.
2. Place the patient in the lateral decubitus position close to the edge of the bed or table. The patient (held by an assistant, if possible) should be positioned with her knees pulled up toward the stomach and head flexed onto the chest. This enhances flexion of the vertebral spine and widens the interspaces between the spinous processes. Place a pillow beneath the patient's side to prevent sagging and ensure alignment of the spinal column. In an obese patient or a patient with arthritis or scoliosis, the sitting position, leaning forward, may be preferred.
3. Palpate the supracristal plane (see above) and carefully determine the location of the L4–L5 interspace.

4. Open the kit, put on sterile gloves, and prep the area with povidone-iodine solution, working in a circular fashion and covering several interspaces. Next, drape the patient.

5. With a 25-gauge needle and lidocaine, raise a skin wheal over the L4–L5 interspace. Anesthetize the deeper structures with a 22-gauge needle.

6. Examine the spinal needle with stylet for defects, then insert it into the skin wheal and into the spinous ligament. Hold the needle between your index and middle fingers with your thumb holding the stylet in place. Direct the needle cephalad at a 30- to 45-degree angle, in the midline and parallel to the bed.

7. Advance the needle through the major structures and "pop" it through the dura into the subarachnoid space. An experienced operator can feel these layers, but an inexperienced physician may need to remove the obturator periodically to look for return of fluid. It is important always to replace the obturator prior to advancing the spinal needle. The needle may be withdrawn with the obturator removed, however. This technique may be useful if the needle has passed through the back wall of the canal. Direct the bevel of the needle parallel to the long axis of the body so that the dural fibers are separated rather than sheared. This method helps to cut down on "spinal headaches."

8. If no fluid returns, it is sometimes helpful to rotate the needle slightly. If still no fluid appears, and you think you are within the subarachnoid space, 1 cc of air can be injected since it is not uncommon for a piece of tissue to clog the needle. **Never** inject saline or distilled water. If no air returns and if spinal fluid cannot be aspirated, the bevel of the needle probably lies in the epidural space; advance it with the stylet in place.

9. When fluid returns, attach a manometer and stopcock and measure the pressure. Normal opening pressure is 70–180 mm H_2O in the lateral position. Increased pressure may be due to a tense patient, congestive heart failure (CHF), ascites, subarachnoid hemorrhage, infection, or a space-occupying lesion. Decreased pressure may be due to needle position or obstructed flow (you may need to leave the needle in for a myelogram since, if it is moved, the subarachnoid space may be lost).

10. Collect 0.5–2 mL samples in serial labeled containers. Send them to the lab in this order:
    a. First tube for bacteriology: gram stain, routine culture and sensitivity (C&S), acid-fast bacilli (AFB), and fungal cultures and stains.
    b. Second tube for glucose and protein.
    c. Third tube for cell count: CBC with differential.
    d. Fourth tube for special studies: VDRL test for syphilis, counterimmunoelectrophoresis (CIEP), etc.
    Note: Some physicians prefer to send the first and last tubes for

CBC since this practice permits better differentiation between a **subarachnoid hemorrhage** and a **traumatic tap.** In a traumatic tap, the number of red blood cells should be much higher in the first tube than in the last one. In subarachnoid hemorrhage, the cell counts should be equal and the fluid should be **xanthochromic,** indicating the presence of old blood.

11. Withdraw the needle and place a dry sterile dressing over the site.
12. Instruct the patient to remain recumbent for 6–12 hours and encourage increased fluid intake to help prevent "spinal headaches."
13. Interpret the results based on Table 3–9.

Complications:
1. Spinal headache, the most common complication (about 20%), appears within the first 24 hours after the puncture. It goes away when the patient is lying down and is aggravated when the patient sits up. It is usually characterized by a severe, throbbing pain in the occipital region and can last a week. It is thought to be caused by intracranial traction resulting from the acute volume depletion of CSF and by persistent leakage from the puncture site. To help prevent spinal headaches, keep the patient recumbent for 6–12 hours, encourage intake of fluids, use the smallest needle possible, and keep the bevel of the needle parallel to the long axis of the body to help prevent a persistent CSF leak.
2. Trauma to nerve roots or to the conus medullaris is much less frequent (some anatomic variation does exist, but it is very rare for the cord to end below L3). If the patient suddenly complains of paresthesias (numbness or shooting pains in the legs), the procedure should be stopped.
3. Herniation of either the cerebellum or the medulla occurs rarely during or after a spinal tap, usually in a patient with increased intracranial pressure. This complication can often be reversed medically if it is recognized early.
4. Meningitis.
5. Bleeding in the subarachnoid or subdural space can occur with resulting paralysis, especially if the patient is receiving anticoagulant therapy or has severe liver disease with a coagulopathy.

22. ORTHOSTATIC BLOOD PRESSURE MEASUREMENT

Indications:
To evaluate syncope, dizziness, volume depletion, hemorrhage.

Materials:
Blood pressure cuff and stethoscope.

Procedure:
Changes in blood pressure and pulse when a patient moves from the

TABLE 3–9. DIFFERENTIAL DIAGNOSIS OF CEREBROSPINAL FLUID.

Condition	Color	Opening Pressure (mm H_2O)	Protein (mg/100 mL)	Glucose (mg/100 mL)	Cells (#/mm³)
Adult (normal)	Clear	70–180	15–45	45–80	0–5 lymphs
Newborn (normal)	Clear	70–180	20–120	⅔ serum glucose	40–60 lymphs
Viral infection	Clear or opalescent	Normal or slightly increased	Normal or slightly increased	Normal	10–500 lymphs (polys early)
Bacterial infection	Opalescent yellow, may clot	Increased	50–1500	Decreased, usually < 20	25–10,000 polys
Granulomatous (TB, fungal)	Clear or opalescent	Often increased	Increased, but usually < 500	Decreased, usually 20–40	10–500 lymphs
Subarachnoid hemorrhage	Bloody or xanthochromic after 2–8 h	Usually increased	Increased	Normal	WBC/RBC ratio same as blood

WBC = white blood cell; RBC = red blood cell.
From Gomella LG (ed): Clinician's Pocket Reference, 7th ed. Norwalk, Connecticut, Appleton & Lange, 1992.

381

supine to the upright position are very sensitive guides for detecting early volume depletion. Even before a person becomes overtly tachycardic or hypotensive because of volume loss, the demonstration of orthostatic hypotension aids in the diagnosis.

1. Have the patient lie down for 5–10 minutes. Determine the blood pressure and pulse.
2. Then have the patient stand up. If she is unable to stand, have her sit at the bedside with legs dangling.
3. After about 1 minute, determine the blood pressure and pulse again.

Complications:
None.

Interpretation:
A drop in systolic blood pressure > 10 mm Hg or an increase in pulse rate > 10 suggests **volume depletion.** A change in heart rate is more sensitive and occurs with a lesser degree of volume depletion. Other causes include peripheral vascular disease, surgical sympathectomy, diabetes, and medications (prazosin, hydralazine, or reserpine).

23. PELVIC EXAMINATION

Indications:
Evaluation of female patient.

Materials:
1. Gloves.
2. Vaginal speculum and lubricant.
3. Slides, fixative, cotton swab, and cervical wooden spatula prepared for a Pap smear.
4. Materials for other diagnostic tests: culture media to test for gonorrhea, *Chlamydia,* herpes; sterile cotton swabs, plain glass slides, KOH and normal saline solutions as needed.

Procedure:
1. The pelvic exam should be carried out in a comfortable fashion for both the patient and physician. An assistant **must** be present for the procedure, and a female assistant **must** be present if the examiner is a male. The patient should be draped appropriately and her feet placed in the stirrups on the examining table. A low stool, a good light source, and all needed supplies should be assembled before the exam begins.
2. Inform the patient of each move in advance. Glove your hands before proceeding.

General Inspection
1. Observe the skin of the perineum for swelling, ulcers, condylomas (venereal warts), or color changes.
2. Separate the labia to examine the clitoris and vestibule. Multiple

clear vesicles on an erythematous base on the labia suggest herpes.
3. Observe the urethral meatus for developmental abnormalities, discharge, neoplasm, and abscess of Bartholin's gland at the 4 or 8 o'clock position.
4. Inspect the vaginal orifice for discharge or for protrusion of the walls (cystocele, rectocele, urethral prolapse).
5. Note the condition of the hymen.

Speculum Examination
1. Use a speculum moistened with warm water, **not** with lubricant (lubricant will interfere with Pap tests and slide studies). Check the temperature on the patient's leg to see if the speculum is comfortable.
2. Because the anterior wall of the vagina is close to the urethra and bladder, do not exert pressure in this area. Pressure should be placed on the posterior surface of the vagina. With the speculum directed at a 45-degree angle to the floor, spread the labia and insert the speculum fully, pressing posteriorly. The cervix should pop into view with some manipulation as the speculum is opened.
3. Inspect the cervix and vagina for color, lacerations, growths, nabothian cysts, and evidence of atrophy.
4. Inspect the cervical os for size, shape, color, and discharge.
5. Inspect the vagina for secretions and obtain specimens for a Pap smear, other smear, or culture (see tests for vaginal infections and Pap smear below).
6. Inspect the vaginal wall; rotate the speculum as you draw it out, to see the entire canal.

Bimanual Examination
1. For this part, stand up. It is best to use whichever hand is comfortable to do the internal vaginal exam. Remove the glove from the hand that will examine the abdomen.
2. Place lubricant on the first and second gloved fingers, and then, keeping pressure on the posterior fornix, introduce them into the vagina.
3. Palpate the tissue at 5 and 7 o'clock between the first and second fingers and the thumb to rule out any abnormality of Bartholin's gland. Likewise, palpate the urethra and paraurethral (Skene's) gland.
4. Place the examining fingers on the posterior wall of the vagina to further open the introitus. Ask the patient to bear down. Is there evidence of prolapse, rectocele, or cystocele?
5. Palpate the cervix. Note the size, shape, consistency, and motility, and test for tenderness (the so-called **chandelier sign** or marked cervical tenderness, which is positive in pelvic inflammatory disease).

6. With your fingers in the vagina posterior to the cervix and your hand placed on the abdomen just above the symphysis, the corpus of the uterus can be forced between the two examining hands. Note size, shape, consistency, position, and motility.

7. Move the fingers in the vagina to one or the other fornix and place the hand on the abdomen in a more lateral position to bring the adnexal areas under examination. Palpate the ovaries, if possible, for any masses, consistency, and motility. Unless the fallopian tubes are diseased, they usually are not palpable.

Rectovaginal Examination

1. Insert your index finger into the vagina and place the well-lubricated middle finger in the rectum.

2. Palpate the posterior surface of the uterus and the broad ligament for nodularity, tenderness, or other masses. Examine the uterosacral and rectovaginal septum. Nodularity here may represent endometriosis.

3. It may also be helpful to do a test for occult blood if a stool specimen is available.

Papanicolaou (Pap) Smear. The Pap smear is helpful in the early detection of cervical dysplasia, neoplasia, and cervical carcinoma. Annual Pap smears are recommended.

1. With the unlubricated speculum in place, use a wooden cervical spatula to obtain a scraping from the squamocolumnar junction. Rotate the spatula 360 degrees around the external os. Smear the specimen on a frosted slide that has the patient's name written on it in pencil. Fix the slide either in a bottle of fixative or with commercially available spray fixative. The slide must be fixed within 10 seconds or there will be drying artifact.

2. Next, obtain a specimen from the endocervical canal; use a cotton swab and prepare the slide as noted above.

3. Using a wooden spatula, obtain an additional specimen from the posterior/lateral vaginal pool of fluid and smear it on a slide.

4. Complete the appropriate lab slips. Forewarn the patient that she may experience some spotty vaginal bleeding following the Pap smear.

Tests for Cervical or Vaginal Infections

1. **GC (gonococcal) culture:** Use a sterile cotton swab to obtain a specimen from the endocervical canal and plate it out on **Thayer-Martin** medium.

2. **Wet Mount:** See Procedure 32, page 397.

3. **Gram stain:** Gram-negative intracellular diplococci ("GNIDs") are pathognomonic of *Neisseria gonorrhoeae*. The most commonly found bacteria in gram stains are large gram-positive rods (lactobacilli), which are normal vaginal flora.

4. **Herpes cultures:** A routine Pap smear of the cervix or a Pap

smear of the herpetic lesion (multiple clear vesicles on a painful erythematous base) may demonstrate herpes inclusion bodies. A herpes culture may be done by taking a viral culture swab of the suspicious lesion or of the endocervix.
5. **Chlamydia cultures:** Special swabs can be obtained for *Chlamydia* cultures.

Complications:
Bleeding from:
1. Tumor.
2. Placenta previa (contraindicated).
3. Rupture of membranes.

24. PERITONEAL (ABDOMINAL) PARACENTESIS

Indications:
1. To determine the cause of ascites.
2. To determine if intra-abdominal bleeding is present or if a viscus has ruptured (diagnostic peritoneal lavage is considered a more accurate test).
3. Therapeutic removal of fluid when distention is pronounced or there is respiratory distress associated with it (acute treatment only).

Contraindications:
1. Abnormal coagulation factors.
2. Uncertainty whether distention is due to peritoneal fluid or to a cystic structure (ultrasound can help here).

Materials:
1. Minor procedure tray.
2. Angiocaths or Jelcos (18- to 20-gauge with a 1 ½-inch needle).
3. 20–60 mL syringe.
4. Sterile specimen containers.

Procedure:
Peritoneal paracentesis is surgical puncture of the peritoneal cavity for aspiration of fluid. The presence of ascitic fluid is indicated by abdominal distention, shifting dullness, and a palpable fluid wave.

1. Have the patient sign informed consent if she is able. Have the patient empty the bladder, or place a Foley catheter if she is unable to void or if significant mental status changes are present.
2. The entry site is usually the midline 3–4 cm below the umbilicus. Avoid old surgical scars since the bowel may be adherent to the abdominal wall. Alternatively, the entry site can be in the left or right lower quadrant midway between the umbilicus and the anterior superior iliac spine or in the patient's flank, depending on the percussion of the fluid wave.
3. Prep and drape the patient appropriately. Raise a skin wheal with lidocaine over the proposed entry site.

4. With the catheter mounted on the syringe, advance it through the anesthetized area carefully while gently aspirating. You will meet some resistance as you enter the fascia. When fluid returns freely, leave the catheter in place, remove the needle, and begin to aspirate. Sometimes it is necessary to reposition the catheter because of abutting bowel.

5. Aspirate the amount needed for tests (20–30 mL). For a therapeutic tap, do not remove more than 500 mL in 10 minutes. One liter is the maximum that should be removed at one time; this volume permits fluids and electrolytes to equilibrate. In cirrhotic patients without edema, never withdraw more than 1 L; in cirrhotics with edema, several liters can be removed with relative safety.

6. Quickly remove the needle, apply a sterile 4 × 4 gauze square, and apply pressure with tape.

7. Depending on the clinical picture, send samples for total protein, specific gravity, lactate dehydrogenase (LDH), amylase, cytology, culture, stains, CBC, or food fibers.

Complications:
Peritonitis, perforated viscus, hemorrhage, precipitation of hepatic coma if the patient has severe liver disease, oliguria, hypotension.

Interpretation:
Transudative ascites is found with cirrhosis, nephrosis, and congestive heart failure. **Exudative ascites** is found with tumors, peritonitis (tuberculosis, perforated viscus), and hypoalbuminemia. See Table 3–10 to interpret the results of fluid analysis.

25. PHOSPHATIDYLGLYCEROL (PG) TEST

Indications:
To evaluate fetal lung maturity.

Materials:
Amniostat-FLM agglutination test: 2 mL of amniotic fluid.

Procedure:
1. Label four test tubes: "Patient," "Negative," "Positive," and "Strong Positive."
2. Centrifuge 1.5 mL of amniotic fluid and obtain the supernatant.
3. In the tube labeled "Patient," add 0.025 mL of the supernatant amniotic fluid.
4. Add 0.025 mL of reagent A to each tube.
5. Add 0.025 mL of buffer to each tube.
6. Mix well.
7. Add 0.025 mL of reagent B to each ring on the agglutination slide provided.

TABLE 3–10. DIFFERENTIAL DIAGNOSIS OF ASCITIC OR PLEURAL FLUID.

Lab Value	Transudate	Exudate
Specific gravity	< 1.016	> 1.016
Absolute protein	< 3 g/100 mL	> 3 g/100 mL
Protein (ascitic or pleural to serum ratio)	< 0.5	> 0.5
LDH (ascitic or pleural to serum ratio)	< 0.6	> 0.6
Absolute LDH	< 200 IU	> 200 IU
Glucose (serum to ascitic or pleural ratio)	< 1	> 1
Fibrinogen (clot)	No	Yes
WBC (ascitic)	< 500/mm³	> 1000/mm³
WBC (pleural)	Very low	> 2500/mm³
Differential (pleural)		Polys early, monos later
RBC (ascitic)		> 100 RBC/mm³

Other selected tests:

Cytology. Bizarre cells with large nuclei may represent reactive mesothelial cells and **not a** malignancy. Malignant cells suggest a tumor.

pH (pleural). Generally > 7.3. If between 7.2 and 7.3, suspect TB or malignancy. If < 7.2, suspect empyema.

Glucose (pleural). Normal pleural fluid glucose is ⅔ serum glucose. Pleural fluid glucose is **much** lower than serum glucose in effusions due to rheumatoid arthritis (0–16 mg/100 mL).

Triglycerides and positive Sudan stain (pleural fluid). Chylothroax.
Food fibers (ascitic). Perforated viscus.

From Gomella LG (ed): Clinician's Pocket Reference, 7th ed. Norwalk, Connecticut, Appleton & Lange, 1992.

8. Pipet 0.010 mL from each tube into appropriately marked rings on the slide.
9. Rotate at 60 rpm for 9 minutes.
10. Compare the patient's slide to the three other slides.

Complications:
None.

Interpretation:
A "strong positive" should display relatively large white particles against an absolutely clear background. The "negative" should display a uniform gray-white background with only a grainy appearance.

26. SCALP pH

Indications:
Fetal scalp blood pH determination should be considered to clarify fetal heart rate tracings suggestive of hypoxia. Specific clinical situations may include the following:

1. Confusing or difficult to interpret pattern (eg, fetal arrhythmia).
2. Absent beat-to-beat variability, unrelated to narcotic or sedative drugs, with no ominous periodic changes.
3. Late decelerations with good beat-to-beat variability with vaginal delivery anticipated within 60–90 minutes.
4. Severe variable decelerations with good beat-to-beat variability.
5. Mild to moderate variable decelerations associated with decreased or absent beat-to-beat variability.

Contraindications:
1. Known or suspected fetal blood dyscrasias (von Willebrand's disease or hemophilia).
2. Inaccessibility to 24-hour microblood gas analysis or excessive laboratory turnaround time (> 10–15 minutes).
3. Chorioamnionitis (relative contraindication).
4. Maternal viral infection (ie, HIV or HSV).

Materials:
1. Light source.
2. Micro blood gas analyzer.
3. Fetal blood sampling tray.
4. Conical polypropylene endoscope.
5. Metal fleas.
6. Magnet.
7. Sealant and/or caps for capillary tubes.
8. Lancet with 2 mm blade and long handle.
9. Capillary tubes (300 µL heparinized).
10. Silicone gel.
11. Cotton swabs or sponges.

Procedure:
1. Place the patient in the dorsal lithotomy position or lateral Sims position.
2. Prep the perineum with povidone-iodine and drape with sterile towels.
3. Insert the conical endoscope into the vagina and place it against the presenting part, usually the vertex. The presenting breech may be sampled, but avoid the brow, face, and genitals.
4. The light source should be connected to the endoscope. If not available, an over-shoulder light source may be utilized.
5. Clean the area to be sampled with a cotton swab. Part the hair to clear a space for sampling the scalp.
6. Spray ethyl chloride onto the sample site to induce local hyperemia for enhanced blood collection.
7. Apply silicone gel to the puncture area using a cotton swab.
8. Use the lancet to puncture the skin to a maximum depth of 2 mm.
9. Collect blood into the heparinized capillary tube by capillary action.

10. Introduce the metal flea into the capillary tube and maneuver it with the magnet to admix the blood with heparin.
11. Occlude the capillary tube with either sealant or plastic caps prior to transfer to the laboratory.
12. Use a cotton swab to apply pressure to the sample site for one full contraction. Prior to completion of the procedure, observe for bleeding during the subsequent contraction.

Interpretation:
1. If the pH is normal (> 7.25), the patient may be observed and the procedure repeated later if obstetrically indicated.
2. If the pH demonstrates preacidosis (7.20–7.25), make preparations for cesarean delivery and repeat the procedure within 30 minutes. If evidence of metabolic acidosis exists, immediate delivery should be considered.
3. If the pH suggests frank acidosis (< 7.20), immediate delivery is indicated.

Complications:
Maternal complications of fetal scalp blood sampling are virtually nonexistent. Fetal complications are also rare but may include:

1. Fetal exsanguination secondary to large puncture site(s) or undiagnosed coagulopathy.
2. Scalp infection, which may occur in < 1% of procedures.
3. Blade breakage.

27. SIGMOIDOSCOPY

Indications:
1. Tumor staging.
2. Rectal bleeding.
3. Cancer screening.

Materials:
1. Examination gloves.
2. Lubricant.
3. Occult blood stool test kit (Hemoccult paper and developer).
4. Sigmoidoscope with obturator and light source.
5. Insufflation bag.
6. Tissues.
7. Long (rectal) swabs and a suction catheter.
8. Proctologic examination table (helpful but not essential).

Procedure:
There are several techniques for examining the distal large bowel. These include **sigmoidoscopy** (endoscopic examination of the last 25 cm of the GI tract), **flexible sigmoidoscopy** (examination up to 40 cm from the end of the GI tract), **proctoscopy** (roughly synonymous with

sigmoidoscopy, but technically means examination of the last 12 cm), and **anoscopy** (examination of the anus and most distal rectum).

1. Enemas and cathartics are not routinely given before sigmoidoscopy, although some physicians prefer to give a mild prep such as a fleet enema just before the exam. Have the patient sign a consent form.
2. Sigmoidoscopy can be performed with the patient in bed lying on her side in the knee-chest position, but the best results are obtained with the patient in the "jackknife" position on the procto table. Do not position the patient until all materials are at hand and you are ready to start.
3. Converse with the patient to create distraction and to relieve apprehension. Announce each maneuver in advance. Glove before proceeding.
4. Observe the anal region for skin tags, hemorrhoids, fissures, etc. Do a careful rectal exam with a gloved finger and plenty of lubricant and check for occult blood (**Hemoccult test**) on the stool recovered on the glove.
5. Lubricate the sigmoidoscope well and insert it with the obturator in place. Aim toward the patient's umbilicus initially. Advance 2–3 cm past the internal sphincter and remove the obturator.
6. Always advance under direct vision and make sure the lumen is always visible. **Insufflation** (introducing air) may be used to help visualize the lumen, but remember that this may be painful. It is necessary to follow the curve of the sigmoid toward the sacrum by directing the scope more posteriorly toward the back. A change from smooth mucosa to concentric rings signifies entry into the sigmoid colon. The scope should reach 15 cm with ease. Use suction and the rectal swabs as needed to clear the way.
7. At this point, the sigmoid curves to the patient's left. Warn the patient that she may feel a cramping sensation. If you ever have difficulty negotiating a curve, do not force it.
8. After advancing as far as possible, slowly remove the scope; use a small rotary motion to view all surfaces. Observation here is critical. Remember to release the air from the colon before withdrawing the scope.
9. Inform the patient that she may experience mild cramping after the procedure.

Complications:
Bleeding (rare), perforation (rare).

28. SKIN TESTING

Indications:
1. Screening for a current or past infectious agent (tuberculosis, coccidioidomycosis, etc).

2. Screening for immune competency (so-called anergy screen) in debilitated patients.

Materials:
1. Appropriate antigen (usually 0.1 mL).
2. A small, short needle (25-, 26-, or 27-gauge).
3. 1 mL syringe.
4. Alcohol swab.

Procedure:
Skin tests for **delayed type hypersensitivity (type IV, tuberculin)** are the most commonly administered and interpreted; allergy tests (immediate wheal and flare) are rarely performed by the student or house officer. Delayed hypersensitivity (so called because there is a 12- to 36-hour lag time until a reaction occurs) is caused by activation of sensitized lymphocytes after contact with an antigen. The inflammatory reaction results from direct cytotoxicity and the release of lymphokines.

1. The most commonly used site is the flexor surface of the forearm approximately 4 inches below the elbow crease.
2. Prep the area with alcohol. With the bevel up, introduce the needle into the upper layers of skin but **not** into the subcutis. Inject 0.1 mL of antigen. The goal is to inject the antigen intradermally. If done properly, you will raise a discrete white bleb approximately 10 mm in diameter. The bleb should disappear soon, and no dressing is needed.
3. Mark the test site with a pen and document the site in the patient's chart. If multiple tests are being administered, identify each one.

Specific Skin Tests

Tuberculosis (PPD or Mantoux)
1. The solution of **purified protein derivative (PPD)** comes in three tuberculin unit (TU) "strengths": 1 TU ("first"), 5 TU ("intermediate"), and 250 TU ("second"). 1 TU is used if the patient is expected to be hypersensitive (history of a positive skin test); 5 TU is the standard initial screening test. A patient who has a negative response to a 5 TU test dose may react to the 250 TU solution. A patient who does not respond to 250 TU is considered nonreactive to PPD. A patient may not react if she has never been exposed to the antigen or if she is anergic and unable to respond to any antigen challenge.
2. To interpret the PPD skin test, examine the injection site at 24, 48, and 72 hours. Measure the area of induration (the firm, raised area), not the erythematous area:

0–5 mm induration: a negative response

> 10 mm induration: a positive response

3. An equivocal PPD test may represent infection with an atypical species of mycobacteria. It is important to check the PPD test at intervals. If the patient develops a severe reaction to the skin test, apply hydrocortisone cream to prevent skin sloughing.

Tine Test. The tine test for tuberculosis is useful only as a mass screening procedure. The PPD is a much more sensitive and specific test and should be used on all hospitalized patients. A positive tine test is the presence of vesicles.

Anergy Screen (Anergy Battery). An anergy screen is based on the assumption that a patient has been exposed in the past to certain common antigens and a healthy patient is able to mount a reaction to them. To perform the screen, one can use an assortment of antigens such as mumps, *Candida,* or *Trichophyton* (positive test is an area of erythema > 1.5 cm). These are generally applied and read just like the PPD test.

Anergy screens are used to evaluate a patient's immunologic status or her ability to withstand the stresses of surgery. They are also used in specific situations: if you suspect that a patient is PPD-positive but she does not react to the test, do an anergy screen along with the PPD test to see if she can mount any response at all.

Complications:
Anaphylaxis or local reaction in patients with previous exposure or active disease.

29. SUCTION CURETTAGE

Indications:
1. Termination of pregnancy.
2. Endometrial sampling.
3. Evacuation of hydatidiform molar pregnancy.

Materials:
1. Speculum.
2. Antiseptic such as iodine or chlorhexidine.
3. Tenaculum.
4. Uterine sound.
5. Uterine curet.
6. Formalin.
7. Suction machine.
8. Laminaria.
9. Cervical dilators.

Procedure:
1. Dilate the cervix with hydrophilic laminariae prior to the procedure.

2. Careful pelvic exam should precede endometrial biopsy. In patients who may be pregnant, appropriate testing should precede biopsy.
3. Obtain informed consent, then prep the vagina with antiseptic such as iodine or chlorhexidine.
4. Induce paracervical anesthesia with 1% or 2% lidocaine.
5. Apply the tenaculum to the cervix.
6. Dilate the cervix with dilators if laminariae are not used.
7. Sound the uterus.
8. Place an appropriate size suction catheter into the uterus.
9. Attach it to the suction machine (negative pressure range 30–50 cm Hg) (Figure 3–11).
10. Pass the catheter with suction through all quadrants of the uterus.
11. Send tissue to the pathology lab.

Complications:
Bleeding, infection, uterine perforation, bladder and bowel injury.

30. THORACENTESIS

Indications:
1. To determine the cause of a pleural effusion.
2. To remove pleural fluid therapeutically in the event of respiratory distress.

Contraindications:
None are absolute: pneumothorax, hemothorax, or any major respiratory impairment on the contralateral side, or coagulopathy.

Materials:
1. Prepackaged thoracentesis kit or minor procedure tray.
2. Stopcock.
3. Hemostat.

Procedure:
Thoracentesis is surgical puncture of the chest wall to aspirate fluid or air from the pleural cavity. The area of pleural effusion will be dull to percussion with decreased whisper or breath sounds. Pleural fluid will cause blunting of the costophrenic angles on chest x-ray. Blunting usually indicates that at least 300 mL of fluid is present. If you suspect that the amount of fluid is < 300 mL or that the fluid is loculated (trapped and not free flowing), a lateral decubitus film is helpful. Loculated effusions will not layer out. Thoracentesis can be done safely on fluid visualized on a lateral decubitus film if at least 10 mm of fluid is measurable on the decubitus x-ray.

1. Obtain an informed consent. Have the patient sit up comfortably, preferably leaning forward slightly on a bedside tray table. Have her practice increasing intrathoracic pressure using the Valsalva maneuver or by humming.

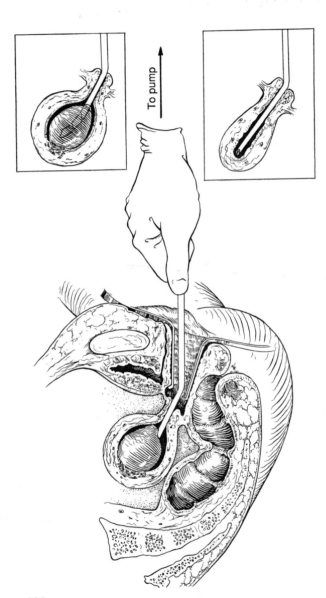

Figure 3-11. Suction method for induced abortion. (*From Pernoll ML, Benson RC [eds]: Current Obstetric and Gynecologic Diagnosis and Treatment, 6th ed. Norwalk, Connecticut, Appleton & Lange, 1987.*)

To pump

2. The usual site for thoracentesis is the posterolateral aspect of the back over the diaphragm but under the fluid level. Confirm the site by counting the ribs, based on the x-ray, and percussing out the fluid level.

3. Sterile technique should be used including gloves, povidone-iodine prep, and drapes. Thoracentesis kits come with an adherent drape with a hole in it.

4. Make a skin wheal over the proposed site with a 25-gauge needle and lidocaine. Change to a 22-gauge, 1 ½-inch needle and infiltrate up and over the rib; try to anesthetize the deeper structures and the pleura. During this time, you should be aspirating back for pleural fluid. Once fluid returns, note the depth of the needle and mark it with a hemostat. This gives you an approximate depth. Remove the needle.

5. Measure the 15- to 18-gauge thoracentesis needle to the same depth as the first needle with the hemostat. Penetrate through the anesthetized area with the thoracentesis needle. **Make sure you "march" over the top of the rib** to avoid the neurovascular bundle that runs below the rib. Attach the three-way stopcock and tubing and aspirate the amount needed. Turn the stopcock and evacuate the fluid through the tubing. The lung may have difficulty reexpanding with more than 1000 mL per tap.

6. Have the patient hum or do the Valsalva maneuver as you withdraw the needle. This maneuver increases intrathoracic pressure and decreases the chance of a pneumothorax. Bandage the site.

7. Obtain a chest x-ray to evaluate the fluid level and to rule out a pneumothorax. An expiratory film may be best because it helps to reveal a small pneumothorax.

8. Distribute specimens in containers, label slips, and send them to the lab. Always order pH, specific gravity, protein, lactate dehydrogenase (LDH), cell count and differential, glucose, gram stain and cultures, acid-fast cultures and smears, and fungal cultures and smears. Optional lab studies are cytology if you suspect a malignancy, amylase if you suspect an effusion secondary to pancreatitis (usually on the left), and a Sudan stain and triglycerides if chylothorax is a possibility.

Complications:
Pneumothorax, hemothorax, infection, pulmonary laceration, hypotension.

Interpretation:
Transudate is usually associated with nephrosis, congestive heart failure (CHF), or cirrhosis; an **exudate** is associated with infection (pneumonia, tuberculosis), malignancy, empyema, peritoneal dialysis, pancreatitis, or chylothorax.

31. URINARY TRACT PROCEDURES

Bladder Catheterization

Indications:
1. To relieve urine retention.
2. To collect an uncontaminated urine specimen for diagnostic purposes.
3. To monitor urine output in critically ill patients.
4. To perform bladder tests (cystogram, cystometrogram).

Contraindication:
Urethral disruption associated with pelvic fracture.

Materials:
1. Prepackaged bladder catheter tray (may or may not include a Foley catheter).
2. Catheter of choice:
    a. **Foley Catheter:** This type has a balloon at the tip to keep it in the bladder. Use a 16–18 French for adults (the higher the number, the larger the diameter). Irrigation catheters ("three-way Foley") should be larger (20–22 French).
    b. **Red rubber catheter:** This is a plain rubber or latex catheter without a balloon, usually used for "in and out catheterization" in which the urine is removed and the catheter is not left indwelling.

Procedure:
1. Each insertion of a catheter implants bacteria into the bladder, so strict aseptic technique is mandatory.
2. Have the patient lie supine in a well-lighted area with knees flexed wide and heels together to get adequate exposure of the meatus.
3. Open the kit and put on the gloves. Get all the materials ready before you attempt to insert the catheter. Open the prep solution and soak the cotton balls. Apply the sterile drapes.
4. Inflate and deflate the balloon of the Foley catheter to assure its proper function. Coat the end of the catheter with lubricant jelly.
5. Use one gloved hand to prep the urethral meatus, working from the pubis toward the anus; hold the labia apart with the other gloved hand.
6. After inflation, pull the catheter back so that the balloon will come to rest on the bladder neck. There should be good urine return when the catheter is in place. If a large amount of lubricant jelly was placed into the urethra, the catheter may need to be flushed with sterile saline to clear excess lubricant. **A catheter that will not irrigate is in the urethra, not the bladder.**
7. The catheter may be taped to the patient's leg. The catheter is usually attached to a gravity drainage bag or some device for

measuring the amount of urine. Many new kits come with the catheter already secured to the drainage bag. These systems are considered "closed systems" and should not be opened if at all possible.

"In and Out" Catheterized Urine. If urine is needed for analysis or for culture and sensitivity, a so-called in and out cath can be done. This is also useful for measuring residual urine. The incidence of inducing infection with this procedure is about 3%.

The procedure is identical to that for bladder catheterization. The main difference is that a red rubber catheter (no balloon) is often used, and is removed immediately after the specimen is collected.

Clean-Catch Urine Specimen. A clean-catch urine is useful for routine urinalysis, but is only fair for culturing urine because of the potential for contamination.

1. Separate the labia widely to expose the urethral meatus; keep the labia spread throughout the procedure.
2. Cleanse the urethral meatus with povidone-iodine solution from front to back and rinse with sterile water.
3. Catch the midstream portion of the urine in a sterile container.

32. WET MOUNT

Indication:
Evaluation of vaginal discharge.

Material:
1. Two microslides with cover slips.
2. 10% KOH.
3. Normal saline.
4. Microscope.
5. Speculum and cotton-tipped applicator.

Procedure:
1. Place a bivalve speculum in the vaginal vault.
2. Place 1 drop of normal saline on slide A and 1 drop of KOH on slide B.
3. With the cotton-tipped applicator, obtain a sample of the discharge and add it to the normal saline and KOH droplet.
4. Evaluate under the microscope after attaching a cover slip.
5. Identify organisms (ie, *Candida albicans* or flagellated *Trichomonas vaginalis*) or clue cells (*Gardnerella vaginalis*).

Complications:
None.

4   Fluids and Electrolytes

ORDERING IV FLUIDS

The following are general guidelines to ordering maintenance and replacement fluids in patients. Clinical judgement is needed to modify these appropriately.

Maintenance Fluids

D5¼NS with KCl 20 meq/L. Determine the 24-hour water requirement by the following formula, called the Kg method, and divide by 24 hours to determine the hourly rate.

Kg Method

- For the first 10 kg of body weight: 100 mL/kg/day **plus**
- For the second 10 kg of body weight: 50 mL/kg/day **plus**
- For weight above 20 kg: 20 mL/kg/day

Pediatric Patients:
Use the same solution, but determine the daily fluid requirements by either of the following:

Kg Method. As outlined above.

Meter-Squared Method. Maintenance fluids are 1500 mL/m²/day. Divide by 24 to get the flow rate per hour. To calculate surface area, use the body surface area charts in the Appendix.

Specific Replacement Fluids

Table 4–1 gives general guidelines to the daily production of various body fluids.

Gastric (NG Tube, Emesis):
D5½NS with KCl 20 meq/L.

Diarrhea:
D5LR with KCl 15 meq/L. Use body weight as a replacement guide (about 1 L for each 1 kg, or 2.2 lb, lost).

Bile:
D5LR with HCO_3^- 25 meq/L (½ ampule).

Pancreatic:
D5LR with HCO_3^- 50 meq/L (1 ampule).

TABLE 4–1. COMPOSITION AND DAILY PRODUCTION OF BODY FLUIDS.

	Electrolytes (meq/L)				Average Daily Production[a] (in mL)
Fluid	Na⁺	Cl⁻	K⁺	HCO₃⁻	
Sweat	50	40	5	0	Varies
Saliva	60	15	26	50	1500
Gastric juice	60–100	100	10	0	1500–2500
Duodenum	130	90	5	0–10	300–2000
Bile	145	100	5	15	100–800
Pancreatic juice	140	75	5	115	100–800
Ileum	140	100	2–8	30	100–9000
Diarrhea	120	90	25	45	—

[a]In adults.

From Gomella LG (ed): Clinician's Pocket Reference, 7th edition. Norwalk, Connecticut, Appleton & Lange, 1992.

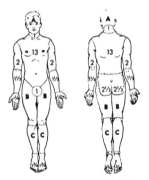

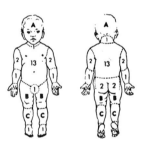

Relative Percentages of Areas Affected by Growth

	Age		
Area	10	15	Adult
A = half of head	5 ½	4 ½	3 ½
B = half of one thigh	4 ¼	4 ½	4 ¾
C = half of one leg	3	3 ¼	3 ½

Relative Percentages of Areas Affected by Growth

	Age		
Area	0	1	5
A = half of head	9 ½	8 ½	6 ½
B = half of one thigh	2 ¾	3 ¼	4
C = half of one leg	2 ½	2 ½	2 ¾

FIGURE 4–1. Tables for estimating the extent of burns in adults and children. In adults, a reasonable system for calculating the percentage of body burned is the rule of nine's: each arm equals 9%, the head equals 9%, the anterior and posterior trunk each equal 18%, each leg equals 18%, and the perineum equals 1%. (*From Way LW [ed]: Current Surgical Diagnosis and Treatment, 8th ed. San Mateo, CA, Appleton & Lange, 1988.*)

TABLE 4–2. COMPOSITION OF COMMONLY USED CRYSTALLOIDS. [a]

Fluid	Glucose (g/L)	Na+	Cl-	K+	Ca+2	HCO3- [b]	Mg+2	HPO4-2	kcal (per liter)
D5W (5% dextrose in water)	50	—	—	—	—	—	—	—	170
D10W (10% dextrose in water)	100	—	—	—	—	—	—	—	340
D20W (20% dextrose in water)	200	—	—	—	—	—	—	—	680
D50W (50% dextrose in water)	500	—	—	—	—	—	—	—	1700
½ NS (0.45% NaCl)	—	77	77	—	—	—	—	—	—
3% NS	—	513	154	—	—	—	—	—	—
NS (0.9% NaCl)	—	154	154	—	—	—	—	—	—
D5% ¼ NS	50	38	38	—	—	—	—	—	170
D5% NS (0.9% NaCl)	50	154	154	—	—	—	—	—	170
D5LR (5% dextrose in lactated Ringer's)	50	130	110	4	3	27	—	—	180
Lactated Ringer's	—	130	110	4	3	27	—	—	<10
Ionosol MB	50	25	22	20	—	23	3	3	170
Normosol M	50	40	40	13	—	16	3	—	170

[a]Electrolyte values are in meq/L.
[b]HCO3 is administered in these solutions as lactate that is converted to bicarbonate.
NS = normal saline.
From Gomella LG (ed): Clinician's Pocket Reference, 7th edition. Norwalk, Connecticut, Appleton & Lange, 1992.

COMPOSITION OF PARENTERAL FLUIDS

Parenteral fluids are generally classified based on molecular weight and oncotic pressure. Colloids (albumin, blood, dextran, hetastarch, plasma protein fraction) are generally > 8000 dalton molecular weight and have high oncotic pressure. Crystalloids (most IV fluids) are < 8000 dalton molecular weight and have low oncotic pressure (Table 4–2).

BURN PATIENTS

See Figure 4–1. Use the Parkland formula: total fluid required during the first 24 hours = (% body burn) × (body weight in kg) × 4 mL. Replace with lactated Ringer's solution over 24 hours. Use:

- ½ total over first 8 hours (from time of burn)
- ¼ total over second 8 hours
- ¼ total over third 8 hours

5 Blood Component Therapy

Type and Cross (T&C):
The blood bank will ABO and Rh type and antibody screen the patient's blood and match the patient with specific donor units.

Type and Hold (Type and Screen):
The blood bank will ABO and Rh type the patient and screen for antibodies. No units will be set up until needed.

Products:
Table 5–1 describes blood bank products and gives common indications for their use.

Transfusion Procedure

1. When the blood products become available, make sure the patient has good venous access for the transfusion (18-gauge or larger is preferred in an adult).
2. Remember to verify with another person, such as a nurse, the information on the request slip, blood bag, and the patient's identification (ID) bracelet. Many hospitals have defined protocols for this procedure. Ask the patient to give her name, and do not ask "are you Jane Doe?" since many patients will respond "yes" automatically.
3. Blood products to be transfused may only be mixed with isotonic normal saline. Using hypotonic products such as D5W can result in hemolysis of the blood in the tubing. Lactated Ringer's should not be used because the calcium chelates the anticoagulant citrate.
4. When transfusing large volumes of packed red cell (PRBC) blood (> 6 to 8 units), some physicians advocate periodic transfusion of platelets and fresh-frozen plasma (FFP). Also, a calcium replacement is sometimes needed, since the preservative used in the blood is a calcium binder and hypocalcemia can result after large amounts of blood are transfused. In massive transfusions, the blood should be warmed to prevent hypothermia and cardiac arrhythmias.

Emergency Transfusions

Transfusing non-cross-matched blood is rarely indicated since most blood banks can do a routine cross-match within 1 hour. In cases of

TABLE 5–1. BLOOD COMPONENT THERAPY PRODUCTS, DESCRIPTIONS, AND COMMON INDICATIONS.

Product	Description	Common Indications
Whole blood	No elements removed 1 unit = 450 mL ± 45 mL Contains red cells, white cells, plasma, and platelets (platelets may be nonfunctional)	Not for routine use Acute, massive bleeding Open heart surgery Neonatal total exchange
Packed red cells (PRBC)	Most plasma removed 1 unit = 250–300 mL 1 unit should raise Hct 3% in most adults	Replacement in chronic and acute blood loss, GI bleeding, trauma, surgery
Universal pedi-packs	250–300 mL divided into 3 bags Contains red cells, some white cells, some plasma and platelets	Transfusion of infants
Platelets	1 "pack" should raise count by 6000 "6-pack" means a pool of platelets from 6 units of blood 1 pack = about 50 mL	Plaelets < 20,000 in nonbleeding patient, < 50,000 in preop patient, < 50,000 in actively bleeding patient Nondestructive thrombocytopenia; not in idiopathic thrombocytopenic purpura (ITP) or thrombotic thrombocytopenic purpura (TTP) or DIC unless bleeding and count < 20,000
Leukocyte-poor red cells	Most WBC removed to make it less antigenic 1 unit = 200–250 mL	Potential renal transplant patients Previous febrile transfusion reactions Patients requiring multiple transfusions (leukemia, etc)
Washed RBCs	Like leukocyte-poor red cells but WBC almost completely removed 1 unit = 300 mL	As for leukocyte-poor red cells but very expensive and much more purified
Deglycerolized RBCs (frozen-thawed RBCs)	Frozen for up to 3 years in a glycerol preparation	Useful for autotransfusions and storing extremely rare blood types Lymphoid cells destroyed to decrease likelihood of graft-vs.-host reaction; used typically in transplant recipients
Granulocyte concentrate		Granulocytopenia with sepsis absolute granulocyte count < 500/mm2 on at least 2 counts) not responsive to antibiotics

TABLE 5–1. BLOOD COMPONENT THERAPY PRODUCTS, DESCRIPTIONS, AND COMMON INDICATIONS.

Product	Description	Common Indications
Cryoprecipitated antihemophilic factor (Cryo)	Contains Factor VIII, Factor XIII, von Willebrand's factor, and fibrinogen 1 unit = 10 mL	Hemophilia A (Factor VIII deficiency), von Willebrand's disease, and fibrinogen deficiency
Fresh, frozen plasma (FFP)	Contains Factors II, VII, IX, X, XI, XII, XIII, and heat-labile V and VII About 1 hour to thaw 1 unit = 150–250 mL	Undiagnosed bleeding disease with active bleeding When transfusing > 6–8 units of blood Patient with liver disease Immune globulin deficiency
Single donor plasma	Like FFP but lacks Factors V and VIII About 1 hour to thaw 1 unit = 150–200 mL	Plasma replacement Stable clotting factor replacement Reversal of Coumadin, hemophilia B
Rho Gam (Rho D immune globulin)	Antibody against Rh factor	Rh– mother with Rh+ baby, within 72 hours of delivery

All of the aforementioned items usually require a "clot tube" to be sent for typing. The following products are usually dispensed by most hospital pharmacies and are ordered as a medication.

Product	Description	Common Indications
Factor VIII (purified antihemophilic factor)	From pooled plasma, pure Factor VIII Increased hepatitis risk	Routine for hemophilia A (Factor VIII deficiency)
Factor IX concentrate (prothrombin complex)	Increased hepatitis risk Factors II, VII, IX, and X Equivalent to 2 units of plasma	Active bleeding in Christmas disease (Factor IX deficiency)
Immune serum globulin	Precipitate from plasma "Gamma globulin"	Immune globulin deficiency Disease prophylaxis (hepatitis A, measles, etc)
5% Albumin or 5% plasma protein fraction	Precipitate from plasma (see Chapter 7)	Plasma volume expanders in acute blood loss
25% Albumin	Precipitate from plasma Draws extravascular fluid into circulation	Hypoalbuminemia, volume expander, burns

From Gomella LG (ed): Clinician's Pocket Reference, *7th ed. Norwalk, Connecticut, Appleton & Lange, 1992.*

TABLE 5–2. FREQUENCY OF ABO AND RH BLOOD GROUPINGS AND GENERAL COMPATIBILITY GUIDELINES.

Type (ABO/Rh)	Occurrences	Can Usually Receive Blood From
O+	1 in 3	O (+/–)
O–	1 in 15	O (–)
A+	1 in 3	A (+/–) or O (+/–)
A–	1 in 16	A (–) or O (–)
B+	1 in 12	B (+/–) or O (+/–)
B–	1 in 67	B (–) or O (–)
AB+	1 in 29	AB, A, B or O (all + or –)
AB–	1 in 167	AB, A, B or O (all –)

From Gomella LG (ed): Clinician's Pocket Reference, 7th ed. Norwalk, Connecticut, Appleton & Lange, 1992.

massive exsanguinating hemorrhage, type-specific blood (ABO and Rh matched only), usually available in 10 minutes, can be used. If this is too long, type O, Rh negative, PRBC blood can be used as a last resort.

Transfusion Reactions

Over 85% of adverse hemolytic transfusion reactions relate to clerical error (see Problem 71, page 270).

Blood Groups (Table 5–2)

O– is the universal donor and AB+ is the universal recipient.

Transfusion Formula

To estimate the volume of whole blood or PRBC needed to raise a hematocrit to a known amount, use the following formula:

$$\text{Volume of cells} = \frac{\text{Total blood volume of patient} \times (\text{Desired HCT} - \text{Actual HCT})}{\text{Hematocrit of transfusion product}}$$

- Total blood volume = 70 mL/kg in adults, 80 mL/kg in children
- Hematocrit of packed red cells = approximately 70
- hematocrit of whole blood = approximately 40

Example: What volume of PRBC is needed to raise the hematocrit of a 50 kg adult from 20 to 30?

$$\text{Volume PRBC} = \frac{50 \text{ kg } (70 \text{ mL/kg}) \times (30 - 20)}{70} = 500 \text{ mL}$$

6 Ventilator Management

Indications and Setup	Hypoxemia
Routine Modification of Settings	Hypercapnia
Troubleshooting Agitation	High Peak Pressures
	Weaning

INDICATIONS AND SETUP

I. Indications

A. Ventilatory failure. This is judged by the degree of hypercapnia. A $PaCO_2 > 50$ mm Hg indicates ventilatory failure; however, many patients will have chronic ventilatory failure with renal compensation (retaining HCO_3^-) to adjust the pH toward normal. Thus, absolute pH is often a better guide to determine the need for ventilatory assistance than $PaCO_2$. Respiratory acidosis with a rapidly falling pH or an absolute pH < 7.24 is an indication for ventilatory support. The prototype of pure ventilatory failure is the drug overdose patient in whom there is sudden loss of central respiratory drive with uncontrolled hypercapnia. Patients with sepsis, neuromuscular disease, or chronic obstructive pulmonary disease (COPD) may also have hypercapnic ventilatory failure.

B. Hypoxemic respiratory failure. Inability to oxygenate is an important indication for ventilatory support. A $PaO_2 < 60$ mm Hg on $\geq 50\%$ inspired oxygen fraction (FiO_2) constitutes hypoxemic respiratory failure. Although these patients can sometimes be managed with higher FiO_2 delivery systems, such as partial or nonrebreather masks or continuous positive airway pressure (CPAP) delivered by mask, they are at high risk for respiratory arrest and should be closely monitored in an intensive care unit. Worsening of the respiratory status necessitates prompt intubation and ventilatory support. The prototype disease for hypoxemic respiratory failure is adult respiratory distress syndrome (ARDS), in which the high shunt fraction leads to refractory hypoxemia.

C. **Mixed respiratory failure.** Most patients actually have failure of both ventilation and oxygenation. The indications for ventilatory support remain the same as listed earlier. The threshold for initiating ventilatory support will be even lower with these patients since oxygen management may further compound hypercapnia. An example of mixed respiratory failure is COPD with acute bronchitis. Bronchospasm alters the ventilation/perfusion ratio (V/Q) relationships, leading to worsening hypoxemia. Bronchospasm and accumulated secretions result in a high work of breathing and consequent hypercapnia.

D. **Neuromuscular failure.** This is actually a category of ventilatory failure but deserves special mention because of its differing management. Hypercapnia occurs just before arrest, and thus criteria other than arterial blood gases (ABGs) are needed.

1. In progressive tachypnea, breath rates higher than 24/min are an early sign of respiratory failure. A progressive rise in the breath rate or sustained breath rates higher than 35/min are an indication for ventilatory support.

2. Abdominal paradox indicates dyssynergy between chest wall muscles and the diaphragm and impending respiratory failure. It is manifested by inward movement of the abdominal wall during inspiration rather than the normal outward motion.

3. A vital capacity < 15 mL/kg (1000 mL for a person of normal body size) is associated with acute respiratory arrest as well as inability to clear secretions. Similarly, a negative inspiratory force below –25 cm H_2O implies impending respiratory arrest. Guillain-Barré syndrome is the prototype of a neuromuscular disease in which the preceding criteria need strict attention. A patient with Guillain-Barré syndrome should be closely observed and followed with frequent vital capacity (VC) determinations. A rapidly falling VC or VC < 1000 mL requires initiation of respirator support.

II. **Tracheal Intubation** (See Procedure 13, Endotracheal Intubation, page 363.)
Endotracheal intubation is actually the most difficult and most complication-ridden part of ventilator initiation. Skill and experience are required for correct placement. Aspiration, esophageal intubation, and intubation of the right mainstem bronchus are common complications. Bilateral breath sounds always need to be confirmed by chest auscultation in each axilla. A portable chest x-ray should be obtained immediately after intubation. Intubation can be accomplished by three routes.

A. Nasotracheal intubation. This can be accomplished blind in an awake patient. It requires experience and adequate local anesthesia. Complications include esophageal intubation, nosebleeds, kinking of the endotracheal tube (ETT), and postobstructive sinusitis. A smaller ETT is usually required for nasotracheal versus orotracheal intubation; this leads to a higher work of breathing because of increased resistance, difficulties with adequate suctioning, and higher ventilation pressures. Nasotracheal ETTs are more comfortable than orotracheal ETTs and are less damaging to the larynx because of better stabilization in the airway.

B. Orotracheal intubation. Placement of orotracheal tubes requires normal neck mobility to allow hyperextension of the neck for direct visualization of the vocal cords. Larger ETTs can be placed by this route. Adequate local anesthesia or sedation is necessary for safe placement without aspiration.

C. Tracheostomy. Tracheostomy is a surgical procedure most often done acutely for upper airway obstruction; however, in patients who require more than 14–21 days of ventilatory support, a tracheostomy is recommended. Tracheostomy tubes facilitate the weaning process by decreasing tube resistance since the tube is shorter and of greater radius. Patients are able to eat, and find the tubes more comfortable.

III. Ventilator Setup

A. The ventilator. Almost all modern ventilators are time- and volume-cycled. Elaborate alarm systems are present to alert personnel to inadequate ventilation, high pressure, disconnection of the ETT, and so forth. Effective ventilation is measured by changes in $PaCO_2$. Minute ventilation (V_e) is tidal volume × breath rate. Thus, ventilation may be adjusted by changing the breath rate, the tidal volume, or both. Tidal volumes above 12 mL/kg may cause overdistention of alveoli and increase the risk of pneumothorax. Most initial tidal volumes are therefore set at 10–12 mL/kg. Oxygenation is adjusted by changing FiO_2. Prolonged $FiO_2 > 60\%$ may cause pulmonary fibrosis. Thus, downward adjustment to "safe levels" sufficient to maintain O_2 saturation > 90% should be attempted if indicated by ABGs. If an O_2 saturation > 90% cannot be maintained when decreasing the $FiO_2 < 60\%$, other means such as positive end-expiratory pressure (PEEP) can be used. The mode of ventilation should be specified.

1. Control mode delivers a set rate and tidal volume irrespective of patient efforts.

2. **Assist control (AC) mode** allows patient triggering of machine breaths once a threshold of inspiratory flow or effort is attained. It also supplies a backup rate in case of apnea or paralysis.

3. **Intermittent mandatory ventilation (IMV)** provides a set number of machine breaths per minute and allows the patient to make spontaneous breaths as well. **Synchronized intermittent mandatory ventilation (SIMV)** allows synchronization of the IMV breaths with patient efforts. As the rate is turned down, the patient assumes more and more of the work of breathing.

4. **Continuous positive airway pressure (CPAP)** allows completely spontaneous respirations while the patient is still connected to the ventilator. A set amount of continuous pressure may be applied as well (from 0 to 30 cm H_2O). Initial ventilator settings should be dictated by the underlying condition as well as previous blood gas results. An example of settings for a patient status post respiratory arrest would be:

- FiO_2 1.0
- AC mode
- Rate 14
- Tidal volume 800 mL

An attempt should be made to supply the patient with at least as much minute ventilation as was required prior to intubation. Thus, patients with pulmonary edema, ARDS, or neuromuscular disease may require minute ventilation rates of 14–22 L/min. The AC mode will generally be more comfortable and will alleviate the work of breathing to a large extent. Sample settings might be:

- FiO_2 1.0
- AC mode
- Rate 18
- Tidal volume 750 mL

The patient with COPD, on the other hand, should not be overventilated initially. Such patients may have a chronically high bicarbonate level because of renal compensation, and overventilation could cause a severe alkalosis. Sample settings might be:

- FiO_2 0.5
- SIMV mode
- Pressure support 15 cm
- Rate 12
- Tidal volume 800 mL

B. Additional setup requirements

1. Restrain the patient's hands, since a natural reaction to the ETT upon awakening is to pull it out.
2. Place a nasogastric tube to decompress the stomach and to continue essential oral medications.
3. Obtain a stat portable chest x-ray to confirm ETT placement and to reassess any underlying pulmonary disease.
4. Treat any underlying pulmonary disease (maximize bronchodilators in status asthmaticus or vasodilators and diuretics in pulmonary edema).
5. Consider prophylactic measures. Heparin 5000 U SQ q12h may reduce the incidence of pulmonary embolism while the patient is on bed rest. Bleeding from stress ulceration can be prevented with antacids, ranitidine (Zantac), or sucralfate (Carafate).
6. Order other medications as needed, such as morphine for pain, lorazepam (Ativan) for restlessness, or haloperidol (Haldol) for agitation.

ROUTINE MODIFICATION OF SETTINGS

Arterial blood gases should be monitored and adjusted to a normal pH (7.37–7.44) and $PaO_2 > 60$ mm Hg on < 60% O_2. Tachypnea should be investigated for adequacy of ventilation or for any new cause, such as fever, prior to sedating the patient.

I. Adjusting PaO_2

A. To decrease: FiO_2 should be decreased in increments of 10–20% with either ABGs or oximetry checked in between. The "rule of sevens" states that there will be a 7 mm Hg fall in PaO_2 for each 1% decrease in FiO_2.

B. To increase

1. Ventilation has some effect on PaO_2 (as shown by the alveolar air equation); therefore, correction of the respiratory acidosis will improve oxygenation.
2. Positive end-expiratory pressure can be added in increments of 2–4 cm H_2O. PEEP recruits previously collapsed alveoli, holds them open, and restores functional residual capacity (FRC) to a more physiologic level. It counteracts pulmonary shunts and will raise PaO_2. PEEP increases intrathoracic pressure and may thus impede venous return and decrease cardiac output. This is particularly true in the presence of volume depletion and shock. If PEEP levels > 12–14 cm H_2O are needed, placement of a Swan-Ganz

catheter is recommended to monitor mixed venous oxygen levels and cardiac output.

II. Adjusting PaCO$_2$

A. To decrease
1. Increase the rate.
2. Check for leaks in the system.

B. To increase
1. Decrease the rate.
2. You may have to switch from AC mode to SIMV mode to eliminate patient-driven central hyperventilation.
3. An old (but tried and true!) method is to place increased exhalation tubing to increase dead space and actually have the patient rebreathe CO_2.

TROUBLESHOOTING

Agitation

I. **Problem.** A patient on a ventilator becomes agitated, constantly struggling, trying to pull out all tubes, and actively fighting the respirator.

II. Immediate Questions

A. **Is the patient still properly connected?** Hypoxemia or hypercapnia resulting from the patient's becoming disconnected from the respirator may result in agitation.

B. **What were the most recent arterial blood gases (ABGs)?** Again, hypoxemia or hypercapnia can cause agitation. Adjusting the settings can correct either problem.

C. **What does the chest x-ray show?** Atelectasis from mucus plugging or pneumothorax, which can occur spontaneously in asthmatics or as a result of barotrauma, can lead to hypoxemia or hypercapnia.

D. **What is the underlying diagnosis? What are the current medications and intravenous fluids?** Agitation may be related to the underlying diagnosis or a medication, and unrelated to the respiratory status. Cimetidine (Tagamet) and narcotics can cause confusion, especially in the elderly. Numerous metabolic disturbances such as hyponatremia and hypernatremia can lead to confusion and possibly agitation.

E. **What are the ventilator settings?** The ventilator may have been set incorrectly, resulting in hypoxemia or hypercapnia. Barotrauma leading to pneumothorax is associated with high PEEP settings.

III. Differential Diagnosis

A. Causes of respiratory decompensation
1. **Worsening of underlying pulmonary disease.**
2. **Pneumothorax.**
3. **Endotracheal tube (ETT) displacement.** The tube can migrate out of the trachea, high in the glottis, or down the right mainstem bronchus.
4. **Mucus plugs.** These can result in atelectasis and hypoxemia.
5. **Ventilator malfunction.**
6. **Pulmonary embolism (PE).** Immobilization is a major risk for PE.
7. **Aspiration.**
8. **Inadequate oxygenation or respiratory muscle fatigue.**

B. Sepsis.

C. ICU psychosis.

D. Medications. Numerous medications such as digoxin (Lanoxin), lidocaine, theophylline, imipenem-cilastatin (Primaxin), diazepam (Valium), and cimetidine may cause psychosis, especially in high doses or with decreased clearance states.

E. Electrolyte imbalance. Hyponatremia, hypernatremia, hypercalcemia, hypocalcemia, and hypophosphatemia can cause confusion which may lead to agitation.

IV. Database

A. Physical examination key points
1. **Endotracheal tube.** Carefully check the patency, position, and function of the ETT.
2. **Vital signs.** Tachypnea may suggest hypoxemia. Tachycardia and hypertension can result from agitation or be associated with respiratory failure or an underlying problem such as myocardial infarction. Hypotension implies sepsis, cardiogenic shock, or possible tension pneumothorax or massive pulmonary embolism. An elevated temperature suggests sepsis or possibly a pulmonary infection. Tachycardia, tachypnea, and fever may be associated with PE. A pulsus paradoxus > 20 mm Hg implies severe respiratory distress or pericardial tamponade.
3. **HEENT.** Check for distended neck veins which can result

from pericardial tamponade. Tracheal deviation may be caused by a tension pneumothorax.

4. **Chest.** Auscultate for bilateral breath sounds. Absent breath sounds on one side suggest pneumothorax or an improperly placed ETT. Bilaterally absent breath sounds can be secondary to either bilateral pneumothoraces or severe respiratory failure.

5. **Extremities.** Check for cyanosis.

6. **Skin.** Palpate for subcutaneous emphysema, which can result from a very high PEEP or may be seen in asthmatics.

B. **Laboratory data**

1. **Arterial blood gases.** Obtain ABGs to rule out hypoxemia and hypercapnia as well as severe acidosis and alkalosis.

2. **Electrolyte panel.** Determine levels of electrolytes, including calcium and phosphorus.

C. **Radiologic and other studies.** Obtain a chest x-ray to rule out atelectasis and pneumothorax and to evaluate underlying pulmonary disease.

V. Plan

A. **Emergency management**

1. Examine the patient as outlined earlier. Carefully check ETT function, ventilator connections, and the chart for medications, history, lab values, and previous settings.

2. Suction the patient vigorously. This confirms tube patency and clears out any mucus plugs.

3. Manually bag the patient to check for ease of ventilation. Marked difficulty can be seen with tension pneumothorax.

4. Obtain ABGs, electrolyte panel, and stat chest x-ray.

5. If the patient appears cyanotic or "air hungry," turn the inspired oxygen fraction (FiO_2) to 1.0 and the ventilator mode to assist control.

6. If hypotension and unilateral breath sounds are found concomitantly, consider chest tube insertion for tension pneumothorax. Patients on ventilators can rapidly die of tension pneumothorax.

7. If ICU psychosis is suspected, reassure the patient and have family members help to reorient her. Often a familiar voice will work wonders! Ask the nurses to move the patient to a room with a window; this has been shown to reduce ICU psychosis.

8. Check the ventilator settings. Perhaps too much effort is required to open the valves or to initiate a breath.

9. If everything else is stable and the patient is endangering herself, sedate the patient. Haloperidol (Haldol) 0.5–2.0 mg

IM or IV and lorazepam (Ativan) 0.5–2.0 mg IV are the currently recommended agents.

Hypoxemia

I. Problem. A patient on a respirator requires $\geq 60\%$ FiO_2 to maintain $PaO_2 > 60$ mm Hg.

II. Immediate Questions

A. What is the sequence of arterial blood gases (ABGs)? In other words, is this an acute or a slowly developing change? Rapid deterioration implies an immediately life-threatening process such as tension pneumothorax or massive pulmonary embolism (PE).

B. What is the underlying diagnosis? A patient with long bone fractures may develop fat embolus syndrome, a patient with sepsis may develop adult respiratory distress syndrome (ARDS), and a patient with head injury might develop neurogenic pulmonary edema.

C. What are the ventilator settings? Has a change been made recently? An error may have been made with the ventilator settings, or recent changes may have been made too aggressively in an attempt to wean the patient from the ventilator.

III. Differential Diagnosis

A. Shunts secondary to alveolar filling or to obstructed bronchi with consequent collapse
  1. **Pneumonia.**
  2. **Pulmonary contusion.**
  3. **Atelectasis.** The endotracheal tube (ETT) may be too far in the right mainstem bronchus, or there may be mucus plugs.
  4. **ARDS or cardiogenic pulmonary edema.**

B. Shunt at the cardiac level. An acute ventricular septal defect may develop, especially in the setting of acute myocardial infarction (MI). Sudden pulmonary hypertension will occasionally lead to a patent foramen ovale and physiologic shunt at the atrial level. A tip-off to this situation is a worsening shunt and PaO_2 as positive end-expiratory pressure (PEEP) is increased.

C. Shunts secondary to pneumothorax

D. Ventilation/perfusion (V/Q) mismatch
  1. **Bronchospasm.**
  2. **Pulmonary embolism.**

3. **Aspiration.** This is still possible, even when an ETT is in place.

E. **Inadequate ventilation**
   1. **Ventilator disconnection or malfunction.**
   2. **Wrong settings.** Has the patient recently been changed to intermittent mandatory ventilation (IMV) which has resulted in hypoventilation?
   3. **Sedatives.** Sedation can result in hypoxemia secondary to hypoventilation. These drugs should be used cautiously, especially during weaning.
   4. **Neuromuscular disease.** Hypophosphatemia or aminoglycosides can cause neuromuscular weakness, which can lead to hypoxemia secondary to hypoventilation and lack of sighing.

IV. Database
A. **Physical examination key points**
   1. **Endotracheal tube.** Confirm proper ETT position and listen for any leaks.
   2. **Vital signs.** Tachypnea implies worsening of the respiratory status. Tachycardia can be associated with a variety of conditions including PE, sepsis, MI, and worsening of underlying pulmonary disease. Fever can be seen with PE or an infection.
   3. **Neck.** Stridor suggests upper airway obstruction.
   4. **Chest.** Check for bilateral breath sounds, signs of consolidation, or new onset of wheezing. Unilateral breath sounds suggest a pneumothorax or possibly displacement of the ETT in one of the mainstem bronchi. Palpate the chest for new subcutaneous emphysema, which can occur in asthmatics or as a result of high PEEP.
   5. **Heart.** New murmurs or a new third (S3) or fourth (S4) heart sound may be present with an MI.
   6. **Extremities.** Check nail beds for cyanosis from worsening of the pulmonary status. Also check legs for unilateral edema or other signs of phlebitis, which point to PE.
   7. **Skin.** Check for new rashes to suggest a drug or anaphylactic reaction.

B. **Laboratory data**
   1. Repeat ABGs or check oximetry to assess the accuracy of initial ABGs and progression of deterioration.
   2. Sputum appearance and gram stain can direct antibiotic therapy if pneumonia is present.
   3. A Swan-Ganz catheter will have to be in place to measure mixed venous oxygen saturation (MVO_2). MVO_2 is a direct

reflection of oxygen delivery to the tissues and extraction of oxygen. It can be used to determine the presence of an intracardiac shunt.

C. Radiologic and other studies

1. **Stat chest x-ray.** Obtain a chest film to rule out atelectasis and pneumothorax and to evaluate underlying pulmonary disease.
2. **Electrocardiogram.** An evolving MI may be evident. New right axis deviation, right bundle branch block, P pulmonale, or the combination of an S wave in lead I, Q wave in lead III, and T wave in lead III ($S_1Q_3T_3$) imply PE; however, these characteristic findings are often absent. Sinus tachycardia is the most common electrocardiographic finding with PE.
3. **Ventilation/perfusion scan.** A V/Q scan should be obtained if clinical suspicion is high for PE.
4. **Swan-Ganz catheter.** This is placed to measure PaO_2 and exclude a cardiac shunt as well as to measure cardiac output and MVO_2.

V. Plan

A. Suction. Vigorously suction the patient to prove patency of the ETT and dislodge mucus plugs.

B. Correct anemia. Oxygen delivery to tissue depends on the hemoglobin level as well as cardiac output and PaO_2.

C. Treat underlying disorders

1. Insert a chest tube for pneumothorax.
2. Reassess antibiotic choices. A pneumonia secondary to *Legionella* requires erythromycin.
3. Consider more vigorous chest physical therapy or even bronchoscopy for recalcitrant mucus plugging or atelectasis.
4. Maximize the use of bronchodilators if bronchospasm is the problem. Corticosteroids such as hydrocortisone 125–500 mg or methylprednisolone 60–200 mg should be added and dosed every 4 hours. Aerosolized albuterol (Ventolin) or metaproterenol (Alupent) should likewise be given at least every 4 hours.
5. Cardiogenic pulmonary edema should be vigorously treated with afterload reduction and diuresis.

D. Optimize ventilator settings

1. Correct any hypoventilation. This may mean giving up on weaning and using the assist control (AC) mode with the patient essentially controlled on a high minute ventilation.
2. Increase FiO_2 to 100%. Your first priority is to prevent anoxic

brain or cardiac damage. You may then reduce the FiO_2 as other maneuvers further improve the pO_2.

3. PEEP will recruit unused, collapsed, or partially collapsed alveoli to overcome pulmonary shunts. It should be added in 2- to 4-cm increments while monitoring cardiac output and blood pressure.

4. As a last resort, oxygen consumption (VO_2) can be markedly reduced by administering a neuromuscular blocking agent. Vecuronium bromide (Norcuron) may be given as a 5–15 mg bolus and then a continuous drip of 4–12 mg/h. Norcuron is preferred over pancuronium because it has a shorter half-life and does not cause tachycardia. Remember to continue medications for pain and sedation since these agents do not block sensations.

E. Optimize hemodynamics

1. Consider placing a Swan-Ganz catheter when high levels of PEEP are in use, when shock of unclear cause is present, when a cardiac shunt is suspected, or when volume status is unclear.

2. Correct volume excess because it will obviously make congestive heart failure and ARDS much worse.

3. Likewise, volume depletion will alter both cardiac output and V/Q ratios and may adversely affect oxygen delivery. A fall in blood pressure with the addition of PEEP almost always means volume depletion.

4. Correct anemia so as to maximize O_2 delivery. If ARDS is present, red blood cell transfusions should either be washed or given through leukocyte removal filters to prevent an exacerbation of the disease from the transfusion.

5. Correct low cardiac output to maximize O_2 delivery. Administer positive inotropic agents such as dobutamine and drugs for afterload reduction such as intravenous nitroglycerin or nitroprusside.

Hypercapnia

I. **Problem.** $PaCO_2$ remains > 40 mm Hg in a patient on a ventilator. $PaCO_2$ is a direct reflection of both CO_2 production and alveolar ventilation. $PaCO_2$ increases when ventilation/perfusion (V/Q) mismatch worsens or dead space increases.)

II. Immediate Questions

A. **What is the sequence of arterial blood gases (ABGs)? In other words, is this an acute or a slowly developing change?** Rapid deterioration implies an immediately life-threatening process such as tension pneumothorax or massive pulmonary embolism (PE).

B. What is the underlying diagnosis? Worsening of underlying pulmonary disease (pneumonia, atelectasis, or bronchospasm) can cause hypoventilation. Long bone fractures may be complicated by fat emboli. A patient with sepsis may develop adult respiratory distress syndrome, and head injury may be complicated by neurogenic pulmonary edema.

III. Differential Diagnosis

A. Inadequate minute ventilation (V_e)
1. **Too low a rate, inadequate tidal volume, or both.**
2. **Patient tiring during synchronized intermittent mandatory ventilation (SIMV) or weaning.**
3. **Endotracheal tube (ETT) leak.**
4. **Worsening bronchospasm.**
5. **Pulmonary embolism.** Remember that immobilization is a major risk factor.

B. Increased CO_2 production
1. **High-carbohydrate feedings.**
2. **Increased metabolism.** This includes hyperthyroidism, fever, sepsis, and high work of breathing as well as rewarming after surgical procedures, a common but frequently overlooked cause of CO_2 production.

C. Oversedation. Excessive sedation decreases central ventilatory drive.

IV. Database

A. Physical examination key points
1. **Endotracheal tube.** Check the position of the tube and look for a leak.
2. **Vital signs.** Tachycardia can be associated with fever, sepsis, worsening bronchospasm, PE, and hyperthyroidism. Tachypnea can be seen with PE, worsening bronchospasm, or sepsis. Fever suggests infection but can also be seen with hyperthyroidism and PE.
3. **Chest.** Auscultate to look for new onset of wheezes or a change in the equality of breath sounds.
4. **Heart.** Listen for a new loud pulmonic second sound (P2), which suggests a PE.
5. **Extremities.** Check the legs for unilateral edema or other signs of phlebitis.
6. **Musculoskeletal examination.** Check for signs of respira-

tory fatigue: abdominal paradox or accessory muscle use is seen with severe respiratory failure.

B. Laboratory data
1. **Arterial blood gases.** Repeat ABGs or check oximetry to assess the accuracy of initial ABGs and progression of deterioration.
2. **Complete blood count with differential.** An elevated white count with increase in banded neutrophils suggests infection or sepsis.

C. Radiologic and other studies. With a chest x-ray, proper ETT position can be ensured and new pulmonary infiltrates can be ruled out.

V. Plan

A. Check the position and function of the ETT. If there is a persistent leak, replace the tube.

B. Verify proper ventilator function. Check especially for leaky connections.

C. Drugs. Verify that the sedation medications ordered are those that have actually been given and note when they were last administered. If the patient is oversedated, you can either increase the minute ventilation or reverse narcotic sedation with naloxone (Narcan) 0.4 mg IV.

D. Look for a source of sepsis. Adjust antibiotics as indicated. Lower oxygen consumption (VO_2) by treating fever with Tylenol or a cooling blanket.

E. Review ventilator settings. If the tidal volume is too low, dead space ventilation will be present. Correct this by raising the tidal volume. If the patient is tiring on a low SIMV rate, switch either to a higher rate or back to assist control (AC) mode.

F. Review the nutrition regimen in use. If the patient is critically ill with bronchospasm or ARDS, you may be forced to reduce CO_2 production. To do this, decrease the D25W in hyperalimentation fluids to D15W or D10W. The caloric difference can be made up with lipids; as much as 500 mL of 20% intralipids can be given IV daily.

High Peak Pressures

I. Problem. The ventilator peak pressures remain consistently above 50 cm H_2O.

II. Immediate Questions

A. **Is this a new problem or has it developed progressively?** The answer to this question will be readily available on the respiratory therapy bedside flow sheet.

B. **What is the underlying diagnosis?** Severe underlying pulmonary disease can cause high ventilatory peak pressures.

C. **What are the most recent arterial blood gases?** A decrease in pO_2, increase in pCO_2, or combination of both may point to worsening of the underlying pulmonary disease.

D. **Has endotracheal tube function or position changed? Is it possible to suction the patient?** The tube could be kinked or plugged with secretions.

III. Differential Diagnosis

A. **Endotracheal tube**
   1. The ETT is too small or is obstructed with secretions.
   2. The tube is kinked, especially if nasotracheally placed.
   3. The tube has migrated down the right mainstem bronchus so that the entire tidal volume is going into one lung. This also increases coughing and anxiety.

B. **Incorrect ventilator settings**
   1. **High tidal volume.** Tidal volumes > 12 mL/kg may tremendously increase distention pressure.
   2. **High positive end-expiratory pressure.** PEEP should always be used at the lowest possible level.
   3. **High minute ventilation.** A high minute ventilation may lead to the phenomenon of "auto PEEP," in which inadequate time to exhale leads to "stacked breaths."

C. **Worsening lung disease.** All of these following conditions show concomitant falls in lung compliance:
   1. Severe status asthmaticus.
   2. Adult respiratory distress syndrome.
   3. Cardiogenic pulmonary edema.
   4. Interstitial lung disease.

D. **Uncooperative or agitated patient**
   1. Biting the ETT.
   2. Fighting the ventilator.
   3. Coughing.

E. **Abdominal distention**

F. **Tension pneumothorax.** It is always imperative to exclude pneumothorax as a cause of new onset of high peak pressures because death can occur quickly.

IV. Database

A. Physical examination key points

1. **Endotracheal tube.** Verify the patency of the ETT and check its position to rule out migration down the right mainstem bronchus.

2. **Vital signs.** Tachycardia and tachypnea can occur with worsening of the underlying pulmonary disease and with agitation. Hypotension and tachycardia suggest tension pneumothorax.

3. **HEENT.** An increase in jugular venous distention (JVD) implies congestive heart failure. Tracheal deviation can be seen with tension pneumothorax.

4. **Chest.** Absent breath sounds, especially with hypotension, and unilateral hyperresonance to percussion point to tension pneumothorax. Rales suggest congestive heart failure.

5. **Heart.** A third heart sound (S3) implies left ventricular dysfunction or congestive heart failure.

6. **Abdomen.** Examine for tenderness and distention.

7. **Extremities.** New cyanosis is consistent with worsening of the underlying pulmonary disease. Edema will be seen with biventricular or right-sided heart failure.

8. **Skin.** Check for subcutaneous emphysema, which can be associated with barotrauma or seen with severe asthma.

B. Laboratory data

1. **Arterial blood gases.** Repeat ABGs or check oximetry to assess the accuracy of initial AGBs and progression of deterioration.

2. **Complete blood count with differential.** An elevated white count with increase in banded neutrophils suggests infection or sepsis.

C. Radiologic and other studies.
Use a stat portable chest x-ray to check the position of the ETT, rule out kinking, rule out pneumothorax, and assess any change in underlying pulmonary disease.

V. Plan

A. Try to suction the patient.
If the patient is biting down on the ETT, insert an oral airway or sedate her. If she is not biting down but the suction tube will not pass, the ETT is kinked or blocked and must be replaced.

B. Ventilate the patient with an ambu bag and confirm equal breath sounds.
Unequal breath sounds could result from tension pneumothorax or from improper positioning of the ETT. Reposition the tube if necessary. In an average-sized person, an oral ETT should not be in farther than 24 cm at the lip; however,

there is considerable variability among patients and the chest x-ray should always be reviewed. If there is considerable resistance to bagging, a tension pneumothorax may be present.

C. Place a chest tube if pneumothorax is present.

D. Adjust the ventilator. Try to reduce PEEP to the minimum needed for adequate oxygenation. Try reducing high tidal volumes to 10 mL/kg. Increase FiO_2 as needed to ensure adequate oxygenation.

E. Sedation may have to be increased.

F. Adjustment of alarms. If all possibilities have been evaluated, alarms may be increased to higher levels; however, the risk of an acute tension pneumothorax will increase with higher peak pressures.

WEANING

I. **Requirements.** Once the underlying cause of respiratory failure has been corrected, it is time for the most arduous task of all: weaning the patient from the respirator.

A. **Stabilization.** The underlying disease must be under optimum control.

B. **Initiation of weaning.** The process is begun in the early morning. Patients like to rest rather than work all night—just like doctors! Criteria for initiating weaning are listed in Table 6–1.

II. **Techniques**

A. **T-Piece (or T-tube bypass).** The patient is taken off the respira-

TABLE 6–1. CRITERIA FOR WEANING FROM MECHANICAL VENTILATION.

Parameter	Value
Pulmonary mechanics	
Vital capacity	> 10–15 mL/kg
Resting minute ventilation (tidal volume × rate)	> 10 L/min
Spontaneous respiratory rate	< 30 breaths/min
Negative inspiratory forces	> –25 cm H_2O
Oxygenation	
A-a gradient	< 300–500 mm Hg
Shunt fraction	< 15%
PO_2 (on 40% FIO_2)	> 70 mm Hg
PCO_2	< 45 mm Hg

From Gomella LG (ed): Clinician's Pocket Reference, 7th ed. Norwalk, Connecticut, Appleton & Lange, 1992.

tor for a limited period and the endotracheal tube (ETT) is connected to a constant flow of O_2 (usually 40%). If the patient tolerates breathing independently, the length of time off the respirator is progressively increased. This is a tried and true method. It is particularly easy to use in patients with no underlying lung disease, such as those recovering from a drug overdose.

There are several drawbacks to this technique. No alarms are available since the patient is totally disconnected from the ventilator. It is time consuming for the respiratory therapists and nurses. Perhaps most importantly, it is much more work than spontaneously breathing without an ETT. This is due to the relatively small diameter of the tube: remember, resistance increases by the fourth power of the radius.

B. **Synchronized intermittent mandatory ventilation (SIMV).** In this method, fewer and fewer machine breaths are given as the patient begins taking spontaneous breaths in between. For example, a patient breathing at a rate of 14 in assist control mode is switched to SIMV mode, rate 14. The rate is then decreased to 10, to 6, to 4, and then to 0. Most physicians either place the patient on continuous positive airway pressure (CPAP) mode at this juncture or observe the patient briefly on a T-piece.

This method has several theoretical advantages over T-piece weaning. Backup alarms, including automatic rates in case of apnea, are in place. A graded assumption of work is done, allowing "retraining" of respiratory muscles. This method has never been proven clearly superior to T-piece weaning, however. Moreover, the work of breathing is still high because of ETT resistance as well as the inherent resistance of the SIMV circuit valves. One way to decrease the work of breathing with the SIMV weaning technique is to add pressure support (PS) to the system. Pressure support is a positive pressure boost that is initiated when the respirator senses a certain liter flow rate during inspiration. The respirator then supplies a set amount of positive pressure (and, by Boyle's law, it also supplies some tidal volume). A PS level of 10–15 cm H_2O will overcome the increased work caused by ETT resistance.

C. **Continuous positive airway pressure and pressure support.** With this method the patient is switched to the spontaneous breathing mode, which in modern ventilators is the CPAP mode. In current usage, CPAP is equivalent to positive end expiratory pressure (PEEP) except that it is used exclusively in spontaneously breathing mode. Anywhere from 0 to 30 cm H_2O pressure may be used, but generally the lowest level possible (usually 0–5 cm) is preferred. Pressure support may be used concomitantly to augment the patient's spontaneous breaths. It can then be progressively decreased as the patient increases tidal volumes. For example, PS levels of 25, then 20, then 15, and finally 10 can be used while monitoring the patient's breath rate, tidal volumes, and arterial blood gases (ABGs). This method requires an alert, cooperative patient who is spontaneously breathing (and if you do not have that, why wean anyway?). Machine backup functions remain in place in case of apnea or other inadequate parameters.

III. **Timing.** Deciding when to extubate the patient is part of the art of medicine. Still, fulfilling certain criteria ensures success:

A. Breath rate is < 30/min.

B. ABGs show a pH > 7.35 and adequate oxygenation.

C. The patient is awake and alert.

D. A normal gag reflex is present.

E. The stomach is not distended.

IV. **Postextubation.** After extubation, it is important that the patient be encouraged to cough frequently and forcefully. Respiratory therapy treatments should be continued. During waking hours, incentive spirometry should be used several times an hour to encourage deep breathing. The patient must be carefully observed for stridor, respiratory muscle fatigue, or other signs of failure. Oxygen should be continued at the same level or at a level slightly higher than was given via the respirator prior to intubation. ABGs should be checked 2–4 hours after extubation to confirm the adequacy of ventilation and oxygenation.

REFERENCES

Burns DM: Mechanical ventilation: devices and methods. In Bordow RA, Moser KM (eds): *Manual of Clinical Problems in Pulmonary Medicine,* 2nd ed. Boston, Little, Brown, 1985, pp 238–241.

Burns DM: Mechanical ventilation: weaning and complications. In Bordow RA, Moser KM (eds): *Manual of Clinical Problems in Pulmonary Medicine,* 2nd ed. Boston, Little, Brown, 1985, pp 241–244.

Glauser FL, Polatty C, Sessler CN. Worsening oxygenation in the mechanically ventilated patient: causes, mechanisms and early detection. *Am Rev Respir Dis* 138:458, 1988.

Luce JM et al: Intermittent mandatory ventilation. *Chest* 79:678, 1981.

MacIntyre NR: Weaning from mechanical ventilatory support: volume-assisting intermittent breaths versus pressure-assisting every breath. *Respir Care* 33:121, 1988.

Spragg RC, Krieger BP: Airway control. In Bordow RA, Moser KM (eds): *Manual of Clinical Problems in Pulmonary Medicine,* 2nd ed. Boston, Little, Brown, 1985, pp 235–238.

7 Commonly Used Medications

Generic Drugs: General Classification	Cephalosporins
Generic Drugs: Indications and Dosages	Nonsteroidal Anti-inflammatory Agents
Antipseudomonal Penicillins	Oral Contraceptives
Antistaphylococcal Penicillins	Sulfonylureas
Beta Blocking Agents	Breast Feeding and Medications
	Therapeutic Drug Levels
	Aminoglycoside Dosing

This section is designed to serve as a quick reference to commonly used medications in obstetric and gynecologic patients. You should be familiar with all the indications, contraindications, and side effects of any medications that you prescribe. Such detailed information is beyond the scope of this manual and can be found in the package insert, *Physicians' Desk Reference* (*PDR*), or the *American Hospital Formulary Service*.

Drugs in this section are listed in alphabetical order by generic name. Some of the more common trade names are listed for each medication. Drugs under the control of the Drug Enforcement Agency (Schedule II–V controlled substances) are indicated by the symbol [C].

The FDA Pregnancy Category is included for most of the listed medications.

Category A: **Controlled studies show no risk.** Adequate, well-controlled studies in pregnant women have failed to demonstrate risk to the fetus.

Category B: **No evidence of risk in humans.** Either animal findings show risk but human findings do not or, if no adequate human studies have been done, animal findings are negative.

Category C: **Risk cannot be ruled out.** Human studies are lacking, and animal studies are either positive for fetal risk or lacking as well. However, potential benefits may justify the potential risk.

Category D: **Positive evidence of risk.** Investigational or postmarketing data show risk to the fetus. Nevertheless, potential benefits may outweigh the potential risk.

Category X: **Contraindicated in pregnancy.** Studies in animals or humans, or investigational or postmarketing reports, have shown fetal risk which clearly outweighs any possible benefit to the patient.

GENERIC DRUGS: GENERAL CLASSIFICATION

Analgesic/Anti-inflammatory/Antipyretic

Acetaminophen
Acetaminophen with butalbital and caffeine
Acetaminophen with codeine
Aspirin
Aspirin with butalbital and caffeine
Aspirin with codeine
Buprenorphine
Butorphanol
Codeine
Diclofenac sodium
Diflunisal
Fenoprofen
Flurbiprofen
Hydromorphone
Ibuprofen
Indomethacin
Ketoprofen
Ketorolac
Levorphanol
Meperidine
Methadone
Morphine sulfate
Nalbuphine
Naproxen
Oxycodone
Pentazocine
Piroxicam
Propoxyphene
Sulindac
Tolmetin

Antacid/Anti-Gas

Aluminum carbonate
Aluminum hydroxide
Aluminum hydroxide with magnesium hydroxide
Aluminum hydroxide with magnesium hydroxide and simethicone
Aluminum hydroxide with magnesium trisilicate and alginic acid
Calcium carbonate
Dihydroxyaluminum sodium carbonate
Magaldrate
Simethicone

Antianxiety

Alprazolam
Chlordiazepoxide
Clorazepate
Diazepam
Doxepin
Halazepam
Hydroxyzine
Lorazepam
Meprobamate
Oxazepam
Prazepam

Antiarrhythmic

Amiodarone
Bretylium
Disopyramide
Encainide
Flecainide
Lidocaine
Mexiletine
Procainamide
Quinidine
Tocainide

Antibiotic

Amikacin
Amoxicillin
Amoxicillin and potassium
  clavulanate
Ampicillin
Ampicillin and sulbactam
Azithromycin
Aztreonam
Carbenicillin
Cefaclor
Cefadroxil
Cefamandole
Cefazolin
Cefixime
Cefmetazole
Cefonicid
Cefoperazone
Ceforanide
Cefotaxime
Cefotetan
Cefoxitin
Cefprozil
Ceftazidime
Ceftizoxime
Ceftriaxone
Cefuroxime
Cefuroxime axetil
Cephalexin
Cephalothin
Cephapirin
Cephradine
Chloramphenicol
Ciprofloxacin
Clarithromycin
Clindamycin
Cloxacillin
Demeclocycline
Dicloxacillin
Doxycycline
Erythromycin
Ethambutol
Gentamicin
Imipenem and cilastatin
Isoniazid
Methicillin

Metronidazole
Mezlocillin
Minocycline
Nafcillin
Neomycin sulfate
Netilmicin
Norflaxacin
Ofloxacin
Oxacillin
Penicillin G aqueous
Penicillin G benzathine
Penicillin G procaine
Penicillin V potassium
Pentamidine
Piperacillin
Rifampin
Silver sulfadiazine
Streptomycin
Sulfamethoxazole
Sulfasalazine
Sulfisoxazole
Tetracycline
Ticarcillin
Ticarcillin and potassium clavulanate
Tobramycin
Trimethoprim and sul-
  famethoxazole
Vancomycin

Anticoagulant/Thrombolytic and Related Agents

Alteplase, recombinant
Aminocaproic acid
Anistreplase
Antihemophilic factor (Factor VIII)
Dipyridamole
Heparin
Pentoxifylline
Protamine sulfate
Streptokinase
Urokinase
Warfarin

Anticonvulsant

Carbamazepine
Clonazepam

Diazepam
Ethosuximide
Lorazepam
Pentobarbital
Phenobarbital
Phenytoin
Valproic acid

Antidepressant

Amitriptyline
Amoxapine
Doxepin
Imipramine
Nortriptyline
Sertraline
Trazodone

Antidiabetic

Acetohexamide
Chlorpropamide
Glipizide
Glyburide
Insulins
Tolazamide
Tolbutamide

Antidiarrheal

Diphenoxylate with atropine
Kaolin and pectin
Lactobacillus
Loperamide
Opium, camphorated tincture
Opium, tincture

Antiemetic/Emetic

Benzquinamide
Buclizine
Chlorpromazine
Cyclizine
Dimenhydrinate
Dronabinol
Droperidol
Gallium nitrate
Ipecac syrup
Meclizine

Metoclopramide
Ondansetron
Prochlorperazine
Promethazine
Thiethylperazine
Trimethobenzamide

Antifungal

Amphotericin B
Butoconazole
Clotrimazole
Clotrimazole and betamethasone
Econazole
Fluconazole
Flucytosine
Griseofulvin
Ketoconazole
Miconazole
Nystatin
Terconazole
Tioconazole

Antihistamine

Astemizole
Azatadine
Brompheniramine
Chlorpheniramine
Clemastine fumarate
Cyproheptadine
Diphenhydramine
Promethazine
Terfenadine
Trimeprazine
Triprolidine

Antihyperlipidemic

Cholestyramine
Colestipol
Gemfibrozil
Lovastatin
Niacin
Pravastatin
Probucol
Simvastatin

Antihypertensive

Acebutolol
Atenolol
Captopril
Clonidine
Diazoxide
Diltiazem
Enalapril
Felodipine
Guanabenz
Guanadrel
Guanethidine
Guanfacine
Hydralazine
Isradipine
Labetalol
Lisinopril
Methyldopa
Metoprolol
Minoxidil
Nadolol
Nicardipine
Nifedipine
Nitroglycerin
Nitroprusside
Penbutolol
Pindolol
Prazosin
Propranolol
Quinapril
Terazosin
Timolol
Trimethaphan camsylate
Verapamil

Antineoplastic

Altretamine
Bleomycin
Carboplatin
Chlorambucil
Cisplatin
Cyclophosphamide
Dacarbazine
Dactinomycin
Diethylstilbestrol
Doxorubicin
Etoposide
Fluorouracil
Hydroxyurea
Ifosfamide
Interferon alfa
Leucovorin
Leuprolide
Medroxyprogesterone
Megestrol acetate
Melphalan
Mesna
Methotrexate
Mitomycin
Nitrogen mustard
Plicamycin
Tamoxifen citrate
Triethylene-thiophosphoramide
Vinblastine
Vincristine

Antipsychotic

Chlorpromazine
Haloperidol
Lithium carbonate
Molindone
Perphenazine
Prochlorperazine
Thioridazine
Thiothixene
Trifluoperazine

Antitussive/Decongestant/ Expectorant/Mucolytic

Acetylcysteine
Benzonatate
Codeine
Dextromethorphan
Guaifenesin
Pseudoephedrine

Antiviral

Acyclovir
Amantadine
Foscarnet

Ganciclovir
Vidarabine
Zidovudine (AZT)

Bronchodilator

Albuterol
Aminophylline
Bitolterol
Ephedrine sulfate
Epinephrine
Isoetharine
Isoproterenol
Metaproterenol
Oxtriphylline
Terbutaline
Theophylline

Cardiovascular

Acebutolol
Amrinone
Atenolol
Atropine
Carteolol
Digoxin
Diltiazem
Dipyridamole
Dobutamine
Dopamine
Edrophonium
Ephedrine sulfate
Epinephrine
Esmolol
Isoproterenol
Isosorbide dinitrate
Isosorbide monohydrate
Labetalol
Metoprolol
Nadolol
Nicardipine
Nifedipine
Nitroglycerin
Norepinephrine
Penbutolol
Phenylephrine
Pindolol
Propranolol

Sodium polystyrene sulfonate
Timolol
Verapamil

Cathartic/Laxative

Bisacodyl
Docusate calcium
Docusate potassium
Docusate sodium
Glycerin suppositories
Lactulose
Magnesium citrate
Magnesium hydroxide
Mineral oil
Polyethylene glycol–electrolyte
  solution
Psyllium
Sorbitol

Diuretic

Acetazolamide
Amiloride
Bumetanide
Chlorothiazide
Chlorthalidone
Ethacrynic acid
Furosemide
Hydrochlorothiazide
Hydrochlorothiazide and amiloride
Hydrochlorothiazide and spirono-
  lactone
Hydrochlorothiazide and
  triamterene
Indapamide
Mannitol
Metolazone
Spironolactone
Triamterene

Emetic
(see Antiemetic/Emetic)

Estrogen

Estradiol, topical
Estradiol transdermal system
Estrogen, conjugated

Estrogen, conjugated with
  methyltestosterone
Estrogen, esterified
Estrogen, esterified with
  methyltestosterone
Ethinyl estradiol

Gastrointestinal

Belladonna tincture
Cimetidine
Dicyclomine
Famotidine
Hyoscyamine sulfate
Mesalamine enema
Metoclopramide
Misoprostol
Nizatidine
Omeprazole
Pancreatin
Pancrelipase
Propantheline
Ranitidine
Sucralfate
Vasopressin

Hormone/Synthetic Substitute

Cortisone
Desmopressin
Desoxycorticosterone acetate
  (DOCA)
Dexamethasone
Fludrocortisone acetate
Glucagon
Gonadorelin
Hydrocortisone
Leuprolide
Levonorgestrel implants
Medroxyprogesterone
Methylprednisolone
Metyrapone
Nafarelin
Norethindrone
Prednisolone
Prednisone

Progesterone in oil
Vasopressin

Immunosuppressive

Antithymocyte globulin (ATG)
Azathioprine
Cyclosporine
Steroids

Local Anesthetic

Anusol
Lidocaine

Muscle Relaxant

Carisoprodol
Chlorzoxazone
Cyclobenzaprine
Diazepam
Methocarbamol
Pancuronium
Vecuronium

Narcotic Antagonist

Naloxone

Oral Contraceptive

See Table 7–11

Ovulation Stimulant

Chorionic gonadotropin
Clomiphene citrate
Menotropins
Urofollitropin

Oxytocic

Methylergonovine
Oxytocin

Plasma Volume Expander

Albumin
Dextran 40
Hetastarch
Plasma protein fraction

Respiratory Inhalant

Acetylcysteine
Beclomethasone
Cromolyn sodium
Flunisolide
Ipratropium bromide

Sedative/Hypnotic

Diphenhydramine
Flurazepam
Hydroxyzine
Lorazepam
Pentobarbital
Phenobarbital
Secobarbital
Temazepam
Triazolam

Supplement

Calcium salts
Cholecalciferol
Cyanocabalamin
Ferrous sulfate
Folic acid
Iron dextran
Magnesium oxide
Magnesium sulfate
Phytonadione (vitamin K)
Potassium supplements
Pyridoxine
Sodium bicarbonate
Thiamine

Thyroid/Antithyroid

Levothyroxine
Liothyronine
Liotrix
Methimazole
Propylthiouracil
SSKI (saturated solution of potassium iodide)

Tocolytic

Magnesium sulfate
Ritodrine
Terbutaline

Toxoid/Vaccine/Serum

Hepatitis B immune globulin
Hepatitis B vaccine
Immune globulin, intravenous
Pneumococcal vaccine polyvalent
Tetanus immune globulin
Tetanus toxoid

Urinary Tract Agent

Belladonna and opium suppositories
Bethanechol
Flavoxate
Hyoscyamine sulfate
Methenamine mandelate and hippurate
Nalidixic acid
Neomycin-polymyxin bladder irrigant
Nitrofurantoin
Oxybutynin
Phenazopyridine
Trimethoprim

Vaginal Preparation

Amino-Cerv pH 5.5 cream
Butoconazole
Estradiol, topical
Miconazole
Nystatin
Terconazole
Tioconazole
Triple sulfa cream

Miscellaneous

Beractant
Bromocriptine
Charcoal, activated
Colfosceril palmitate
Crotamiton
Disulfiram
Epoetin alfa (erythropoietin)

Lindane (gamma benzene
   hexachloride)
Midazolam
Nicotine transdermal

Permethrin
Physostigmine
Probenecid
Progestin levonorgestrel

GENERIC DRUGS: INDICATIONS AND DOSAGES

Acebutolol (Sectral) (see Table 7–6, page 571)

Acetaminophen (Tylenol, others)

Category: B

Indications: Mild pain, headache, fever

Actions: Nonnarcotic analgesic, antipyretic

Dosage: 650–1000 mg PO or PR q4–6h

Supplied: Tablets 325 mg, 500 mg; elixir 120 mg/5 mL; suppositories 325, 650 mg

Notes: Overdose causes hepatotoxicity—treat with *N*-acetylcysteine (charcoal not usually recommended); unlike aspirin, has no anti-inflammatory or platelet-inhibiting action

Acetaminophen with Butalbital and Caffeine (Fioricet)

Category: C

Indications: Mild pain, headache, especially with associated stress

Actions: Nonnarcotic analgesic

Dosage: 1–2 tablets or capsules PO q4–6h prn

Supplied: Each tablet or capsule contains 325 mg acetaminophen, 40 mg caffeine, and 50 mg butalbital

Acetaminophen with Codeine (Tylenol No. 1, 2, 3, 4) [C]

Category: C

Indications: Relief of mild to moderate pain

Actions: Combined effects of acetaminophen and a narcotic analgesic

Dosage: 1–2 tablets q3–4h prn

Supplied: Tablets; capsules; elixir containing acetaminophen 120 mg and codeine 12 mg per 5 mL

Notes: Codeine in No. 1 = 7.5 mg, No. 2 = 15 mg, No. 3 = 30 mg, No. 4 = 60 mg

Acetazolamide (Diamox)

Category: C

Indications: Diuresis, glaucoma, alkalinization of urine

Actions: Carbonic anhydrase inhibitor

Dosage:
  Diuretic: 250–375 mg IV or PO qd
  Glaucoma: 250 mg PO qd–qid; maximum of 1000 mg/d

Supplied: Tablets 125 mg, 250 mg; SR capsules 500 mg; injection 500 mg per vial

Notes: Contraindicated in renal failure, sulfa hypersensitivity; follow Na^+ and K^+; watch for metabolic acidosis

Acetohexamide (Dymelor) (see Table 7–12, page 578)

Acetylcysteine (Mucomyst)

Indications: Mucolytic agent as adjuvant therapy for chronic broncho-pulmonary diseases and cystic fibrosis; as antidote to acetaminophen hepatotoxicity within 24 hours of ingestion

Actions: Splits disulfide linkages between mucoprotein molecular complexes; protects the liver by restoring glutathione levels in acetaminophen overdose

Dosage:
  Nebulizer: 3–5 mL of 20% solution diluted with equal volume of water or normal saline, administred tid–qid
  Antidote, PO or NG: 140 mg/kg diluted 1 : 4 in carbonated beverage as loading dose, then 70 mg/kg q4h for 17 doses

Supplied: Solution 10%, 20%

Notes: Watch for bronchospasm when used by inhalation in asthmatics; activated charcoal will adsorb acetylcysteine when given orally for acute acetaminophen ingestion/toxicity

Acyclovir (Zovirax)

Category: C

Indications: Treatment and prevention of herpes simplex, herpes zoster, and varicella-zoster viral infections

Actions: Inhibits viral DNA replication

Dosage:

Topical: Apply 0.5 inch ribbon q3h

Oral:

- *Initial therapy for genital herpes:* 200 mg po q4h while awake, for total of 5 capsules per day for 10 days
- *Chronic suppression:* 200 mg PO tid for up to 6 months
- *Intermittent therapy:* As for initial therapy, except treat for 5 days beginning at the earliest prodrome
- *Herpes zoster:* 800 mg 5 times per day

Intravenous: 5 mg/kg IV q8h for 5–7 days

Supplied: Ointment 5%; capsules 200 mg; injection 500 mg per vial

Notes: Adjust the dosage in renal failure

Adenosine (Adenocard)

Category: C

Indications: Paroxysmal supraventricular tachycardia, including that associated with Wolff-Parkinson-White syndrome

Actions: Class 4 antiarrhythmic; slows conduction time through the AV node

Dosage: 6 mg rapid IV bolus; may be repeated in 1–2 minutes at 12 mg IV if no response

Supplied: Injection 6 mg/2 mL

Notes: Doses > 12 mg are not recommended; caffeine and theophylline antagonize its effects

Albumin (Albuminar, Albutein, Buminate, others)

Indications: Plasma volume expansion for shock resulting from burns, surgery, hemorrhage, or other trauma

Actions: Maintenance of plasma colloid oncotic pressure

Dosage: 25 g IV initially; subsequent infusions should depend upon clinical situation and response

Supplied: Solution 5%, 25%

Notes: Contains 130–160 meq Na^+/L

Albuterol (Proventil, Ventolin)

Category: C

Indications: Treatment of bronchospasm in reversible obstructive airway disease; prevention of exercise-induced bronchospasm

Actions: Beta-adrenergic sympathomimetic bronchodilator

Dosage: 2–4 inhalations q4–6h; 1 Rotacap q4–6h; 2–4 mg PO tid–qid

Supplied: Tablets 2 mg, 4 mg; syrup 2 mg/5 mL; metered-dose inhaler; solution for nebulization 0.083%, 0.5%; Rotacap 200 µg

Alprazolam (Xanax) [C]

Category: D

Indications: Management of anxiety disorders, anxiety associated with depression

Actions: Benzodiazepine

Dosage: 0.25–0.5 mg PO tid (maximum 4 mg/d)

Supplied: Tablets 0.25 mg, 0.5 mg, 1.0 mg

Notes: Reduce the dosage in elderly and debilitated patients

Alteplase, Recombinant (Activase)

Category: C

Indications: Treatment of acute myocardial infarction

Actions: Tissue plasminogen activator; causes thrombolysis

Dosage: 100 mg IV over 3 hours

Supplied: Powder for injection 20 mg, 50 mg

Notes: Bleeding is an adverse effect

Altretamine (Hexalen)

Category: D

Indications: Ovarian cancer

Actions: Unknown

Dosage: Varies with protocol

Supplied: Capsules 50 mg

Notes: Can cause nausea, vomiting, bone marrow suppression, and peripheral neuropathy

Aluminum Carbonate (Basaljel)

Indications: Hyperacidity (peptic ulcer, hiatal hernia, etc), supplement to management of hyperphosphatemia

Actions: Neutralizes gastric acid

Dosage: 2 capsules or tablets or 10 mL (in water) q2h prn

Supplied: Capsules, tablets, suspension

Aluminum Hydroxide (ALternaGEL, Amphojel)

Indications: Hyperacidity (peptic ulcer, hiatal hernia, etc), supplement to management of hyperphosphatemia

Actions: Neutralizes gastric acid

Dosage: 10–30 mL or 1–2 tablets (0.6 g) PO 4–6 times daily

Supplied: Tablets 300 mg, 600 mg; chewable tablets 500 mg; suspension 320 mg/5 mL, 600 mg/5 mL

Notes: May be used in renal insufficiency; can cause constipation

Aluminum Hydroxide with Magnesium Hydroxide (Maalox)

Indications: Hyperacidity (peptic ulcer, hiatal hernia, etc)

Actions: Neutralizes gastric acid

Dosage: 10–60 mL or 2–4 tablets PO qid or prn

Supplied: Tablets, suspension

Notes: Doses qid best given after meals and at bedtime; use with caution in renal failure; can cause hypermagnesemia, especially with renal insufficiency

Aluminum Hydroxide with Magnesium Hydroxide and Simethicone (Maalox Plus, Mylanta, Mylanta II)

Indications: Hyperacidity with bloating (peptic ulcer, etc)

Actions: Neutralizes gastric acid

Dosage: 10–60 mL or 2–4 tablets PO qid or prn

Supplied: Tablets, suspension

Notes: Use with caution in renal insufficiency (can cause hypermagnesemia); Mylanta II contains twice the amount of aluminum and magnesium hydroxide as Mylanta

Aluminum Hydroxide with Magnesium Trisilicate and Alginic Acid (Gaviscon)

Indications: Symptomatic relief of heartburn, hiatal hernia

Actions: Neutralizes gastric acid

Dosage: 2–4 tablets or 15–30 mL PO qid followed by water

Supplied: Tablets, suspension

Amantadine (Symmetrel)

Category: C

Indications: Treatment or prophylaxis of influenza A viral infection

Actions: Prevents release of infectious viral nucleic acid into the host cell

Dosage: 200 mg PO qd or 100 mg PO bid

Supplied: Capsules 100 mg; syrup 50 mg/5 mL

Notes: Reduce the dosage in renal failure

Amikacin (Amikin)

Category: D

Indications: Short-term therapy for serious infections due to gram-negative aerobes and staphylococci

Actions: Aminoglycoside antibiotic

Dosage: 15 mg/kg/24h IV divided q8–12h or based on renal function; refer to **Aminoglycoside Dosing,** page 567.

Supplied: Injection 100 mg/2 mL, 500 mg/2 mL

Notes: Not a first-line drug; may be effective against gram-negative bacteria resistant to gentamicin or tobramycin; monitor renal function carefully for dosage adjustments

Amiloride (Midamor)

Category: B

Indications: Hypertension, congestive heart failure

Actions: Potassium-sparing diuretic

Dosage: 5 mg PO qd; increase to 10 mg qd if needed

Supplied: Tablets 5 mg

Notes: Hyperkalemia may occur; monitor serum potassium

Aminocaproic Acid (Amicar)

Category: C

Indications: Treatment of excessive bleeding resulting from systemic hyperfibrinolysis and urinary fibrinolysis

Actions: Inhibits fibrinolysis via inhibition of plasminogen activator substances

Dosage: 100 mg/kg IV, then 1 g/m^2/h to maximum of 18 g/m^2/d or 100 mg/kg/dose q8h

Supplied: Tablets 500 mg; syrup 250 mg/mL; injection 250 mg/mL

Notes: Administer for 8 hours or until bleeding is controlled; contraindicated in disseminated intravascular coagulation (DIC); **not for upper urinary tract bleeding**

Amino-Cerv pH 5.5 Cream

Indications: Mild cervicitis, postpartum cervicitis or cervical tears, and following cauterization, cryosurgery, and conization

Dosage:
Mild cervicitis: 1 applicatorful intravaginally qhs for 2 weeks
Postpartum (after bleeding has subsided): 1 applicatorful intravaginally qhs for 4 weeks
Postcauterization, postcryosurgery, postconization: 1 applicatorful intravaginally qhs for 2–4 weeks

Supplied: Vaginal cream

Notes: Contains 8.34% urea, 0.5% sodium propionate, 0.83% methionine, 0.35% cystine, 0.83% inositol, benzalkonium chloride

Aminophylline

Category: C

Indications: Asthma, bronchospasm

Actions: Relaxes smooth muscle of the bronchi and pulmonary blood vessels

Dosage:
Acute Asthma Attack: Load 6 mg/kg IV, then 0.4–0.9 mg/kg/h IV
Chronic asthma: 24 mg/kg/d PO or PR divided q6h

Supplied: Tablets 100 mg, 200 mg; solution 105 mg/5 mL; suppositories 250 mg, 500 mg; injection 25 mg/mL

Notes: Individualize dosage; signs of toxicity include nausea, vomiting, irritability, tachycardia, ventricular arrhythmias, and seizures; following serum levels is necessary (see Table 7–14, Drug Levels; aminophylline is about 85% theophylline); rectal doses are absorbed erratically

Amiodarone (Cordarone)

Category: D

Indications: Treatment of recurrent ventricular fibrillation or hemodynamically unstable ventricular tachycardia

Actions: Class 3 antiarrhythmic

Dosage:
Loading dose: 800–1600 mg PO qd for 1–3 weeks
Maintenance: 600–800 mg PO qd for 1 month, then 200–400 mg qd

Supplied: Tablets 200 mg

Notes: Average half-life is 53 days; potentially toxic effects leading to pulmonary fibrosis, liver failure, ocular opacities, as well as exacerbation of arrhythmias; **patient must be hospitalized during loading;** response requires 1 month as a rule

Amitriptyline (Elavil, others)

Category: D

Indications: Depression, peripheral neuropathy, chronic pain, cluster and migraine headaches

Actions: Tricyclic antidepressant

Dosage: Initially, 50–100 mg PO qhs; may increase to 300 mg qhs

Supplied: Tablets 10 mg, 25 mg, 50 mg, 75 mg, 100 mg, 150 mg; injection 10 mg/mL

Notes: Has strong anticholinergic side effects; can cause urine retention, sedation

Amoxapine (Asendin)

Category: C

Indications: Depression, anxiety

Actions: Tricyclic antidepressant

Dosage: Initially, 150 mg PO qhs or 50 mg PO tid; increase to 300 mg qd

Supplied: Tablets 25 mg, 50 mg, 100 mg, 150 mg

Notes: Reduce dosage in the elderly; taper slowly when discontinuing therapy

Amoxicillin (Amoxil, Larotid, Polymox, others)

Category: B

Indications: Treatment of susceptible gram-negative bacteria (*H. influenzae, E. coli, P. mirabilis, N. gonorrhoeae*) and gram-positive bacteria (streptococci)

Actions: Inhibits cell wall synthesis

Dosage: 250–500 mg PO q8h

Supplied: Capsules 250 mg, 500 mg; suspension 50 mg/5 mL, 125 mg/5 mL, 250 mg/5 mL

Notes: Has cross-hypersensitivity with penicillin; can cause diarrhea, but less frequently than with ampicillin; skin rash is common; many hospital strains of *E. coli* are now resistant

Amoxicillin and Potassium Clavulanate (Augmentin)

Category: B

Indications: Treatment of beta-lactamase-producing strains of *H. influenzae, S. aureus, E. coli,* and *Klebsiella pneumoniae*

Actions: Combination of beta-lactam antibiotic and beta-lactamase inhibitor

Dosage: 250–500 mg as amoxicillin PO q8h

Supplied: Amoxicillin/potassium clavulanate combination: tablets 250/125 mg, 500/125 mg; suspension 125/31.25 mg per 5 mL, 250/62.5 mg per 5 mL

Notes: Do not substitute two 250 mg tablets for one 500 mg tablet or an overdose of clavulanic acid will occur; GI intolerance is the most common side effect

Amphotericin B (Fungizone)

Category: B

Indications: Severe systemic fungal infections

Actions: Binds to sterols in the fungal membrane, altering membrane permeability

Dosage: Test dose of 1 mg IV, then gradually increase as tolerated to 0.25–0.5 mg/kg/24h IV over 6 hours; total dose varies with indication; doses often range from 35–50 mg qd or every other day

Supplied: Powder for injection 50 mg per vial

Notes: Severe side effects occur with IV infusion; monitor liver and renal function; hypokalemia and hypomagnesemia may be seen from renal wasting; pretreatment with aspirin or acetaminophen and antihistamines (Benadryl, etc) helps to minimize adverse effects; small amounts of heparin (1 U/mL) and hydrocortisone (1 mg per milligram amphotericin) added to the infusate may help to minimize phlebitis

Ampicillin (Amcill, Omnipen, others)

Category: B

Indications: Treatment of susceptible gram-negative bacteria (*Shigella, Salmonella, E. coli, H. influenzae, P. mirabilis, N. gonorrhoeae*) and gram-positive bacteria (streptococci)

Actions: Beta-lactam antibiotic; inhibits cell wall synthesis

Dosage: 500 mg–2 g IM or IV q6h or 250–500 mg PO qid

Supplied: Capsules 250 mg, 500 mg; suspension 100 mg/mL, 125 mg/5 mL, 250 mg/5 mL, 500 mg/5 mL; powder for injection

Notes: Has cross-hypersensitivity with penicillin; can cause diarrhea and skin rash; many hospital strains of *E. coli* are resistant

Ampicillin and Sulbactam (Unasyn)

Category: B

Indications: Treatment of beta-lactamase-producing strains of *S. aureus, H. influenzae, Klebsiella* species, *P. mirabilis*, and *Bacteroides* species

Actions: Combination of beta-lactam antibiotic and beta-lactamase inhibitor

Dosage: 1.5–3.0 g (2 : 1 ampicillin sodium : sulbactam) IM or IV q6h

Supplied: Powder for injection 1.5 g, 3.0 g vials

Notes: Ampicillin and sulbactam are in a 2:1 ratio; adjust dosage in renal failure; observe for hypersensitivity reactions

Amrinone (Inocor)

Category: C

Indications: Short-term management of congestive heart failure

Actions: Positive inotrope with vasodilating activity

Dosage: Initially give IV bolus of 0.75 mg/kg over 2–3 minutes followed by maintenance dose of 5–10 µg/kg/min

Supplied: Injection 5 mg/mL

Notes: Not to exceed 10 mg/kg/d; incompatible with dextrose-containing solutions; monitor for fluid and electrolyte changes and renal function during therapy

Anistreplase (Eminase)

Category: C

Indications: Acute myocardial infarction

Actions: Thrombolytic agent

Dosage: 30 units IV over 2–5 minutes

Supplied: Vials containing 30 units

Notes: Clearance is approximately 90 minutes after rapid infusion; can cause bleeding; **do not** use after recent streptococcal infections

Antihemophilic Factor [Factor VIII] (Monoclate-P)

Category: C

Indications: Treatment of classic hemophilia A

Actions: Replacement of clotting Factor VIII

Dosage: 1 AHF unit/kg increases Factor VIII concentration in the body by approximately 2%

Units required = kg × desired Factor VIII increase as % of normal × 0.5

Supplied: Check each vial for the number of units contained in the vial

Notes: Patient's % of normal Factor VIII concentration must be ascertained prior to dosing for these calculations; not effective for controlling bleeding in von Willebrand's disease

Anti-thymocyte Globulin [ATG] (Atgam)

Category: C

Indications: Management of allograft rejection in renal transplant patients

Actions: Reduces the number of circulating thymus-dependent lymphocytes

Dosage: 10–30 mg/kg/d IV

Supplied: Injection 50 mg/mL

Notes: Do not administer to a patient with prior history of severe systemic reaction to any other equine gamma globulin preparation; discontinue treatment if severe, unremitting thrombocytopenia or leukopenia occurs

Anusol, Anusol-HC

Category: C

Indications: Symptomatic relief of pain from external and internal hemorrhoids

Actions: Local anesthetic

Dosage: 1 suppository qAM, qhs, and following each bowel movement; apply cream freely to anal area q6–12h

Supplied: Suppository, cream, ointment

Notes: Anusol-HC also contains hydrocortisone for anti-inflammatory effect

Aspirin (Bayer, others)

Category: D

Indications: Mild pain, headache, fever, inflammation, prevention of emboli, prevention of myocardial infarction (MI)

Actions: Prostaglandin inhibitor

Dosage:
Pain, fever: 325–650 mg q4–6h PO or PR
Rheumatoid arthritis: 3–6 g PO qd
Platelet inhibitory action: 325 mg PO qd
Prevention of MI: 325 mg PO qd

Supplied: Tablets 325 mg, 500 mg; enteric coated tablets 325 mg, 500 mg, 650 mg, 975 mg; SR tablets 650 mg, 800 mg; suppositories 60 mg, 120 mg, 125 mg, 130 mg, 195 mg, 200 mg, 300 mg, 325 mg, 600 mg, 650 mg, 1.2g

Notes: GI upset and erosion are common adverse reactions; may be prevented by ingestion with food

Aspirin with Butalbital and Caffeine (Fiorinal) [C]

Category: D

Indications: Mild pain, headache, especially with associated stress

Actions: Nonnarcotic analgesic

Dosage: 1–2 tablets or capsules PO q4–6h prn

Supplied: Each capsule or tablet contains 325 mg aspirin, 40 mg caffeine, and 50 mg butalbital

Notes: Also available with codeine: No. 1 = 7.5 mg; No. 2 = 15 mg; No. 3 = 30 mg; significant drowsiness is associated with use

Aspirin with Codeine (Empirin No. 1, No. 2, No. 3, No. 4) [C]

Category: C

Indications: Relief of mild to moderate pain

Actions: Combined effects of aspirin and a narcotic analgesic

Dosage: 1–2 tablets PO q3–4h prn

Supplied: Tablets 325 mg and codeine as below

Notes: Codeine in No. 1 = 7.5 mg, No. 2 = 15 mg, No. 3 = 30 mg, No. 4 = 60 mg

Astemizole (Hismanal)

Category: C

Indications: Allergic rhinitis

Actions: Antihistamine

Dosage: 10 mg PO qd

Supplied: Tablets 10 mg

Notes: Nonsedating; take on an empty stomach; can affect allergy skin testing for weeks after one dose

Atenolol (Tenormin) (see Table 7–6, page 571)

Atropine

Category: C

Indications: Symptomatic bradycardia, parkinsonism, relief of pylorospasm

Actions: Antimuscarinic agent

Dosage:
Emergency Cardiac Care: 0.5 mg IV q15min, up to 2.0 mg total

Supplied: Tablets 0.3 mg, 0.4 mg, 0.6 mg; injection 0.05 mg/mL, 0.1 mg/mL, 0.3 mg/mL, 0.4 mg/mL, 0.5 mg/mL, 0.8 mg/mL, 1.0 mg/mL

Notes: Can cause blurred vision, urine retention, dry mucous membranes

Azatadine (Optimine)

Category: B

Indications: Hay fever, allergic rhinitis, chronic urticarcia

Actions: Antihistamine

Dosage: 1–2 mg PO bid

Supplied: Tablets 1 mg

Notes: Has many anticholinergic side effects

Azathioprine (Imuran)

Category: D

Indications: Adjunct for the prevention of rejection in renal transplantation; rheumatoid arthritis; systemic lupus erythematosus

Actions: Immunosuppressive agent

Dosage: 1–3 mg/kg/d PO or IV

Supplied: Tablets 50 mg; injection 100 mg/20 mL

Notes: May cause GI intolerance; injection should be handled as with any antineoplastic agent

Azithromycin (Zithromax)

Category: C

Indications: Treatment of upper and lower respiratory tract infections due to *Streptococcus, H. influenzae,* and *M. catarrhalis;* nongonococcal urethritis and cervicitis due to *Chlamydia trachomatis*

Actions: Macrolide antibiotic; inhibits 50S ribosome

Dosage:
Respiratory tract: Load 500 mg, then 250 mg PO qd for 4 days (total of 5 days of therapy)
Chlamydia: 1 g PO as single dose

Supplied: Capsules 250 mg

Notes: Increases theophylline levels; used to treat various opportunistic infections in AIDS patients under protocol

Aztreonam (Azactam)

Category: B

Indications: Treatment of aerobic gram-negative bacteria including *Pseudomonas aeruginosa*

Actions: Monobactam antibiotic; inhibits cell wall synthesis

Dosage: 1–2 g IV or IM q6–12h

Supplied: Powder for injection 500 mg, 1 g, 2 g

Notes: Not effective against gram-positive or anaerobic bacteria; may be given to penicillin-allergic patients

Beclomethasone Nasal Inhaler (Beconase, Vancenase)

Category: C

Indications: Allergic rhinitis refractory to conventional therapy with antihistamines and decongestants

Actions: Inhaled corticosteroid

Dosage: 1 spray intranasally bid–qid

Supplied: Nasal inhaler

Notes: Nasal spray delivers 42 μg per dose

Beclomethasone Oral Inhaler (Beclovent, Vanceril)

Category: C

Indications: Chronic asthma

Actions: Inhaled corticosteroid

Dosage: 2 inhalations tid–qid (maximum, 20 per day)

Supplied: Oral inhaler

Notes: Not effective for acute asthma attacks; an anti-inflammatory topical steroid, can cause oral thrush

Belladonna and Opium Suppositories (B & O Supprettes) [C]

Category: C

Indications: Treatment of bladder spasms; moderate to severe pain

Actions: Antispasmodic agent

Dosage: Insert 1 suppository rectally q4–6h prn

Supplied: Suppositories 15A, 16A: 15A = 30 mg powdered opium with 16.2 mg belladonna extract; 16A = 60 mg powdered opium with 16.2 mg belladonna extract

Notes: Has anticholinergic side effects; caution subjects about sedation, urine retention, constipation

Belladonna, Tincture

Category: C

Indications: Adjunctive therapy in peptic ulcer disease, spastic colon, diarrhea

Actions: Antimuscarinic/antispasmodic agent

Dosage: 0.6–1.0 mL PO tid–qid

Supplied: Liquid with 27–33 mg of belladonna alkaloids per 100 mL

Notes: Liquid contains 65–70% alcohol; has anticholinergic side effects; use with caution in patients with narrow-angle glaucoma

Benazepril (Lotensin)

Category: D

Indications: Treatment of hypertension

Actions: Angiotensin-converting enzyme (ACE) inhibitor

Dosage: 10–40 mg PO qd

Supplied: Tablets 5 mg, 10 mg, 20 mg, 40 mg

Notes: Can cause symptomatic hypotension in patients taking diuretics; may cause a nonproductive cough

Bepridil (Vascor)

Category: C

Indications: Treatment of chronic stable angina

Actions: Calcium channel blocking agent

Dosage: 200–400 mg PO qd

Supplied: Tablets 200 mg, 300 mg, 400 mg

Notes: Can cause serious ventricular arrhythmias (including torsades de pointes) and agranulocytosis

Benzonatate (Tessalon Perles)

Category: C

Indications: Symptomatic relief of nonproductive cough

Actions: Anesthetizes stretch receptors in the respiratory passages

Dosage: 100 mg PO tid

Supplied: Capsules 100 mg

Notes: Can cause sedation

Benzquinamide (Emete-con)

Category: C

Indications: Nausea and vomiting

Actions: Antiemetic

Dosage: 50 mg IM q3–4h prn

Supplied: Powder for injection 50 mg per vial

Notes: Alternative antiemetic when phenothiazines or antihistamines are contraindicated

Beractant (Survanta)

Category: C

Indications: Prevention and treatment of respiratory distress syndrome in premature infants

Actions: Replacement of pulmonary surfactant

Dosage: 4 mL/kg

Supplied: Suspension containing 25 mg phospholipid per milliliter

Notes: Administered via endotracheal tube

Bethanechol (Duvoid, Urecholine, others)

Category: C

Indications: Neurogenic atony of the bladder with urine retention; **not** to be used when obstruction is present

Actions: Stimulates the parasympathetic nervous system

Dosage: 10–50 mg PO tid–qid or 5 mg SQ tid–qid and prn

Supplied: Tablets 5 mg, 10 mg, 25 mg, 50 mg; injection 5 mg/mL

Notes: Contraindicated in bladder outlet obstruction, asthma, heart disease; **do not** administer IM or IV

Bisacodyl (Dulcolax)

Indications: Constipation, bowel prep

Actions: Stimulant laxative

Dosage: 5–10 mg PO or 10 mg PR prn

Supplied: Enteric coated tablets 5 mg; suppositories 10 mg

Notes: **Do not** use with acute abdomen or bowel obstruction; **do not** chew tablets; **do not** give within 1 hour of antacids or milk

Bitolterol (Tornalate)

Category: C

Indications: Prophylaxis and treatment of asthma and reversible bronchospasm

Actions: Sympathomimetic bronchodilator

Dosage: 2 inhalations q8h

Supplied: Aerosol 0.8%

Bleomycin (Blenoxane)

Category: D

Indications: Cervical and germ cell ovarian cancer

Actions: Antibiotic; inhibits DNA and protein synthesis, especially in the G_2 and M phases

Dosage: Varies with protocol

Supplied: Injection 15 units

Notes: Causes nausea, vomiting, fever, mucositis, and anaphylaxis

Bretylium (Bretylol)

Category: C

Indications: Acute treatment of ventricular arrhythmias unresponsive to conventional therapy

Actions: Class 3 antiarrhythmic

Dosage: 5 mg/kg IV over 1 minute; may repeat q15–30min with 10 mg/kg (maximum, 30 mg/kg); maintenance, 1–2 mg/min IV infusion

Supplied: Injection 50 mg/mL

Notes: Nausea and vomiting are associated with rapid IV push; should gradually reduce dose and discontinue in 3–5 days; effects are seen within first 10–15 minutes; a transient rise in blood pressure is seen initially; hypotension is the most frequent adverse effect and occurs within the first hour of treatment

Bromocriptine (Parlodel)

Category: C

Indications: Hyperprolactinemia, prevention of lactation

Actions: Direct acting on the striatal dopamine receptors

Dosage:
Hyperprolactinemia: 5–7.5 mg PO qd
Lactation: 2.5 mg PO qd–tid

Supplied: Tablets 2.5 mg; capsules 5 mg

Notes: Nausea and vertigo are common side effects

Brompheniramine (Dimetane, others)

Category: C

Indications: Allergic reactions

Actions: Antihistamine

Dosage: 4–8 mg PO tid–qid or 10 mg IM q6–12h

Supplied: Tablets 4 mg; SR tablets 8 mg, 12 mg; elixir 2 mg/5 mL; injection 10 mg/mL, 100 mg/mL

Notes: Has anticholinergic side effects

Buclizine (Bucladin-S Softabs)

Category: C

Indications: Control of nausea, vomiting, dizziness, or motion sickness

Actions: Centrally acting antiemetic

Dosage: 50 mg dissolved in the mouth bid; 50 mg PO prophylactically 30 minutes prior to travel

Supplied: Tablets 50 mg

Notes: Not safe in pregnancy; contains tartrazine, observe patient for allergic reaction

Bumetanide (Bumex)

Category: C

Indications: Edema from congestive heart failure, hepatic cirrhosis, and renal disease

Actions: Loop diuretic

Dosage: 0.5–2.0 mg PO qd or 0.5–1.0 mg IV q8–24h

Supplied: Tablets 0.5 mg, 1.0 mg; injection 0.25 mg/mL

Notes: Monitor fluid and electrolyte (K^+) status during treatment

Buprenorphine (Buprenex)

Category: C

Indications: Relief of moderate to severe pain

Actions: Narcotic agonist-antagonist

Dosage: 0.3 mg IM or slow IV push q6h prn

Supplied: Injection 0.324 mg/mL (equal to 0.3 mg buprenorphine)

Notes: Can induce withdrawal syndrome in opioid-dependent patients

Buspirone (BuSpar)

Category: B

Indications: Short-term relief of anxiety

Actions: Antianxiety agent

Dosage: 5–10 mg PO tid

Supplied: Tablets 5 mg, 10 mg

Notes: No abuse potential; no physical or psychological dependence

Butoconazole (Femstat)

Category: C

Indications: Vaginal fungal infections

Actions: Topical antifungal

Dosage: 1 applicatorful intravaginally qhs for 3–6 days

Supplied: Vaginal cream 2%

Notes: For pregnant patients, use in second and third trimesters only

Butorphanol (Stadol)

Category: B

Indications: Analgesic for moderate to severe pain

Actions: Narcotic agonist-antagonist

Dosage: 2 mg IM or 1 mg IV q3–4h prn

Supplied: Injection 1 mg/mL, 2 mg/mL

Notes: Can induce withdrawal syndrome in opioid-dependent subjects

Calcium Carbonate (Alka-Mints, Tums)

Indications: Hyperacidity (peptic ulcer, hiatal hernia, etc)

Actions: Neutralizes gastric acid

Dosage: 500 mg–1.5 g PO prn

Supplied: Chewable tablets 350 mg, 420 mg, 500 mg, 550 mg, 750 mg, 850 mg; suspension

Calcium Salts [Chloride, Gluconate, others]

Indications: Calcium replacement, ventricular fibrillation, electromechanical dissociation

Actions: Dietary supplement; increases myocardial contractility

Dosage:
Replacement: 1–2 g PO qd
Cardiac emergencies: Calcium chloride 0.5–1.0 g IV q10min **or** calcium gluconate 1.0–2.0 g IV q10min

Supplied: Oral; injections of the various salts

Notes: Calcium chloride contains 270 mg (13.6 meq) elemental calcium per gram; calcium gluconate contains 90 mg (4.5 meq) elemental calcium per gram

Captopril (Capoten)

Category: D

Indications: Hypertension, congestive heart failure (CHF)

Actions: Angiotensin-converting enzyme (ACE) inhibitor

Dosage:
Hypertension: Initially, 25 mg PO bid–tid; titrate to maintenance dose q1–2 wk by 25 mg increments per dose (maximum, 450 mg/d) to desired effect
CHF: Initially, 6.25–12.5 mg PO tid; titrate to desired effect

Supplied: Tablets 12.5 mg, 25 mg, 50 mg, 100 mg

Notes: Use with caution in renal failure; give 1 hour before meals; can cause rash, proteinuria, and cough

Carbamazepine (Tegretol)

Category: C

Indications: Epilepsy, trigeminal neuralgia

Actions: Anticonvulsant

Dosage: 200 mg PO bid initially; increase by 200 mg/d; usual, 800–1200 mg/d

Supplied: Tablets 200 mg; chewable tablets 100 mg; suspension 100 mg/5 mL

Notes: Can cause severe hematologic side effects; monitor CBC; monitor serum levels (see Table 7–14, Drug Levels, page 585); generic products are **not** interchangeable

Carbenicillin (Geocillin, Geopen, Pyopen) (see Table 7–4, page 569)

Carboplatin (Paraplatin)

Category: D

Indications: Cervical and ovarian cancer

Actions: Nonspecific alkylating agent, causing interstrand DNA cross-linking

Dosage: Varies with protocol

Supplied: Injection 50 mg, 150 mg, 450 mg

Notes: Causes nausea, vomiting, bone marrow suppression, peripheral neuropathy

Carisoprodol (Soma)

Indications: Adjunct to sleep and physical therapy for relief of painful musculoskeletal conditions

Actions: Centrally acting muscle relaxant

Dosage: 350 mg PO qid

Supplied: Tablets 350 mg

Notes: Avoid alcohol and other CNS depressants

Carteolol (Cartrol) (see Table 7–6, page 571)

Cefaclor (Ceclor) (see Table 7–7, page 572)

Cefadroxil (Duricef, Ultracef) (see Table 7–7, page 572)

Cefamandole (Mandol) (see Table 7–8, page 573)

Cefazolin (Ancef, Kefzol) (see Table 7–7, page 572)

Cefixime (Suprax) (see Table 7–9, page 574)

Cefmetazole (Zefazone) (see Table 7–8, page 573)

Cefonicid (Monocid) (see Table 7–8, page 573)

Cefoperazone (Cefobid) (see Table 7–9, page 574)

Ceforanide (Precef) (see Table 7–8, page 573)

Cefotaxime (Claforan) (see Table 7–9, page 574)

Cefotetan (Cefotan) (see Table 7–9, page 574)

Cefoxitin (Mefoxin) (see Table 7–8, page 573)

Cefprozil (Cefzil) (see Table 7–8, page 573)

Ceftazidime (Fortaz, Tazidime, Tazicef) (see Table 7–9, page 574)

Ceftizoxime (Cefizox) (see Table 7–9 , page 574)

Ceftriaxone (Rocephin) (see Table 7–9, page 574)

Cefuroxime (Zinacef) (see Table 7–8, page 573)

Cefuroxime Axetil (Ceftin) (see Table 7–8, page 573)

Cephalexin (Keflex) (see Table 7–7, page 572)

Cephalothin (Keflin) (see Table 7–7, page 572)

Cephapirin (Cefadyl) (see Table 7–7, page 572)

Cephradine (Velosef, Anspor) (see Table 7–7, page 572)

Charcoal, Activated (Actidose, Liqui-Char, Superchar)

Indications: Emergency treatment in poisoning by most drugs and chemicals

Actions: Adsorbent detoxicant

Dosage:
Acute intoxication: 30–100 g
Gastrointestinal dialysis: 25–50 g q4–6h

Supplied: Powder, liquid

Notes: Administer with a cathartic; liquid dosage forms are in a sorbitol base; protect the airway in lethargic or comatose patients

Chlorambucil (Leukeran)

Category: D

Indications: Ovarian cancer

Actions: Nonspecific alkylating agent that causes cytotoxic cross-linking

Dosage: Varies with protocol

Supplied: Tablets 2 mg

Notes: Causes bone marrow suppression, GI distress, dermatitis, hepatotoxicity

Chloramphenicol (Chloromycetin)

Category: C

Indications: Serious infections caused by gram-positive and gram-negative aerobic and anaerobic bacteria

Actions: Interferes with protein synthesis

Dosage: 50–100 mg/kg/d PO or IV in 4 divided doses

Supplied: Capsules 250 mg, 500 mg; suspension 150 mg/5 mL; powder for injection

Notes: Aplastic anemia has been associated with use of this agent; monitor hematology studies carefully; reduce the dosage with hepatic impairment; oral agents should be used whenever possible (the oral products are more bioavailable than the injection); *Pseudomonas aeruginosa* is almost always resistant

Chlordiazepoxide (Librium) [C]

Category: D

Indications: Anxiety, tension, alcohol withdrawal

Actions: Benzodiazepine, sedative, antianxiety agent

Dosage:
Mild anxiety, tension: 5–10 mg PO tid–qid or prn
Severe anxiety, tension: 25–50 mg IM or IV tid–qid or prn
Alcohol withdrawal: 50–100 mg IM or IV; repeat in 2–4 hours if needed, up to 300 mg in 24 hours; gradually taper daily dosage

Supplied: Capsules and tablets 5 mg, 10 mg, 25 mg; powder for injection 100 mg per ampule

Notes: Reduce dosage in the elderly; absorption of IM doses can be erratic

Chlorothiazide (Diuril)

Category: D

Indications: Hypertension, edema, congestive heart failure

Actions: Thiazide diuretic

Dosage: 500 mg–1.0 g PO or IV qd–bid

Supplied: Tablets 250 mg, 500 mg; suspension 250 mg/5 mL; powder for injection 500 mg per vial

Notes: Contraindicated in anuria

Chlorpheniramine (Chlor-Trimeton, others)

Category: B

Indications: Allergic reactions

Actions: Antihistamine

Dosage: 4 mg PO q4–6h prn; 8–12 mg PO bid of sustained release

Supplied: Tablets 4 mg; chewable tablets 2 mg; SR tablets 8 mg, 12 mg; syrup 2 mg/5 mL; injection 10 mg/mL, 100 mg/mL

Notes: Anticholinergic side effects; sedation

Chlorpromazine (Thorazine)

Category: C

Indications: Psychotic disorders, apprehension, intractable hiccups, control of nausea and vomiting

Actions: Phenothiazine antipsychotic, antiemetic

Dosage:
Acute anxiety, agitation: 10–25 mg PO or PR bid–tid

Severe symptoms: 25 mg IM; may repeat in 1 hour, then 25–50 mg PO or PR tid
Outpatient antipsychotic: 10–25 mg PO bid–tid
Hiccups: 25–50 mg PO bid–tid

Supplied: Tablets 10 mg, 25 mg, 50 mg, 100 mg, 200 mg; SR capsules 30 mg, 75 mg, 150 mg, 200 mg, 300 mg; syrup 10 mg/5 mL; concentrate 30 mg/mL, 100 mg/mL; suppositories 25 mg, 100 mg; injection 25 mg/mL

Notes: Beware of extrapyramidal side effects, sedation; has alpha-adrenergic blocking properties

Chlorpropamide (Diabinese) (see Table 7–12, page 578)

Chlorthalidone (Hygroton, others)

Category: D

Indications: Hypertension; edema associated with congestive heart failure, steroid and estrogen therapy

Actions: Thiazide diuretic

Dosage: 50–100 mg PO qd

Supplied: Tablets 25 mg, 50 mg, 100 mg

Notes: Contraindicated in anuria

Chlorzoxazone (Paraflex, Parafon Forte DSC)

Category: C

Indications: Adjunct to rest and physical therapy for the relief of discomfort associated with acute, painful musculoskeletal conditions

Actions: Centrally acting skeletal muscle relaxant

Dosage: 250–500 mg PO tid–qid

Supplied: Tablets 250 mg, caplets 500 mg

Cholecalciferol [Vitamin D$_3$] (Delta D)

Category: C

Indications: Dietary supplement for treatment of vitamin D deficiency

Actions: Enhances intestinal calcium absorption

Dosage: 400–1000 IU PO qd

Supplied: Tablets 400 IU, 1000 IU

Notes: 1 mg cholecalciferol = 40,000 IU of vitamin D activity

Cholestyramine (Questran)

Category: C

Indications: Adjunctive therapy for reduction of serum cholesterol in patients with primary hypercholesterolemia; relief of pruritus associated with partial biliary obstruction

Actions: Binds bile acids in the intestine to form an insoluble complex

Dosage: Individualized to 4 g 1–6 times daily

Supplied: 4 g cholestyramine resin/9 g of powder

Notes: Mix 4 g cholestyramine in 2–6 oz of noncarbonated beverage

Chorionic Gonadotropin [HCG] (Chorex, Profasi HP)

Category: C

Indications: Induction of ovulation

Actions: Identical action to pituitary luteinizing hormone

Dosage: 1000–10,000 units IM as a single dose

Supplied: Powder for injection

Cimetidine (Tagamet)

Category: B

Indications: Duodenal ulcer; ulcer prophylaxis in hypersecretory states such as trauma, burns, surgery, Zollinger-Ellison syndrome, etc

Actions: Histamine H_2 receptor antagonist

Dosage:
    Active ulcer: 2400 mg/d IV as continuous infusion or 300 mg IV q6–8h; 400 mg PO bid or 800 mg PO qhs
    Maintenance therapy: 400 mg PO qhs

Supplied: Tablets 200 mg, 300 mg, 400 mg, 800 mg; liquid 300 mg/5 mL; injection 300 mg/2 mL

Notes: Extend the dosing interval to q12h with creatinine clearance < 30 mL/min; decrease dosage in the elderly (may cause confusion); has drug interactions with theophylline, digoxin, and possibly others

Ciprofloxacin (Cipro)

Category: C

Indications: Broad-spectrum activity against a variety of gram-positive and gram-negative aerobic bacteria

Actions: DNA gyrase inhibitor; interferes with DNA synthesis

Dosage: 250–750 mg PO q12h, or 200–400 mg IV q12h

Supplied: Tablets 250 mg, 500 mg, 750 mg; injection 200 mg, 400 mg

Notes: Not active against streptococci; drug interaction with theophylline increases theophylline serum levels; absorption inhibited by antacids; nausea, diarrhea, vomiting, abdominal discomfort are common side effects

Cisplatin (Platinol)

Category: D

Indications: Cervical and germ cell cancer

Actions: Nonspecific alkylating agent producing interstrand and intrastrand cross-links in DNA

Dosage: Varies with protocol

Supplied: Injection 1 mg/mL

Notes: Hydrate the patient; causes nephrotoxicity, nausea, vomiting, bone marrow suppression, ototoxicity, neurotoxicity

Clarithromycin (Biaxin)

Category: C

Indications: Treatment of upper and lower respiratory tract infections due to *Streptococcus, H. influenzae, M. catarrhalis,* or *Mycoplasma;* treatment of skin and skin structure infections

Actions: Macrolide antibiotic; inhibits 50S ribosome

Dosage: 250–500 mg PO bid for 7–14 days

Supplied: Tablets 250 mg, 500 mg

Notes: Increases theophylline and carbamazepine levels; may be effective in treating MAC infections in AIDS patients

Clemastine Fumarate (Tavist)

Category: B

Indications: Allergic rhinitis

Actions: Antihistamine

Dosage: 1.34 mg PO bid to 2.68 mg PO tid (maximum, 8.04 mg/d)

Supplied: Tablets 1.34 mg, 2.68 mg; syrup 0.67 mg/5 mL

Clindamycin (Cleocin)

Category: B

Indications: Susceptible strains of streptococci, pneumococci, staphylococci, and gram-positive and gram-negative anaerobes; no activity against gram-negative aerobes

Actions: Bacteriostatic; interferes with protein synthesis

Dosage: 150–450 mg PO qid; 300–600 mg IV q6h or 900 mg IV q8h

Supplied: Capsules 75 mg, 150 mg; suspension 75 mg/5 mL; injection 300 mg/2 mL

Notes: Beware of severe diarrhea, which may represent pseudomembranous colitis caused by *C. difficile*

Clomiphene Citrate (Clomid, Serophene)

Category: X

Indications: Ovulatory failure

Actions: Mediates ovulation through increased output of pituitary gonadotropins

Dosage: 50–100 mg PO qd for 5 days

Supplied: Tablets 50 mg

Notes: Not effective in patients with primary pituitary or ovarian failure; carries risk of multiple births; common reactions include hot flashes, bloating, breast discomfort, headache, nausea and vomiting

Clonazepam (Klonopin) [C]

Category: C

Indications: Lennox-Gastaut syndrome, akinetic and myoclonic seizures, absence seizures

Actions: Benzodiazepine anticonvulsant

Dosage: 1.5 mg PO qd in 3 divided doses; increase by 0.5–1.0 mg/d q3d prn up to 20 mg/d

Supplied: Tablets 0.5 mg, 1.0 mg, 2.0 mg

Notes: Has CNS side effects including sedation

Clonidine (Catapres)

Category: C

Indications: Hypertension; opioid and tobacco withdrawal

Actions: Centrally acting alpha-adrenergic stimulant

Dosage: 0.10 mg PO bid adjusted daily by 0.10–0.20 mg increments (maximum, 2.4 mg/d)

Supplied: Tablets 0.1 mg, 0.2 mg, 0.3 mg

Notes: Dry mouth, drowsiness, sedation occur frequently; more effective for hypertension when combined with a diuretic; rebound hypertension can occur with abrupt cessation at doses above 0.2 mg bid

Clonidine Transdermal (Catapres TTS)

Category: C

Indications: Hypertension

Actions: Centrally acting alpha-adrenergic stimulant

Dosage: Apply 1 patch q7d to a hairless area on the upper arm or torso; titrate according to individual therapeutic requirements

Supplied: TTS-1, TTS-2, TTS-3 (programmed to deliver 0.1, 0.2, or 0.3 mg of clonidine per day for 1 week)

Notes Doses above 2 TTS-3 are usually not associated with increased efficacy

Clorazepate (Tranxene) [C]

Category: D

Indications: Acute anxiety disorders; acute alcohol withdrawal symptoms; adjunctive therapy in partial seizures

Actions: Benzodiazepine

Dosage: 15–60 mg PO qd in single or divided doses

Supplied: Capsules and tablets 3.75 mg, 7.5 mg, 15 mg

Notes: Monitor patients with renal and hepatic impairment (drug may accumulate); has CNS depressant effects

Clotrimazole (Lotrimin, Mycelex)

Category: C

Indications: Treatment of candidiasis and tinea infections

Actions: Antifungal; alters cell membrane permeability

Dosage:
  Oral: 1 troche dissolved slowly in the mouth 5 times a day for 14 days
  Vaginal Cream: 1 applicatorful qhs for 7–14 days
  Vaginal tablets: 100 mg vaginally qhs for 7 days or 200 mg (2 tablets) vaginally qhs for 3 days or single dose of one 500 mg tablet vaginally hs
  Topical: Apply 3–4 times daily for 10–14 days

Supplied: Cream 1%; solution 1%; lotion 1%; troche 10 mg; vaginal tablets 100 mg, 500 mg; vaginal cream 1%

Notes: Oral prophylaxis is commonly used in immunosuppressed patients

Clotrimazole and Betamethasone Cream (Lotrisone)

Category: B

Indications: Relief of inflammatory and pruritic manifestations

Actions: Topical antifungal–corticosteroid combination

Dosage: Apply to affected area a few times a day

Supplied: Topical cream

Cloxacillin (Cloxapen, Tegopen) (see Table 7–5, page 570)

Codeine [C]

Category: C

Indications: Mild to moderate pain; symptomatic relief of cough

Actions: Narcotic analgesic; depresses the cough reflex

Dosage:
  Analgesic: 15–60 mg PO or IM qid prn
  Antitussive: 5–15 mg PO q4h prn

Supplied: Tablets 15 mg, 30 mg, 60 mg; injection 30 mg/mL, 60 mg/mL

Notes: Most often used in combination with acetaminophen or other agents such as terpin hydrate or guaifenesin; 120 mg is equivalent to 10 mg morphine IM

Colestipol (Colestid)

Category: C

Indications: Adjunctive therapy for reduction of serum cholesterol in patients with primary hypercholesterolemia

Actions: Binds bile acids in the intestine to form an insoluble complex

Dosage: 15–30 PO qd divided into 2–4 doses

Supplied: 5 g packets, 500 g bottles

Notes: Do not use dry powder; mix with beverages, soups, cereals, etc

Colfosceril Palmitate (Exosurf Neonatal)

Indications: Prophylaxis and treatment of respiratory distress syndrome in infants

Actions: Synthetic lung surfactant

Dosage: 5 mL/kg/dose administered through the endotracheal tube as soon after birth as possible and again at 12 and 24 hours

Supplied: Injection 100 mg

Notes: Monitor pulmonary compliance and oxygenation carefully; can cause pulmonary hemorrhage in infants weighing < 700 g at birth; may cause mucus plugging of the endotracheal tube

Corticosteroids (see Steroids)

Cortisone (see Steroids and Table 7–3, page 552)

Cromolyn Sodium (Intal, Nasalcrom, Opticrom)

Category: B

Indications: Adjunct to the treatment of asthma; **not** for an acute attack; prevention of exercise-induced asthma; allergic rhinitis; ophthalmic allergic manifestations

Actions: Antiasthmatic, antiallergic, and mast cell stabilizer

Dosage:
Inhalation: 20 mg (as powder in capsule) inhaled qid; aerosol, inhale 2 puffs qid
Nasal instillation: Spray once in each nostril 2–6 times daily
Ophthalmic: 1–2 drops in each eye 4–6 times daily

Supplied: Capsules for inhalation 20 mg; solution for nebulization 20 mg/2 mL; metered-dose inhaler; nasal solution 40 mg/mL; ophthalmic solution 4%.

Notes: Inhalation of dry powder can cause cough, bronchospasm; may need to switch to metered-dose inhaler; can require 2–4 weeks for maximal effect in perennial allergic disorders

Crotamiton (Eurax)

Category: C

Indications: Eradication of scabies and symptomatic relief of pruritic skin

Actions: Scabicidal; antipruritic

Dosage: Apply and massage into skin; repeat in 24 hours

Supplied: Cream 10%, lotion 10%

Notes: Keep away from eyes and mouth

Cyanocobalamin [Vitamin B$_{12}$]

Category: A

Indications: Pernicious anemia and other B$_{12}$ deficiency states

Actions: Dietary replacement of vitamin B$_{12}$

Dosage: 100 μg IM or SQ qd for 1 week, then 100 μg IM twice a week for 1 month, then 100 μg IM monthly

Supplied: Tablets 25 μg, 50 μg, 100 μg, 250 μg, 500 μg, 1000 μg; injection 30 μg/mL, 100 μg/mL, 1000 μg/mL

Notes: Oral absorption is highly erratic, altered by many drugs and not recommended

Cyclizine (Marezine)

Category: B

Indications: Prevention and treatment of nausea, vomiting, and dizziness of motion sickness

Actions: Antiemetic, anticholinergic, and antihistaminic properties

Dosage: 50 mg PO 30 minutes prior to travel; may repeat q4–6h to maximum of 200 mg/d; 50 mg IM q4–6h

Supplied: Tablets 50 mg; injection 50 mg/mL

Notes: Anticholinergic and sedative side effects are common

Cyclobenzaprine (Flexeril)

Category: B

Indications: Adjunct to rest and physical therapy for relief of muscle spasm associated with acute painful musculoskeletal conditions

Actions: Centrally acting skeletal muscle relaxant

Dosage: 10 mg PO tid

Supplied: Tablets 10 mg

Notes: Do not use for longer than 2–3 weeks; has sedative and anticholinergic properties

Cyclophosphamide (Cytoxan)

Category: D

Indications: Breast and ovarian cancer, soft tissue sarcoma

Actions: Alkylating agent

Dosage: Varies with protocol

Supplied: Tablets 25 mg; powder for injection 100 mg, 200 mg, 500 mg, 1 g, 2 g

Notes: Causes nausea, vomiting, bone marrow suppression, hemorrhagic cystitis, alopecia

Cyclosporine (Sandimmune)

Category: C

Indications: Prophylaxis of organ rejection in kidney, liver, and heart allogeneic transplants in conjunction with adrenal corticosteroids

Actions: Reversibly inhibits immunocompetent lymphocytes

Dosage:
 Oral: 15 mg/kg/d beginning 12 hours prior to transplant; after 2 weeks, taper dose by 5 mg per week to 5–10 mg/kg/d
 IV: If patient is unable to take orally, give ⅓ the oral dose IV

Supplied: Oral solution 100 mg/mL; injection 50 mg/mL

Notes: Should **not** be administered with any other immunosuppressive agents except adrenal corticosteroids; can elevate BUN and creatinine, which may be confused with renal transplant rejection; has many drug interactions; should be administered in glass containers

Cyproheptadine (Periactin)

Category: B

Indications: Allergic reactions; especially good for itching

Actions: Phenothiazine antihistamine

Dosage: 4 mg PO tid (maximum, 0.5 mg/kg/d)

Supplied: Tablets 4 mg; syrup 2 mg/5 mL

Notes: Anticholinergic side effects and drowsiness are common; can stimulate the appetite in some patients

Dacarbazine (DTIC-Dome)

Category: C

Indications: Soft tissue and uterine sarcomas

Actions: Inhibits DNA synthesis by acting as a purine analog

Dosage: Varies with protocol

Supplied: Injection 100 mg/10 mL

Notes: Can cause nausea, vomiting, bone marrow suppression, flulike syndrome, anaphylaxis

Dactinomycin (Cosmegen)

Category: C

Indications: Choriocarcinoma, germ cell and soft tissue sarcoma

Actions: Antibiotic; inhibits messenger RNA synthesis, active in the G_1 phase

Dosage: Varies with protocol

Supplied: Injection 0.5 mg

Notes: Causes nausea, vomiting, flulike syndrome, anaphylaxis

Demeclocycline (Declomycin)

Category: D

Indications: Treatment of SIADH, infections

Actions: Bacteriostatic antimicrobial agent of the tetracycline family; inhibits protein synthesis

Dosage:
   SIADH: 300–600 mg PO q12h
   Antimicrobial: 150 mg PO q6h or 300 mg PO q12h

Supplied: Capsules 150 mg; tablets 150 mg, 300 mg

Notes: Reduce dosage in renal failure; can cause diabetes insipidus

Desmopressin (DDAVP, Stimate)

Category: B

Indications: Diabetes insipidus (intranasal and parenteral); bleeding due to hemophilia A and type I von Willebrand's disease (parenteral)

Actions: Synthetic analog of vasopressin, a naturally occurring human antidiuretic hormone; increases Factor VIII

Dosage:
Diabetes insipidus:
- *Intranasal:* 0.1–0.4 mL (10–40 µg) qd as a single dose or in 2–3 divided doses
- *Parenteral:* 0.5–1 mL (2–4 µg) qd in 2 divided doses; if converting from intranasal to parenteral dosing, use 1/10 of the intranasal dose

Hemophilia A and von Willebrand's disease: 0.3 µg/kg diluted to 50 mL with normal saline, infused slowly over 15–30 minutes

Supplied: Injection 4 µg/mL; nasal solution 0.1 µg/mL

Notes: In the elderly, adjust fluid intake to avoid water intoxication and hyponatremia

Desoxycorticosterone Acetate [DOCA] (Percorten)

Category: C

Indications: Partial treatment for adrenocortical insufficiency

Actions: Adrenal corticosteroid with potent mineralocorticoid activity

Dosage:
Injection: 2–5 mg/d IM into upper outer quadrant of the gluteal region
Pellets: By surgical implantation

Supplied: Injection 5 mg/mL; repository injection 25 mg/mL; pellets 125 mg

Notes: Must be used in conjunction with a glucocorticoid

Dexamethasone (Decadron) (see Steroids and Table 7–3, page 552)

Dextran 40 (Rheomacrodex)

Indications: Plasma expander for adjunctive therapy in shock

Actions: Plasma volume expander

Dosage:
Shock: 10 mL/kg infused rapidly with maximum dose of 20 mL/kg in the first 24 hours; total daily dosage beyond 24 hours should not exceed 10 mL/kg and should be discontinued after 5 days

Deep vein thrombosis: 500–1000 mL on day of surgery, then 500 mL/d for 2–5 days

Supplied: 10% dextran 40 in 0.9% saline or 5% dextrose solution; dextran 70 can be used for prophylaxis of deep vein thrombosis

Notes: Observe for hypersensitivity reactions; monitor renal function and electrolytes

Dextromethorphan (Benylin DM, Mediquell)

Category: C

Indications: Control of nonproductive cough

Actions: Depresses the cough center

Dosage: 10–20 mg PO q4h prn

Supplied: Chewy squares 15 mg; lozenges 5 mg; syrup 5 mg/5 mL, 7.5 mg/5 mL, 10 mg/5 mL, 15 mg/5 mL; sustained-action liquid 30 mg/5 mL

Dezocine (Dalgan)

Category: C

Indications: Management of pain

Actions: Narcotic agonist-antagonist

Dosage: 5–20 mg IM or 2.5–10 mg IV q2–4h prn

Supplied: Injection 5 mg/mL, 10 mg/mL, 15 mg/mL

Notes: May cause withdrawal in patients dependent on narcotics

Diazepam (Valium) [C]

Category: D

Indications: Anxiety, alcohol withdrawal, muscle spasm, status epilepticus, preoperative sedation

Actions: Benzodiazepine

Dosage:
Status epilepticus: 0.2–0.5 mg/kg/dose IV q15–30min to maximum of 30 mg
Anxiety, muscle spasm: 2–10 mg PO or IM q3–4h prn
Preoperative: 5–10 mg PO or IM 20–30 minutes before the procedure; may be given IV just prior to the procedure
Alcohol withdrawal: Initially 2–5 mg IV; repeat q3–4h prn

Supplied: Tablets 2 mg, 5 mg, 10 mg; SR capsules 15 mg; solution 5 mg/5 mL, 5 mg/mL; injection 5 mg/mL

Notes: Do not exceed 5 mg/min IV (respiratory arrest can occur); absorption of IM dose can be erratic

Diazoxide (Hyperstat, Proglycem)

Category: C

Indications: Hypertensive emergencies; management of hypoglycemia due to hyperinsulinism

Actions: Relaxes smooth muscle in the peripheral arterioles; inhibits pancreatic insulin release

Dosage:
Hypertensive crisis: 1–3 mg/kg/dose IV up to maximum of 150 mg IV; may repeat at 15-minute intervals until desired effect is achieved
Hyperinsulinemic hypoglycemia: 3–8 mg/kg/24h PO divided q8–12h

Supplied: Capsules 50 mg; oral suspension 50 mg/mL; injection 300 mg/20 mL

Notes: Cannot be titrated

Diclofenac Sodium (Voltaren) (see Table 7–10, page 575)

Dicloxacillin (Dycill, Dynapen) (see Table 7–5, page 570)

Dicyclomine (Bentyl)

Category: B

Indications: Treatment of functional or irritable bowel syndromes

Actions: Smooth muscle relaxant

Dosage: 20 mg PO qid initially, increased to 160 mg/d; or 20 mg IM q6h

Supplied: Tablets 20 mg; capsules 10 mg, 20 mg; syrup 10 mg/5 mL; injection 10 mg/mL

Notes: Anticholinergic effects may limit dosage

Didanosine (Videx)

Category: B

Indications: Treatment of HIV infection in patients intolerant to zidovudine (AZT)

Actions: Antiviral agent; inhibits viral DNA replication

Dosage:

	Tablets	Powder
50–70 kg	300 mg bid	375 mg bid
50–74 kg	200 mg bid	250 mg bid
35–49 kg	125 mg bid	167 mg bid

Supplied: Chewable tablets 25 mg, 50 mg, 100 mg, 150 mg; powder packets 100 mg, 167 mg, 250 mg, 375 mg; powder for oral solution

Notes: Adult patients should take **two** tablets for each dose to have adequate buffering to prevent drug degradation; side effects include peripheral neuropathy, pancreatitis, and headache; there is an increased incidence of pancreatitis when used concomitantly with ganciclovir induction

Diethylstilbestrol [DES]

Category: X

Indications: Breast cancer, Prevent pregnancy in rape victim

Actions: Hormone; estrogen supplementation

Dosage: Varies with protocol

Supplied: Tablets 1 mg, 2.5 mg, 5 mg; enteric coated tablets 1 mg, 5 mg

Notes: Causes nausea, vomiting, thrombosis, hypertension, gynecomastia

Diflunisal (Dolobid) (see Table 7–10, page 575)

Digoxin (Lanoxicaps, Lanoxin)

Category: C

Indications: Congestive heart failure, atrial fibrillation and flutter, paroxysmal atrial tachycardia

Actions: Positive inotrope; increases the refractory period of the atrioventricular node

Dosage:
> *PO digitalization:* 0.50–0.75 mg PO, then 0.25 mg PO q6–8h to a total dose of 1.0–1.5 mg
> *IV or IM digitalization:* 0.25–0.50 mg IM or IV, then 0.25 mg q4–6h to total dose of about 1 mg
> *Daily maintenance:* 0.125–0.50 mg PO, IM, or IV qd (average daily dose, 0.125–0.25 mg)

Supplied: Tablets 0.125 mg, 0.25 mg, 0.5 mg; capsules 0.05 mg, 0.1 mg, 0.2 mg; elixir 0.05 mg/mL; injection 0.1 mg/mL, 0.25 mg/mL

Notes: Can cause heart block; low potassium can potentiate toxicity; reduce the dosage in renal failure; symptoms of toxicity include nausea, vomiting, headache, fatigue, visual disturbances (yellow-green halos around lights), cardiac arrhythmias (see Table 7–14, Drug Levels, page 585); IM injection can be painful and has erratic absorption

Dihydroxyaluminum Sodium Carbonate (Rolaids)

Indications: Heartburn, gastroesophageal reflux, acid indigestion

Actions: Neutralizes gastric acid

Dosage: 1–2 tablets PO prn

Supplied: Chewable tablets 334 mg

Diltiazem (Cardizem)

Category: C

Indications: Treatment of angina pectoris, prevention of reinfarction, hypertension; IV: atrial fibrillation or flutter and paroxysmal supraventricular tachycardia

Actions: Calcium channel blocking agent

Dosage:
> *Oral:* 30 mg PO qid initially; titrate to 180–360 mg/d in divided doses

as needed; or sustained release 60–120 mg PO bid titrated to effect (maximum 360 mg/d); **or** continuous dosage 180–300 mg PO qd
Intravenous: 0.25 mg/kg IV bolus over 2 minutes; may repeat dose in 15 minutes at 0.35 mg/kg

Supplied: Tablets 30 mg, 60 mg, 90 mg, 120 mg; SR capsules 60 mg, 90 mg, 120 mg; CD capsules 180 mg, 240 mg, 300 mg; injection 5 mg/mL

Notes: Contraindicated in sick sinus syndrome, atrioventricular block, hypotension

Dimenhydrinate (Dramamine)

Category: B

Indications: Prevention and treatment of nausea, vomiting, dizziness, or vertigo of motion sickness

Actions: Antiemetic

Dosage: 50–100 mg PO q4–6h (maximum, 400 mg/d); 50 mg IM or IV prn

Supplied: Tablets 50 mg; chewable tablets 50 mg; capsules 50 mg; liquid 12.5 mg/4 mL; injection 50 mg/mL

Notes: Has anticholinergic side effects

Diphenhydramine (Benadryl, others)

Category: B

Indications: Allergic reactions, motion sickness, potentiation of narcotics, sedation, cough suppression, treatment of extrapyramidal reactions

Actions: Antihistamine; antiemetic

Dosage: 25–50 mg PO or IM bid–tid

Supplied: Tablets and capsules 25 mg, 50 mg; elixir 12.5 mg/5 mL; syrup 12.5 mg/5 mL; injection 10 mg/mL, 50 mg/mL

Notes: Anticholinergic side effects including dry mouth, urine retention; causes sedation; increase the dosing interval in moderate to severe renal failure

Diphenoxylate with Atropine (Lomotil) [C]

Category: C

Indications: Diarrhea

Actions: A constipating meperidine congener

Dosage: Initially 5 mg PO tid or qid until under control; then 2.5–5.0 mg PO bid

Supplied: Tablets 2.5 mg diphenoxylate/0.025 mg atropine; liquid 2.5 mg diphenoxylate/0.025 mg atropine per 5 mL

Notes: Atropine-type side effects

Dipyridamole (Persantine)

Category: B

Indications: Prevention of postoperative thromboembolic disorders; chronic angina pectoris

Actions: Dilates coronary arteries; antiplatelet activity

Dosage:
  Antiplatelet effect: 75–100 mg PO tid–qid
  Angina: 50 mg PO tid

Supplied: Tablets 25 mg, 50 mg, 75 mg

Notes: Aspirin potentiates the antiplatelet effect; can cause nausea and vomiting

Disopyramide (Napamide, Norpace)

Category: C

Indications: Suppression and prevention of premature ventricular contractions

Actions: Class 1A antiarrhythmic

Dosage: 400–800 mg PO qd, divided q6h for regular capsules or q12h for sustained-release capsules

Supplied: Capsules 100 mg, 150 mg; SR capsules 100 mg, 150 mg

Notes: Has anticholinergic side effects (urine retention); negative inotropic properties may induce congestive heart failure; decrease the dosage in impaired hepatic function

Disulfiram (Antabuse)

Category: C

Indications: Deterrent to alcohol consumption

Actions: Blocks oxidation of alcohol to produce an unpleasant reaction when alcohol is consumed

Dosage: 500 mg PO qd for 1–2 weeks, then 250 mg PO qd

Supplied: Tablets 250 mg, 500 mg

Notes: Patients must avoid all hidden forms of alcohol (cough syrup, sauces, etc); CBC and liver function tests should be checked periodically

Dobutamine (Dobutrex)

Category: C

Indications: Short-term use in patients with cardiac decompensation secondary to depressed contractility

Actions: Positive inotropic agent

Dosage: Continuous IV infusion of 2.5–10 µg/kg/min; rarely 40 µg/kg/min may be required; titrate according to response

Supplied: Injection 250 mg/20 mL

Notes: Monitor ECG for increase in heart rate and ectopic activity; monitor blood pressure; monitor pulmonary wedge pressure and cardiac output if possible

Docusate Calcium (Surfak, others)

Docusate Potassium (Dialose)

Docusate Sodium (Colace, Doss, others)

Category: C

Indications: Constipation-prone patient; adjunct to painful anorectal conditions (hemorrhoids)

Actions: Stool softener

Dosage: 50–500 mg PO qd

Supplied:
Calcium: Capsules 50 mg, 240 mg
Potassium: Capsules 100 mg, 240 mg
Sodium: Tablets 50 mg, 100 mg; capsules 50 mg, 60 mg, 100 mg, 240 mg, 250 mg, 300 mg; syrup 50 mg/15 mL, 60 mg/15 mL; liquid 150 mg/15 mL; solution 50 mg/mL

Notes: Has no significant side effects; no laxative action

Dopamine (Dopastat, Intropin)

Category: C

Indications: Short-term use in patients with cardiac decompensation secondary to decreased contractility; to increase organ perfusion

Actions: Positive inotropic agent

Dosage: 5 µg/kg/min by continuous IV infusion, titrated by increments of 5 µg/kg/min to maximum of 50 µg/kg/min based on effect

Supplied: Injection 40 mg/mL, 80 mg/mL, 160 mg/mL

Notes: Dosage greater than 10 µg/kg/min can decrease renal perfusion; monitor urine output; monitor ECG for increase in heart rate and ectopic activity; monitor blood pressure; monitor PCWP and cardiac output if possible

Doxepin (Adapin, Sinequan)

Category: C

Indications: Depression or anxiety

Actions: Tricyclic antidepressant

Dosage: 50–150 mg PO qd, usually qhs but can be in divided doses

Supplied: Capsules 10 mg, 25 mg, 50 mg, 75 mg, 100 mg, 150 mg; oral concentrate 10 mg/mL

Notes: Has anticholinergic, CNS, and cardiovascular side effects

Doxorubicin (Adriamycin)

Category: D

Indications: Breast, endometrial, and ovarian cancer

Actions: Anthracycline antibiotic; inhibits nucleic acid synthesis

Dosage: Varies with protocol

Supplied: Injection 10 mg, 20 mg, 50 mg, 100 mg

Notes: Causes nausea, vomiting, bone marrow suppression, alopecia, cardiotoxicity, red urine; tissue necrosis occurs with extravasation

Doxycycline (Vibramycin)

Category: D

Indications: Broad-spectrum antibiotic including activity against *Rickettsiae, Chlamydia,* and *Mycoplasma pneumoniae*

Actions: Tetracycline; interferes with protein synthesis

Dosage: 100 mg PO q12h the first day, then 100 mg PO qd–bid or 100 mg IV q12h

Supplied: Tablets 50 mg, 100 mg; capsules 50 mg, 100 mg; syrup 50 mg/5 mL; powder for oral suspension 25 mg/5 mL; powder for injection 100 mg, 200 mg per vial

Notes: Useful for chronic bronchitis; the tetracycline of choice for patients with renal impairment

Dronabinol (Marinol) [C]

Category: B

Indications: Nausea and vomiting associated with cancer chemotherapy

Actions: Antiemetic

Dosage: 5–15 mg/m^2 PO q4–6h prn

Supplied: Capsules 2.5 mg, 5 mg, 10 mg

Notes: The principal psychoactive substance present in marijuana; many CNS side effects

Droperidol (Inapsine)

Category: C

Indications: Nausea and vomiting

Actions: Tranquilization, sedation, and antiemetic

Dosage: 1.25–2.5 mg IV prn

Supplied: Injection 2.5 mg/mL

Notes: Can cause drowsiness, moderate hypotension, and occasionally tachycardia

Econazole (Spectazole)

Category: C

Indications: Treatment of most tinea, cutaneous *Candida,* and tinea versicolor infections

Actions: Topical antifungal

Dosage: Apply to affected areas bid (qd for tinea versicolor) for 2–4 weeks

Supplied: Topical cream 1%

Notes: Relief of symptoms and clinical improvement may be seen early in treatment, but the full course of therapy should be carried out to avoid recurrence

Edrophonium (Tensilon)

Category: C

Indications: Diagnosis of myasthenia gravis; treatment of acute myasthenic crisis; curare antagonist; paroxysmal atrial tachycardia (PAT)

Actions: Anticholinesterase

Dosage:
Test for myasthenia gravis: 2 mg IV in 1 minute; if tolerated, give 8 mg IV; a positive test is a brief increase in strength
PAT: 10 mg IV to maximum of 40 mg

Supplied: Injection 10 mg/mL

Notes: Can cause severe cholinergic effects; keep atropine available

Enalapril (Vasotec)

Category: D

Indications: Hypertension, congestive heart failure

Actions: Angiotensin-converting enzyme (ACE) inhibitor

Dosage: 2.5–5 mg PO qd, titrated by effect to 10–40 mg qd as 1–2 divided doses; **or** 1.25 mg IV q6h

Supplied: Tablets 2.5 mg, 5 mg, 10 mg, 20 mg; injection 1.25 mg/mL

Notes: Initial dose could produce symptomatic hypotension, especially with diuretics; discontinue diuretic for 2–3 days before beginning therapy if possible; monitor closely for increases in serum potassium; can cause a nonproductive cough

Ephedrine Sulfate

Category: C

Indications: Acute bronchospasm, nasal congestion, hypotension, narcolepsy, enuresis, myasthenia gravis

Actions: Sympathomimetic that stimulates both alpha and beta receptors

Dosage: 25–50 mg IM or IV q10min to maximum of 150 mg/d **or** 25–50 mg PO q3–4h prn

Supplied: Capsules 25 mg, 50 mg; syrup 11 mg/5 mL, 20 mg/5 mL; injection 25 mg/mL, 50 mg/mL

Epinephrine (Adrenalin, Sus-Phrine, others)

Category: C

Indications: Cardiac arrest, anaphylactic reaction, acute asthma

Actions: Beta-adrenergic agonist with alpha effects

Dosage:
Emergency cardiac care: 0.5–1.0 mg (5–10 mL of 1 : 10,000) IV q5min to response
Anaphylaxis: 0.3–0.5 mL of 1 : 1000 dilution SQ; may repeat q10–15min to maximum of 1 mg/dose and 5 mg/d
Asthma: 0.3–0.5 mL of 1: 1000 dilution SQ, repeated at 20-minute to 4-hour intervals; **or** 1 inhalation (metered-dose) repeated in 1–2 minutes; **or** suspension 0.1–0.3 mL SQ for extended effect

Supplied: Injection 1 : 1000, 1 : 10,000, 1 : 100,000; suspension for injection 1 : 200; aerosol; solution for nebulization

Notes: Sus-Phrine offers sustained action; in acute cardiac settings may be given via endotracheal tube if a central line is not available

Epoetin alfa [Erythropoietin] (Epogen, Procrit)

Category: C

Indications: Anemia associated with chronic renal failure and zidovudine (AZT) treated HIV-infected patients

Actions: Erythropoietin supplementation

Dosage: 50–100 units/kg 3 times weekly; adjust dose q4–6wk prn

Supplied: Injection 2000 units, 4000 units, 10,000 units

Notes: Can cause hypertension, headache, tachycardia, nausea and vomiting

Erythromycin (E-Mycin, ERYC-250, Erythrocin, Ilosone, others)

Category: B

Indications: Group A streptococci (*S. pyogenes*), alpha-hemolytic streptococci and *N. gonorrhoeae* infections in penicillin-allergic patients, *S. pneumoniae, Mycoplasma pneumoniae,* Legionnaire's disease, and soft tissue infection caused by *S. aureus*

Actions: Bacteriostatic; interferes with protein synthesis

Dosage: 250–500 mg PO qid or 500 mg–1 g IV qid

Supplied:
   Powder for injection as lactobionate and gluceptate salts: 250 mg, 500 mg, 1 g
   Base: Tablets 250 mg, 333 mg, 500 mg; capsules 125 mg, 250 mg
   Estolate: Chewable tablets 125 mg, 250 mg; capsules 125 mg, 250 mg; drops 100 mg/mL; suspension 125 mg/5 mL, 250 mg/5 mL
   Stearate: Tablets 250 mg, 500 mg
   Ethylsuccinate: Chewable tablets 200 mg; tablets 400 mg; suspension 200 mg/5 mL, 400 mg/5mL

Notes: Frequent mild GI disturbances; estolate salt is associated with cholestatic jaundice; erythromycin base is not well absorbed from the GI tract; some forms such as Eryc are better tolerated with respect to GI irritation

Esmolol (Brevibloc)

Category: C

Indications: Supraventricular tachycardia, noncompensatory sinus tachycardia

Actions: Beta-adrenergic blocking agent

Dosage: Initiate treatment with 500 µg/kg load over 1 minute, then 50 µg/kg/min for 4 minutes; if response is inadequate, repeat loading dose and follow with maintenance infusion of 100 µg/kg/min for 4 minutes; continue titration process by repeating loading dose followed by incremental increases in the maintenance dose of 50 µg/kg/min every 4 minutes until desired heart rate is reached or decrease in blood pressure occurs; average dose is 100 µg/kg/min

Supplied: Injection 10 mg/mL, 250 mg/mL

Notes: Monitor closely for hypotension; decreasing or discontinuing the infusion will reverse hypotension in approximately 30 minutes

Estazolam (ProSom) [C]

Category: X

Indications: Insomnia

Actions: Benzodiazepine; sedative-hypnotic

Dosage: 1–2 mg PO qhs prn

Supplied: Tablets 1 mg, 2 mg

Estradiol, Topical (Estrace)

Category: X

Indications: Atrophic vaginitis and kraurosis vulvae associated with menopause

Actions: Estrogen supplementation

Dosage: 2–4 g daily for 2 weeks, then 1 g 1–3 times a week

Supplied: Vaginal cream

Estradiol Transdermal System (Estraderm)

Category: X

Indications: Severe vasomotor symptoms associated with menopause; female hypogonadism

Actions: Hormone replacement

Dosage: Apply one 0.05 system patch twice weekly; adjust dose as necessary to control symptoms

Supplied: Transdermal patches 0.05 mg, 0.1 mg (delivering 0.05 mg or 0.1 mg per 24 hours)

Estrogen, Conjugated (Premarin)

Category: X

Indications: Moderate to severe vasomotor symptoms associated with menopause; atrophic vaginitis; prevention of estrogen deficiency induced osteoporosis

Actions: Hormone replacement

Dosage: 0.3–1.25 mg PO qd cyclically

Supplied: Tablets 0.3 mg, 0.625 mg, 0.9 mg, 1.25 mg, 2.5 mg; injection 25 mg/mL

Notes: Do not use in pregnancy; associated with increased risk of endometrial carcinoma, gallbladder disease, thromboembolism, and possibly breast cancer

Estrogen, Conjugated with Methyltestosterone (Premarin with Methyltestosterone)

Category: X

Indications: Moderate to severe vasomotor symptoms associated with menopause; postpartum breast engorgement

Actions: Estrogen and androgen combination

Dosage: 1 tablet PO qd for 3 weeks, then 1 week off

Supplied: Tablets (estrogen/methyltestosterone) 0.625 mg/5 mg, 1.25 mg/10 mg

Estrogen, Esterified (Estratab, Menest)

Category: X

Indications: Vasomotor symptoms, atrophic vaginitis, or kraurosis vulvae associated with menopause; female hypogonadism

Actions: Estrogen supplementation

Dosage:
  Menopause: 0.3–1.25 mg qd
  Hypogonadism: 2.5 mg PO qd–tid

Supplied: Tablets 0.3 mg, 0.625 mg, 1.25 mg, 2.5 mg

Estrogen, Esterified with Methyltestosterone (Estratest)

Category: X

Indications: Moderate to severe vasomotor symptoms associated with menopause; postpartum breast engorgement

Actions: Estrogen and androgen supplementation

Dosage: 1 tablet PO qd for 3 weeks, then 1 week off

Supplied: Tablets (estrogen/methyltestosterone) 0.625 mg/1.25 mg, 1.25 mg/2.5 mg

Ethacrynic Acid (Edecrin)

Category: B

Indications: Edema, congestive heart failure, ascites, any time rapid diuresis is desired

Actions: Loop diuretic

Dosage: 50–200 mg PO qd **or** 50 mg IV prn

Supplied: Tablets 25 mg, 50 mg; powder for injection 50 mg

Notes: Contraindicated in anuria; has many severe side effects

Ethambutol (Myambutol)

Category: B

Indications: Pulmonary tuberculosis

Actions: Inhibits cellular metabolism

Dosage: 15 mg/kg PO qd as single dose

Supplied: Tablets 100 mg, 400 mg

Notes: Can cause vision changes and GI upset

Ethinyl Estradiol (Estinyl, Feminone)

Category: X

Indications: Vasomotor symptoms associated with menopause; female hypogonadism

Actions: Estrogen supplementation

Dosage: 0.02–1.5 mg PO daily divided qd–tid

Supplied: Tablets 0.02 mg, 0.05 mg, 0.5 mg

Ethosuximide (Zarontin)

Category: C

Indications: Absence seizures

Actions: Anticonvulsant

Dosage: 500 mg PO qd initially; increase by 250 mg/d q4–7d prn

Supplied: Capsules 250 mg; syrup 250 mg/5 mL

Notes: Blood dyscrasias and CNS and GI side effects can occur; use with caution in patients with renal or hepatic impairment; see Table 7–14, Drug Levels, page 585.

Etidronate Disodium (Didronel)

Category: B

Indications: Treatment of hypercalcemia of malignancy

Actions: Inhibits bone resorption

Dosage: 7.5 mg/kg/d IV or PO for 3 days; retreatment may be necessary

Supplied: Tablets 200 mg, 400 mg; injection 300 mg/6 mL

Etoposide (VePesid)

Category: D

Indications: Gestational trophoblastic disease and ovarian germ cell cancer

Actions: Mitotic inhibitor; inhibits DNA synthesis in the G_2 portion of the cell cycle

Dosage: Varies with protocol

Supplied: Capsules 50 mg; injection 20 mg/mL

Notes: Causes nausea, vomiting, bone marrow suppression, diarrhea, fever, peripheral neuropathy, hypotension

Famotidine (Pepcid)

Category: B

Indications: Short-term treatment of active duodenal ulcer and benign gastric ulcer, maintenance therapy for duodenal ulcer, hypersecretory conditions

Actions: Histamine H_2 antagonist

Dosage:
  Ulcer: 20–40 mg PO qhs **or** 20 mg IV q12h
  Hypersecretory conditions: 20–160 mg PO q6h

Supplied: Tablets 20 mg, 40 mg; suspension 40 mg/5 mL; injection 10 mg/mL

Notes: Decrease the dosage in severe renal failure

Felodipine (Plendil)

Category: C

Indications: Treatment of hypertension

Actions: Calcium channel blocking agent

Dosage: 5–20 mg PO qd

Supplied: Extended release tablets 5 mg, 10 mg

Notes: Closely monitor the blood pressure of elderly patients and patients with impaired hepatic function; doses of < 10 mg should not be used in these patient groups

Fenoprofen (Nalfon) (see Table 7–10, page 575)

Ferrous Sulfate

Indications: Iron deficiency anemia; iron supplementation

Actions: Dietary supplementation

Dosage: 100–200 mg PO qd of elemental iron divided tid–qid

Supplied: Tablets 195 mg, 300 mg, 325 mg; SR capsules 150 mg, 250 mg; drops 75 mg/0.6 mL, 125 mg/mL; elixir 220 mg/5 mL; Syrup 90 mg/5 mL

Notes: Will turn stools and urine dark; can cause GI upset, constipation; vitamin C taken with ferrous sulfate will increase the absorption of iron, especially in patients with atrophic gastritis

Flavoxate (Urispas)

Category: B

Indications: Symptomatic relief of dysuria, urgency, nocturia, suprapubic pain, urinary frequency, and incontinence

Actions: Counteracts smooth muscle spasm of the urinary tract

Dosage: 100–200 mg PO tid–qid

Supplied: Tablets 100 mg

Notes: Can cause drowsiness, blurred vision, dry mouth

Flecainide (Tambocor)

Category: C

Indications: Life-threatening ventricular arrhythmias

Actions: Class 1C antiarrhythmic

Dosage: 100 mg PO q12h; increase in increments of 50 mg q12h every 4 days to maximum of 400 mg/d

Supplied: Tablets 100 mg

Notes: May cause new or worsened arrhythmias; therapy should be initiated in the hospital; may dose q8h if patient is intolerant or uncontrolled at q12h interval; has drug interactions with propranolol, digoxin, verapamil, and disopyramide; can cause congestive heart failure

Fluconazole (Diflucan)

Category: C

Indications: Treatment of oropharyngeal and esophageal candidiasis; serious infections caused by *Candida* spp including pneumonia, urinary tract infections, and peritonitis; maintenance therapy for cryptococcal meningitis in patients with AIDS

Actions: Antifungal; inhibits fungal cytochrome P-450 and sterol demethylation

Dosage: 100–400 mg PO or IV qd

Supplied: Tablets 50 mg, 100 mg, 200 mg; injection 2 mg/mL

Notes: Adjust the dosage in renal insufficiency

Flucytosine (Ancobon)

Category: C

Indications: Serious infections caused by susceptible strains of *Candida* or *Cryptococcus*

Actions: Antifungal

Dosage: 50–150 mg/kg PO daily divided q6h

Supplied: Capsules 250 mg, 500 mg

Notes: Can cause nausea, vomiting, diarrhea; take capsules a few at a time over 15 minutes

Fludrocortisone Acetate (Florinef)

Category: C

Indications: Partial treatment for adrenocortical insufficiency

Actions: Mineralocorticoid replacement

Dosage: 0.05–0.1 mg/24h PO

Supplied: Tablets 0.1 mg

Notes: Must be used in conjunction with a glucocorticoid; dosage changes are based on plasma reinin activity; can cause congestive heart failure

Flunisolide (AeroBid)

Category: C

Indications: Bronchial asthma in patients requiring chronic corticosteroid therapy

Actions: Topical corticosteroid

Dosage: 2–4 inhalations twice daily

Supplied: Aerosol delivering 250 mg per actuation

Notes: Can cause thrush; **not** for acute asthma attack

Fluorouracil (Adrucil)

Category: D

Indications: Breast and ovarian cancer

Actions: Antimetabolite; inhibits DNA synthesis and to a lesser extent inhibits formation of RNA

Dosage: Varies with protocol

Supplied: Injection 50 mg/mL

Notes: Causes nausea, vomiting, diarrhea, bone marrow suppression, mucositis

Flurazepam (Dalmane) [C]

Category: D

Indications: Insomnia

Actions: Benzodiazepine

Dosage: 15–30 mg PO qhs prn

Supplied: Capsules 15 mg, 30 mg

Flurbiprofen (Ansaid) (see Table 7–10, page 575)

Folic Acid

Category: A

Indications: Macrocytic (folate deficiency) anemia

Actions: Dietary supplementation

Dosage:
Supplement: 0.4 mg PO qd
Folate deficiency: 1.0 mg PO qd–tid

Supplied: Tablets 0.1 mg, 0.4 mg, 0.8 mg, 1.0 mg; injection 5 mg/mL, 10 mg/mL

Foscarnet (Foscavir)

Category: C

Indications: Treatment of CMV retinitis in patients with AIDS

Actions: Inhibits viral DNA polymerase and reverse transcriptase

Dosage:
Induction: 60 mg/kg IV q8h
Maintenance: 90–120 mg/kg IV qd

Supplied: Injection 24 mg/mL

Notes: Dosage **must** be adjusted for renal function; is nephrotoxic; causes electrolyte abnormalities, monitor ionized calcium closely; administer through a central line

Fosinopril (Monopril)

Category: D

Indications: Treatment of hypertension

Actions: Angiotensin-converting enzyme (ACE) inhibitor

Dosage: Initially 10 mg PO qd; may be increased to a maximum of 80 mg/ PO daily divided qd–bid

Supplied: Tablets 10 mg, 20 mg

Notes: Decrease dosage in the elderly; do **not** need to adjust dose for renal insufficiency; may cause a nonproductive cough and dizziness

Furosemide (Lasix)

Category: C

Indications: Edema, hypertension, congestive heart failure

Actions: Loop diuretic

Dosage: 20–80 mg PO or IV qd–bid

Supplied: Tablets 20 mg, 40 mg, 80 mg; solution 10 mg/mL, 40 mg/5 mL; injection 10 mg/mL

Notes: Monitor for hypokalemia; use with caution in hepatic disease

Gallium Nitrate (Ganite)

Category: X

Indications: Treatment of hypercalcemia of malignancy

Actions: Inhibits resorption of calcium from the bones

Dosage: 100–200 mg/m^2/d for 5 days

Supplied: Injection 25 mg/mL

Notes: Can cause renal insufficiency; < 1% of patients develop acute optic neuritis

Ganciclovir (Cytovene)

Category: C

Indications: Retinitis caused by cytomegalovirus (CMV)

Actions: Inhibits viral DNA synthesis

Dosage: 5 mg/kg IV q12h for 14–21 days, then 5 mg/kg/d IV for 7 days a week or 6 mg/kg/d IV for 5 days of every week

Supplied: Powder for injection 500 mg

Notes: **Not** a cure for CMV; granulocytopenia and thrombocytopenia are the major toxicities; a potential carcinogen

Gemfibrozil (Lopid)

Category: B

Indications: Hypertriglyceridemia (types IV and V hyperlipoproteinemia)

Actions: Lipid-regulating agent

Dosage: 1200 mg PO qd in 2 divided doses 30 minutes before the morning and evening meals

Supplied: Tablets 600 mg; capsules 300 mg

Notes: Monitor liver function tests and serum lipids during therapy; cholelithiasis can occur secondary to treatment; may enhance effect of warfarin

Gentamicin (Garamycin)

Category: C

Indications: Serious infections caused by susceptible *Pseudomonas, Proteus, E. coli, Klebsiella, Enterobacter,* and *Serratia,* and for initial treatment of gram-negative sepsis

Actions: Bactericidal; interferes with protein synthesis

Dosage: Based on renal function and desired serum concentration; refer to **Aminoglycoside Dosing,** page 567

Supplied: Injection 2 mg/mL, 10 mg/mL, 40 mg/mL

Notes: Nephrotoxic and ototoxic; decrease the dosage in renal insufficiency; monitor creatinine clearance and serum concentration for dosage adjustments; see Table 7–14, Drug Levels, page 585

Glipizide (Glucotrol) (see Table 7–12, page 578)

Glucagon

Category: B

Indications: Treatment of severe hypoglycemic reactions in diabetic patients with sufficient liver glycogen stores

Actions: Accelerates liver glycogenolysis

Dosage: 0.5–1.0 mg SQ, IM, or IV, repeated after 20 minutes prn

Supplied: Powder for injection 1 mg, 10 mg

Notes: Administration of IV glucose is necessary if the patient fails to respond to glucagon; ineffective in states of starvation, adrenal insufficiency, or chronic hypoglycemia

Glyburide (DiaBeta, Micronase) (see Table 7–12, page 578)

Glycerin Suppository

Category: C

Indications: Constipation

Actions: Hyperosmolar laxative

Dosage: 1 suppository PR prn

Supplied: Suppositories; liquid 4 mL per applicatorful

Gonadorelin (Lutrepulse)

Category: B

Indications: Primary hypothalamic amenorrhea

Actions: Stimulates the pituitary to release luteinizing hormone and follicle-stimulating hormone

Dosage: 5–20 μg IV q90min for 21 days using a reservoir and pump

Supplied: Injection 0.8 mg, 3.2 mg

Notes: Risk of multiple pregnancies

Griseofulvin (Fulvicin, Grifulvin, Grisactin, Gris-PEG)

Category: C

Indications: Treatment of ringworm infections of the skin, hair, and nails which will not respond to topical agents alone

Actions: Inhibits fungal cell division

Dosage:
Tinea corporis, tinea crusris: 330–375 mg PO qd for 2–4 weeks
Tinea capitis: 330–375 mg PO qd for 4–6 weeks
Tinea pedis: 660–750 mg PO qd for 4–8 weeks

Tinea unguium: 600–750 mg PO qd for 4–8 months

Supplied:
Microsize: Tablets 250 mg, 500 mg; capsules 125 mg, 250 mg; suspension 125 mg/5 mL
Ultramicrosize: Tablets 125 mg, 165 mg, 250 mg, 330 mg

Notes: Patients on extended therapy should be monitored for renal, hepatic, and hematopoietic function; beneficial effect may not be apparent for some time; patient should continue entire course of therapy; GI absorption is improved when taken with food

Guaifenesin (Robitussin, others)

Category: C

Indications: Symptomatic relief of dry, nonproductive cough

Actions: Expectorant

Dosage: 100–400 mg PO q3–6h prn

Supplied: Tablets 100 mg, 200 mg; SR tablets 600 mg; capsules 200 mg; SR capsules 300 mg; syrup 67 mg/5 mL, 100 mg/5 mL, 200 mg/5 mL

Guanabenz (Wytensin)

Category: C

Indications: Hypertension

Actions: Central alpha-adrenergic agonist

Dosage: Initially 4 mg PO bid; increase by 4 mg/d increments at 1–2 week intervals up to maximum of 32 mg bid

Supplied: Tablets 4 mg, 8 mg

Notes: Sedation, dry mouth, dizziness, and headache are common

Guanadrel (Hylorel)

Category: B

Indications: Hypertension

Actions: Inhibits norepinephrine release from peripheral storage sites

Dosage: 5 mg PO bid initially; increase by 10 mg/d increments at weekly intervals up to maximum of 75 mg PO bid

Supplied: Tablets 10 mg, 25 mg

Notes: Has drug interactions with tricyclic antidepressants; fewer orthostatic changes and less impotence than with guanethidine

Guanethidine (Ismelin)

Category: C

Indications: Hypertension

Actions: Inhibits release of norepinephrine from peripheral storage sites

Dosage: Initially 10–25 mg PO qd; increase dose based on response

Supplied: Tablets 10 mg, 25 mg

Notes: Can produce profound orthostatic hypotension, especially with diuretic use; can potentiate effects of vasopressor agents; interaction with tricyclic antidepressants reduces the effectiveness of guanethidine; increased bowel movements and explosive diarrhea are possible

Guanfacine (Tenex)

Category: B

Indications: Hypertension

Actions: Centrally acting alpha-adrenergic agonist

Dosage: 1 mg PO qhs initially; increase by 1 mg/24h increments to maximum of 3 mg/24h; split dose bid if blood pressure increases at the end of the dosing interval

Supplied: Tablets 1 mg

Notes: Use with a thiazide diuretic is recommended; sedation and drowsiness are common; rebound hypertension can occur with abrupt cessation of therapy

Halazepam (Paxipam) [C]

Category: D

Indications: Anxiety disorders

Actions: Benzodiazepine

Dosage: 20–40 mg PO tid–qid

Supplied: Tablets 20 mg, 40 mg

Notes: Reduce dosage in the elderly

Haloperidol (Haldol)

Category: C

Indications: Management of psychotic disorders; agitation

Actions: Antipsychotic, neuroleptic

Dosage:
Moderate symptoms: 0.5–2.0 mg PO bid–tid
Severe symptoms or agitation: 3–5 mg PO bid–tid **or** 1–5 mg IM q4h prn (maximum, 100 mg/d)

Supplied: Tablets 0.5 mg, 1 mg, 2 mg, 5 mg, 10 mg, 20 mg; liquid concentrate 2 mg/mL; injection 5 mg/mL; decanoate 50 mg/mL

Notes: Can cause extrapyramidal symptoms, hypotension; reduce dosage in the elderly

Heparin Sodium

Category: C

Indications: Venous thrombosis, prevention of venous thrombosis and pulmonary emboli, atrial fibrillation with emboli formation, acute arterial occlusion

Actions: Acts with antithrombin III to inactivate thrombin and inhibit thromboplastin formation

Dosage:
Prophylaxis: 5000 units SQ q8–12h
Treatment of thrombosis: Loading dose of 50–75 units/kg IV, then 10–20 units/kg/h IV (adjust dose based on partial thromboplastin time (PTT))

Supplied: Injection 10 units mL, 100 units/mL, 1000 units/mL, 5000 units/mL, 10,000 units/mL, 20,000 units/mL, 40,000 units/mL

Notes: Follow PTT, thrombin time, or activated clotting time to assess effectiveness; heparin has little effect on prothrombin time; for full anticoagulation, PTT should be 1 ½–2 times control; follow platelet counts (can cause thrombocytopenia)

Hepatitis B Immune Globulin (H-BIG, Hep-B-Gammagee, HyperHep)

Category: C

Indications: Exposure to HB_sAg-positive patients through blood, plasma, or serum (accidental needle-stick, mucous membrane contact, oral ingestion)

Actions: Passive immunization

Dosage: 0.06 mL/kg IM, to maximum of 5 mL, within 24 hours of exposure; repeat at 1 month after exposure

Supplied: Injection in 1 mL, 4 mL, and 5 mL vials

Notes: Administered in gluteal or deltoid muscle; if exposure continues, the patient should receive hepatitis B vaccine

Hepatitis B Vaccine (Engerix-B, Recombivax HB)

Category: C

Indications: Prevention of type B hepatitis

Actions: Active immunization

Dosage: Three IM doses of 1 mL each, the first two given 1 month apart, the third 6 months after the first

Supplied:
Engerix-B: Injection 20 mg/mL
Recombivax HB: Injection 10 µg/mL

Notes: IM injections for adults should be administered in the deltoid; can cause fever, injection site soreness; derived from recombinant DNA technology

Hetastarch (Hespan)

Category: C

Indications: Plasma volume expansion as an adjunct in treatment of shock due to hemorrhage, surgery, burns, other trauma

Actions: Synthetic colloid with properties similar to albumin

Dosage: 500–1000 mL (maximum, 1500 mL/d) IV at a rate not to exceed 20 mL/kg/h

Supplied: Injection 30 g/500 mL in 0.9% saline solution

Notes: Not a substitute for blood or plasma; contraindicated in patients with severe bleeding disorders, severe congestive heart failure, or renal failure with oliguria or anuria

Hydralazine (Apresoline)

Category: C

Indications: Moderate to severe hypertension

Actions: Peripheral vasodilator

Dosage: Begin at 10 mg PO qid, then increase to 25 mg qid to maximum of 300 mg/d; for rapid control of pressure, 10–40 mg IM prn

Supplied: Tablets 10 mg, 25 mg, 50 mg, 100 mg; injection 20 mg/mL

Notes: Use with caution in impaired hepatic function or coronary artery disease; compensatory sinus tachycardia can be eliminated with addition of propranolol; chronically high doses can cause an SLE-like syndrome; supraventricular tachycardia can occur following IM administration

Hydrochlorothiazide (Esidrix, HydroDIURIL, others)

Category: B

Indications: Edema, hypertension, congestive heart failure

Actions: Thiazide diuretic

Dosage: 25–100 mg PO qd in single or divided doses

Supplied: Tablets 25 mg, 50 mg, 100 mg; oral solution 50 mg/5 mL, 100 mg/mL

Notes: Hypokalemia is frequent; hyperglycemia, hyperuricemia, hyperlipidemia, and hyponatremia are common side effects

Hydrochlorothiazide and Amiloride (Moduretic)

Category: B

Indications: Hypertension, adjunctive therapy for congestive heart failure

Actions: Combined effects of thiazide diuretic and potassium-sparing diuretic

Dosage: 1–2 tablets PO qd

Supplied: Tablets (amiloride/hydrochlorothiazide) 5 mg/50 mg

Notes: Should not be given to diabetics or patients with renal failure

Hydrochlorothiazide and Spironolactone (Aldactazide)

Category: D

Indications: Edema (from congestive heart failure, cirrhosis), hypertension

Actions: Combined effects of thiazide diuretic and potassium-sparing diuretic

Dosage: 25–200 mg each component PO qd in divided doses

Supplied: Tablets (hydrochlorothiazide/spironolactone) 25 mg/25 mg, 50 mg/50 mg

Hydrochlorothiazide and Triamterene (Dyazide, Maxzide)

Category: D

Indications: Edema, hypertension

Actions: Combined effects of thiazide diuretic and potassium-sparing diuretic

Dosage:
Dyazide: 1–2 capsules PO qd–bid
Maxzide: 1 tablet/PO qd

Supplied:
Dyazide capsules: 50 mg triamterene/25 mg hydrochlorothiazide (HCTZ)
Maxzide-25MG tablets: 37.5 mg triamterene/25 mg HCTZ
Maxzide tablets: 75 mg triamterene/50 mg HCTZ

Notes: The HCTZ component in Maxzide is more bioavailable than that in Dyazide; can cause hyperkalemia as well as hypokalemia; follow serum potassium

Hydrocortisone (see Steroids and Table 7–3, page 552)

Hydromorphone (Dilaudid) [C]

Category: C

Indications: Moderate to severe pain

Actions: Narcotic analgesic

Dosage: 1–4 mg PO, IM, IV or PR q4–6h prn

Supplied: Tablets 1 mg, 2 mg, 3 mg, 4 mg; injection 1 mg/mL, 2 mg/mL, 3 mg/mL, 4 mg/mL, 10 mg/mL; suppositories 3 mg

Notes: 1.5 mg IM is equivalent to 10 mg morphine IM

Hydroxyurea (Hydrea)

Category: D

Indications: Cervical and ovarian cancer

Actions: Immediate inhibition of DNA synthesis without affecting the synthesis of RNA or protein

Dosage: Varies with protocol

Supplied: Capsules 500 mg

Notes: Causes nausea, vomiting, bone marrow suppression, anorexia

Hydroxyzine (Atarax, Vistaril)

Category: C

Indications: Anxiety, tension, sedation, itching

Actions: Antihistamine, antianxiety

Dosage:
Anxiety or sedation: 50–100 mg PO or IM qid or prn (maximum, 600 mg/d)
Itching: 25–50 mg PO or IM tid–qid

Supplied: Tablets 10 mg, 25 mg, 50 mg, 100 mg; capsules 25 mg, 50 mg, 100 mg; syrup 10 mg/5 mL; injection 25 mg/mL, 50 mg/mL

Notes: Useful in potentiating the effects of narcotics; **not** for IV use; drowsiness and anticholinergic effects are common

Hyoscyamine Sulfate (Anaspaz, Cytospaz, Levsin)

Category: C

Indications: Control of gastric secretion, visceral spasm, spastic bladder, pylorospasm

Actions: Anticholinergic, antispasmodic

Dosage:
Oral: 0.125–0.25 mg PO tid–qid
Parenteral: 0.25–0.5 mg SQ, IM, or IV bid–qid prn

Supplied: Tablets 0.125 mg, 0.15 mg; timed-release capsules 0.375 mg; solution 0.125 mg/mL; elixir 0.125 mg/5 mL; injection 0.5 mg/mL

Notes: Can cause dizziness, blurred vision, dry mouth, difficulty with urination

Ibuprofen (Advil, Motrin, Rufen, others) (see Table 7–10 page 575)

Ifosfamide (Ifex)

Category: D

Indications: Breast and ovarian cancer

Actions: Alkylating agent related to nitrogen mustards: interacts with DNA

Dosage: Varies with protocol

Supplied: Injection 1 g, 3 g

Notes: Use with mesna; causes hemorrhagic cystitis, nausea, vomiting, bone marrow suppression, alopecia

Imipenem and Cilastatin (Primaxin)

Category: C

Indications: Treatment of serious infections caused by a wide variety of susceptible bacteria; inactive against *S. aureus,* group A and B streptococci, and others

Actions: Bactericidal, interferes with cell wall synthesis

Dosage: 250–500 mg (imipenem) IV q6h

Supplied: Injection (imipenem/cilastatin) 250mg/250mg, 500 mg/500 mg

Notes: Seizures can occur if the drug accumulates; adjust dosage for renal insufficiency to avoid drug accumulation if calculated creatinine clearance is < 70 mL/min

Imipramine (Tofranil)

Category: B

Indications: Depression

Actions: Tricyclic antidepressant

Dosage:
Hospitalized patient: Start at 100 mg/24h PO or IV in divided doses; may increase over several weeks to 250–300 mg/24h
Outpatient: Maintenance of 50–150 mg PO qhs, not to exceed 200 mg/24h

Supplied: Tablets 10 mg, 25 mg, 50 mg; capsules 75 mg, 100 mg, 125 mg, 150 mg; injection 12.5 mg/mL

Notes: Do not use with MAO inhibitors; produces less sedation than amitriptyline

Immune Globulin, Intravenous (Gamimune N, Gammagard, Sandoglobulin)

Category: C

Indications: IgG antibody deficiency diseases such as congenital agammaglobulinemia, common variable hypogammaglobulinemia; idiopathic thrombocytopenic purpura (ITP)

Actions: IgG supplementation

Dosage:
Immunodeficiency: 100–200 mg/kg IV monthly at a rate of 0.01–0.04 mL/kg/min, up to a maximum of 400 mg/kg/dose
ITP: 400 mg/kg/dose IV qd for 5 days

Supplied: Injection 50 mg/mL; powder for injection 0.5 g, 1 g, 2.5g, 3 g, 5 g, 6 g, 10 g vials

Notes: Adverse effects are associated mostly with rate of infusion

Indapamide (Lozol)

Category: B

Indications: Hypertension, congestive heart failure

Actions: Thiazide diuretic

Dosage: 2.5–5.0 mg PO qd

Supplied: Tablets 2.5 mg

Notes: Doses > 5 mg do not have additional effects on lowering blood pressure

Indomethacin (Indocin) (see Table 7–10, page 575)

Insulin

Category: B

Indications: Diabetes mellitus that cannot be controlled by diet, oral hypolycemic agents, or a combination of both

Actions: Insulin supplementation

Dosage: Based on serum glucose levels; usually given SQ, may also be given IV or IM

Supplied: See Table 7–1, page 502.

Notes: The highly purified insulins provide an increase in free insulin; monitor patients closely for several weeks when changing doses

Interferon Alfa (Intron A, Roferon-A, Alferon–N)

Category: C

Indications: Hairy cell leukemia, condyloma acuminata

TABLE 7–1. COMPARISON OF INSULINS.

Type of Insulin	Onset (h)	Peak (h)	Duration (h)
Rapid			
Regular Iletin II	0.25–0.5	2.0–4.0	5–7
Humulin R	0.5	2.0–4.0	6–8
Novolin R	0.5	2.5–5.0	5–8
Intermediate			
NPH Iletin II	1.0–2.0	6–12	18–24
Lente Iletin II	1.0–2.0	6–12	18–24
Humulin N	1.0–2.0	6–12	14–24
Novolin L	2.5–5.0	7–15	18–24
Novolin 70/30	0.5	7–12	24
Prolonged			
Ultralente	4.0–6.0	14–24	28–36
Humulin U	4.0–6.0	8–20	24–28

Fron Gomella LG (ed): Clinician's Pocket Reference, *7th ed. Norwalk, Connecticut, Appleton & Lange, 1992.*

Actions: Direct antiproliferative action against tumor cells and modulation of the host immune response

Dosage:
Alfa-2a: 3 million IU daily SQ or IM for 16–24 weeks
Alfa-2b: 2 million IU/m^2 IM or SQ 3 times a week for 2–6 months
Alfa–n3: 250,000 IU per wart intralesional, twice weekly for 8 weeks

Supplied: Injection

Notes: Is being used in many investigational protocols; flulike symptoms are a common reaction

Ipecac Syrup

Category: C

Indications: Treatment of drug overdose and certain cases of poisoning

Actions: Irritation of GI mucosa and stimulation of the chemoreceptor trigger zone

Dosage: 15–30 mL PO followed by 200–300 mL water; if no emesis occurs in 20 minutes, may repeat once

Supplied: Syrup 15 mL, 30 mL

Notes: Do not use for ingestion of petroleum distillates or of strong acid, base, or other corrosive or caustic agents; not for use in comatose or unconscious patients; use with caution in CNS depressant overdoses

Ipratropium Bromide Inhalant (Atrovent)

Category: B

Indications: Bronchospasm associated with chronic obstructive pulmonary disease

Actions: Synthetic anticholinergic agent similar to atropine

Dosage: 2–4 puffs qid

Supplied: Metered-dose inhaler 18 µg/dose

Notes: Not for initial treatment of acute episodes of bronchospasm

Iron Dextran (Imferon)

Category: C

Indications: Iron deficiency when oral supplementation is not possible

Actions: Parenteral iron supplementation

Dosage: Based on estimate of iron deficiency (see package insert)

Supplied: Injection containing 50 mg iron per milliliter

Notes: Must give a test dose (anaphylaxis is common); may be given deep IM using "Z-track" technique, although the IV route is preferred

Isoetharine (Bronkosol, Bronkometer)

Category: C

Indications: Bronchial asthma and reversible bronchospasm

Actions: Sympathomimetic bronchodilator

Dosage:
  Nebulization: 0.25–1.0 mL diluted 1 : 3 with saline q4–6h
  Metered-dose inhaler: 1–2 inhalations q4h

Supplied: Metered-dose inhaler 340 µg/dose; solution for inhalation

Isoniazid [INH]

Category: C

Indications: Active tuberculosis and prevention of tuberculosis

Actions: Bactericidal; interferes with lipid and nucleic acid biosynthesis

Dosage:
Active TB: 5 mg/kg/24h PO or IM (usually 300 mg/d)
Prophylaxis: 300 mg PO qd for 6–12 months

Supplied: Tablets 50 mg, 100 mg, 300 mg; syrup 50 mg/5 mL; injection 100 mg/mL

Notes: Can cause severe hepatitis; give with other antituberculosis drugs for active TB; IM and IV routes are rarely used; to prevent peripheral neuropathy, may give pyridoxine 50–100 mg/qd

Isoproterenol (Isuprel, Medihaler-Iso)

Category: C

Indications: Shock, cardiac arrest, atrioventricular (AV) nodal block, asthma

Actions: Beta-1 and beta-2 receptor stimulant

Dosage:
Emergency cardiac care: 2–20 µg/min IV infusion, titrated to effect
Shock: 1–4 µg/min IV infusion, titrated to effect
AV nodal block: 20–60 µg IV push; may repeat q3–5min; 1–5 µg/min IV infusion for maintenance
Asthma: 1–2 inhalations 4–6 times daily

Supplied: Aerosol 80 µg/dose, 125 µg/dose; solution for nebulization; injection 200 µg/mL

Notes: Contraindications include tachycardia; pulse > 130 bpm can induce ventricular arrhythmias

Isosorbide Dinitrate (Isordil)

Category: C

Indications: Angina pectoris

Actions: Relaxation of vascular smooth muscle

Dosage:
Acute angina: 2.5–10.0 mg PO (chewable tablet) or SL q5–10min prn;
> 3 doses should not be given in 15- to 30-minute period
Angina prophylaxis: 5–60 mg PO tid

Supplied: Tablets 5 mg, 10 mg, 20 mg, 30 mg, 40 mg; SR tablets 40 mg; sublingual tablets 2.5 mg, 5 mg, 10 mg; chewable tablets 5 mg, 10 mg; capsules 40 mg; SR capsules 40 mg

Notes: Nitrates should not be given on a chronic q6h or qid basis (tolerance can develop); can cause headaches; usually need to give a higher oral dose to achieve same results as with sublingual forms; can be given with hydralazine to treat congestive heart failure

Isosorbide Monohydrate (ISMO)

Category: C

Indications: Prevention of angina pectoris

Actions: Relaxes vascular smooth muscle

Dosage: 20 mg PO bid with the two doses given 7 hours apart

Supplied: Tablets 20 mg

Isradipine (DynaCirc)

Category: C

Indications: Hypertension

Actions: Calcium channel blocking agent

Dosage: 2.5–5.0 mg PO bid

Supplied: Capsules 2.5 mg, 5.0 mg

Kaolin and Pectin (Kaopectate, others)

Indications: Treatment of diarrhea

Actions: Adsorbent demulcent

Dosage: 60–120 mL PO after each loose stool or q3–4h prn

Supplied: Oral suspension

Ketoconazole (Nizoral)

Category: C

Indications: Treatment of systemic fungal infections: candidiasis, chronic mucocutaneous candidiasis, oral thrush, blastomycosis, coccidioidomycosis, histoplasmosis, paracoccidioidomycosis; topical cream for localized fungal infections due to dermatophytes and yeast

Actions: Inhibits fungal cell wall synthesis

Dosage:
Oral: 200 mg qd; increase to 400 mg qd for very serious infections
Topical: Apply to affected area once daily

Supplied: Tablets 200 mg; suspension 100 mg/5 mL; topical cream 2%

Notes: Associated with severe hepatotoxicity; monitor liver function tests closely throughout the course of therapy; **drug interaction** with any agent that increases gastric pH will prevent absorption of ketoconazole; can enhance oral anticoagulants; can react with alcohol to produce disulfiram-like reaction

Ketoprofen (Orudis) (see Table 7–10, page 575)

Ketorolac (Toradol) (see Table 7–10, page 575)

Labetalol (Normodyne, Trandate) (also see Table 7–6, page 571)

Category: C

Indications: Hypertension, hypertensive emergencies

Actions: Alpha- and beta-adrenergic blocking agent

Dosage:
Hypertension: 100 mg PO bid initially, then 200–400 mg PO bid
Hypertensive emergency: 20–80 mg IV bolus, then 2 mg/min IV infusion titrated to effect

Supplied: Tablets 100 mg, 200 mg, 300 mg; injection 5 mg/mL

Lactobacillus Granules (Lactinex)

Indications: Control of diarrhea, especially after antibiotic therapy

Actions: Replacement of intestinal flora

Dosage: 1 packet, 2 capsules, or 4 tablets with meals or liquids PO tid

Supplied: Chewable tablets; capsules; powder in 1 g packets

Lactulose (Cephulac, Chronulac)

Category: B

Indications: Hepatic encephalopathy, laxative

Actions: Acidifies the colon, allowing ammonia to diffuse into the colon

Dosage:
Acute hepatic encephalopathy: 30–45 mL PO tid–qid
Chronic laxative therapy: 30–45 mL PO tid–qid; adjust dosage q1–2d to produce 2–3 soft stools daily

Supplied: Syrup 10 g/15 mL

Notes: Can cause severe diarrhea resulting in hypernatremia

Leucovorin Calcium (Wellcovorin)

Category: C

Indications: Overdose of folic acid antagonist

Actions: Circumvents the action of folate reductase inhibitors

Dosage: 10–100 mg/m^2 IV or PO q3–6h

Supplied: Tablets 5 mg, 25 mg; solution 1 mg/mL; injection 5 mg/mL, 10 mg/mL

Notes: Many different dosing schedules exist for "leucovorin rescue" following methotrexate therapy

Leuprolide (Lupron)

Category: X

Indications: Endometriosis; breast, ovarian, and endometrial cancer

Actions: Luteinizing hormone releasing hormone (LH-RH) agonist, inhibits gonadotropin secretion

Dosage: Varies with protocol

Supplied: Injection 5 mg/mL; depot suspension 3.75 mg/mL, 7.5 mg/mL

Notes: Causes hot flashes, edema, ECG changes

Levonorgestrel Implants (Norplant)

Category: X

Indications: Prevention of pregnancy

Dosage: Implant 6 capsules in the midforearm

Supplied: Kits containing 6 implantable capsules, each containing 36 mg

Notes: Prevents pregnancy for up to 5 years; capsules may be removed if pregnancy is desired

Levorphanol (Levo-Dromoran) [C]

Category: C

Indications: Moderate to severe pain

Actions: Narcotic analgesic

Dosage: 2 mg PO or SQ prn

Supplied: Tablets 2 mg; injection 2 mg/mL

Levothyroxine (Synthroid)

Category: A

Indications: Hypothyroidism

Actions: Supplementation of T_4

Dosage: 25–50 µg PO or IV qd initially; increase by 25–50 µg/d every month; usual dose, 100–150 µg/qd

Supplied: Tablets 0.025 mg, 0.05 mg, 0.075 mg, 0.1 mg, 0.112 mg, 0.125 mg, 0.15 mg, 0.175 mg, 0.2 mg, 0.3 mg; injection 0.2 mg, 0.5 mg

Notes: Titrate dosage based on clinical response and thyroid function tests; dosage may be increased more rapidly in young to middle-aged patients; elderly patients may require only 50–100 µg/d; in patients with possible coronary artery disease, start with 12.5–25 µg/d

Lidocaine (Xylocaine)

Category: B

Indications: Treatment of cardiac arrhythmias; local anesthetic

Actions: Class 1B antiarrhythmic

Dosage:
  Arrhythmias: 1 mg/kg (50–100 mg) IV bolus, then 2–4 mg/min IV infusion; repeat bolus after 5 minutes
  Local anesthetic: Infiltrate a few milliliters of 0.5–1.0% solution (maximum, 4.5 mg/kg or about 28 mL of 1% solution in a 70 kg adult)

Supplied: Injection 0.5%, 1%, 2%, 4%, 10%, 20%

Notes: Epinephrine may be added to injectable forms for local anesthesia to prolong effect and help decrease bleeding; for IV forms, dosage reduction is required with liver disease and congestive heart failure; dizziness, paresthesias, and convulsions are associated with toxicity

Lindane [Gamma Benzene Hexachloride] (Kwell)

Category: B

Indications: Head lice, crab lice, scabies

Actions: Ectoparasiticide and ovicide

Dosage:
Cream or lotion: Apply thin layer after bathing and leave in place for 24 hours; pour on laundry
Shampoo: Apply 30 mL and develop lather with warm water for 4 minutes; comb out nits

Supplied: Cream 1%; lotion 1%; shampoo 1%

Notes: Caution with overuse (may be absorbed into blood)

Liothyronine (Cytomel)

Category: A

Indications: Hypothyroidism

Actions: T_3 replacement

Dosage: Initial dose of 25 μg/24h PO, then titrate q1–2wk according to clinical response and thyroid function tests to maintenance of 25–75 μg PO qd

Supplied: Tablets 5 μg, 25 μg, 50 μg

Notes: Reduce dosage in the elderly

Liotrix (Euthroid, Thyrolar)

Category: A

Indications: Hypothyroidism

Actions: Mixture of T_4 and T_3 in a 4 : 1 ratio

Dosage: 15–30 mg PO qd

Supplied: Tablets (thyroid equivalent) 15 mg, 30 mg, 60 mg, 120 mg, 180 mg

Lisinopril (Prinivil, Zestril)

Category: D

Indications: Hypertension

Actions: Angiotensin-converting enzyme (ACE) inhibitor

Dosage: 5–40 mg PO qd

Supplied: Tablets 5 mg, 10 mg, 20 mg

Notes: Side effects include dizziness, headache, cough

Lithium Carbonate (Eskalith, others)

Category: D

Indications: Manic episodes of bipolar illness; maintenance therapy in recurrent disease

Actions: Effects a shift toward intraneuronal metabolism of catecholamines

Dosage:
Acute mania: 600 mg PO tid **or** 900 mg SR bid
Maintenance: 300 mg PO tid–qid

Supplied: Tablets 300 mg; SR tablets 300 mg, 450 mg; capsules 150 mg, 300 mg, 600 mg; syrup 300 mg/5 mL

Notes: Dosage must be titrated; follow serum levels (see Table 7–14, Drug Levels, page 585); common side effects are polyuria, tremor; contraindicated in severe renal impairment; sodium retention or diuretic use may potentiate toxicity

Loperamide (Imodium)

Category: B

Indications: Diarrhea

Actions: Slows intestinal motility

Dosage: 4 mg PO initially, then 2 mg after each loose stool; up to 16 mg/d

Supplied: Capsules 2 mg; liquid 1 mg/5 mL

Notes: Do not use in acute diarrhea caused by *Salmonella, Shigella,* or *C. difficile*

Lorazepam (Ativan, others) [C]

Category: D

Indications: Anxiety and anxiety mixed with depression; insomnia; control of status epilepticus

Actions: Benzodiazepine

Dosage:
Anxiety: 0.5–1 mg PO bid–tid
Insominia: 2–4 mg PO qhs
Status epilepticus: 2.5–10 mg/dose IV; repeat at 15- to 20-minute intervals for 2 doses prn

Supplied: Tablets 0.5 mg, 1 mg, 2 mg; injection 2 mg/mL, 4 mg/mL

Notes: Decrease dosage in the elderly

Lovastatin (Mevacor)

Category: X

Indications: Adjunct to the diet for reduction of elevated total and LDL cholesterol levels in patients with primary hypercholesterolemia (types IIa and IIb)

Actions: Reduces production and increases catabolism of LDL cholesterol

Dosage: 20 mg PO qd with the evening meal; may increase at 4-week intervals to maximum of 80 mg/d taken with meals

Supplied: Tablets 20 mg

Notes: Patient should be maintained on a standard cholesterol-lowering diet throughout treatment; monitor liver function tests q6wk during the first year of therapy and do annual ophthalmic exams for opacities; headache and GI intolerance are common

Magaldrate (Lowsium, Riopan)

Indications: Hyperacidity associated with peptic ulcer, gastritis, and hiatal hernia

Actions: Low-sodium antacid

Dosage: 1–2 tablets PO or 5–10 mL PO between meals and hs

Supplied: Tablets; suspension

Notes: Contains < 0.3 mg sodium per tablet or teaspoonful; do not use in renal insufficiency

Magnesium Citrate

Indications: Vigorous bowel prep; constipation

Actions: Saline laxative

Dosage: 120–240 mL PO prn

Supplied: Effervescent solution

Notes: Do not use in renal insufficiency or intestinal obstruction

Magnesium Hydroxide (Milk of Magnesia)

Indications: Constipation

Actions: Saline laxative

Dosage: 15–30 mL **or** 1 tablet PO prn

Supplied: Tablets 325 mg; suspension 8%

Notes: Do not use in renal insufficiency or intestinal obstruction

Magnesium Oxide (Mag-Ox 400, Maox, Uro-Mag)

Indications: Replacement for low plasma levels

Actions: Magnesium supplementation

Dosage: 400–840 mg/d divided qd–qid

Supplied: Tablets 400 mg, 420 mg; capsules 140 mg

Notes: Doses may be higher in patients previously receiving cisplatin; may cause diarrhea

Magnesium Sulfate

Category: A

Indications: Replacement for low plasma levels (alcoholism, hyperalimentation); refractory hypocalcemia; preeclampsia and premature labor

Actions: Magnesium supplementation

Dosage:
Supplement: 1–2 g IM or IV; repeat dosing based on response and continued hypomagnesemia
Preeclampsia: 2–4 g/h IV loading dose
Premature labor: 4–6 g/h IV loading dose

Supplied: Injection 100 mg/mL, 125 mg/mL, 250 mg/mL, 500 mg/mL

Notes: Reduce dosage with low urine output or renal insufficiency

Mannitol

Category: C

Indications: Osmotic diuresis (cerebral edema, oliguria, anuria, myoglobinuria, etc)

Actions: Osmotic diuretic

Dosage:
Diuresis: Test dose of 0.2 g/kg/dose IV over 3–5 minutes; if no diuresis within 2 hours, discontinue
Cerebral edema: 0.25 g/kg/dose IV push, repeated at 5-minute intervals prn; increase incrementally to 1 g/kg/dose prn for intracranial hypertension

Supplied: Injection 5%, 10%, 15%, 20%, 25%

Notes: Use with caution in congestive heart failure or volume overload

Meclizine (Antivert)

Category: B

Indications: Motion sickness, vertigo associated with diseases of the vestibular system

Actions: Antiemetic, anticholinergic, and antihistaminic properties

Dosage: 25 mg PO tid–qid prn

Supplied: Tablets 12.5 mg, 25 mg, 50 mg; chewable tablets 25 mg; capsules 25 mg

Notes: Drowsiness, dry mouth, and blurred vision commonly occur

Medroxyprogesterone (Provera)

Category: D

Indications: Secondary amenorrhea and abnormal uterine bleeding due to hormonal imbalance; endometrial cancer

Actions: Progestin supplementation

Dosage:
Secondary amenorrhea: 5–10 mg PO qd for 5–10 days
Abnormal uterine bleeding: 5–10 mg PO qd for 5–10 days beginning on day 16 or 21 of the menstrual cycle
Cancer: 400–1000 mg IM per week

Supplied: Tablets 2.5 mg, 5.0 mg, 10 mg; depot injection 100 mg/mL, 400 mg/mL

Notes: Contraindicated with past thromboembolic disorders or hepatic disease

Megestrol Acetate (Megace)

Category: X

Indications: Breast and endometrial cancer

Actions: Hormone; antiluteinizing effect

Dosage: Varies with protocol

Supplied: Tablets 20 mg, 40 mg

Notes: Can cause nausea, vomiting, abdominal pain, breast tenderness

Melphalan (Alkeran)

Category: D

Indications: Breast and ovarian cancer

Actions: Nitrogen mustard-like bifunctional alkylating agent

Dosage: Varies with protocol

Supplied: Tablets 2 mg

Notes: Can cause nausea and bone marrow suppression

Menotropins (Pergonal)

Category: X

Indications: Induction of ovulation

Actions: Gonadotropin supplementation

Dosage: 75–150 IU qd IM for 9–12 days

Supplied: Injection (follicle-stimulating hormone/luteinizing hormone) 75 IU/75 IU, 150 IU/150 IU

Notes: Should be given with human chorionic gonadotropin; risk of multiple births

Meperidine (Demerol) [C]

Category: B

Indications: Relief of moderate to severe pain

Actions: Narcotic analgesic

Dosage: 50–100 mg PO or IM q3–4h prn

Supplied: Tablets 50 mg, 100 mg; syrup 50 mg/5 mL; injection 10 mg/mL, 25 mg/mL, 50 mg/mL, 75 mg/mL, 100 mg/mL

Notes: 75 mg IM is equivalent to 10 mg morphine IM; beware of respiratory depression

Meprobamate (Equanil, Miltown)

Category: D

Indications: Short-term relief of symptoms of anxiety

Actions: Mild tranquilizer, antianxiety agent

Dosage: 200–400 mg PO tid–qid; sustained-release 400–800 mg PO bid

Supplied: Tablets 200 mg, 400 mg; 600 mg; SR capsules 200 mg, 400 mg

Notes: Can cause drowsiness

Mesalamine (Rowasa)

Category: B

Indications: Treatment of mild to moderate distal ulcerative colitis, proctosigmoiditis, or proctitis

Actions: Unknown; may topically inhibit prostaglandins

Dosage: Retention enema ghs

Supplied: Rectal suspension 4 g/60 mL

Mesna (MESNEX)

Category: B

Indications: Prevention of ifosfamide-induced hemorrhagic cystitis

Actions: Detoxifying agent

Dosage: 240 mg/m^2 infused at 0, 4, and 8 hours after ifosfamide administration

Supplied: Injection 100 mg/mL

Notes: Can cause altered taste and diarrhea

Metaproterenol (Alupent, Metaprel)

Category: C

Indications: Bronchodilator for asthma and reversible bronchospasm

Actions: Sympathomimetic bronchodilator

Dosage:
Inhalation: 2–3 inhalations q3–4h to maximum of 12 per 24 hours
Oral: 20 mg q6–8h

Supplied: Tablets 10 mg, 20 mg; syrup 10 mg/5 mL; metered-dose inhaler 650 µg/dose; solution for inhalation 0.4%, 0.6%

Notes: Fewer beta-1 effects and longer acting than isoproterenol

Methadone (Dolophine) [C]

Category: B

Indications: Severe pain; detoxification and maintenance in narcotic addiction

Actions: Narcotic analgesic

Dosage: 2.5–10 mg IM q4h or 5–15 mg PO q8h (titrate as needed)

Supplied: Tablets 5 mg, 10 mg; oral solution 5 mg/5 mL, 10 mg/5 mL; injection 10 mg/mL

Notes: Equianalgesic with parenteral morphine; has a long half-life, increase dosage slowly to avoid respiratory depression

Methenamine Hippurate (Hiprex, Urex)

Methenamine Mandelate (Mandelamine, others)

Category: C

Indications: Suppression of chronic urinary tract infection

Actions: Bactericidal; converted to formaldehyde in acid urine

Dosage: 1 g PO bid

Supplied: Tablets 1 g

Notes: For maximum effect, urinary pH should be < 5.5; use oral vitamin C or ammonium chloride to acidify urine; GI distress and urinary tract irritation are common

Methicillin (Staphcillin) (see Table 7–5, page 570)

Methimazole (Tapazole)

Category: D

Indications: Hyperthyroidism; prep for thyroid surgery or radiation

Actions: Blocks formation of T_3 and T_4

Dosage: Initially 15–60 mg PO qd divided tid; maintenance, 5–15 mg PO qd

Supplied: Tablets 5 mg, 10 mg

Notes: Follow the patient clinically and with thyroid function tests

Methocarbamol (Robaxin)

Indications: Relief of discomfort associated with painful musculoskeletal conditions

Actions: Centrally acting skeletal muscle relaxant

Dosage: 1.5 g PO qid for 2–3 days, then 1 g PO qid maintenance therapy; IV form is rarely indicated

Supplied: Tablets 500 mg, 750 mg; injection 100 mg/mL

Notes: Can discolor urine; can cause drowsiness or GI upset; contraindicated in myasthenia gravis

Methotrexate (Folex)

Category: D

Indications: Breast and ovarian cancer, gestational trophoblastic disease

Actions: Antimetabolite; inhibits dihydrofolic acid reductase

Dosage: Varies with protocol

Supplied: Tablets 2.5 mg; injection 2.5 mg/mL, 25 mg/mL; preservative-free injection 25 mg/mL

Notes: Can cause nausea, vomiting, bone marrow suppression, fever, mucositis; may be administered intrathecally

Methyldopa (Aldomet)

Category: B

Indications: Essential hypertension

Actions: Centrally acting antihypertensive agent

Dosage: 250–500 mg PO bid–tid (maximum, 2–3 g/d) **or** 250 mg–1 g IV q4–8h

Supplied: Tablets 125 mg, 250 mg, 500 mg; oral suspension 250 mg/5 mL; injection 250 mg/5 mL

Notes: Do not use in liver disease; can discolor urine; initial transient sedation or drowsiness occurs frequently

Methylergonovine (Methergine)

Category: C

Indications: Postpartum atony and hemorrhage

Actions: Induces rapid and sustained tetanic uterotonic effect

Dosage:
IM: 0.2 mg after delivery of the placenta; may repeat at 2–4-hour intervals
Oral: 0.2 mg tid–qid for maximum of 1 week

Supplied: Tablets 0.2 mg; injection 0.2 mg/mL

Note: Contraindicated in preeclampsia, eclampsia, and hypertension

Methylprednisolone (Solu-Medrol) (see Steroids and Table 7–3, page 552)

Metoclopramide (Reglan)

Category: B

Indications: Relief of diabetic gastroparesis, symptomatic gastroesophageal reflux, relief of chemotherapy-induced nausea and vomiting

Actions: Stimulates motility of the upper GI tract

Dosage:
Diabetic Gastroparesis: 10 mg PO 30 minutes before meals and qhs; or the same dose given IV for 10 days, then switch to PO
Gastroesophageal reflux: 10–15 mg PO 30 minutes before meals and qhs
Antiemetic: 1–3 mg/kg slow IV 30 minutes prior to antineoplastic agent, then q2h for two doses, then q3h for three doses

Supplied: Tablets 5 mg, 10 mg; syrup 5 mg/5 mL; injection 5 mg/mL

Notes: Dystonic reactions are common with high doses and may be treated with Benadryl 50 mg IV; can also be used to facilitate small bowel intubation and radiologic evaluation of the upper GI tract

Metolazone (Diulo, Zaroxolyn)

Category: B

Indications: Mild to moderate essential hypertension, edema secondary to renal disease or cardiac failure

Actions: Thiazide-like diuretic

Dosage:
Hypertension: 2.5–5 mg PO qd
Edema: 5–20 mg PO qd

Supplied: Tablets 2.5 mg, 5 mg, 10 mg

Notes: Monitor fluids and electrolytes

Metoprolol (Lopressor) (see Table 7–6, page 571)

Metronidazole (Flagyl)

Category: B

Indications: Amebiasis, trichomoniasis, *C. difficile,* and anaerobic infections

Actions: Interferes with DNA synthesis

Dosage:
Anaerobic infections: 500 mg IV q6–8h
Amebic Dysentery: 750 mg PO qd for 5–10 days
Trichomoniasis: 2 g PO in 1 dose or 250 mg PO tid for 7 days
C. difficile: 500 mg PO q8h for 7–10 days

Supplied: Tablets 250 mg, 500 mg; injection 500 mg

Notes: For *Trichomonas* infections, also treat the partner; reduce dosage in hepatic failure; has no activity against aerobic bacteria; use in combination in serious mixed infections or infections of unknown cause

Metyrapone (Metopirone)

Category: C

Indications: Diagnostic test for hypothalamic-pituitary adrenocorticotrophic hormone (ACTH) function

Actions: Inhibits endogenous adrenal corticosteroid synthesis

Dosage:
Day 1 (Control period): Collect 24-hour urine to measure 17-hydroxycorticosteroids (17-OHCS) or 17-ketogenic steroids (17-KGS)
Day 2: For ACTH test, infuse 50 units ACTH over 8 hours and measure 24-hour urinary steroids
Days 3–4: Rest period
Day 5: Administer metyrapone 750 mg PO q4h for 6 doses with milk or snack
Day 6: Determine 24-hour urinary steroids

Supplied: Tablets 250 mg

Notes: Normal 24-hour 17-OHCS level is 3–12 mg and increases to 15–45 mg/24h following ACTH; normal response to metyrapone is a 2- to 4-fold increase in 17-OHCS excretion; drug interactions with phenytoin, cyproheptadine, and estrogens may lead to subnormal response

Mexiletine (Mexitil)

Category: C

Indications: Suppression of symptomatic ventricular arrhythmias

Actions: Class 1B antiarrhythmic

Dosage: 200–300 mg q8h, not to exceed 1200 mg/d; administer with food or antacids

Supplied: Capsules 150 mg; 200 mg, 250 mg

Notes: Not to be used in cardiogenic shock or in second- or third-degree atrioventricular block if no pacemaker; can worsen severe arrhythmias; monitor liver function during therapy; drug interactions with hepatic enzyme inducers and suppressors require dosage changes

Mezlocillin (Mezlin) (see Table 7–4, page 569)

Miconazole (Monistat)

Category: C

Indications: Severe systemic fungal infections including coccidioidomycosis, candidiasis, and *Cryptococcus;* various tinea forms, cutaneous candidiasis, vulvovaginal candidiasis, tinea versicolor

Actions: Fungicidal; alters permeability of the fungal cell membrane

Dosage:
Systemic: Dosage range is from 200–3600 mg/24h IV based on diagnosis, divided tid
Topical: Apply to affected area bid for 2–4 weeks
Intravaginal: Insert 1 applicatorful or suppository qhs for 7 days

Supplied: Injection 10 mg/mL; topical cream 2%; lotion 2%; powder 2%; spray 2%; vaginal suppositories 200 mg; vaginal cream 2%

Notes: Antagonistic to amphotericin B in vivo; rapid IV infusion can cause tachycardia or arrhythmias; can potentiate warfarin drug activity

Midazolam (Versed) [C]

Category: D

Indications: Preoperative sedation, conscious sedation for short procedures

Actions: Short-acting benzodiazepine

Dosage: 1–5 mg IV or IM, titrated to effect

Supplied: Injection 1 mg/mL, 5 mg/mL

Notes: Monitor patient for respiratory depression; can produce hypotension during conscious sedation

Milk of Magnesia (see Magnesium hydroxide)

Mineral Oil

Category: C

Indications: Constipation

Actions: Emollient laxative

Dosage: 15–30 mL PO prn

Supplied: Liquid

Minocycline (Minocin)

Category: D

Indications: Infections caused by susceptible strains of many gram-positive and gram-negative bacteria, *Rickettsiae, Mycoplasma pneumoniae, Chlamydia,* syphilis, gonorrhea

Actions: Bacteriostatic; interferes with protein synthesis

Dosage: 50 mg PO qid **or** 100 mg PO or IV bid

Supplied: Capsules and tablets 50 mg, 100 mg; suspension 50 mg/5 mL; injection 100 mg

Notes: A tetracycline antibiotic

Minoxidil (Loniten, Rogaine)

Category: C

Indications: Severe hypertension, treatment of female pattern baldness

Actions: Peripheral vasodilator, stimulates vertex hair growth

Dosage:
Oral: 2.5–10 mg bid–qid
Topical: Apply twice daily

Supplied: Tablets 2.5 mg, 10 mg; topical solution 2%

Notes: Pericardial effusion and volume overload can occur; hypertrichosis can develop with chronic use

Misoprostol (Cytotec)

Category: X

Indications: Prevention of NSAID-induced gastric ulcers

Actions: Synthetic prostaglandin with both antisecretory and mucosal protective properties

Dosage: 200 μg PO qid

Supplied: Tablets 200 µg

Notes: **Do not** take if pregnant (can cause miscarriage with potentially dangerous bleeding); GI side effects are common

Mitomycin (Mutamycin)

Category: D

Indications: Breast, cervical, and ovarian cancer

Actions: Antibiotic; inhibits DNA synthesis

Dosage: Varies with protocol

Supplied: Injection 5 mg, 20 mg, 40 mg

Notes: Can cause nausea, vomiting, bone marrow suppression, mucositis, nephrotoxicity

Molindone (Moban)

Category: C

Indications: Management of psychotic disorders

Actions: Piperazine phenothiazine

Dosage: 5–100 mg PO tid–qid

Supplied: Tablets 5 mg, 10 mg, 25 mg, 50 mg, 100 mg; concentrate 20 mg/mL

Morphine Sulfate [C]

Category: C

Indications: Relief of severe pain

Actions: Narcotic analgesic

Dosage:
Oral: 10–30 mg q4h prn; sustained-release 30–60 mg q8–12h
IM: 5–20 mg q4h prn
IV: 2.5–15 mg q4h prn given over 4–5 minutes
Epidural: By experienced anesthesiologist

Supplied: Tablets 10 mg, 15 mg, 30 mg; SR tablets 15 mg, 30 mg, 60 mg; solution 10 mg/5 mL, 20 mg/5 mL, 100 mg/5 mL; suppositories 5 mg, 10 mg, 20 mg; injection 2 mg/mL, 4 mg/mL, 5 mg/mL, 8 mg/mL, 10 mg/mL, 15 mg/mL; preservative-free injection 0.5 mg/mL, 1 mg/mL

Notes: Has large number of narcotic side effects; may require scheduled dosing to relieve severe chronic pain

Muromonab-CD3 (Orthoclone OKT3)

Category: C

Indications: Treatment of acute rejection following organ transplantation

Actions: Blocks T-cell function

Dosage: 5 mg IV qd for 10–14 days

Supplied: Injection 5 mg/5 mL

Notes: Is a murine antibody; may cause significant fever and chills after the first dose

Nadolol (Corgard) (see Table 7–6, page 571)

Nafarelin (Synarel)

Category: X

Indications: Endometriosis

Actions: Semisynthetic gonadotropin-releasing hormone analog

Dosage: 200 µg sprayed intranasally bid

Supplied: Intranasal spray 200 µg/spray

Notes: Can cause hot flashes, decreased libido, vaginal dryness, mood changes, headaches

Nafcillin (Nafcil, Unipen) (see Table 7–5, page 570)

Nalbuphine (Nubain)

Category: B

Indications: Moderate to severe pain

Actions: Narcotic agonist-antagonist

Dosage: 10–20 mg IM or IV q4–6h prn

Supplied: Injection 10 mg/mL, 20 mg/mL

Notes: Causes CNS depression and drowsiness

Nalidixic Acid (NegGram)

Category: B

Indications: Urinary tract infections caused by susceptible strains of *Proteus, Klebsiella, Enterobacter,* and *E. coli*

Actions: Interferes with DNA polymerization

Dosage: 1 g PO qid for 7–14 days

Supplied: Tablets 250 mg, 500 mg, 1 g; suspension 250 mg/5 mL

Notes: Resistance emerges within 48 hours in a significant percentage of trials; can enhance the effect of oral anticoagulants; can cause CNS adverse effects which reverse upon discontinuation of the drug

Naloxone (Narcan)

Category: B

Indications: Complete or partial reversal of narcotic depression

Actions: Narcotic antagonist

Dosage: 0.4–2.0 mg IV, IM, or SQ q5min, to maximum total dose of 10 mg

Supplied: Injection 0.4 mg/mL, 1.0 mg/mL; neonatal injection 0.02 mg/mL

Notes: Can precipitate acute withdrawal in addicts; if no response after 10 mg, suspect a nonnarcotic cause

Naproxen (Anaprox, Naprosyn) (see Table 7–10, page 575)

Neomycin-Polymyxin Bladder Irrigant (Neosporin G.U. Irrigant)

Category: D

Indications: Continuous irrigant for prophylaxis against bacteriuria and gram-negative bacteremia associated with use of an indwelling catheter

Actions: Bactericidal

Dosage: 1 mL irrigant added to 1 L 0.9% saline solution; continuous irrigation of the bladder with 1–2 L of solution per day

Supplied: Ampules 1 mL, 20 mL

Notes: Potential for bacterial or fungal superinfection; possibility for neomycin-induced ototoxicity or nephrotoxicity

Neomycin Sulfate

Category: C

Indications: Hepatic coma

Actions: Suppresses GI bacterial flora

Dosage: 1–4 g PO qid

Supplied: Tablets 500 mg; oral solution 125 mg/5 mL

Netilmicin (Netromycin)

Category: D

Indications: Serious infections caused by susceptible gram-negative organisms

Actions: Aminoglycoside; interferes with protein synthesis

Dosage: Normal renal function: 6.0 mg/kg/d in 3 divided doses; dosage must be adjusted in renal failure. The standard aminoglycoside dosing guides appearing in Tables 7–14 and 7–15 at the end of this chapter **cannot** be used to adjust the dose

Supplied: Injection 100 mg/mL

Notes: Nephrotoxic and ototoxic; decrease the dosage in renal insufficiency

Niacin (Nicobid)

Category: A

Indications: Adjunctive therapy in patients with significant hyperlipidemia who do not respond adequately to diet and weight loss

Actions: Inhibits lipolysis, decreases esterification of triglyceride, increases lipoprotein lipase activity

Dosage: 1–2 g PO tid with meals; up to 8 g/d

Supplied: SR capsules 125 mg, 250 mg, 300 mg, 400 mg, 500 mg; tablets 20 mg, 25 mg, 50 mg, 100 mg, 500 mg; elixir 50 mg/5 mL

Notes: Upper body and facial flushing and warmth can occur after a dose; can cause GI upset

Nicardipine (Cardene)

Category: C

Indications: Treatment of chronic stable angina and hypertension

Actions: Calcium channel blocking agent

Dosage:
Oral: 20–40 mg tid **or** sustained release 30–60 mg bid
Intravenous: 0.5–2.2 mg/h continuous infusion

Supplied: Capsules 20 mg, 30 mg; SR capsules 30 mg, 45 mg, 60 mg; injection 2.5 mg/mL

Notes: Oral to IV conversion: 20 mg tid = 0.5 mg/h, 30 mg tid = 1.2 mg/h, 40 mg tid = 2.2 mg/h

Nicotine Transdermal System (Habitrol, Nicoderm, Nicotrol, Prostep)

Category: X

Indications: Aid to smoking cessation for the relief of nicotine withdrawal

Actions: Provides systemic delivery of nicotine

Dosage: Individualize the dosage to the patient's needs and the transdermal system used; see package insert for detailed dosing information on each formula

Agent	Patch Size (cm^2)	Nicotine Dose/Patch	Recommended Duration (wk)
Habitrol	30	21 mg/24h	4–8
	20	14 mg/24h	2–4
	10	7 mg/24h	2–4
Nicoderm	22	21 mg/24h	4–8
	15	14 mg/24h	2–4
	7	7 mg/24th	2–4
Nicotrol	30	15 mg/16h[a]	4–12
	20	10 mg/16h	2–4
	10	5 mg/16h	2–4
PROSTEP	7	22 mg/24h	4–8
		11 mg/24h	2–4

[a]Nicotrol patch is worn 16 hours to mimic the natural smoking pattern. All others are worn 24 hours.

Supplied: Transdermal patch (see above)

Notes: Patient must stop smoking and use behavioral modification for transdermal systems to be effective

Nifedipine (Adalat, Procardia)

Category: C

Indications: Vasospastic or chronic stable angina, hypertensive crisis

Actions: Calcium channel blocking agent

Dosage: 10–30 mg PO q8h (maximum, 180 mg/d); sustained-release 30–90 mg PO qd

Supplied: Capsules 10 mg, 20 mg; SR tablets 30 mg, 60 mg, 90 mg

Notes: Headaches are common on initial treatment; reflex tachycardia can occur

Nitrofurantoin (Furadantin, Macrodantin)

Category: B

Indications: Urinary tract infections

Actions: Baceriostatic; interferes with carbohydrate metabolism

Dosage:
Suppression: 50–100 mg PO qd
Usual dose: 50–100 mg PO qid

Supplied: Capsules and tablets 50 mg, 100 mg; suspension 25 mg/ 5 mL

Notes: GI side effects are common; should be taken with food, milk, or antacid; macrocrystals (Macrodantin) cause less nausea than other forms of the drug

Nitrogen Mustard (Mustargen)

Category: D

Indications: Ovarian cancer

Actions: Polyfunctional alkylating agent

Dosage: Varies with protocol

Supplied: Injection 10 mg

Notes: May cause nausea, vomiting, bone marrow suppression, alopecia, skin necrosis

Nitroglycerin (Nitrolingual, Nitro-Bid Ointment, Nitro-bid IV, Nitrodisc, Transderm-Nitro, Tridil, others)

Category: C

Indications: Angina pectoris (acute and prophylactic therapy), congestive heart failure, blood pressure control

Actions: Relaxation of vascular smooth muscle

Dosage:
Sublingual: 1 tablet q5min prn for 3 doses
Translingual: 1–2 metered doses sprayed onto oral mucosa
Oral: 2.5–9.0 mg tid
Intravenous: 5–20 μg/min, titrated to effect

Topical: Apply 1–2 inches of ointment to the chest wall q6h, then wipe off at night
Transdermal: One 5–20 cm patch qd

Supplied: Sublingual tablets 0.15 mg, 0.3 mg, 0.4 mg, 0.6 mg; translingual spray 0.4 mg/dose; SR capsules 2.5 mg, 6.5 mg, 9 mg; SR tablets 2.6 mg, 6.5 mg, 9.0 mg; injection 0.5 mg/mL, 0.8 mg/mL, 5 mg/mL, 10 mg/mL; ointment 2%; transdermal patches delivering 2.5, 5, 7.5, 10, or 15 mg/24h

Notes: Tolerance to nitrates will develop with chronic use after 1–2 weeks and can be avoided by providing a nitrate-free period each day; shorter-acting nitrates should be used on a tid basis, and long-acting patches and ointment should be removed before bedtime to prevent development of tolerance

Nitroprusside (Nipride)

Category: C

Indications: Hypertensive emergency, aortic dissection, pulmonary edema

Actions: Reduces systemic vascular resistance

Dosage: 0.5–10 µg/kg/min IV infusion, titrated to desired effect

Supplied: Injection 50 mg per vial

Notes: Thiocyanate, the metabolite, is excreted by the kidney; thiocyanate toxicity occurs at plasma levels of 5–10 mg/dL; if used to treat aortic dissection, a beta blocker must be used concomitantly

Nizatidine (Axid)

Category: C

Indications: Treatment of duodenal ulcers

Actions: Histamine antagonist H_2

Dosage:
  Active ulcer: 150 mg PO bid or 300 mg PO qhs
  Maintenance: 150 mg PO qhs

Supplied: Capsules 150 mg, 300 mg

Norepinephrine (Levophed)

Category: C

Indications: Acute hypotensive states

Actions: Peripheral vasoconstrictor acting on both the arterial and venous beds

Dosage: Initially 8–12 µg/min IV; titrate to response

Supplied: Injection 1 mg/mL

Notes: Correct blood volume depletion as much as possible prior to initiation of vasopressor therapy; drug interaction with tricyclic antidepressants can lead to severe, prolonged hypertension; infuse into a large vein to avoid extravasation; inject phentolamine 5–10 mg in 10 mL normal saline locally as antidote to extravasation

Norethindrone (Aygestin, Norlutate, Norlutin)

Category: X

Indications: Amenorrhea, abnormal uterine bleeding, endometriosis

Actions: Progestin supplementation

Dosage:
Amenorrhea: 2.5–20 mg PO qd, starting on day 5 of the menstrual cycle and ending on day 25
Endometriosis: 5–10 mg PO qd for 2 weeks; increasing to 15–30 mg/d

Supplied: Tablets 5 mg

Notes: The acetate salt is approximately twice as potent

Norfloxacin (Noroxin)

Category: C

Indications: Treatment of complicated and uncomplicated urinary tract infections due to a wide variety of pathogens including *E. coli, Enterobacter cloacae, Proteus mirabilis,* indole-positive *Proteus* species, *Pseudomonas aeruginosa, S. aureus, S. epidermidis*

Actions: Quinolone antibiotic; inhibits DNA gyrase

Dosage: 400 mg PO bid

Supplied: Tablets 400 mg

Notes: Not for use in pregnancy; should be taken 1 hour before or 2 hours after meals; do not take with antacids

Nortriptyline (Aventyl, Pamelor)

Category: D

Indications: Endogenous depression

Actions: Tricyclic antidepressant

Dosage: 25 mg PO tid–qid (maximum, 100 mg/d)

Supplied: Capsules 10 mg, 25 mg, 75 mg; solution 10mg/5 mL

Notes: Has many anticholinergic side effects including blurred vision, urine retention, dry mouth

Nystatin (Mycostatin, Nilstat)

Category: B

Indications: Treatment of *Candida* infections (thrush, vaginitis)

Actions: Alters membrane permeability

Dosage:
  Oral: 400,000–600,000 units 4–5 times daily
  Vaginal: 1 tablet qd
  Topical: Apply 2–3 times daily

Supplied: Oral suspension 100,000 units/mL; oral tablets 500,000 units; troches 200,000 units; vaginal tablets 100,000 units; topical cream, ointment, and powder 100,000 units/g

Notes: Not absorbed orally, therefore not effective for systemic infections

Ofloxacin (Floxin)

Category: C

Indications: Treatment of infections of the lower respiratory tract, skin and skin structures, and urinary tract, uncomplicated gonorrhea, and *Chlamydia* infections

Actions: Bactericidal; inhibits DNA gyrase

Dosage: 200–400 mg PO or IV q12h

Supplied: Tablets 200 mg, 400 mg; injection 200 mg; 400 mg

Notes: Can cause nausea, vomiting, diarrhea, and headache; drug interactions with antacids, sucralfate, and iron- and zinc-containing products that decrease its absorption; may increase theophylline levels

Olsalazine (Dipentum)

Category: C

Indications: Maintenance of remission of ulcerative colitis

Actions: Anti-inflammatory activity

Dosage: 500 mg PO bid

Supplied: Capsules 250 mg

Notes: Take with food; can cause diarrhea

Omeprazole (Prilosec)

Category: C

Indications: Treatment of duodenal ulcers

Actions: Proton pump inhibitor

Dosage: 20–40 mg PO qd

Supplied: Capsules 20 mg

Notes: Patients must not crush or chew tablets

Ondansetron (Zofran)

Category: B

Indications: Prevention of nausea and vomiting associated with chemotherapy

Actions: Antiemetic; serotonin antagonist

Dosage: 0.15 mg/kg IV 30 minutes prior to chemotherapy, then again in 4 and 8 hours

Supplied: Injection 2 mg/mL

Notes: Diarrhea and headache are common side effects

Opium, Camphorated Tincture (Paregoric) [C]

Category: B

Indications: Diarrhea, relief of severe pain in place of morphine, sedative-hypnotic

Actions: Antispasmodic; narcotic analgesic

Dosage: 5–10 mL PO up to qid

Supplied: Liquid

Notes: Has CNS depressant activity due to its morphine content (2 mg/5 mL)

Opium, Tincture [C]

Category: B

Indications: Diarrhea, relief of severe pain in place of morphine, sedative-hypnotic

Actions: Antispasmodic; narcotic analgesic

Dosage: 0.6 mL PO qid

Supplied: Liquid 10% opium

Notes: Has CNS depressant activity due to its morphine content (0.6 mL = 6 mg)

Oxacillin (Bactocill, Prostaphlin) (see Table 7–5, page 570)

Oxazepam (Serax) [C]

Category: D

Indications: Anxiety, acute alcohol withdrawal

Actions: Benzodiazepine

Dosage:
  Anxiety: 10–15 mg PO tid–qid
  Alcohol withdrawal: 15–30 mg PO tid–qid

Supplied: Tablets 15 mg; capsules 10 mg, 15 mg, 30 mg

Oxtriphylline (Choledyl)

Category: C

Indications: Asthma, bronchospasm

Actions: Relaxes smooth muscle of the bronchi and pulmonary blood vessels

Dosage: 200 mg PO qid; SR tablets 400–600 mg PO q12h

Supplied: Tablets 100 mg, 200 mg; SR tablets 400 mg, 600 mg; elixir 100 mg/5 mL

Notes: Contains 64% theophylline

Oxybutynin (Ditropan)

Category: B

Indications: Symptoms associated with neurogenic or reflex neurogenic bladder

Actions: Antispasmodic

Dosage: 5 mg PO bid–qid

Supplied: Tablets 5 mg; syrup 5 mg/5 mL

Notes: Anticholinergic side effects

Oxycodone (Percocet, Percodan, Tylox) [C]

Category: C

Indications: Moderate to moderately severe pain

Actions: Narcotic analgesic

Dosage: 1–2 tablets or capsules PO q4–6h prn

Supplied:
Percocet tablet: 5 mg oxycodone/325 mg acetaminophen
Percodan tablet: 4.5 mg oxycodone/325 mg aspirin
Tylox capsule: 5 mg oxycodone/500 mg acetaminophen

Oxytocin (Pitocin, Syntocinon)

Indications: Initiate or improve uterine contractions, control postpartum bleeding

Actions: Uterine stimulant, especially on the gravid uterus

Dosage: 1–2 mU/min IV; increase to maximum of 20 mU/min

Supplied: Injection 10 units/mL

Pamidronate Disodium (Aredia)

Category: C

Indications: Treatment of hypercalcemia of pregnancy

Actions: Inhibits bone resorption

Dosage: 60–90 mg IV infused over 24 hours

Supplied: Injection 30 mg

Notes: Allow 7 days to elapse before retreatment

Pancrelipase (Cotazym, Pancrease)

Category: C

Indications: For patients deficient in pancreatic exocrine enzymes (cystic fibrosis, chronic pancreatitis, other pancreatic insufficiency) and for steatorrhea of malabsorption syndrome

Actions: Supplementation of pancreatic enzymes

Dosage: 1–3 tablets PO after meals

Supplied: Tablets

Notes: Avoid antacids; can cause nausea, abdominal cramps, or diarrhea; patients should not crush or chew enteric coated products

Pancuronium (Pavulon)

Category: C

Indications: Aid in management of patients on mechanical ventilation

Actions: Nondepolarizing muscle relaxant

Dosage: 2–4 mg IV q2–4h prn

Supplied: Injection 1 mg/mL, 2 mg/mL

Notes: Patient must be intubated and on controlled ventilation; use adequate amount of sedation or analgesia (morphine, etc)

Penbutolol (Levatol) (see Table 7–6, page 571)

Penicillin G (Potassium or Sodium) Aqueous (Pentids, Pfizerpen)

Category: B

Indications: Most gram-positive infections (except penicillin-resistant staphylococci) including streptococci, clostridia, corynebacteria, and some coliform bacteria; also syphilis

Actions: Inteferes with cell wall synthesis

Dosage:
Oral: 400,000–800,000 units qid
Intravenous: Dosage varies greatly depending on indications, with range from 1.2–24 million units per day

Supplied: Tablets 200,000 units, 250,000 units, 400,000 units, 500,000 units, 800,000 units; powder for oral suspension 200,000 units/5 mL, 400,000 units/5 mL; powder for injection

Notes: Beware of hypersensitivity reactions; the drug of choice for group A steptococcal, pneumococcal, and syphilis infections

Penicillin G Benzathine (Bicillin)

Category: B

Indications: Useful as a single-dose treatment regimen for streptococcal pharyngitis, rheumatic fever and glomerulonephritis prophylaxis, and syphilis

Actions: Interferes with cell wall synthesis

Dosage: 1.2–2.4 million units deep IM injection

Supplied: Injection 300,000 units/mL, 600,000 units/mL

Notes: Sustained action with detectable levels for up to 4 weeks; the drug of choice for treatment of noncongenital syphilis; Bicillin L-A contains the benzathine salt only; Bicillin C-R contains a combination of benzathine and procaine salts and is used for most acute strep infections (300,000 units procaine with 300,000 units benzathine/mL or 900,000 units benzathine with 300,000 units procaine/2 mL)

Penicillin G Procaine (Wycillin, others)

Category: B

Indications: Moderately severe infection caused by penicillin-sensitive organisms that respond to low persistent serum levels (syphilis and uncomplicated pneumococcal pneumonia)

Actions: Interferes with cell wall synthesis

Dosage: 2.4–4.8 million units IM and 1 g of probenecid PO

Supplied: Injection 300,000 units/mL, 500,000 units/mL, 600,000 units/mL

Notes: A long-acting parenteral penicillin; blood levels last up to 15 hours; give probenecid at least 30 minutes prior to administration to prolong its action

Penicillin V (Pen-Vee K, V-Cillin K, others)

Category: B

Indications: Most gram-positive infections (except penicillin-resistant staphylococci) including streptococci, clostridia, corynebacteria, and some coliform bacteria; also syphilis

Actions: Interferes with cell wall synthesis

Dosage: 250–500 mg PO qid

Supplied: Tablets 125 mg, 250 mg, 500 mg; powder for oral suspension 125 mg/5 mL, 250 mg/5 mL

Notes: A well-tolerated oral penicillin; 250 mg is equal to 400,000 units of penicillin G

Pentamadine Isethionate (NebuPent, Pentam 300)

Category: C

Indications: Treatment and prevention of *Pneumocystis carinii* pneumonia

Actions: Inhibits the synthesis of DNA, RNA, phospholipids, and protein synthesis

Dosage:
Parenteral: 4 mg/kg IV or deep IM injection daily
Inhalation: 300 mg once every 4 weeks, administered via Respirgard II nebulizer

Supplied: Injection 300 mg per vial; aerosol 300 mg

Notes: Monitor the patient for severe hypotension following IV or IM dosing; is associated with pancreatic islet cell necrosis leading to hyperglycemia or hypoglycemia; monitor hematology studies for leukopenia and thrombocytopenia; IM dosing may result in sterile abscess formation

Pentazocine (Talwin) [C]

Category: C

Indications: Moderate to severe pain

Actions: Narcotic agonist-antagonist

Dosage: 30 mg IM or IV; 50–100 mg PO q3–4h prn

Supplied: Tablets 50 mg (with naloxone 0.5 mg); injection 30 mg/mL

Notes: 30–60 mg IM is equianalgesic to 10 mg morphine IM; associated with considerable dysphoria

Pentobarbital (Nembutal, others) [C]

Category: D

Indications: Insomnia, convulsions, induced coma following severe head injury

Actions: Barbiturate

Dosage:
Sedative: 20–40 mg PO q6–12h
Hypnotic: 100–200 mg PO qhs
Induced coma: Load 3–5 mg/kg IV for single dose; maintenance, 2–3.5 mg/kg/dose hourly prn to keep level at 25–40 µg/mL

Supplied: Capsules 50 mg, 100 mg; elixir 20 mg/5 mL; suppositories 30 mg, 60 mg, 120 mg, 200 mg; injection 50 mg/mL

Notes: Can cause respiratory depression; can produce profound hypotension when given rapidly to induce coma; tolerance to sedative-hypnotic effect is acquired within 1–2 weeks

Pentoxifylline (Trental)

Category: C

Indications: Intermittent claudication

Actions: Lowers blood viscosity by restoring erythrocyte flexibility

Dosage: 400 mg PO tid with meals

Supplied: Tablets 400 mg

Notes: Treat for at least 8 weeks to see full effect

Permethrin (Nix)

Category: B

Indications: Eradication of lice

Actions: Pediculocide

Dosage: Saturate hair and scalp, allow to remain in hair for 10 minutes before rinsing out

Supplied: Liquid 1%

Perphenazine (Trilafon)

Category: C

Indications: Psychotic disorders, intractable hiccups, severe nausea

Actions: Phenothiazine; antipsychotic, antiemetic

Dosage:
Antipsychotic: 4–8 mg PO tid (maximum, 64 mg/d)
Hiccups: 5 mg IM q6h prn **or** 1 mg IV at not less than 1–2 mg/min intervals up to 5 mg

Supplied: Tablets 2 mg, 4 mg, 8 mg, 16 mg; oral concentrate 16 mg/5 mL; injection 5 mg/mL

Phenazopyridine (Pyridium, others)

Category: B

Indications: Symptomatic relief of discomfort from lower urinary tract irritation

Actions: Local anesthetic effect on urinary tract mucosa

Dosage: 200 mg PO tid

Supplied: Tablets 100 mg, 200 mg

Notes: Causes GI disturbances; colors urine red-orange, which can stain clothing

Phenobarbital [C]

Category: D

Indications: Seizure disorders, insomnia, anxiety

Actions: Barbiturate

Dosage:
Sedative-hypnotic: 30–120 mg PO or IM qd prn
Anticonvulsant: Loading dose of 10–12 mg/kg in 3 divided doses, then 1–3 mg/kg/24h PO or IV

Supplied: Tablets 8 mg, 16 mg, 32 mg, 65 mg, 100 mg; elixir 20 mg/5 mL; injection 30 mg/mL, 60 mg/mL, 65 mg/mL, 130 mg/mL

Notes: Tolerance develops to sedation; long half-life allows single daily dosing (see Table 7–14, Drug Levels, page 585)

Phenylephrine (Neo-Synephrine)

Category: C

Indications: Treatment of vascular failure in shock, anaphylaxis, or drug-induced hypotension; nasal congestion; mydriatic

Actions: Postsynaptic alpha-receptor stimulant

Dosage:
Mild to moderate hypotension: 2–5 mg IM or SQ elevates blood pressure (BP) for 2 hours; 0.1–0.5 mg IV elevates BP for 15 minutes.
Severe hypotension or shock: Initiate continuous infusion at 100–180 µg/min; after BP is stabilized, maintain at 40–60 µg/min
Mydriasis: 1–2 drops in the eye
Intranasal: 1–2 sprays in each nostril

Supplied: Injection 10 mg/mL; nasal solution 0.125%, 0.16%, 0.2%, 0.25%, 0.5%, 1%; ophthalmic solution 0.12%, 2.5%, 10%

Notes: Promptly restore blood volume if loss has occurred; use with extreme caution in hyperthyroidism, bradycardia, partial heart block, myocardial disease, or severe arteriosclerosis; use large veins for infusion to avoid extravasation; inject phentolamine 10 mg in 10–15 mL normal saline locally as antidote for extravasation; activity is potentiated by oxytocin, MAOIs, and tricyclic antidepressants

Phenytoin (Dilantin)

Category: D

Indications: Tonic-clonic and partial seizures

Actions: Inhibits spread of seizures in the motor cortex

Dosage:
Loading: 15–20 mg/kg IV at a maximum infusion rate of 25 mg/min **or** orally in 400 mg doses at 4-hour intervals
Maintenance: 200 mg PO or IV bid or 300 mg qhs initially, then follow plasma concentrations

Supplied: Capsules 30 mg, 100 mg; chewable tablets 50 mg; oral suspension 30 mg/5 mL, 125 mg/5 mL; injection 50 mg/mL

Notes: Beware of cardiac depressant side effects, especially with IV administration; follow levels as needed (see Table 7–14, Drug Levels, page 585); nystagmus and ataxia are early signs of toxicity; gum hyperplasia occurs with long-term use; avoid use of oral suspension if possible (absorption is erratic); avoid in pregnancy

Physostigmine (Antilirium)

Category: C

Indications: Antidote for tricyclic antidepressant, atropine, or scopolamine overdose

Actions: Reversible cholinesterase inhibitor

Dosage: 2 mg IM or slow IV q15min

Supplied: Injection 1 mg/mL

Notes: Rapid IV administration is associated with convulsions; has cholinergic side effects; can cause asystole

Phytonadione [Vitamin K] (AquaMEPHYTON, others)

Category: C

Indications: Coagulation disorders caused by faulty formation of Factors II, VII, IX, and X; hyperalimentation

Actions: Supplementation; needed for the production of Factors II, VII, IX, and X

Dosage:
Anticoagulant-induced prothrombin deficiency: 2.5–10.0 mg PO or IV **slowly**

Hyperalimentation: 10 mg IM or IV every week

Supplied: Tablets 5 mg; injection 2 mg/mL, 10 mg/mL

Notes: With parenteral treatment, usually see first change in prothrombin in 12–24 hours; anaphylaxis can result from IV dosage; should be administered slowly IV

Pindolol (Visken) (see Table 7–6, page 571)

Piperacillin (Pipracil) (see Table 7–4, page 569)

Piroxicam (Feldene) (see Table 7–10, page 575)

Plasma Protein Fraction (Plasmanate, others)

Category: C

Indications: Shock and hypotension

Actions: Plasma volume expansion

Dosage: 250–500 mL IV initially (not > 10 mL/min); subsequent infusions should depend upon clinical response

Supplied: Injection 5%

Notes: Hypotension is associated with rapid infusion; contains 130–160 meq sodium per liter

Plicamycin (Mithracin)

Category: X

Indications: Treatment of hypercalcemia of malignancy

Actions: Antibiotic; inhibits DNA-dependent RNA synthesis, rendering osteoclasts unable to respond to parathyroid hormone

Dosage: 25 µg/kg/d IV for 3–4 days

Supplied: Injection 2500 µg

Notes: Can cause nausea, vomiting, diarrhea, stomatitis

Pneumococcal Vaccine, Polyvalent (Pneumovax)

Category: C

Indications: Immunization against pneumococcal infections in patients predisposed to or at high risk of acquiring these infections

Actions: Active immunization

Dosage: 0.5 mL IM

Supplied: Injection containing 25 µg each of 23 polysaccharide isolates per 0.5 mL dose

Notes: Do not vaccinate during immunosuppressive therapy

Polyethylene Glycol–Electrolyte [PEG] Solution (Colyte, GoLYTELY)

Category: C

Indications: Bowel cleansing prior to examination

Actions: Osmotic cathartic

Dosage: Following 3–4 hour fast, drink 240 mL of solution q10min until 4 L is consumed

Supplied: Powder for reconstitution to 4 L in container

Notes: First bowel movement should occur in approximately 1 hour; may cause some cramping or nausea

Potassium Supplements

Category: A

Indications: Prevention or treatment of hypokalemia

Actions: Supplementation of potassium

Dosage: 16–24 meq/d PO divided qd–bid (Table 7–2)

Notes: Can cause GI irritation; powder and liquids must be mixed with beverage (unsalted tomato juice is very palatable); use cautiously in renal insufficiency and along with NSAIDs and ACE inhibitors

Pravastatin (Pravastatin)

Category: C

Indications: Reduction of elevated cholesterol levels

Actions: HMG-CoA reductase inhibitor

Dosage: 10–40 mg PO qhs

Supplied: Tablets 10 mg, 20 mg

Prazepam (Centrax) [C]

Category: D

Indications: Anxiety disorders

Actions: Benzodiazepine

TABLE 7–2. ORAL POTASSIUM SUPPLEMENTS.

Brand Name	Salt	Form	meq Potassium/Dosing Unit
Kaochlor 10%	KCl	Liquid	20 meq/15 mL
Kaochlor S-F 10% (sugar-free)	KCl	Liquid	20 meq/15 mL
Kaon Elixir	K⁺ gluconate	Liquid	20 meq/15 mL
Kaon	K⁺ gluconate	Tablets	5 meq/tablet
Kaon-Cl	KCl	Tablet, SR	6.67 meq/tablet
Kaon-Cl 20%	KCl	Liquid	40 meq/15 mL
Kay Ciel	KCl	Liquid	20 meq/15 mL
K-Lor	KCl	Powder	15 or 20 meq/packet
Klorvess	KCl	Liquid	20 meq/15 mL
Klotrix	KCl	Tablet, SR	10 meq/tablet
K-Lyte	K⁺ bicarbonate	Effervescent tablet	25 meq/tablet
K-Tab	KCl	Tablet, SR	10 meq/tablet
Micro-K	KCl	Capsules	8 meq/capsule
Slow-K	KCl	Tablet, SR	8 meq/tablet

From Gomella LG (ed): Clinician's Pocket Reference, 7th ed. Norwalk, Connecticut, Appleton & Lange, 1992.

Dosage: 5–10 mg PO tid–qid, or 20–50 mg PO qhs to minimize daytime drowsiness

Supplied: Tablets 10 mg; capsules 5 mg, 10 mg, 20 mg

Prazosin (Minipress)

Category: C

Indications: Hypertension

Actions: Peripherally acting alpha-adrenergic blocker

Dosage: 1 mg PO tid; may increase to total daily dose of 5 mg qid

Supplied: Capsules 1 mg, 2 mg, 5 mg

Notes: Can cause orthostatic hypotension, so patient should take first dose at bedtime; tolerance develops to this effect; tachyphylaxis can result

Prednisolone (see Steroids and Table 7–3, page 552)

Prednisone (see Steroids and Table 7–3, page 552)

Probenecid (Benemid, others)

Category: B

Indications: Gout; maintenance of serum levels of penicillins or cephalosporins

Actions: Renal tubular blocking agent

Dosage:
Gout: 0.25 g bid for 1 week, then 0.5 g PO bid
Antibiotic effect: 1–2 g PO 30 minutes prior to dose of antibiotic

Supplied: Tablets 500 mg

Probucol (Lorelco)

Category: B

Indications: Adjunctive therapy for reduction of serum cholesterol

Actions: Lowers serum cholesterol

Dosage: 500 mg PO bid with morning and evening meals

Supplied: Tablets 250 mg, 500 mg

Notes: Can cause prolongation of QT interval on ECG; diarrhea or loose stools are common; can also lower HDL

Procainamide (Procan, Pronestyl)

Category: C

Indications: Treatment of supraventricular and ventricular arrhythmias

Actions: Class 1A antiarrhythmic

Dosage:
Emergency cardiac care: 100–200 mg/dose IV q5min until dysrhythmia resolves, hypotension ensues, or dose totals 1 g; then maintenance of 1–4 mg/min IV infusion
Chronic dosing: 50 mg/kg/d PO in divided doses q4–6h

Supplied: Tablets and capsules 250 mg, 375 mg, 500 mg; SR tablets 250 mg, 500 mg, 750 mg, 1000 mg; injection 100 mg/mL, 500 mg/mL

Notes: Can cause hypotension and a lupus-like syndrome; dosage adjustment required with renal impairment; see Table 7–14, Drug Levels, page 585

Prochlorperazine (Compazine)

Category: C

Indications: Nausea, vomiting, agitation, psychotic disorders

Actions: Phenothiazine antiemetic, antipsychotic

Dosage:
  Antiemetic: 5–10 mg PO tid–qid, **or** 25 mg PR bid, **or** 5–10 mg deep
  IM q4–6h
  Antipsychotic: 10–20 mg IM acutely **or** 5–10 mg PO tid–qid for maintenance

Supplied: Tablets 5 mg, 10 mg, 25 mg; SR capsules 10 mg, 15 mg, 30
mg; syrup 5 mg/5 mL; suppositories 2.5 mg, 5 mg, 25 mg; injection 5
mg/mL

Notes: A much larger dose may be required for antipsychotic effect;
extrapyramidal side effects are common; treat acute extrapyramidal reactions with diphenhydramine

Progesterone in Oil (Gesterol 50, Progestaject)

Category: X

Indications: Amenorrhea, abnormal uterine bleeding

Actions: Progestin supplementation

Dosage: 5–10 mg IM qd for 6–8 days

Supplied: Injection 50mg/mL

Promethazine (Phenergan)

Category: C

Indications: Nausea, vomiting, motion sickness

Actions: Phenothiazine antihistamine, antiemetic

Dosage: 12.5–50 mg PO, PR, or IM bid–qid prn

Supplied: Tablets 12.5 mg, 25 mg, 50 mg; syrup 6.25 mg/mL, 25
mg/mL; suppositories 12.5 mg, 25 mg, 50 mg; injection 25 mg/mL, 50
mg/mL

Notes: High incidence of drowsiness

Propafenone (Rythmol)

Category: C

Indications: Treatment of life-threatening ventricular arrhythmias

Actions: Class 1C antiarrhythmic

Dosage: 150–300 mg PO q8h

Supplied: Tablets 150 mg, 300 mg

Notes: Can cause dizziness, unusual taste, and first-degree heart block

Propantheline (Pro-Banthine)

Category: C

Indications: Symptomatic treatment of small intestine hypermotility, spastic colon, ureteral spasm, bladder spasm, pylorospasm

Actions: Antimuscarinic agent

Dosage: 15 mg PO before meals and 30 mg PO hs

Supplied: Tablets 7.5 mg, 15 mg

Notes: Anticholinergic side effects such as dry mouth, blurred vision, etc, are common

Propoxyphene (Darvocet, Darvon) [C]

Category: C

Indications: Mild to moderate pain

Actions: Narcotic analgesic

Dosage: 32–65 mg PO q4h prn

Supplied:
Darvon (propoxyphene HCl): 32 mg, 65 mg
Darvon-N (propoxyphene napsylate): 100 mg, equivalent to 65 mg propoxyphene HCl
Darvocet-N: Propoxyphene napsylate/acetaminophen
Darvon compound: Propoxyphene HCl/aspirin/caffeine

Notes: Intentional overdose can be lethal

Propranolol (Inderal) (see Table 7–6, page 571)

Propylthiouracil [PTU]

Category: D

Indications: Hyperthyroidism

Actions: Inhibits production of T_3 and T_4 and conversion of T_4 to T_3

Dosage: Begin at 100 mg PO q8h (may need up to 1200 mg/d for control); after patient is euthyroid (6–8 weeks), taper dose by 1/3 q4–6wk to maintenance dose of 50–150 mg/24h; treatment can usually be discontinued in 2–3 years

Supplied: Tablets 50 mg

Notes: Follow patient clinically; monitor thyroid function tests

Protamine Sulfate

Category: C

Indications: Reversal of heparin effect

Actions: Neutralizes heparin

Dosage: Based on amount of heparin reversal desired; given slow IV, 1 mg will reverse approximately 100 units of heparin administered in the preceding 3–4 hours to a maximum dose of 50 mg

Supplied: Injection 10 mg/mL

Notes: Follow coagulation studies; can have anticoagulant effect if given without heparin

Pseudoephedrine (Afrinol, Novafed, Sudafed, others)

Category: C

Indications: Decongestant

Actions: Sympathomimetic

Dosage: 30–60 mg PO q6–8h; sustained-release 120 mg PO q12h

Supplied: Tablets 30 mg, 60 mg; SR capsules 120 mg; liquid 15 mg/5 mL; syrup 30 mg/5 mL

Notes: Contraindicated in hypertension or coronary artery disease and in patients taking MAO inhibitors; an ingredient in many cough and cold preparations

Psyllium (Effer-syllium, Metamucil, Serutan)

Indications: Constipation, diverticular disease of the colon

Actions: Bulk laxative

Dosage: 1 teaspoon (7 g) in a glass of water qd–tid

Supplied: Granules 4 g/tsp, 25 g/tsp; powder 3.5 g per packet

Notes: Do not use if bowel obstruction is suspected; one of the safest laxatives; psyllium in effervescent form (Effer-Syllium) usually contains potassium and should be used with caution in renal failure

Pyridoxine [Vitamin B$_6$]

Category: A

Indications: Treatment and prevention of vitamin B$_6$ deficiency

Actions: Supplementation of vitamin B_6

Dosage:
Deficiency: 2.5–10.0 mg PO qd
Drug-induced neuritis: 50 mg PO qd

Supplied: Tablets 10 mg, 25 mg, 50 mg, 100 mg, 200 mg, 250 mg, 500 mg; injection 100 mg/mL

Quazepam (Doral) [C]

Category: X

Indications: Insomnia

Actions: Benzodiazepine

Dosage: 7.5–15 mg PO qhs prn

Supplied: Tablets 7.5 mg, 15 mg

Notes: Reduce dosage in the elderly

Quinapril (Accupril)

Category: D

Indications: Treatment of hypertension

Actions: Angiotensin converting enzyme (ACE) inhibitor

Dosage: 10–80 mg PO once daily

Supplied: Tablets 5 mg, 10 mg, 20 mg, 40 mg

Quinidine (Quinaglute, Quinidex)

Category: C

Indications: Prevention of tachydysrhythmias

Actions: Class 1A antiarrhythmic

Dosage:
Premature atrial or ventricular contractions (PACs, PVCs): 200–300 mg PO tid–qid
Conversion of atrial fibrillation or flutter: Use after digitalization, 200 mg q2–3h for 8 doses; then increase daily dose to maximum of 3–4 g or until normal rhythm is restored

Supplied:
Sulfate: Tablets 100 mg, 200 mg, 300 mg; capsules 200 mg, 300 mg; SR tablets 300 mg; injection 200 mg/mL
Gluconate: SR tablets 324 mg, 330 mg; injection 80mg/mL

Notes: Contraindicated in digitalis toxicity, atrioventricular block; follow serum levels if available (see Table 7–14, Drug Levels, page 585); extreme hypotension can occur with IV administration; the sulfate salt contains 83% quinidine, the gluconate salt 62% quinidine

Ramipril (Altace)

Category: D

Indications: Treatment of hypertension

Actions: Angiotensin-converting enzyme (ACE) inhibitor

Dosage: 2.5–20 mg PO daily divided qd–bid

Supplied: Capsules 1.25 mg, 2.5 mg, 5 mg, 10 mg

Notes: May use in combination with diuretics; can cause a nonproductive cough

Ranitidine (Zantac)

Category: B

Indications: Duodenal ulcer, active benign ulcer, hypersecretory conditions, gastroesophageal reflux

Actions: Histamine H_2 receptor antagonist

Dosage:
Ulcer: 150 mg PO bid, 300 mg PO qhs, **or** 50 mg IV q6–8h; **or** 400 mg IV/d continuous infusion
Maintenance: 150 mg PO qhs
Hypersecretion: 150 mg PO bid

Supplied: Tablets 150 mg, 300 mg; syrup 15 mg/mL; injection 25 mg/mL

Notes: Reduce the dosage in renal failure; note that oral and parenteral doses differ

Rifampin (Rifadin)

Category: C

Indications: Tuberculosis; treatment and prophylaxis of *N. meningitidis, H. influenzae,* or *S. aureus* carriers

Actions: Inhibits DNA-dependent RNA polymerase activity

Dosage:
N. meningitidis and H. influenzae carriers: 600 mg PO qd for 4 days
Tuberculosis: 600 mg PO or IV qd **or** twice weekly with combination-therapy regimen

Supplied: Capsules 150 mg, 300 mg; injection 600 mg

Notes: Has multiple side effects; causes orange-red discoloration of bodily secretions including tears; is never used as a single agent to treat active tuberculosis infections

Ritodrine (Yutopar)

Category: B

Indications: Management of preterm labor

Actions: Beta-receptor agonist

Dosage: 0.15–0.35 mg/min IV continuous infusion, then 10 mg q2h for 24 hours, then 10–20 mg q4–6h

Supplied: Tablets 10 mg; injection 10 mg/15 mL

Secobarbital (Seconal) [C]

Category: D

Indications: Insomnia

Actions: Rapidly acting barbiturate

Dosage: 100 mg PO or IM qhs prn

Supplied: Tablets 100 mg; capsules 50 mg, 100 mg; injection 50 mg/mL

Notes: Beware of respiratory depression; tolerance is acquired within 1–2 weeks

Sertraline (Zoloft)

Category: B

Indications: Treatment of depression

Actions: Inhibits neuronal uptake of serotonin

Dosage: 50–200 mg PO qd

Supplied: Tablets 50 mg, 100 mg

Notes: May cause activation of manic/hypomanic state; has caused weight loss in clinical trials

Silver Sulfadiazine (Silvadene)

Category: B

Indications: Prevention of sepsis in second- and third-degree burns

Actions: Bactericidal

Dosage: Aseptically cover affected area with 1/16-inch coating bid

Supplied: Cream 1%

Notes: Can have systemic absorption with extensive application

Simethicone (Mylicon)

Category: C

Indications: Symptomatic treatment of flatulence

Actions: Defoaming action

Dosage: 40–125 mg PO after meals and hs prn

Supplied: Tablets 40 mg, 80 mg, 125 mg; capsules 125 mg; drops 40 mg/0.6 mL

Simvastatin (Zocor)

Category: C

Indications: Reduction of elevated cholesterol levels

Actions: HMG-CoA reductase inhibitor

Dosage: 5–40 mg PO qd in the evening

Supplied: Tablets 5 mg, 10 mg, 20 mg, 40 mg

Sodium Bicarbonate

Indications: Alkalinization of urine, treatment of metabolic acidosis

Dosage: Titrate to effect based on blood gases or urine pH

Supplied: Tablets 325 mg, 650 mg; injection 0.5 meq/mL, 1 meq/mL

Notes: One gram neutralizes 12 meq of acid

Sodium Polystyrene Sulfonate (Kayexalate)

Category: C

Indications: Treatment of hyperkalemia

Actions: Sodium and potassium ion-exchange resin

Dosage: 15–60 g PO or 30–60 g PR q6h based on serum K^+

Supplied: Powder; suspension 15 g/60 mL sorbitol

Notes: Can cause hypernatremia; give with an agent such as sorbitol to promote movement through the bowel

Sorbitol

Indications: Constipation

Actions: Laxative

Dosage: 30–60 mL of 20–70% solution prn

Supplied: Liquid 70%

Spironolactone (Aldactone)

Category: D

Indications: Treatment of hyperaldosteronism, essential hypertension, edematous states (congestive heart failure, cirrhosis)

Actions: Aldosterone antagonist, potassium-sparing diuretic

Dosage: 25–100 mg PO qid

Supplied: Tablets 25 mg, 50 mg, 100 mg

Notes: Can cause hyperkalemia and gynecomastia; avoid prolonged use; the diuretic of choice for cirrhotic edema and ascites

SSKI (Saturated Solution of Potassium Iodide)

Category: D

Indications: As an expectorant to help thin tenacious mucus in various chronic pulmonary conditions; thyroid storm

Actions: Enhances secretion of respiratory fluids, thus decreasing mucus viscosity; iodine supplementation

Dosage: 0.3–0.6 mL (300–600 mg) tid–qid diluted in water; maximum, 6 mL (6 g) per day

Supplied: Solution 1000 mg/mL

Notes: Not for use during pregnancy (can lead to fetal goiter); drug interaction with lithium and antithyroid agents enhances hypothyroid effects; thyroid function tests may be altered; watch for chronic iodine poisoning

Steroids

The following relates only to the commonly used systemic glucocorticoids

Category: C

Indications: Endocrine disorders (adrenal insufficiency), rheumatoid disorders, collagen vascular diseases, dermatologic diseases, allergic states, edematous states (cerebral, nephrotic syndrome), immunosuppression for transplantation, hypercalcemia, malignancies (breast, lymphomas)

Dosage:
Varies with indications and institutional protocols. Some commonly used dosages are:

Acute adrenal insufficiency (Addisonian crisis): Hydrocortisone 100 mg IV q6h
Chronic adrenal insufficiency: Hydrocortisone 20 mg PO qAM, 10 mg PO qPM; may need mineralocorticoid supplementation such as desoxycorticosterone acetate (DOCA)
Hypercalcemia of malignancy: Hydrocortisone 250–500 mg PO or IV initially, then prednisone 10–30 mg PO qd
Cerebral edema: dexamethasone 10 mg IV, then 4–6 mg IV q4–6h

Notes: See Table 7–3. All can cause hyperglycemia and adrenal suppression; never stop steroids acutely, especially during chronic treatment; taper dose

Streptokinase (Kabikinase, Streptase)

Category: C

Indications: Coronary artery thrombosis, acute massive pulmonary embolism, deep vein thrombosis

TABLE 7–3. COMPARISON OF GLUCOCORTICOIDS.

Drug (Brand Name)	Equivalent Dose (mg)	Relative Mineralocorticoid Activity	Duration (h)	Route
Cortisone (Cortone)	25.00	2	8–12	PO, IM
Dexamethasone (Decadron)	0.75	0	36–72	PO, IV
Hydrocortisone (Solu-Cortef)	20.00	2	8–12	PO, IM, IV
Methylprednisolone (Depo-Medrol, Solu-Medrol)	4.00	0	36–72	PO, IM, IV
Prednisolone (Delta-Cortef)	5.00	1	12–36	PO, IM, IV
Prednisone (Deltasone)	5.00	1	12–36	PO

From Gomella LG (ed): Clinician's Pocket Reference, *7th ed. Norwalk, Connecticut, Appleton & Lange, 1992.*

Actions: Activates plasminogen to plasmin, which degrades fibrin

Dosage:
Thrombosis or embolism: Loading dose of 250,000 IU through a peripheral vein over 30 minutes IV, then 100,000 IU/h IV for 24–72 hours
Transmural MI: 1,500,000 IU over 60 minutes IV

Supplied: Powder for injection

Notes: If maintenance infusion is not adequate to maintain thrombin clotting time at 2–5 times control, refer to the package insert, *Physicians' Desk Reference,* or *American Hospital Formulatory Service* for adjustments; heparinization is required following streptokinase administration

Streptomycin

Category: D

Indications: Tuberculosis, bacterial endocarditis

Actions: Aminoglycoside antibiotic; interferes with protein synthesis

Dosage: 1–4 g IM qd divided bid–qid

Supplied: Injection 400 mg/mL; powder for injection 1 g, 5 g

Notes: Nephrotoxic, ototoxic; decrease the dosage in renal impairment

Sucralfate (Carafate)

Category: B

Indications: Treatment of duodenal ulcer, gastric ulcer

Actions: Forms ulcer-adherent complex that protects the lesion against acid, pepsin, and bile salts

Dosage: 1 g PO qid

Supplied: Tablets 1 g

Notes: Administer 1 hour prior to meals and hs; antacids may also be used if taken 30 minutes after sucralfate; continue treatment for 4–8 weeks unless healing is demonstrated by x-ray or endoscopy; constipation is the most frequent side effect

Sulfamethoxazole
(see Trimethoprim and sulfamethoxazole)

Sulfasalazine (Azulfidine)

Category: B

Indications: Ulcerative colitis

Actions: Sulfonamide antibiotic

Dosage: 500 mg–1 g PO bid–qid

Supplied: Tablets 500 mg; enteric coated tablets 500 mg; oral suspension 250 mg/5 mL

Notes: Can cause severe GI upset; discolors urine

Sulfinpyrazone (Anturane)

Category: B

Indications: Chronic gouty arthritis

Actions: Inhibits renal tubular absorption of uric acid

Dosage: 100–200 mg PO bid

Supplied: Tablets 100 mg; capsules 200 mg

Sulfisoxazole (Gantrisin, others)

Category: C

Indications: Acute uncomplicated urinary tract infections

Actions: Sulfonamide antibiotic

Dosage: 500 mg–1 g PO qid

Supplied: Tablets 500 mg; oral suspension 500 mg/5 mL; syrup 500 mg/5 mL

Notes: Avoid use in last half of pregnancy (causes fetal hyperbilirubinemia)

Sulindac (Clinoril) (see Table 7–10, page 575)

Tamoxifen Citrate (Nolvadex)

Category: D

Indications: Breast and ovarian cancer

Actions: Hormone with potent antiestrogenic properties

Dosage: 10–20 mg PO bid

Supplied: Tablets 10 mg

Notes: Can cause nausea, vomiting, bone pain, hot flashes, weight gain

Temazepam (Restoril) [C]

Category: X

Indications: Insomnia

Actions: Benzodiazepine

Dosage: 15–30 mg PO qhs prn

Supplied: Capsules 15 mg, 30 mg

Notes: Reduce dosage in the elderly

Terazosin (Hytrin)

Category: C

Indications: Hypertension

Actions: Peripherally acting antiadrenergic agent

Dosage: Initially 1 mg PO hs; titrate up to maximum of 5 mg PO qhs

Supplied: Tablets 1 mg, 2 mg, 5 mg

Notes: Hypotension and syncope can occur following first dose; dizziness, weakness, nasal congestion, and peripheral edema are common; must be used with a thiazide diuretic for hypertension

Terbutaline (Brethine, Bricanyl)

Category: B

Indications: Reversible bronchospasm (from asthma, chronic obstructive pulmonary disease); inhibition of premature labor

Actions: Sympathomimetic

Dosage:
Bronchodilator: 2.5–5 mg PO tid; **or** 0.25 mg SQ, may repeat in 15 minutes (maximum, 0.5 mg in 4 hours)
Metered-dose inhaler: 2 inhalations q4–6h
Premature labor: 10–80 µg/min IV infusion for 4 hours, then 2.5 mg PO q4–6h until term

Supplied: Tablets 2.5 mg, 5 mg; injection 1 mg/mL; metered-dose inhaler 0.2 mg/dose

Notes: Use with caution in diabetes, hypertension, hyperthyroidism; high doses can precipitate beta-1 adrenergic effects

Terconazole (Terazol 7)

Category: C

Indications: Vaginal fungal infections

Actions: Topical antifungal

Dosage: 1 applicatorful intravaginally qhs for 7 days

Supplied: Vaginal cream 0.4%

Terfenadine (Seldane)

Category: C

Indications: Seasonal allergic rhinitis

Actions: Relatively nonsedating antihistamine

Dosage: 60 mg PO bid

Supplied: Tablets 60 mg

Tetanus Immune Globulin

Category: C

Indications: Passive immunization against tetanus for any person with a suspected contaminated wound and unknown immunization status

Actions: Passive immunization

Dosage: 250–500 units IM (higher doses if there is a delay in initiation of therapy)

Supplied: Injection 250 unit vial or syringe

Notes: May begin active immunization series at a different injection site if required

Tetanus Toxoid

Category: C

Indications: Protection against tetanus

Actions: Active immunization

Dosage: See Table A–10, page 608, for tetanus prophylaxis

Supplied: Injection: tetanus toxoid, fluid: 4–5 limit flocculation (Lf) units/0.5 mL; tetanus toxoid, adsorbed: 5 Lf units/0.5 mL, 10 Lf units/ 0.5 mL

Tetracycline (Achromycin V, Sumycin)

Category: D

Indications: Broad-spectrum antibiotic active against *Staphylococcus, Streptococcus, Chlamydia, Rickettsia,* and *Mycoplasma*

Actions: Interferes with protein synthesis

Dosage: 250–500 mg PO qid

Supplied: Tablets 250 mg, 500 mg; capsules 100 mg, 250 mg, 500 mg; oral suspension 250 mg/5 mL

Notes: IM and IV routes are not recommended; do not use in impaired renal function (see **Doxycycline**)

Theophylline (Somophyllin, Theo-Dur, Theolair, others)

Category: C

Indications: Asthma, bronchospasm

Actions: Relaxes smooth muscle of the bronchi and pulmonary blood vessels

Dosage: 24 mg/kg/24h PO divided q6h; sustained-release products may be divided q8–12h

Supplied: Elixir 80 mg/15 mL, 150 mg/15 mL; liquid 80 mg/15 mL, 160 mg/15 mL; capsules 100 mg, 200 mg, 250 mg; tablets 100 mg, 125 mg, 200 mg, 225 mg, 250 mg, 300 mg; SR capsules 50 mg, 75 mg, 100 mg, 125 mg, 200 mg, 250 mg, 260 mg, 300 mg; SR tablets 100 mg, 200 mg, 250 mg, 300 mg, 400 mg, 500 mg

Notes: See Table 7–14, Drug Levels, page 585

Thiamine [Vitamin B$_1$]

Category: A

Indications: Thiamine deficiency (beriberi), alcoholic neuritis, Wernicke's encephalopathy

Actions: Dietary supplementation

Dosage:
Deficiency: 100 mg IM qd for 2 weeks, then 5–10 mg PO qd for 1 month
Wernicke's encephalopathy: 100 mg IV for 1 dose, then 100 mg IM qd for 2 weeks

Supplied: Tablets 5 mg, 10 mg, 25 mg, 50 mg, 100 mg, 500 mg; injection 100 mg/mL, 200 mg/mL

Notes: IV thiamine administration is associated with anaphylactic reaction; must be given slowly IV

Thiethylperazine (Torecan)

Indications: Nausea and vomiting

Actions: Antidopaminergic antiemetic

Dosage: 10 mg PO, PR, or IM qd–tid

Supplied: Tablets 10 mg; suppositories 10 mg; injection 5 mg/mL

Notes: Extrapyramidal reactions can occur

Thioridazine (Mellaril)

Category: C

Indications: Psychotic disorders, short-term treatment of depression, agitation, organic brain syndrome

Actions: Phenothiazine antipsychotic

Dosage: Initially 50–100 mg PO tid; maintenance, 10–50 mg PO bid–qid

Supplied: Tablets 10 mg, 15 mg, 25 mg, 50 mg, 100 mg, 150 mg, 200 mg; oral concentrate 30 mg/mL; oral suspension 25 mg/5 mL, 100 mg/5 mL

Notes: Has low incidence of extrapyramidal effects

Thiothixene (Navane)

Category: C

Indications: Psychotic disorders

Actions: Antipsychotic

Dosage:
Mild to moderate psychosis: 2 mg PO tid
Severe psychosis: 5 mg PO bid; increase to maximum of 30 mg tid
IM use: 2 mg 2–5 times per day (maximum, 30 mg/d)

Supplied: Capsules 1 mg, 2 mg, 5 mg, 10 mg, 20 mg; oral concentrate 5 mg/mL; injection 2 mg/mL, 5 mg/mL

Notes: Drowsiness and extrapyramidal side effects are most common

Ticarcillin (Ticar) (see Table 7–4, page 569)

Ticarcillin and Potassium clavulanate (Timentin) (see Table 7–4, page 569)

Timolol (Blocadren, Timoptic) (also see Table 7–6, page 571)

Category: C

Indications: Glaucoma, hypertension, reduction in risk of reinfarction or cardiovascular mortality immediately following acute myocardial infarction

Actions: Beta-adrenergic blocking agent

Dosage:
Glaucoma: 1 gtt of 0.25% or 0.50% solution in each eye bid (Timoptic)
Hypertension and reinfarction: See Table 7–6, page 571

Supplied: Tablets 5 mg, 10 mg, 20 mg; ophthalmic solution 0.25%, 0.5%

Tioconazole (Vagistat)

Category: C

Indications: Vaginal fungal infections

Actions: Topical antifungal

Dosage: 1 applicatorful intravaginally hs (single dose)

Supplied: Vaginal ointment 6.5%

Tobramycin (Nebcin)

Category: D

Indications: Serious gram-negative infections, especially *Pseudomonas*

Actions: Aminoglycoside antibiotic; interferes with protein synthesis

Dosage: Based on renal function; refer to **Aminoglycoside Dosing,** page 567.

Supplied: Injection 10 mg/mL, 40 mg/mL

Notes: Nephrotoxic and ototoxic; decrease the dosage in renal insufficiency; monitor creatinine clearance and serum concentration for dosage adjustments; see Table 7–14, Drug Levels, page 585

Tocainide (Tonocard)

Category: C

Indications: Suppression of ventricular arrhythmias including premature ventricular contractions and ventricular tachycardia

Actions: Class 1B antiarrhythmic

Dosage: 400–600 mg PO q8h

Supplied: Tablets 400 mg, 600 mg

Notes: Has properties similar to lidocaine; reduce the dosage in renal failure; CNS and GI side effects are common

Tolazamide (Ronase, Tolinase, others) (see Table 7–12, page 578)

Tolbutamide (Orinase) (see Table 7–12, page 578)

Tolmetin (Tolectin) (see Table 7–10, page 575)

Trazodone (Desyrel)

Category: C

Indications: Major depression

Actions: Antidepressant

Dosage: 50–150 mg PO qd–qid (maximum, 600 mg/d)

Supplied: Tablets 50 mg, 100 mg, 150 mg

Notes: Can take 1–2 weeks for symptomatic improvement; anticholinergic side effects

Triamterene (Dyrenium)

Category: B

Indications: Edema associated with congestive heart failure, cirrhosis

Actions: Potassium-sparing diuretic

Dosage: 50–100 mg PO qd–bid

Supplied: Capsules 50 mg, 100 mg

Notes: Can cause hyperkalemia; blood dyscrasias, liver damage, and other reactions can occur

Triazolam (Halcion) [C]

Category: X

Indications: Insomnia

Actions: Benzodiazepine

Dosage: 0.125–0.5 mg PO qhs prn

Supplied: Tablets 0.125 mg, 0.25 mg, 0.5 mg

Notes: Produces additive CNS depression with alcohol and other CNS depressants

Triethylenethiophosphoramide (Thiotepa)

Category: D

Indications: Breast and ovarian cancer

Actions: Cell cycle nonspecific alkylating agent

Dosage: Varies with protocol

Supplied: Injection 15 mg

Notes: Can cause nausea, vomiting, bone marrow suppression, headaches

Trifluoperazine (Stelazine)

Category: C

Indications: Psychotic disorders

Actions: Phenothiazine antipsychotic

Dosage: 2–5 mg PO bid

Supplied: Tablets 1 mg, 2 mg, 5 mg, 10 mg; oral concentrate 10 mg/mL; injection 2 mg/mL

Notes: Decrease the dosage in elderly and debilitated patients; oral concentrate must be diluted to 60 mL or more prior to administration

Trimeprazine (Temaril)

Category: C

Indications: Pruritus associated with allergic and nonallergic conditions

Actions: Phenothiazine antihistamine

Dosage: 2.5 mg PO qid prn **or** sustained release 5 mg PO q12h

Supplied: Tablets 2.5 mg; SR capsules 5 mg; syrup 2.5 mg/5 mL

Notes: Extrapyramidal reactions can occur in the elderly

Trimethaphan (Arfonad)

Category: D

Indications: Treatment of hypertensive crisis, treatment of pulmonary edema with pulmonary hypertension associated with systemic hypertension

Actions: Ganglionic blocking agent

Dosage: 0.3–6 mg/min IV infusion, titrated to effect

Supplied: Injection 50 mg/mL

Notes: Has additive effect with other antihypertensive agents; vasopressors may be used to reverse hypotension if required; phenylephrine is the vasopressor of choice for reversal of effects

Trimethobenzamide (Tigan)

Category: C

Indications: Nausea and vomiting

Actions: Anticholinergic antiemetic

Dosage: 250 mg PO or 200 mg PR or IM tid–qid prn

Supplied: Capsules 100 mg, 250 mg; suppositories 100 mg, 200 mg; injection 100 mg/mL

Notes: In the presence of viral infections, can contribute to Reye's syndrome; can cause Parkinson-like syndrome

Trimethoprim (Proloprim, Trimpex)

Category: C

Indications: Urinary tract infections due to susceptible gram-positive or gram-negative organisms

Actions: Inhibits dihydrofolate reductase

Dosage: 100 mg PO bid or 200 mg PO qd

Supplied: Tablets 100 mg, 200 mg

Notes: Reduce the dosage in renal failure; give 1/2 dose if creatinine clearance is 15–30 mL/min; < 15 mL/min is not well studied

Trimethoprim and Sulfamethoxazole (Bactrim, Septra)

Category: C

Indications: Urinary tract infections, otitis media, sinusitis, bronchitis, traveler's diarrhea, *Shigella, Pneumocystis carinii, Nocardia*

Actions: Combined actions of a sulfonamide and trimethoprim

Dosage:
1 double-strength tablet PO bid or 10 mg/kg/24h (based on trimethoprim component) IV in 3–4 divided doses
Pneumocystis carinii: 20 mg/kg/d (trimethoprim component) PO or IV in 3–4 divided doses

Supplied: (Trimethoprim [TMP]/sulfamethoxazole [SMX]) Tablets 80 mg TMP/400 mg SMX; DS tablets 160 mg TMP/800 mg SMX; oral suspension 40 mg TMP/200 mg SMX per 5 mL; injection 80 mg TMP/400 mg SMX per 5 mL

Notes: Reduce the dosage in renal failure; give 1/2 dose if creatinine clearance is 15–30 mL/min; contraindicated if clearance < 15 mL/min

Triple Sulfa Cream (Gyne-Sulf, Sulfa-Gyn, Sultrin)

Category: C

Indications: Treatment of *haemophilus vaginalis* vaginitis

Actions: Topical antibiotic

Dosage: 1 tablet or applicatorful intravaginally bid for 6–10 days

Supplied: Vaginal tablets; vaginal cream

Triprolidine and Pseudoephedrine (Actifed)

Category: C

Indications: Symptomatic relief of allergic and vasomotor rhinitis

Actions: Antihistamine and decongestant combination

Dosage: 1 tablet PO tid–qid or 2 tsp (10 mL) tid–qid

Supplied: Tablets: triprolidine 2.5 mg/pseudoephedrine 60 mg; syrup: triprolidine 1.25 mg/pseudoephedrine 30 mg per 5 mL

Urofollitropin (Metrodin)

Category: X

Indications: Induction of ovulation

Actions: Stimulates ovarian follicular growth

Dosage: 75 IU qd IM for 7–12 days

Supplied: Powder for injection

Notes: Risk of multiple births

Urokinase (Abbokinase)

Category: B

Indications: Pulmonary embolism, coronary artery thrombosis, restoration of patency to IV catheters

Actions: Converts plasminogen to plasmin, which causes clot lysis

Dosage:
Systemic effect: 4400 IU/kg IV over 10 minutes, then 4400 IU/kg/h for 12 hours
Catheter patency: Inject 5000 IU into the catheter and gently aspirate

Supplied: Powder for injection 5000 IU/mL, 250,000 IU/5 mL

Notes: Do not use systemically within 10 days of surgery, delivery, or organ biopsy

Valproic Acid and Divalproex (Depakene and Depakote)

Category: D

Indications: Absence seizures, in combination for tonic/clonic seizures

Actions: Anticonvulsant

Dosage: 15–60 mg/kg/24h PO, divided q8h

Supplied:
Valproic acid: Capsules 250 mg; syrup 250 mg/5 mL
Divalproex: Enteric coated tablets 125 mg, 250 mg, 500 mg

Notes: Monitor liver function tests and follow serum levels (see Table 7–14, Drug Levels, page 585); concurrent use of phenobarbital and phenytoin can alter serum levels of these agents

Vancomycin (Vancocin, Vancoled)

Category: C

Indications: Serious infections due to methicillin-resistant staphylococci and in combination with aminoglycosides for enterococcal endocarditis in penicillin-allergic patients; oral treatment for *C. difficile* pseudomembranous colitis

Actions: Interferes with protein synthesis

Dosage:
Intravenous: 1 g q12h **or** 500 mg q6h
Oral: 250–500 mg PO q6h

Supplied: Capsules 125 mg, 250 mg; powder for oral solution; powder for injection 500 mg, 1000 mg per vial

Notes: Ototoxic and nephrotoxic; not absorbed orally, provides local effect in the gut only; IV dose must be given slowly over 1 hour to prevent "red-man syndrome"; adjust the dosage in renal failure

Vasopressin [Antidiuretic Hormone] (Pitressin)

Category: C

Indications: Treatment of diabetes insipidus, relief of gaseous GI tract distention, severe GI bleeding

Actions: Posterior pituitary hormone; potent GI vasoconstrictor

Dosage:
Diabetes insipidus: 5–10 units SQ or IM tid–qid, or 1.5–5.0 units IM q1–3d of the tannate
GI bleeding: 0.2–0.4 units/min

Supplied: Injection 20 units/mL

Notes: Use with caution in any vascular disease

Vecuronium (Norcuron)

Category: C

Indications: Skeletal muscle relaxation; used in conjunction with mechanical ventilation

Actions: Nondepolarizing neuromuscular blocker

Dosage: 0.08–0.1 mg/kg IV bolus; maintenance of 0.010–0.015 mg/kg after 25–40 minutes followed with additional doses q12–15min

Supplied: Powder for injection 10 mg

Notes: Drug interactions leading to increased effect of vecuronium occur with aminoglycosides, tetracycline, and succinylcholine; has fewer cardiac effects than pancuronium

Verapamil (Calan, Isoptin)

Category: C

Indications: Supraventricular tachyarrhythmias (paroxysmal atrial tachycardia, atrial flutter or fibrillation), vasospastic (Prinzmetal's) and unstable (crescendo, preinfarction) angina, chronic stable angina (classic effort-associated), hypertension

Actions: Calcium channel blocker

Dosage:
  Tachyarrhythmias: 5–10 mg IV over 2 minutes; may repeat in 30 minutes
  Angina: 240–480 mg/24h PO divided tid–qid
  Hypertension: 80–180 mg PO tid or sustained-release 240 mg PO qd

Supplied: Tablets 40 mg, 80 mg, 120 mg; SR tablets 240 mg; injection 5 mg/2 mL

Notes: Use with caution in elderly patients; reduce the dosage in renal failure; constipation is a common side effect

Vidarabine (Vira-A)

Category: C

Indications: Treatment of herpes simplex encephalitis

Actions: Antiviral agent

Dosage: 15 mg/kg/24h by slow IV infusion over 12–24 hours

Supplied: Injection 200 mg/mL

Notes: Early diagnosis and treatment are essential to success of therapy; treat only if patient has positive HSV cell culture; may suppress RBC and platelet counts; avoid administration of allopurinol with vidarabine

Vinblastine (Velban)

Category: D

Indications: Gestational trophoblastic disease, ovarian germ cell cancer

Actions: Mitotic inhibitor; interferes with amino acid metabolic pathways leading from glutamic acid to the citric acid cycle and urea

Dosage: Varies with protocol

Supplied: Injection 1 mg/mL

Notes: Can cause nausea, vomiting, alopecia, bone marrow suppression, SIADH

Vincristine (Oncovin)

Category: D

Indications: Cervical and ovarian germ cell cancer, sarcoma

Actions: Mitotic inhibitor, arrests cell division at the stage of metaphase

Dosage: Varies with protocol

Supplied: Injection 1 mg/mL

Notes: Can cause neurotoxicity, alopecia, constipation, SIADH

Vitamin B$_{12}$ (see Cyanocobalamin)

Vitamin K (see Phytonadione)

Warfarin Sodium (Coumadin)

Category: D

Indications: Prophylaxis and treatment of pulmonary embolism and venous thrombosis, atrial fibrillation with embolization

Actions: Inhibits hepatic production of vitamin K dependent clotting factors in this order: VII, IX, X, II

Dosage: Must be individualized to keep prothrombin time (PT) at 1.12 to 2.0 times control; depending on the indication for use, initially 10–15 mg PO, IM, or IV qd for 1–3 days, then maintenance of 2–10 mg PO, IV, or IM qd; follow daily PT during the initial phase to guide dosage

Supplied: Tablets 2 mg, 2.5 mg, 5 mg, 7.5 mg, 10 mg; powder for injection 50 mg per vial

Notes: PT needs to be checked periodically while on maintenance dose; beware of bleeding caused by excessive anticoagulation (PT > 3 times control); caution patient on effects of taking Coumadin with other medications, especially aspirin; for rapid correction of excessive anticoagulation use vitamin K, fresh-frozen plasma, or both; do not use in pregnancy (highly teratogenic)

Zidovudine [AZT] (Retrovir)

Category: C

Indications: Management of patients with HIV infection

Actions: Antiviral agent

Dosage:
Oral: 100 mg PO 5 times per day
Intravenous: 1–2 mg/kg q4h

Supplied: Capsules 100 mg; syrup 50 mg/5 mL; injection 10 mg/mL

Notes: Not a cure for HIV infection but may extend survival

AMINOGLYCOSIDE DOSING

See Table 7–14, page 585 "Drug Levels: Antibiotics" for the trough and peak levels of the aminoglycosides gentamicin, tobramycin, and amikacin. Peak levels should be drawn 30 minutes after the dose is completely infused; trough levels should be drawn 30 minutes prior to the dose. As a general rule, draw the peak and trough around the time of the fourth maintenance dose.

Therapy can be initiated with the recommended guidelines that follow. **The calculations below are not valid for netilmicin.**

Procedure

1. Calculate the estimated creatinine clearance (CrCl) based on serum creatinine (SCr), age, and weight in kg (a formal creatinine clearance can be ordered instead, if time permits):

$$\text{CrCL: male} = \frac{(140 - \text{age}) \times (\text{Weight in kg})}{(\text{SCr}) \times (72)}$$

$$\text{CrCl: female} = 0.85 \times (\text{CrCl male})$$

2. Select the loading dose:

- Gentamicin: 1.5–2.0 mg/kg
- Amikacin: 5.0–7.5 mg/kg
- Tobramycin: 1.5–2.0 mg/kg

3. By using Table 7–15 you can now select the maintenance dose (as a percentage of the chosen loading dose) most appropriate for the patient's renal function based on CrCl and dosing interval. Shaded areas are the suggested percentages and intervals for any given creatinine clearance.

4. This is only an empirical dose to begin therapy. Serum levels should be monitored routinely for optimal therapy. Use Table 7–14, "Drug Levels: Antibiotics."

TABLE 7-4. ANTIPSEUDOMONAL PENICILLINS. [a]

Drug (Brand Name)	Daily Dosage Range, Adult	Usual Dosing Interval	meq Na+ per Gram	Supplied	Notes
Carbenicillin (Geopen, Pyopen)	8–40 g[b]	4 h	4.7	Injection, oral[c]	1. When used alone, resistant gram (¯) bacteria may occur 2. Hypokalemia and bleeding may occur with high doses
Mezlocillin (Mezlin)	2–24 g[b]	4–6 h	1.85	Injection	1. More active than ticarcillin against Enterobacteriaceae, same activity against *P. aeruginosa*
Piperacillin (Pipracil)	2–24 g[b]	4–6 h	1.85	Injection	1. Good activity against *P. aeruginosa, B. fragillis,* and *Enterobacteriaceae*
Ticarcillin (Ticar)	2–24 g[b]	4–6 h	5.2	Injection	1. See No. 1 above 2. Hypokalemia, bleeding, and Na+ loading less than with carbenicillin
Ticarcillin and potassium clavulanate (Timentin)	9–12 g	4–6 h	4.75	Injection	1. Clavulanate is a beta-lactamase inhibitor

[a]Pregnancy category B.
[b]Reduce the dosage in renal failure.
[c]The oral form of this drug is only to be used for simple urinary tract infections and never for serious infections of any type.
From Gomella LG (ed): Clinician's Pocket Reference, 7th ed. Norwalk, Connecticut, Appleton & Lange, 1992.

TABLE 7–5. ANTISTAPHYLOCOCCAL PENICILLINS. [a]

Drug (Brand Name)	Daily Dosage Range, Adult	Usual Dosing Interval	Supplied	Notes
Cloxacillin (Cloxapen, Tegopen)	1–2 g	6 h	Oral	1. Administer on an empty stomach at least 1 h before 2 h after meals
Dicloxacillin (Dynapen)	0.5–1 g	6 h	Oral	1. See Cloxacillin
Methicillin	4–12 g[b]	4–6	Injection	1. Interstitial nephritis can occur with high doses 2. Use high dose (12–18 g/d) for *Staph.* meningitis
Nafcillin (Unipen)	4–12 g[b]	4–6 h	Injection, oral	1. Poorly absorbed orally, cloxacillin or dicloxacillin better for PO use 2. Injectable form has highest activity against *S. aureus* 3. Can use for *Staph.* meningitis
Oxacillin (Prostaphlin)	4–12 g[b]	4–6 h	Injection, oral	1. Interstitial nephritis can occur with high doses

[a]Pregnancy category B.
[b]Reduce the dosage in renal failure.
From Gomella LG (ed): Clinician's Pocket Reference, 7th ed. Norwalk, Connecticut, Appleton & Lange, 1992.

TABLE 7–6. BETA-ADRENERGIC BLOCKING AGENTS.[a]

Drug (Brand Name)	Receptor Activity	Half-Life	Excretion	Dosing Range and Frequency[b]	
				Angina Pectoris	Hypertension
Acebutolol (Sectral)	β_1	3–4 h	Hepatic, renal	NA	200 mg PO bid or 400 mg PO qd
Atenolol (Tenormin)	β_1	6–9 h	Renal	50–100 mg PO qd[c]	50–100 mg PO qd[c]
Betaxolol (Kerlone)	β_1	14–22 h	Hepatic	NA	10–20 mg PO qd
Carteolol (Cartrol)	β_1, β_2	6 h	Renal	NA	2.5–10 mg PO qd
Labetalol (Normodyne, Trandate)	β_1, β_2, α	6–8 h	Hepatic	NA	100–400 mg PO bid
Metoprolol (Lopressor)	β_1	3–7 h	Hepatic, renal	50–100 PO bid	50–100 PO bid-tid
Nadolol (Corgard)	β_1, β_2	20–40 h	Renal	40–240 mg PO qd[c]	40–320 mg PO qd[c]
Penbutolol (Levatol)	β_1, β_2	5 h	Hepatic, renal	NA	20–40 mg PO qd
Pindolol (Visken)	β_1, β_2	3–4 h	Hepatic, renal	NA	10–40 mg PO bid
Propranolol[d] (Inderal)	β_1, β_2	3–5 h	Hepatic	80–240 mg PO bid-tid	80–480 mg PO bid-tid
Timolol (Blocadren)	β_1, β_2	4 h	Hepatic, renal	10–40 mg PO bid	NA

[a]Pregnancy category C.
[b]Other uses of beta blockers include postmyocardial infarction to reduce mortality, pheochromocytoma, hypertrophic subaortic stenosis.
[c]Reduce the dosage in renal failure.
[d]For arrhythmias, 80–120 mg PO divided tid-qid; migraine, 80–240 mg PO divided bid-tid.
NA = not applicable.
From Gomella LG (ed): Clinician's Pocket Reference, 7th ed. Norwalk, Connecticut, Appleton & Lange, 1992.

TABLE 7–7. FIRST-GENERATION CEPHALOSPORINS.[a]

Drug (Brand Name)	Daily Dosage Adult	Usual Interval	Half-Life	Supplied	Notes
Cefaclor (Ceclor)	0.75–1.5 g[b]	8 h	45 min	Oral	1. High level of activity against *H. influenzae*
Cefadroxil (Duricef, Ultracef)	1–2 g PO[b]	12 h	1.5 h	Oral	1. May be dosed bid
Cefazolin (Ancef, Kefzol)	1.5–12 g[b]	8 h	1.5–2 h	Injection	1. Best of first generation for surgical prophylaxis 2. IM dose fairly well tolerated
Cephalexin (Keflex, Keftab)	1–4 g[b]	6–12 h	45 min–1.5 h	Oral	1. Keftab has better absorption than Keflex
Cephalothin (Keflin)	2–12 g[b]	4–6 h	30–45 min	Injection	1. IV use causes phlebitis; IM use is painful
Cephapirin (Cefadyl)	2–12 g[b]	4–6 h	30–45 min	Injection	1. Possibly less phlebitis and IM use less painful than with cephalothin
Cephradine (Velosef, Anspor)	1–4 g PO[b] or 2–8 g IV[b]	6–12 h	45 min–1.5 h	Oral, injection	1. Less active than cephalothin against *S. aureus*

[a]Pregnancy category B.
[b]Reduce the dosage in renal failure.
From Gomella LG (ed): *Clinician's Pocket Reference, 7th ed. Norwalk, Connecticut, Appleton & Lange, 1992.*

TABLE 7–8. SECOND-GENERATION CEPHALOSPORINS. [a]

Drug (Brand Name)	Daily Dosage Adult	Usual Interval	Half-Life	Supplied	Notes
Cefamandole (Mandol)	3–12 g[b]	4–6 h	30–60 min	Injection	1. High level of activity against *H. influenzae* 2. Disulfiram reaction with alcohol use 3. Monitor PT closely with long-term use
Cefmetazole (Zefazone)	2–8 g[b]	6–12 h	1.2 h	Injection	1. *B. fragilis* coverage
Cefonicid (Monocid)	1–2 g[b]	24 h	4.5 h	Injection	1. Less effective against *S. aureus*
Ceforanide (Precef)	1–2 g[b]	12 h	2.5–3 h	Injection	1. Less effective against *S. aureus*
Cefotetan (Cefotan)	2–6 g[b]	12 h	3–4.6 h	Injection	1. Activity against *B. fragilis* 2. May cause hypoprothrombinemia
Cefoxitin (Mefoxin)	2–12 g[b]	4–6 h	45–60 min	Injection	1. Best cephalosporin against *B. fragilis*, good for mixed aerobic/anaerobic infections in ob/gyn, surgery
Cefprozil (Cefzil)	250–500 mg	12–24 h	5.2–5.9 h	Oral	1. Effective against *Strep., Staph., H. influenzae, M. catarrhalis*
Cefuroxime (Ceftin, Zinacef)	2.25–9 g IV[b] or 500 mg–1 g PO[b]	8 h	1.5 h	Injection, oral	1. Crosses blood-brain barrier; can be used for some organisms in meningitis at higher doses

[a]Pregnancy category B.
[b]Reduce the dosage in renal failure.
From Gomella LG (ed): Clinician's Pocket Reference, 7th ed. Norwalk, Connecticut, Appleton & Lange, 1992.

TABLE 7-9. THIRD-GENERATION CEPHALOSPORINS. [a]

Drug (Brand Name)	Daily Dosage Adult	Usual Interval	Half-Life	Supplied	Notes
Cefixime (Suprax)	400 mg[b]	12–24 h	3–4 h	Oral	1. May cause GI irritation 2. **No** *Staph.* or *Pseudomonas* activity
Cefoperazone (Cefobid)	2–12 g	8–12 h	1.7–2.6 h	Injection	1. Hepatic/renal excretion allows normal dosing in renal failure 2. Disulfiram reactions and hypoprothrombinemia can occur 3. Do not use alone for *Pseudomonas*
Cefotaxime (Claforan)	2–12 g[b]	4–8 h	1 h	Injection	1. Excellent gram (−) activity except for *Pseudomonas* 2. Crosses blood-brain barrier 3. Give ½ dose in CrCl < 20
Ceftazidime (Fortaz)	2–6 g[b]	8–12 h	2 h	Injection	1. Best of third generation against *Pseudomonas* 2. No activity against *B. fragilis*
Ceftizoxime (Cefizox)	2–12 g[b]	8–12 h	1.4–1.9 h	Injection	1. Spectrum similar to cefotaxime 2. Less activity against *B. fragilis*
Ceftriaxone (Rocephin)	1–4 g	24 h	5.8–8.7 h	Injection	1. Long half-life allows once a day dose 2. Home therapy possible 3. No change in renal failure to 2 g/d

[a] Pregnancy category B.
[b] Reduce the dosage in renal failure.
From Gomella LG (ed): Clinician's Pocket Reference, 7th ed. Norwalk, Connecticut, Appleton & Lange, 1992.

TABLE 7–10. NONSTEROIDAL ANTI-INFLAMMATORY AGENTS.[a]

Drug (Brand Name)	Maximum Daily Dose (mg)	Dosing Frequency	Notes
Propionic Acids			
Fenoprofen (Nalfon)	3200	tid, qid	1. Approval for arthritis and analgesia
Flurbiprofen (Ansaid)	300	bid, tid, qid	1. Approval for arthritis
Ibuprofen (Motrin, Rufen)	3200	bid, tid, qid	1. Approval for arthritis, analgesia, and dysmenorrhea 2. Many generic products are available
Ketoprofen (Orudis)	300	tid, qid	1. Approval for arthritis and analgesia
Naproxen (Anaprox, Naprosyn)	1500	bid	1. Approval for arthritis and analgesia 2. Very GI irritating
Indoles			
Indomethacin (Indocin)	200	qd, bid, tid	1. Approval for arthritis 2. SR product available
Ketorolac (Toradol)	120	qid	1. Approval for pain relief 2. Parenteral dosage form
Sulindac (Clinoril)	400	bid	1. Approval for arthritis 2. Least renal toxicity
Tolmetin (Tolectin)	2000	tid, qid	1. Approval for arthritis
Oxicams			
Piroxicam (Feldene)	20	bid	1. Approval for arthritis 2. Very GI irritating
Phenylacetic acids			
Diclofenac (Voltaren)	200	bid, tid	1. Approval for arthritis
Diflunisal (Dolobid)	1500	bid	1. Can prolong prothrombin time
Fenamates			
Meclofenamate (Meclomen)	400	tid, qid	1. Approval for arthritis, analgesia, and dysmenorrhea
Mefenamic acid (Ponstel)	1000	qid	1. Approval for analgesia and dysmenorrhea

[a]Pregnancy category B.
From Gomella LG (ed): Clinician's Pocket Reference, *7th ed. Norwalk, Connecticut, Appleton & Lange, 1992.*

TABLE 7–11. ORAL CONTRACEPTIVES. [a]

Drug	Estrogen (µg)	µg per Month	Progestin (mg)[a]	mg per Month	Cost[b]
Combination					
Loestrin 1/20 21, 28—Parke-Davis	Ethinyl estradiol (20)	420	Norethindrone acetate (1)	21	$15.47
Loestrin 1.5/30 21, 28—Parke-Davis	Ethinyl estradiol (30)	630	Norethindrone acetate (1.5)	31.5	15.47
Nordette 21—Wyeth-Ayerst[c]	Ethinyl estradiol (30)	630	Levonorgestrel (0.15)	3.15	15.23
Levlen 21, 28—Berlex	Ethinyl estradiol (30)	630	Levonorgestrel (0.15)	3.15	13.60
Lo Ovral 21—Wyeth-Ayerst[c]	Ethinyl estradiol (30)	630	Norgestrel (0.3)	6.3	15.94
Triphasil 21—Wyeth-Ayerst[c]	Ethinyl estradiol (30, 40)	680	Levonorgestrel (0.05, 0.075, 0.125)	1.925	14.18
Tri-Levlen 21, 28—Berlex	Ethinyl estradiol (30, 40)	680	Levonorgestrel (0.05, 0.075, 0.125)	1.925	12.98
Brevicon 21, 28—Syntex	Ethinyl estradiol (35)	735	Norethindrone (0.5)	10.5	13.95
Modicon 21—Ortho[c]	Ethinyl estradiol (35)	735	Norethindrone (0.5)	10.5	14.84
Genora 0.5/35 21, 28—Rugby	Ethinyl estradiol (35)	735	Norethindrone (0.5)	10.5	7.44
Nelova 0.5/35 21, 28—Watson	Ethinyl estradiol (35)	735	Norethindrone (0.5)	10.5	9.78
Norinyl 1 + 35 21, 28—Syntex	Ethinyl estradiol (35)	735	Norethindrone (1)	21	13.95
Norethin 1/35 21, 28—Searle	Ethinyl estradiol (35)	735	Norethindrone (1)	21	8.15
Nelova 1/35 21, 28—Watson	Ethinyl estradiol (35)	735	Norethindrone (1)	21	9.78
Genora 1/35 21, 28—Rugby	Ethinyl estradiol (35)	735	Norethindrone (1)	21	11.00
Ortho-Novum 1/35 21—Ortho[c]	Ethinyl estradiol (35)	735	Norethindrone (1)	21	13.64
Tri-Norinyl 21, 28—Syntex	Ethinyl estradiol (35)	735	Norethindrone (0.5, 1.0)	15	13.95
Ortho-Novum 7/7/7 21—Ortho[c]	Ethinyl estradiol (35)	735	Norethindrone (0.5, 0.75, 1.0)	15.75	14.67

Ortho-Novum 10/11 21, 28—Ortho[c]	Ethinyl estradiol (35)	735	Norethindrone (0.5, 1.0)	16	13.58
Nelova 10/11 21, 28—Watson	Ethinyl estradiol (35)	735	Norethindrone (0.5, 1.0)	16	9.78
Ovcon 35 21, 28—Mead Johnson	Ethinyl estradiol (35)	735	Norethindrone (0.4)	8.4	14.68
Demulen 1/35 21, 28—Searle[c]	Ethinyl estradiol (35)	735	Ethynodiol diacetate (1)	21	15.56
Norlestrin 1/50 21, 28—Parke-Davis	Ethinyl estradiol (50)	1050	Norethindrone acetate (1)	21	15.35
Ovcon 50 21, 28—Mead Johnson	Ethinyl estradiol (50)	1050	Norethindrone (1)	21	14.68
Genora 1/50 21, 28—Rugby	Ethinyl estradiol (50)	1050	Norethindrone (1)	21	11.00
Norlestrin 2.5/50 21, 28—Parke-Davis	Ethinyl estradiol (50)	1050	Norethindrone acetate (2.5)	52.5	15.80
Demulen 1/50 21—Searle[c]	Ethinyl estradiol (50)	1050	Ethynodiol diacetate (1)	21	17.32
Ovral 21—Wyeth-Ayerst[c]	Ethinyl estradiol (50)	1050	Norgestrel (0.5)	10.5	18.35
Norinyl 1 + 50 21, 28—Syntex	Mestranol (50)	1050	Norethindrone (1)	21	13.95
Ortho-Novum 1/50 21, 28—Ortho[c]	Mestranol (50)	1050	Norethindrone (1)	21	13.64
Norethin 1/50 21, 28—Searle	Mestranol (50)	1050	Norethindrone (1)	21	8.15
Nelova 1/50 21, 28—Watson	Mestranol (50)	1050	Norethindrone (1)	21	9.78
Progestin only					
Ovrette—Wyeth-Ayerst	None		Norgestrel (0.075)	2.1	15.67
Nor-QD—Syntex	None		Norethindrone (0.35)	9.8	8.34
Micronor—Ortho	None		Norethindrone (0.35)	9.8	17.17

[a] Different progestins cannot be compared on a milligram basis.
[b] Cost to the pharmacist for one month's use, based on manufacturer's listings in *Drug Topics Red Book*, 1988 and October *Update*.
[c] Also available in 28-day regimens at slightly higher cost.
* A representative listing of some commonly used oral contraceptives. Combination pills have the highest reliability for preventing conception; progesterone-only pills are primarily intended for nursing mothers who want to use an oral contraceptive (estrogens are contraindicated during nursing since they decrease lactation).
From The Medical Letter, *Volume 30, page 106, November, 1988. Used with permission.*

TABLE 7–12. SULFONYLUREAS (ORAL HYPOGLYCEMIC AGENTS).[a]

Drug Brand Name	Duration of Activity (h)	Equivalent Dose (mg)	Maximum Daily Dose (mg)
First generation			
Acetohexamide (Dymelor)	12–18	500	1500
Chlorpropamide (Diabinese)	36–60	250	500
Tolazamide (Tolinase)	24	250	1000
Tolbutamide (Orinase)	6–12	1000	3000
Second generation			
Glipizide (Glucotrol)	10–24	5	40
Glyburide (DiaBeta, Micronase)	24	5	20

[a]Contraindicated in pregnancy.
Fron Gomella LG (ed): Clinician's Pocket Reference, *7th ed. Norwalk, Connecticut, Appleton & Lange, 1992.*

TABLE 7–13. BREAST FEEDING AND MEDICATIONS.

Drug or Substance	Compatibility with Breast-Feeding, Effect on Lactation and Adverse Effects on Infant
Acetaminophen	Generally compatible with breast-feeding.
Albuterol	Generally compatible with breast-feeding. Monitor for agitation and spitting up. Use inhaled form to decrease maternal absorption.
Alcohol	Generally compatible with breast-feeding. Monitor for drowsiness, diaphoresis, weakness, and failure to thrive. Intake of 1 g/kg/d may decrease maternal milk ejection reflex.
Amantadine	Contraindicated. Causes release of levodopa in central nervous system.
Amikacin	Generally compatible with breast-feeding. Low concentrations in breast milk because of poor oral absorption.
Aminoglycosides	Generally compatible with breast-feeding. All antibiotics are excreted in breast milk in limited amounts. Apparently safe, not absorbed in newborn gastrointestinal tract. Monitor for diarrhea.
Aminophylline	Generally compatible with breast-feeding. Monitor for irritability.
Amiodarone	Breast-feeding is not recommended because of iodine contained in each dose and possible accumulation of amiodarone in the infant.
Amitriptyline	Generally compatible with breast-feeding.
Amoxapine	Generally compatible with breast-feeding.
Amoxicillin	Generally compatible with breast-feeding. Monitor for diarrhea.
Amphetamine	Generally compatible with breast-feeding. Monitor for irritability, poor sleeping patterns.
Ampicillin	Generally compatible with breast-feeding. Monitor for diarrhea.
Aspartame	Generally compatible with breast-feeding. Use cautiously in carrier of phenylketonuria.
Aspirin	Generally compatible with breast-feeding. Monitor for spitting up or bleeding. Increased risk with high doses used for rheumatoid arthritis (35 g/d).
Atenolol	Generally compatible with breast-feeding.
Atropine	Generally compatible with breast-feeding. No adverse effects reported.
Bethanechol	Generally compatible with breast-feeding. May cause abdominal pain and diarrhea.
Bromides	Breast-feeding not recommended because of possible drowsiness and rash.
Bromocriptine	Contraindicated. Suppresses lactation.
Brompheniramine	Generally compatible with breast-feeding. Monitor for agitation, poor sleeping pattern, feeding problems.
Butorphanol	Generally compatible with breast-feeding.
Caffeine	Generally compatible with breast-feeding. Monitor for irritability, poor sleeping patterns.
Calcitonin	May inhibit lactation.
Captopril	Generally compatible with breast-feeding.
Carbamazepine	Generally compatible with breast-feeding. Risk of bone marrow suppression if taken chronically.
Carbimazole	Generally compatible with breast-feeding. Monitor for goiter.
Cascara sagrada	Generally compatible with breast-feeding. Monitor for diarrhea.

continued

TABLE 7–13. BREAST FEEDING AND MEDICATIONS. (CONTINUED)

Drug or Substance	Compatibility with Breast-Feeding, Effect on Lactation and Adverse Effects on Infant
Cefaclor	Generally compatible with breast-feeding. Monitor for diarrhea.
Cefadroxil	Generally compatible with breast-feeding. Monitor for diarrhea.
Cefamandole	Generally compatible with breast-feeding. Monitor for diarrhea.
Cefazolin	Generally compatible with breast-feeding. Monitor for diarrhea.
Cefonicid	Generally compatible with breast-feeding. Monitor for diarrhea.
Cefoperazone	Generally compatible with breast-feeding. Monitor for diarrhea.
Ceforanide	Generally compatible with breast-feeding. Monitor for diarrhea.
Cefotaxime	Generally compatible with breast-feeding. Monitor for diarrhea.
Ceftizoxime	Generally compatible with breast-feeding. Monitor for diarrhea.
Ceftriaxone	Generally compatible with breast-feeding. Monitor for diarrhea.
Cefuroxime	Generally compatible with breast-feeding. Monitor for diarrhea.
Cephalexin	Generally compatible with breast-feeding. Monitor for diarrhea.
Cephalosporins	Generally compatible with breast-feeding. All antibiotics are excreted in breast milk in limited amounts. Monitor for rash; sensitization possible.
Cephalothin	Generally compatible with breast-feeding. Monitor for diarrhea.
Cephapirin	Generally compatible with breast-feeding. Monitor for diarrhea.
Cephradine	Generally compatible with breast-feeding. Monitor for diarrhea.
Chloral hydrate	Generally compatible with breast-feeding. Monitor for sedation, rash.
Chloramphenicol	Discontinue during breast-feeding. Risk of bone marrow toxicity. Nurse after 24 hours off the drug.
Chloroform	Generally compatible with breast-feeding.
Chloroquine	Generally compatible with breast-feeding.
Chlorothiazide	Generally compatible with breast-feeding but may suppress lactation, especially in first month of lactation. Adverse effects have not been reported, but infant's electrolytes and platelets should be monitored.
Chlorpheniramine	Generally compatible with breast-feeding. Monitor for agitation, poor sleeping pattern, feeding problems.
Chlorpromazine	Generally compatible with breast-feeding. Monitor for sedation.
Chlorpropamide	Contraindicated. Excreted in breast milk and may cause hypolycemia.
Chlortetracycline	Generally compatible with breast-feeding. Monitor for diarrhea.
Chocolate	Generally compatible with breast-feeding. Irritability or increased bowel activity if mother consumes excessive amounts (> 16 oz/d).
Cimetidine	Contraindicated. May suppress gastric acidity in infant, inhibit drug metabolism, and cause CNS stimulation.
Clindamycin	Discontinue during breast-feeding. Risk of gastrointestinal bleeding. Nurse after 24 hours off the drug.
Clonazepam	Generally compatible with breast-feeding. Monitor for respiratory and CNS depression.
Clonidine	Contraindicated. Excreted in breast milk.
Cloxacillin	Generally compatible with breast-feeding. Monitor for diarrhea.
Cocaine	Contraindicated. Causes cocaine intoxication in infant from maternal intranasal use (hypertension, tachycardia, mydriasis, apnea) and from topical use on mother's nipples (apnea and seizures).

TABLE 7–13. BREAST FEEDING AND MEDICATIONS.

Drug or Substance	Compatibility with Breast-Feeding, Effect on Lactation and Adverse Effects on Infant
Codeine	Generally compatible with breast-feeding. Monitor for sedation. Milk ejection reflex (letdown) may be inhibited.
Contraceptives, oral	Contraindicated. Can cause breast enlargement and proliferation of vaginal epithelium in infants.
Coumadin (warfarin, dicumarol)	Generally compatible with breast-feeding.
Cyclophosphamide	Contraindicated. Possible immune suppression. Unknown effect on growth or association with carcinogenesis.
Cyproheptadine	Generally compatible with breast-feeding. Monitor for agitation, poor sleeping pattern, feeding problems.
Desipramine	Generally compatible with breast-feeding.
Dextroamphetamine	Contraindicated. May cause infant stimulation.
Diazepam	Contraindicated. May cause infant sedation.
Diazoxide	Contraindicated. May case hyperglycemia.
Dicumarol	See Coumadin.
Digoxin	Generally compatible with breast-feeding. Monitor for spitting up, diarrhea, heart rate changes.
Diphenhydramine	Generally compatible with breast-feeding. Monitor for agitation, poor sleeping pattern, feeding problems.
Dipyridamole	Generally compatible with breast-feeding.
Disopyramide	Generally compatible with breast-feeding.
Ephedrine	Generally compatible with breast-feeding. Monitor for agitation.
Ergotamine	Contraindicated. Causes vomiting, diarrhea, convulsions.
Erythromycin	Generally compatible with breast-feeding. Monitor for diarrhea.
Ethambutol	Generally compatible with breast-feeding.
Ethanol	See Alcohol.
Ethosuximide	Generally compatible with breast-feeding. Rare occurrence of bone marrow suppression and gastrointestinal upset.
Fava beans	Generally compatible with breast-feeding. Hemolysis in patients with G6PD deficiency.
Fenoprofen	Excreted in breast milk in small quantities.
Folic acid	Generally compatible with breast-feeding.
Gallium-69	Discontinue during breast-feeding. Radioactivity can remain in breast milk for 2 weeks.
Gentamicin	Generally compatible with breast-feeding. Monitor for diarrhea, bloody stools.
Gold salts	Contraindicated. May cause rash, inflammation of kidney and liver.
Guanethidine	Generally compatible with breast-feeding.
Haloperidol	Generally compatible with breast-feeding.
Halothane	Generally compatible with breast-feeding.
Heparin	Generally compatible with breast-feeding.
Heroin	Generally compatible with breast-feeding. Monitor for depression, withdrawal.
Hydralazine	Generally compatible with breast-feeding.
Hydromorphone	Generally compatible with breast-feeding. Monitor for sedation. Milk ejection reflex (letdown) may be inhibited.
Ibuprofen	Generally compatible with breast-feeding. Effects unknown.

continued

TABLE 7–13. BREAST FEEDING AND MEDICATIONS. (CONTINUED)

Drug or Substance	Compatibility with Breast-Feeding, Effect on Lactation and Adverse Effects on Infant
Imipramine	Generally compatible with breast-feeding.
Insulin	Generally compatible with breast-feeding.
Iodine-125	Contraindicated. Risk of thyroid cancer. Radioactivity present in milk for 12 days.
Iodine-131	Contraindicated. Radioactivity in milk for 2–14 days.
Isoniazid	Generally compatible with breast-feeding. Monitor for rash, diarrhea, constipation.
Isoproterenol	Generally compatible with breast-feeding. Monitor for agitation, spitting up. Use aerosol form to decrease maternal absorption.
Isotretinoin	Contraindicated.
Kanamycin	Generally compatible with breast-feeding. Low concentrations in breast milk due to poor oral absorption. Monitor for diarrhea.
Labetalol	Generally compatible with breast-feeding. Monitor for hypotension, bradycardia.
Levodopa	Contraindicated. Inhibitory effect on prolactin release.
Levothyroxine (T_4)	Generally compatible with breast-feeding. Probably does not interfere with neonatal thyroid screening.
Liothyronine (T_3)	Generally compatible with breast-feeding. Probably does not interfere with neonatal thyroid screening.
Lithium	Probably compatible with breast-feeding; however, infant should be monitored for cyanosis, hypotonia, bradycardia, and other lithium toxicities, even though these have not been reported.
Lorazepam	Generally compatible with breast-feeding. Monitor for sedation.
Magnesium sulfate	Generally compatible with breast-feeding.
Meperidine	Generally compatible with breast-feeding. Monitor for sedation. Milk ejection reflex (letdown) may be inhibited.
Mepindolol	Generally compatible with breast-feeding. Monitor for hypotension, bradycardia.
Meprobamate	Generally compatible with breast-feeding but excreted in milk in high amounts. Monitor for sedation.
Metaproterenol	Generally compatible with breast-feeding. Monitor for agitation, spitting up. Use aerosol form to decrease maternal absorption.
Methadone	Generally compatible with breast-feeding. Monitor for sedation, depression, withdrawal on cessation of methadone treatment.
Methimazole	Contraindicated. Potential for interfering with thyroid function.
Methotrexate	Contraindicated. Possible immune suppression. Its effect on growth and association with carcinogenesis are unknown.
Methyldopa	Generally compatible with breast-feeding. Risk of hemolysis, increased liver enzymes.
Methyprylon	Generally compatible with breast-feeding. Monitor for drowsiness.
Metoclopramide	Generally compatible with breast-feeding. Increases milk production.
Metoprolol	Generally compatible with breast-feeding.

TABLE 7–13. BREAST FEEDING AND MEDICATIONS.

Drug or Substance	Compatibility with Breast-Feeding, Effect on Lactation and Adverse Effects on Infant
Metronidazole	Discontinue during breast-feeding. Do not nurse until 12–24 hours after discontinuing to allow excretion of drug.
Minoxidil	Generally compatible with breast-feeding. Monitor for hypotension.
Monosodium glutamate	Generally compatible with breast-feeding.
Morphine	Generally compatible with breast-feeding. Monitor for sedation. Milk ejection reflex (letdown) may be inhibited.
Nadolol	Generally compatible with breast-feeding.
Naproxen	Generally compatible with breast-feeding. Adverse effects unknown.
Nicotine	Generally compatible with breast-feeding. Excessive amounts may cause diarrhea, vomiting, tachycardia, irritability, and decreased milk production.
Nitrofurantoin	Generally compatible with breast-feeding. Excreted in milk in small amounts. Monitor infants with G6PD deficiency for hemolytic anemia.
Oral contraceptives	See Contraceptives, oral.
Oxacillin	Generally compatible with breast-feeding. Monitor for diarrhea.
Oxazepam	Generally compatible with breast-feeding. Monitor for sedation, depression.
Oxprenolol	Generally compatible with breast-feeding. Monitor for hypotension, bradycardia.
Oxycodone (Percodan, Percocet)	Generally compatible with breast-feeding. Monitor for drowsiness.
Penicillins	Generally compatible with breast-feeding. All antibiotics are excreted in breast milk in limited amounts. Monitor for rash, diarrhea, spitting up.
Phencyclidine	Contraindicated. Excreted in high amounts in breast milk.
Phenindione	Contraindicated. Causes hemorrhage in infants.
Phenobarbital	Generally compatible with breast-feeding. Monitor for sucking problems, sedation, rashes.
Phenylbutazone	Generally compatible with breast-feeding.
Phenylpropanolamine	Generally compatible with breast-feeding. Monitor for agitation.
Phenytoin	Generally compatible with breast-feeding. Monitor for methemoglobinuria (rare).
Pindolol	Generally compatible with breast-feeding. Monitor for hypotension, bradycardia.
Potassium iodide	Contraindicated. Goiter and allergic reactions may be seen.
Prednisone	Generally compatible with breast-feeding. Safety of long-term therapy has not been established. If maternal dose is more than 2 times physiologic, avoid breast-feeding.
Primidone	Generally compatible with breast-feeding. Monitor for irritability.
Prochlorperazine	Generally compatible with breast-feeding.
Propoxyphene	Generally compatible with breast-feeding. Monitor for withdrawal after long-term high-dose maternal use.
Propranolol	Generally compatible with breast-feeding. Monitor for hypotension, bradycardia.
Propylthiouracil	Generally compatible with breast-feeding.

continued

TABLE 7–13. BREAST FEEDING AND MEDICATIONS. (CONTINUED)

Drug or Substance	Compatibility with Breast-Feeding, Effect on Lactation and Adverse Effects on Infant
Pseudoephedrine	Generally compatible with breast-feeding. Monitor for agitation.
Pyridoxine	Generally compatible with breast-feeding.
Pyrimethamine	Generally compatible with breast-feeding.
Quinidine	Generally compatible with breast-feeding. Monitor for rash, anemia, arrhythmias. Risk of optic neuritis with chronic use.
Radiopharmaceuticals (generally)	Discontinue during breast-feeding. Consult nuclear medicine physician for selection of radionuclide with shortest excretion time.
Ranitidine	Contraindicated. May decrease infants gastric acidity.
Reserpine	Generally compatible with breast-feeding. Monitor for infantile galactorrhea.
Riboflavin	Generally compatible with breast-feeding.
Rifampin	Generally compatible with breast-feeding.
Saccharin	Generally compatible with breast-feeding.
Secobarbital	Generally compatible with breast-feeding.
Sulfamethoxazole, sulfonamide	Contraindicated. Highly bound drugs can displace bilirubin from protein, increasing risk of kernicterus, without effect on serum bilirubin.
Technetium-99m	Contraindicated. Radioactivity present in breast milk for 15 hours to 3 days.
Terbutaline	Generally compatible with breast-feeding. Monitor for agitation and spitting up. Use inhaled form to decrease maternal absorption if available.
Tetracyclines	Contraindicated. Causes staining of teeth and growth inhibition.
Theophylline	Generally compatible with breast-feeding. Monitor for irritability.
Thiamine	Generally compatible with breast-feeding.
Thioridazine	Generally compatible with breast-feeding.
Thiouracil	Contraindicated. Causes decreased thyroid function. (Does not apply to propylthiouracil.)
Ticarcillin	Generally compatible with breast-feeding. Monitor for diarrhea.
Timolol	Generally compatible with breast-feeding. Monitor for hypotension, bradycardia.
Tobramycin	Generally compatible with breast-feeding. Poor oral absorption. Monitor for diarrhea.
Tolbutamide	Generally compatible with breast-feeding. Monitor for jaundice.
Trifluoperazine	Generally compatible with breast-feeding.
Trimethoprim	Generally compatible with breast-feeding.
Valproic acid	Generally compatible with breast-feeding but carries risk of hepatitis, hemorrhagic pancreatitis.
Vegetarian diet	Generally compatible with breast-feeding. Monitor for vitamin B_{12} deficiency (failure to thrive, psychomotor retardation, megaloblastic anemia).
Vitamin B_{12}	Generally compatible with breast-feeding.
Vitamin D	Generally compatible with breast-feeding. Monitor for increased calcium levels.
Vitamin K	Generally compatible with breast-feeding.
Warfarin	See Coumadin.

From Gomella T (ed): Neonatology, 2nd ed. Norwalk, CT, Appleton & Lange, 1992.

TABLE 7–14. THERAPEUTIC DRUG LEVELS AND GUIDELINES FOR OBTAINING A BLOOD SAMPLE.

Drug	When to Sample	Therapeutic Levels	Usual Half-Life	Potentially Toxic Levels
Antibiotics				
Gentamicin	30 min after 30 min infusion Trough < 0.5 h before next dose	Peak: 4–10 µg/mL Trough: < 2.0 µg/mL	2 h	Peak: > 12 µg/mL Trough: > 2 µg/mL
Tobramycin		Peak: 20–35 µg/mL	2h	Peak: > 35 µg/mL Trough >8 µg/mL
Amikacin		Trough < 8 µg/mL	2h	Peak > 8 µg/mL
Vancomycin	Peak: 1 h after 1 h infusion Trough: < 0.5 h before next dose	Peak: 30–40 µg/mL Trough: 5–10 µg/mL	6–8 h	Trough: > 13 µg/mL
Anticonvulsants				
Carbamazepine	Trough: just before next oral dose in combination with other anticonvulsants	4–12 µg/mL 4–8 µg/mL	15–20 h	>12 µg/mL
Ethosuximide	Trough: just before next oral dose	40–100 µg/mL	30–60 h	>100 µg/mL
Phenobarbital	Trough: just before next dose	15–40 µg/mL	40–120 h	>40 µg/mL
Phenytoin	Trough: just before next dose	10–20 µg/mL	Concentration dependent	>20 µg/mL
Free phenytoin	Draw at same time as total level	1–2 µg/mL		
Primidone	Trough: just before next dose (Note: Primidone is metabolized to phenobarb, order levels separately)	5–12 µg/mL	10–12 h	>12 µg/mL
Valproic acid	Trough: just before next dose	50–100 µg/mL	5–20 h	>100 µg/mL
Bronchodilators				
Aminophylline (IV)	30 min after a loading dose and 24 h after starting or changing a maintenance dose given as a constant infusion	10–20 µg/mL	Nonsmoking adult: 8 h Children and smoking adults: 4 h	>20 µg/mL
Theophylline (PO)	Peak levels: not recommended Trough level: just before next dose	10–20 µg/mL		

continued

TABLE 7–14. THERAPEUTIC DRUG LEVELS AND GUIDELINES FOR OBTAINING A BLOOD SAMPLE. (CONTINUED)

Drug	When to Sample	Therapeutic Levels	Usual Half-Life	Potentially Toxic Levels
Cardiovascular agents				
Digoxin	Trough: just before next dose (levels drawn earlier than 6 h after a dose will be artificially elevated)	0.5–2 ng/mL	36 h	>2 ng/mL
Lidocaine	Steady-state levels are usually achieved after 6–12 h	1.2–5.0 µg/mL	1.5 h	>6 µg/mL
Procainamide	Trough: just before next oral dose IV: 6–12 h after infusion started Combined procainamide plus NAPA	4–10 µg/mL NAPA: 6–10 h 5–30 µg/mL	Procaine: 2.7–5 h > 30 (NAPA + procaine)	>10 µg/mL
Quinidine	Trough: just before next oral dose	23.5 µg/mL	6 h	>10 µg/mL
Other agents				
Amitriptyline plus nortriptyline	Trough: just before next dose	120–250 ng/mL		
Nortriptyline	Trough: just before next dose	50–140 ng/mL		
Lithium	Trough: just before next dose	0.6–1.6 meq/mL	18–20 h	>3 meq/mL
Imipramine plus desipramine	Trough: just before next dose	150–300 ng/mL		
Desipramine	Trough: just before next dose	50–300 ng/mL		
Methotrexate	By protocol	< 0.5 µmol/L after 48 h		
Cyclosporine	Trough: just before next dose	Highly variable Renal: 50–250 ng/mL (RIA) Hepatic: 150–400 ng/mL		

RIA = radioimmunoassay.
From Lance L (ed): Quick Look Drug Reference. Baltimore, LexiComp Williams & Wilkins, 1991. *Used with permission.*

TABLE 7–15. PERCENTAGE OF LOADING DOSE REQUIRED FOR DOSAGE INTERVAL SELECTED.[a]

CrCl (mL/min)	Dosing Interval		
	8 hour	12 hour	24 hour
100	90	—	—
90	88	—	—
70	84	—	—
60	79	91	—
50	74	87	—
40	66	80	—
30	57	72	92
25	51	66	88
20	45	59	83
15	37	50	75
10	29	40	64
7	24	33	55
5	20	28	48
2	14	20	35
0	9	13	25

[a]Shaded areas indicate suggested dosage intervals.
From Hull JH, Sarubbi FA: Gentamicin serum concentrations: pharmacokinetic predictions. Ann Intern Med 85:183, 1976. Used with permission.

Appendix

TABLE A–1. APGAR SCORES.

	Score		
Sign	**0**	**1**	**2**
Appearance (color)	Blue or pale	Pink body with blue extremities	Completely pink
Pulse (heart rate)	Absent	Slow (< 100/min)	> 100/min
Grimace (reflex irritability)	No response	Grimace	Cough or sneeze
Activity (muscle tone)	Limp	Some flexion	Active movement
Respirations	Absent	Slow, irregular	Good, crying

From Gomella LG (ed): Clinician's Pocket Reference, *7th ed. Norwalk, Connecticut, Appleton & Lange, 1992.*

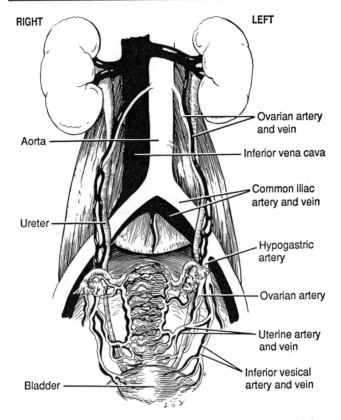

Figure A–1. Blood supply of the pelvis. (*From Pernoll ML, Benson RC [eds]:* Current Obstetric and Gynecologic Diagnosis and Treatment, *6th ed. Norwalk, Connecticut, Appleton & Lange, 1987.*)

BREAST SELF-EXAMINATION

Breast self-examination should be done once a month so you become familiar with the usual appearance and feel of your breasts. Familiarity makes it easier to notice any changes in the breast from one month to another. Early discovery of a change from what is "normal" is the main idea behind BSE. The outlook is much better if you detect cancer in an early stage.

If you menstruate, the best time to do BSE is 2 or 3 days after your period ends, when your breasts are least likely to be tender or swollen. If you no longer menstruate, pick a day such as the first day of the month, to remind yourself it is time to do BSE.

Here is one way to do BSE:

1. Stand before a mirror. Inspect both breasts for anything unusual such as any discharge from the nipples or puckering, dimpling, or scaling of the skin.

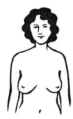

The next two steps are designed to emphasize any change in the shape or contour of your breasts. As you do them, you should be able to feel your chest muscles tighten.

2. Watching closely in the mirror, clasp your hands behind your head and press your hands forward.

3. Next, press your hands firmly on your hips and bow slightly toward your mirror as you pull your shoulders and elbows forward.

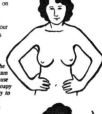

Some women do the next part of the exam in the shower because fingers glide over soapy skin, making it easy to concentrate on the texture underneath.

4. Raise your left arm. Use three or four fingers of your right hand to explore your left breast firmly, carefully, and thoroughly. Beginning at the outer edge, press the flat part of your fingers in small circles, moving the circles slowly around the breast. Gradually work toward the nipple. Be sure to cover the entire breast. Pay special attention to the area between the breast and the underarm, including the underarm itself. Feel for any unusual lump or mass under the skin.

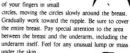

5. Gently squeeze the nipple and look for a discharge. (If you have any discharge during the month— whether or not it is during BSE—see your doctor.) Repeat steps 4 and 5 on your right breast.

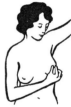

6. Steps 4 and 5 should be repeated lying down. Lie flat on your back with your left arm over your head and a pillow or folded towel under your left shoulder. This position flattens the breast and makes it easier to examine. Use the same circular motion described earlier. Repeat the exam on your right breast.

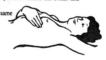

Figure A–2. Breast self-examination. (*From Questions and Answers about Breast Lumps (NIH Publication No. 90–2401). Washington, DC, National Cancer Institute, National Institutes of Health, 1990.*)

TABLE A–2. BODY SURFACE AREA: ADULTS.[a]

Height	Body surface	Mass
cm 120 — 47 in — 46 115 — 45 — 44 110 — 43 — 42 105 — 41 — 40 100 — 39 — 38 95 — 37 — 36 90 — 35 85 — 33 — 32 80 — 31 — 30 75 — 29 — 28 70 — 27 65 — 26 — 25 — 24 60 — 23 — 22 55 — 21 — 20 50 — 19 — 18 45 — 17 — 16 40 — 15 — 14 35 — 13 30 — 12 — 11 cm 25 — 10 in	— 1.10 m² — 1.05 — 1.00 — 0.95 — 0.90 — 0.85 — 0.80 — 0.75 — 0.70 — 0.65 — 0.60 — 0.55 — 0.50 — 0.45 — 0.40 — 0.35 — 0.30 — 0.25 — 0.20 — 0.19 — 0.18 — 0.17 — 0.16 — 0.15 — 0.14 — 0.13 — 0.12 — 0.11 — 0.10 — 0.09 — 0.08 — 0.074 m²	kg 40.0 — 90 lb — 85 35.0 — 80 — 75 30.0 — 70 — 65 25.0 — 60 — 55 — 50 20.0 — 45 — 40 15.0 — 35 — 30 — 25 10.0 — 9.0 — 20 8.0 — 7.0 — 15 6.0 — 5.0 — 4.5 — 10 4.0 — 9 3.5 — 8 3.0 — 7 — 6 2.5 — 5 2.0 — 4 1.5 — 3 kg 1.0 — 2.2 lb

[a]To determine the body surface area in an adult, use a straight edge to connect the height and mass. The point of intersection on the body surface line gives the area in m².
From Lentner C (ed): Geigy Scientific Tables, 8th ed. Basle, CIBA-GEIGY, 1981, vol 1, p 226.

TABLE A–3. BODY SURFACE AREA: CHILDREN.[a]

Height	Body surface	Mass
cm 200 — 79 in 78 195 — 77 76 190 — 75 74 185 — 73 72 180 — 71 70 175 — 69 68 170 — 67 66 165 — 65 64 160 — 63 62 155 — 61 60 150 — 59 58 145 — 57 56 140 — 55 54 135 — 53 52 130 — 51 50 125 — 49 48 120 — 47 46 115 — 45 44 110 — 43 42 105 — 41 40 cm 100 — 39 in	— 2.80 m² — 2.70 — 2.60 — 2.50 — 2.40 — 2.30 — 2.20 — 2.10 — 2.00 — 1.95 — 1.90 — 1.85 — 1.80 — 1.75 — 1.70 — 1.65 — 1.60 — 1.55 — 1.50 — 1.45 — 1.40 — 1.35 — 1.30 — 1.25 — 1.20 — 1.15 — 1.10 — 1.05 — 1.00 — 0.95 — 0.90 — 0.86 m²	kg 150 — 330 lb 145 — 320 140 — 310 135 — 300 130 — 290 125 — 280 120 — 270 — 260 115 — 250 110 — 240 105 — 230 100 — 220 95 — 210 90 — 200 85 — 190 80 — 180 — 170 75 — 70 — 160 — 150 65 — — 140 60 — 130 55 — 120 50 — 110 — 105 45 — 100 — 95 40 — 90 — 85 — 80 35 — 75 — 70 kg 30 — 66 lb

[a]To determine the body surface area in a child, use a straight edge to connect the height and mass. The point of intersection on the body surface line gives the area in m².
From Lentner C (ed): Geigy Scientific Tables, 8th ed. Basle, CIBA-GEIGY, 1981, vol 1, p 227.

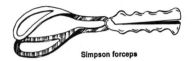

Simpson forceps

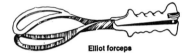

Elliot forceps

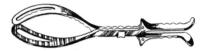

Kielland forceps

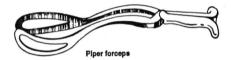

Piper forceps

Figure A–3. Forceps. *continued*

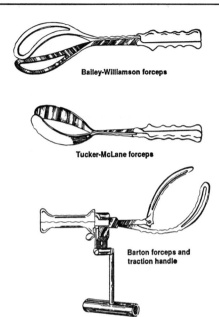

Figure A–3. Continued. (*From Benson RC:* Handbook of Obstetrics & Gynecology, *8th ed. San Mateo, CA, Lange, 1983.*)

TABLE A–4. BISHOP METHOD OF PELVIC SCORING.[a]

Examination	Points		
	1	2	3
Cervical dilatation (cm)	1–2	3–4	5–6
Cervical effacement (%)	40–50	60–70	80
Station of presenting part	–1, –2	0	+1, +2
Consistency of cervix	Medium	Soft	. . .
Position of cervix	Middle	Anterior	. . .

[a]Elective induction of labor may be performed safely when the pelvic score is 9 or more.
Modified and reproduced, with permission, from Bishop EH: Pelvic scoring for elective induction. Obstet Gynecol *24:66, 1964.*

TABLE A–5. CARDIOVASCULAR CHANGES OF PREGNANCY.[a]

Physiologic Variable	Direction and Percent of Change		Time of Onset (wk)	Time of Peak Effect (wk)
Cardiac output	Increased	30–50	±10	20–30
Heart rate	Increased	15–30	10–14	40
Blood volume	Increased	25–50	6–10	32–36
Plasma volume	Increased	40–50	6–10	32
Red cell mass	Increased	20–40	6–10	40
Blood pressure	Decreased early; increased late	No net change	First trimester Third trimester	20 40
Pulmonary and peripheral vascular resistance	Decreased	40–50	6–10	20–24
Oxygen consumption	Increased	15–30	12–16	40
Respiratory rate	Increased	40–50	6–10	40

[a]Greater increase with twin or multiple pregnancy.
From Pernoll ML, Benson RC (eds): Current Obstetric and Gynecologic Diagnosis and Treatment, *6th ed. Norwalk, Connecticut, Appleton & Lange, 1987.*

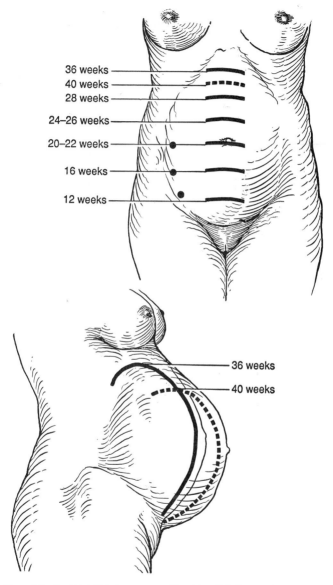

Figure A–4. Fundal height during pregnancy. (*From Pernoll ML, Benson RC [eds]: Current Obstetric and Gynecologic Diagnosis and Treatment, 6th ed. Norwalk, Connecticut, Appleton & Lange, 1987.*)

TABLE A-6. GLASGOW COMA SCALE.

Parameter		Response	Score
Eyes	Open	Spontaneously	4
		To verbal command	3
		To pain	2
	No response		1
Best motor response	To verbal command	Obeys	6
	To painful stimulus	Localizes pain	5
		Flexion-withdrawal	4
		Decorticate (flex)	3
		Decerebrate (extend)	2
		No response	1
Best verbal response		Oriented, converses	5
		Disoriented, converses	4
		Inappropriate responses	3
		Incomprehensible sounds	2
		No response	1

From Gomella LG (ed): Clinician's Pocket Reference, *7th ed. Norwalk, Connecticut, Appleton & Lange, 1992.*

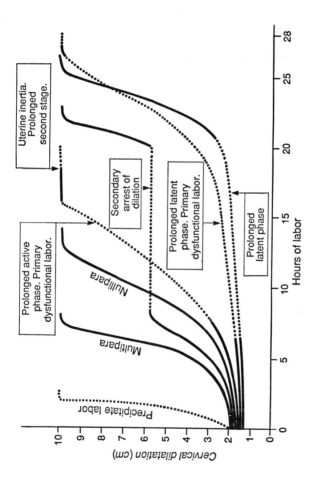

Figure A–5. Labor curves. *(From Pernoll ML, Benson RC [eds]: Current Obstetric and Gynecologic Diagnosis and Treatment, 6th ed. Norwalk, Connecticut, Appleton & Lange, 1987.)*

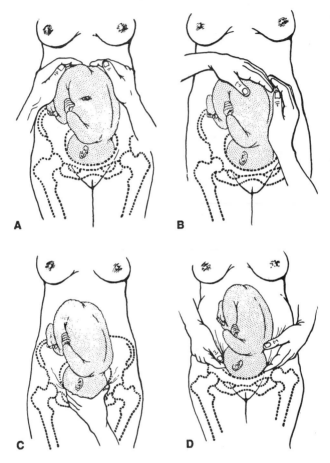

Figure A–6. Leopold's maneuvers. (*From Benson RC:* Handbook of Obstetrics & Gynecology, *8th ed. San Mateo, CA, Lange, 1983.*)

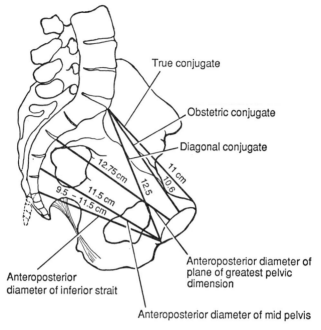

True conjugate

Obstetric conjugate

Diagonal conjugate

12.75 cm

11 cm

12.5

10.6

9.5 – 11.5 cm

11.5 cm

Anteroposterior
diameter of inferior strait

Anteroposterior diameter of
plane of greatest pelvic
dimension

Anteroposterior diameter of mid pelvis

Figure A–7. Pelvic measurements. (*From Benson RC:* Handbook of Obstetrics & Gynecology, *8th ed. San Mateo, CA, Lange, 1983.*)

TABLE A–7. PELVIC CHARACTERISTICS.

	Gynecoid
Widest transverse diameter of inlet	12 cm
Anteroposterior diameter of inlet	11 cm
Side walls	Straight
Forepelvis	Wide
Sacrosciatic notch	Medium
Inclination of sacrum	Medium
Ischial spines	Not prominent
Suprapubic arch	Wide
Transverse diameter of outlet	10 cm
Bone structure	Medium

TABLE A–7. PELVIC CHARACTERISTICS. (CONTINUED)

Android	Anthropoid	Platypelloid
12 cm	< 12 cm	12 cm
11 cm	> 12 cm	10 cm
Convergent	Narrow	Wide
Narrow	Divergent	Straight
Narrow	Backward	Forward
Forward (lower 1/3)	Wide	Narrow
Prominent	Not prominent	Not prominent
Narrow	Medium	Wide
< 10 cm	10 cm	10 cm
Heavy	Medium	Medium

From Pernoll ML, Benson RC (eds): Current Obstetric and Gynecologic Diagnosis and Treatment, 6th ed. Norwalk, Connecticut, Appleton & Lange, 1987.

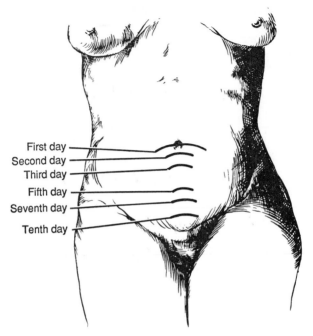

Figure A–8. Postpartum uterine involution. (*From Pernoll ML, Benson RC [eds]:* Current Obstetric and Gynecologic Diagnosis and Treatment, *6th ed. Norwalk, Connecticut, Appleton & Lange, 1987.*)

TABLE A-8. PROPHYLACTIC ANTIBIOTICS IN SURGERY.

Nature of Operation	Likely Pathogens	Recommended Drugs	Adult Dosage before Surgery[a]
CLEAN			
Cardiac			
Prosthetic valve, coronary artery bypass, and other open-heart surgery	*Staphylococcus epidermidis, S. aureus, Corynebacterium,* enteric gram-negative bacilli	Cefazolin *OR* vancomycin[b]	1 gram IV 1 gram IV
Vascular			
Arterial surgery involving the abdominal aorta, a prosthesis, or a groin incision	*S. aureus, S. epidermidis,* enteric gram-negative bacilli	Cefazolin *OR* vancomycin[b]	1 gram IV 1 gram IV
Lower extremity amputation for ischemia	*S. aureus, S. epidermidis,* enteric gram-negative bacilli, clostridia	Cefazolin *OR* vancomycin[b]	1 gram IV 1 gram IV
Neurosurgery			
Craniotomy	*S. aureus, S. epidermidis*	Cefazolin OR vancomycin[b]	1 gram IV 1 gram IV
Orthopedic			
Total joint replacement, internal fixation of fractures	*S. aureus, S. epidermidis*	Cefazolin OR vancomycin[b]	1 gram IV 1 gram IV
Ocular			
	S. aureus, S. epidermidis, streptococci, enteric gram-negative bacilli, *Pseudomonas*	Gentamicin *OR* tobramycin *OR* neomycin–gramicidin–polymyxin B Cefazolin	Multiple drops topically over 2–24 hours 100 mg subconjunctivally at end of procedure

continued

TABLE A–8. PROPHYLACTIC ANTIBIOTICS IN SURGERY. (CONTINUED)

Nature of Operation	Likely Pathogens	Recommended Drugs	Adult Dosage before Surgery[a]
CLEAN-CONTAMINATED			
Head and neck Entering oral cavity or pharynx	*S. aureus*, streptococci, oral anaerobes	Cefazolin *OR* clindamycin	1 gram IV 600 mg IV
Gastroduodenal	Enteric gram-negative bacilli, gram-positive cocci	*High risk, gastric bypass, or percutaneous endoscopic gastrostomy only:* cefazolin	1 gram IV
Biliary tract	Enteric gram-negative bacilli, enterococci, clostridia	*High risk only:* cefazolin	1 gram IV
Colorectal	Enteric gram-negative bacilli, anaerobes	*Oral:* neomycin + erythromycin base[c] *Parenteral:* cefoxitin *OR* cefotetan	
Appendectomy	Enteric gram-negative bacilli, anaerobes	Cefoxitin *OR* cefotetan	1 gram IV 1 gram IV
Vaginal or abdominal hysterectomy	Enteric gram-negative bacilli, anaerobes, group B streptococci, enterococci	Cefazolin	1 gram IV
Cesarean section	Same as for hysterectomy	*High risk only:* cefazolin Aqueous penicillin G	1 gram IV after cord clamping 1 million units IV
Abortion[d]	Same as for hysterectomy	*OR* doxycycline	300 mg PO[d]

606

DIRTY[e]

Ruptured viscus	Enteric gram-negative bacilli, anaerobes, enterococci	Cefoxitin 1 gram IV q6h OR cefotetan 1 gram IV q12h either ± gentamicin 1.5 mg/kg IV q8h OR clindamycin 600 mg IV q6h + gentamicin 1.5 mg/kg IV q8h
Traumatic wound[f]	S. aureus, group A streptococci, clostridia	Cefazolin 1 gram IV q8h

[a]Parenteral prophylactic antimicrobials for clean and clean-contaminated surgery can be given as a single intravenous dose just before the operation. Cefazolin can also be given intramuscularly. For prolonged operations, additional intraoperative doses should be given q4–8h for the duration of the procedure.

[b]For hospitals in which methicillin-resistant S. aureus and S. epidermidis frequently cause wound infection, or for patients allergic to penicillins or cephalosporins. Rapid IV administration may cause hypotension, which could be especially dangerous during induction of anesthesia.

[c]After appropriate diet and catharsis, one gram of each at 1 PM, 2 PM, and 11 PM the day before the operation. An alternative is oral lavage solution (Golytely, and others—Medical Letter, 27:39, 1985) from 1 PM to 6 PM (4–6 hours) until rectal effluent is clear, followed by neomycin 2 grams and metronidazole 2 grams orally at 7 PM and 11 PM (BG Wolff et al, Arch Surg, 1234:895, 1988).

[d]Aqueous penicillin G or doxycycline is recommended for first-trimester abortion in patients considered at high risk for pelvic infection, including those with previous pelvic inflammatory disease, previous gonorrhea, or multiple sex partners. The dosage of doxycycline should be divided into 100 mg one hour before the abortion and 200 mg one half hour after. For mid-trimester abortion, cefazolin, 1 gram IV, is recommended.

[e]For "dirty" surgery, therapy should usually be continued for five to 10 days.

[f]For bite wounds, in which likely pathogens may also include oral anaerobes, Eikenella corrodens (human), and Pasteurella multocida (dog and cat) (DJ Weber and AR Hansen, Infect Dis Clin North Am, 5:663, Sept 1991), some Medical Letter consultants recommend use of amoxicillin-clavulanic acid (Augmentin) or ampicillin–sulbactam (Unasyn).

From The Medical Letter, Volume 34, page 8, January 24, 1992. Used with permission.

TABLE A–9. TETANUS PROPHYLAXIS.

History of Adsorbed Tetanus Toxoid Immunization	Clean, Minor Wounds		All Other Wounds[a]	
	Td	TIG	Td	TIG
Unknown or <3 doses	Yes	No	Yes	Yes
≥3 doses[b]	No[c]	No	No[d]	No

[a]Such as, but not limited to, wounds contaminated with dirt, feces, soil, saliva, etc; puncture wounds; avulsions; and wounds resulting from missiles, crushing, burns, and frostbite.
[b]If only 3 doses of fluid toxoid have been received, then a fourth dose of toxoid, preferably an adsorbed toxoid, should be given.
[c]Yes if more than 10 years since last dose.
[d]Yes if more than 5 years since last dose.
Td = tetanus-diphtheria toxoid (adult type), dose: 0.5 mL IM. For children <7 years of age, DPT (DT, if pertussis vaccine is contraindicated) is preferred to tetanus toxoid alone. For persons ≥7 years of age, Td is preferred to tetanus toxoid alone. **DT = diphtheria-tetanus toxoid (pediatric),** used for those who cannot receive pertussis.
TIG = tetanus immune globulin, dose: 250 units IM.
Based on guidelines from the Centers for Disease Control and reported in *MMWR*, Vol 39, No. 3, 1990.

TABLE A–10. SPECIMEN TUBES FOR VENIPUNCTURE.[a]

Tube Color	Additives	General Use
Red	None	Clot tube to collect serum for chemistry, cross-matching, serology
Red and black (hot pink)	Silicone gel for rapid clot	As above, but not for osmolality or blood bank work
Blue	Sodium citrate (binds calcium)	Coagulation studies (best kept on ice); *not* for fibrin split products
Blue/yellow label		Fibrin split products
Royal blue		Heavy metals, arsenic
Purple	Disodium EDTA (binds calcium)	Hematology; not for lipid profiles
Green	Sodium heparin	Ammonia, cortisol, ionized calcium (best kept on ice)
Green/glass beads		LE prep
Gray	Sodium fluoride	Lactic acid
Yellow	Transport media	Blood cultures

[a]Note: Although the color and type of specimen tubes can vary from one medical center to another, this table lists the types of tubes commonly used and is provided as a general guide.
From Gomella LG (ed): Clinician's Pocket Reference, *7th ed. Norwalk, Connecticut, Appleton & Lange, 1992.*

TABLE A–11. TEMPERATURE CONVERSION.

F	C	C	F
0	−17.7	0	32.0
95.0	35.0	35.0	95.0
96.0	35.5	35.5	95.9
97.0	36.1	36.0	96.8
98.0	36.6	36.5	97.7
98.6	37.0	37.0	98.6
99.0	37.2	37.5	99.5
100.0	37.7	38.0	100.4
101.0	38.3	38.5	101.3
102.0	38.8	39.0	102.2
103.0	39.4	39.5	103.1
104.0	40.0	40.0	104.0
105.0	40.5	40.5	104.9
106.0	41.1	41.0	105.8
	$C = (F - 32) \times \frac{5}{9}$		$F = (C \times \frac{9}{5}) + 32$

F = degrees fahrenheit; C = degrees celsius.
From Gomella LG (ed): Clinician's Pocket Reference, *7th ed. Norwalk, Connecticut, Appleton & Lange, 1992.*

TABLE A–12. WEIGHT CONVERSION.

lb	kg	kg	lb
1	0.5	1	2.2
2	0.9	2	4.4
4	1.8	3	6.6
6	2.7	4	8.8
8	3.6	5	11.0
10	4.5	6	13.2
20	9.1	8	17.6
30	13.6	10	22.0
40	18.2	20	44.0
50	22.7	30	66.0
60	27.3	40	88.0
70	31.8	50	110.0
80	36.4	60	132.0
90	40.9	70	154.0
100	45.4	80	176.0
150	68.2	90	198.0
200	90.8	100	220.0
	kg = lb × 0.454		lb = kg × 2.2

From Gomella LG (ed): Clinician's Pocket Reference, *7th ed. Norwalk, Connecticut, Appleton & Lange, 1992.*

Index

NOTE: Page numbers followed by t and f indicate tables and figures, respectively.